Jenny Stanford Series
on Biocatalysis
Volume 9

Agricultural Biocatalysis

Jenny Stanford Series on Biocatalysis

Series Editor
Peter Grunwald

Titles in the Series

Vol. 1
Industrial Biocatalysis
Peter Grunwald, ed.
2015
978-981-4463-88-1 (Hardcover)
978-981-4463-89-8 (eBook)

Vol. 2
Handbook of Carbohydrate-Modifying Biocatalysts
Peter Grunwald, ed.
2016
978-981-4669-78-8 (Hardcover)
978-981-4669-79-5 (eBook)

Vol. 3
Biocatalysis and Nanotechnology
Peter Grunwald, ed.
2017
978-981-4613-69-9 (Hardcover)
978-1-315-19660-2 (eBook)

Vol. 4
Pharmaceutical Biocatalysis: Fundamentals, Enzyme Inhibitors, and Enzymes in Health and Diseases
Peter Grunwald, ed.
2019
978-981-4800-61-7 (Hardcover)
978-0-429-29503-4 (eBook)

Vol. 5
Pharmaceutical Biocatalysis: Chemoenzymatic Synthesis of Active Pharmaceutical Ingredients
Peter Grunwald, ed.
2019
978-981-4800-80-8 (Hardcover)
978-0-429-35311-6 (eBook)

Vol. 6
Pharmaceutical Biocatalysis: Important Enzymes, Novel Targets, and Therapies
Peter Grunwald, ed.
2021
978-981-4877-13-8 (Hardcover)
978-1-003-04539-7 (eBook)

Vol. 7
Pharmaceutical Biocatalysis: Drugs, Genetic Diseases, and Epigenetics
Peter Grunwald, ed.
2021
978-981-4877-14-5 (Hardcover)
978-1-003-04541-0 (eBook)

Vol. 8
Agricultural Biocatalysis: Theoretical Studies and Photosynthesis Aspects
Peter Jeschke and Evgeni B. Starikov, eds.
2023
978-981-4968-46-1 (Hardcover)
978-1-003-31307-6 (eBook)

Vol. 9
Agricultural Biocatalysis: Enzymes in Agriculture and Industry
Peter Jeschke and Evgeni B. Starikov, eds.
2023
978-981-4968-47-8 (Hardcover)
978-1-003-31310-6 (eBook)

Vol. 10
Agricultural Biocatalysis: Biological and Chemical Applications
Peter Jeschke and Evgeni B. Starikov, eds.
2023
978-981-4968-48-5 (Hardcover)
978-1-003-31314-4 (eBook)

Jenny Stanford Series
on Biocatalysis
Volume 9

Agricultural Biocatalysis
Enzymes in Agriculture and Industry

edited by

Peter Jeschke
Evgeni B. Starikov

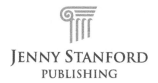

Jenny Stanford
Publishing

Published by

Jenny Stanford Publishing Pte. Ltd.
101 Thomson Road
#06-01, United Square
Singapore 307591

Email: editorial@jennystanford.com
Web: www.jennystanford.com

British Library Cataloguing-in-Publication Data
A catalogue record for this book is available from the British Library.

Agricultural Biocatalysis: Enzymes in Agriculture and Industry

Copyright © 2023 by Jenny Stanford Publishing Pte. Ltd.
All rights reserved. This book, or parts thereof, may not be reproduced in any form or by any means, electronic or mechanical, including photocopying, recording or any information storage and retrieval system now known or to be invented, without written permission from the publisher.

For photocopying of material in this volume, please pay a copying fee through the Copyright Clearance Center, Inc., 222 Rosewood Drive, Danvers, MA 01923, USA. In this case permission to photocopy is not required from the publisher.

ISBN 978-981-4968-47-8 (Hardcover)
ISBN 978-1-003-31310-6 (eBook)

Contents

Preface   xv

Part I   Agricultural Enzymes Market

1. Metagenomics as a Tool to Isolate New Enzymes for Application in Hydrolysis and Synthesis Reactions: The Case of Lipolytic Enzymes   3

Rocío Cuaspa Ropaín, Robson Carlos Alnoch, Patrícia Gruening de Mattos, Janaína Marques de Almeida, David Alexander Mitchell, and Nadia Krieger

1.1	Introduction	4
1.2	Metagenomics as an Enzyme Prospecting Tool	6
1.3	Functional Screening in a Metagenomic Library	19
1.4	Sequence-Based Screening in a Metagenomic Library	21
1.5	Lipolytic Enzymes Isolated from Metagenomic Libraries	23
1.6	The Lipases LipC12, LipG9, and LipMF3: A Case Study	24
1.7	Conclusions	31

2. Plant Pectin Methylesterase: An Insight into Agricultural and Industrial Applications   39

Zeba Khan, Rakesh Srivastava, Sumit K. Bag, and Praveen C. Verma

2.1	Introduction	40
2.2	Pectin Methylesterases Classification	41
2.3	Pectin Methylesterases: An Insight into Their Functions	45
	2.3.1 Role of PMEs in Different Aspects of Plant Development	46
2.4	Role of PMEs in Plant Defense-Related Mechanism	49

2.5	Agriculture and Industrial Applications of PMEs	51
2.6	Conclusion	53

3. Induced Polyphenol Oxidases Are Associated with Laccase Activity in Different Genotypes of Resistant Chickpea Cultivars Infected by *Fusarium oxysporm* f.sp. *ciceris* and Salicylic Acid — **59**

Shivashankar Gayatridevi, Kuruba Sreeramulu, and Senigala K. Jayalakshmi

3.1	Introduction	60
3.2	PPO and Laccase Activity	62
3.3	Detection of PPO and Laccase Isozymes in Native PAGE	64
3.4	Conclusion	69

Part II Plant Enzymes

4. Classification and Evolutionary Landscape of Acid Phosphatase–Encoding Gene Families in Plants — **75**

Amir Feizi, Mohammad Ali Malboobi, Javad Zamani, Tahmineh Lohrasebi, and Shahrokh Kazempour-Osaloo

4.1	Introduction		76
4.2	Plant APase Sequences Retrieval and Comparison		79
4.3	Sequence Alignments, Clustering, and Phylogenetic Analysis		89
4.4	PAP Family		90
	4.4.1	PAP I Subfamily	93
	4.4.2	PAP II Subfamily	95
	4.4.3	PAP III Subfamily	96
	4.4.4	PAP IV Subfamily	96
	4.4.5	PAP V Subfamily	96
4.5	Halo Acid Dehalogenases (HAD)-Related APase Family		97
	4.5.1	HRP I Subfamily	97
	4.5.2	HRP II Subfamily	100
4.6	Phospholipid Phosphatase (PLP) Family		100
4.7	Histidine Acid Phosphatase Family		102

	4.8	Protein E (SurE)-Related Acid Phosphatase Family	104
	4.9	Structural Comparisons of APase Families	106
	4.10	Concluding Remarks	108

5. Acid Phosphatases Roles in Plant Performance — 117

Mohammad Ali Malboobi, Mohammad Sadegh Sabet, Katayoun Zamani, Tahmineh Lohrasebi, Zahra Fathi, and Javad Zamani

5.1	Introduction	118
5.2	Phosphate Ion and Its Significance	119
5.3	Stepwise Plant Response to Available Pi	121
5.4	APases Types and Functions	122
	5.4.1 Purple Acid Phosphatase (PAP) Family	123
	5.4.2 Haloacid Dehalogenase (HAD)-Related Acid Phosphatase (HRP) Family	124
	5.4.3 Phospholipid Phosphatases (PLP) Family	125
	5.4.4 Histidine Acid Phosphatase (HAP) Family	126
	5.4.5 SurE-Related Acid Phosphatase (SAP) Family	127
5.5	Multiple Isoforms and Broad Substrates Range of APases	127
5.6	Tissue-Specific Expression of APases	132
5.7	Responsiveness of APases to Pi Status	135
5.8	Roles of APases in Pi Homeostasis	137
5.9	APases Responsive to Other Stresses	140
5.10	Interplay between APases to Keep Pi Homeostasis	141
5.11	Concluding Remarks	145

6. Superoxide Dismutases in Plants: New Insights into Regulation and Functioning — 159

Ravi Prakash Sanyal, Abiraami T. V., Sabiha Perween, Satish B. Verulkar, Hari S. Misra, and Ajay Saini

6.1	Introduction	160

6.2	Impact of Great Oxygenation Event (GOE) on Cellular Metabolism	161
6.3	Reactive Species: Generation, Molecular Targets, and Scavenging	162
	6.3.1 Superoxide Radical ($O_2^{\cdot-}$)	166
	6.3.2 Hydrogen Peroxide (H_2O_2)	166
	6.3.3 Hydroxyl Radical ($^{\cdot}OH$)	166
	6.3.4 Singlet Oxygen ($^1O_2$)	167
	6.3.5 Other Reactive Species (RNS, RCS, RSS)	167
6.4	Reactive Species and Important Sites of Generation in Plants	168
6.5	Reactive Species: Detrimental and Beneficial Effects	170
6.6	Cellular Antioxidant Defense Systems	172
	6.6.1 Nonenzymatic Antioxidants	173
	6.6.2 Enzymatic Antioxidant Defense System	174
6.7	Multiple SOD Isoforms and Their Need in Biological Systems	176
6.8	Nickel Superoxide Dismutase (Ni SOD)	177
6.9	Cambialistic Superoxide Dismutase (Fe/Mn SOD)	178
6.10	Iron Superoxide Dismutase (Fe SOD)	179
6.11	Manganese Superoxide Dismutase (Mn SOD)	183
6.12	Copper Zinc Superoxide Dismutases (CuZn SODs)	185
6.13	Dynamics of Regulation and Functioning of SODs	188
	6.13.1 *cis* Elements–Mediated Regulation of SODs	188
	6.13.2 MicroRNA miR398–Mediated Regulation of CuZn SODs	191
	6.13.3 Alternative Splicing in Regulation and Functioning of SODs	192
	6.13.4 Copper Chaperone for Superoxide Dismutase (CCS)–Mediated Regulation and Functioning of CuZn SODs	195

		6.13.5	Role of Posttranslational Modifications (PTMs) in SOD Functioning	198
		6.13.6	Genome Duplication–Mediated Copy Number Increase of Plant SOD Genes	201
	6.14		Stress Responsiveness of SODs	203
	6.15		Biotechnological Applications of SODs for Stress Tolerance Enhancement	204
	6.16		Industrial Applications of Plant SODs	208
	6.17		Conclusions	208

7. Peroxisomes from Higher Plants and Their Metabolic Diversity   225

Francisco J. Corpas and José M. Palma

	7.1	Introduction	226
	7.2	Photorespiration	228
	7.3	Fatty Acids β-Oxidation, Glyoxylate Cycle, and Auxin Metabolism	229
	7.4	Biosynthesis of Jasmonic Acid and Polyamine Metabolism	231
	7.5	Metabolism of ROS and RNS	232
	7.6	Pexophagy	235
	7.7	Conclusions and Further Perspectives	235

Part III   Herbicide-Tolerant Traits

8. Oxygenase Enzymes for Agricultural Biotechnology Applications   245

Clayton T. Larue

	8.1	Introduction	246
	8.2	Discovery and Early Development of Herbicide Tolerance Traits	249
	8.3	Dioxygenases for FOP and 2,4-D Tolerance Traits	253
	8.4	Monooxygenase Enzyme for Dicamba Tolerance	257
	8.5	Dioxygenase Enzyme for HPPD Inhibitor Tolerance	260
	8.6	Conclusion	262

Part IV Plant Viruses

9. P1 Leader Proteinases from the *Potyviridae* Family   269
Fabio Pasin and Hongying Shan

9.1	Introduction	270
9.2	P1 Diversity of the *Potyviridae* Genomes	275
9.3	Structural Properties and Proteolytic Activity of P1	276
9.4	P1 Proteins as Viral Suppressors of RNA Silencing	278
9.5	P1 Proteins as Host-Range and Symptom Determinants	280
9.6	Additional P1 Functions	287
9.7	Biotechnologies of P1 Proteinases	288
9.8	Conclusions	290

Part V Soil Enzymes

10. Soil Enzymes: Distribution, Interactions, and Influencing Factors   303
Sesan Abiodun Aransiola, Femi Afolabi, Femi Joseph, and Naga Raju Maddela

10.1	Introduction	304
10.2	Source, Distribution, and Abundance of Soil Enzymes	305
10.3	Ecological Stoichiometry of Plant-Soil-Enzyme Interactions	310
	10.3.1 Role of Plant in Soil Health	311
	10.3.2 Plant-Soil-Enzyme Relationship and Soil Health	312
	10.3.2.1 Soil urease	313
	10.3.2.2 Soil invertase	314
	10.3.2.3 Soil phosphatase	314
10.4	Soil Chemical Properties Versus Soil Enzyme Activities	314
10.5	Impact of Anthropogenic Factors on Soil Enzyme Activities	317
10.6	Conclusions	325

11. **Carbon-, Nitrogen-, Phosphorus-, and Sulfur-Cycling Enzymes and Functional Diversity in Agricultural Systems** — 335

    Avijit Ghosh, Ranjan Paul, Abhijit Sarkar, M. C. Manna, Sudeshna Bhattacharjya, Khurshid Alam, Sourav Choudhury, and Prithusayak Mondal

    11.1 Introduction — 336
    11.2 Carbon-Cycling Enzymes and Their Mechanisms — 337
        11.2.1 Amylase — 337
        11.2.2 β-Glucosidase — 338
        11.2.3 Cellulase and Hemicellulase — 339
        11.2.4 Ligninase — 341
        11.2.5 Invertase — 342
        11.2.6 Laccase — 342
        11.2.7 Pectinase — 342
    11.3 Nitrogen-Cycling Enzymes and Their Mechanisms — 344
        11.3.1 Soil Protease — 344
        11.3.2 Urease — 344
        11.3.3 Chitinase — 345
    11.4 Phosphorus-Cycling Enzymes and Their Mechanisms — 345
        11.4.1 Phosphatase Enzymes — 345
        11.4.2 Phosphomonoesterases — 348
        11.4.3 Phosphodiesterases — 349
        11.4.4 Phosphotriesterases — 350
        11.4.5 Polyphosphates — 351
        11.4.6 Phosphoamidase — 353
    11.5 Sulfur-Cycling Enzymes and Their Mechanisms — 353
        11.5.1 Aryl Sulfatases — 353
    11.6 Microbial Functional Diversity in Agrosystems — 355
    11.7 Conclusions and Future Prospects — 355

Part VI Bioremediation

12. **Bioremediation: Removal of Polycyclic Aromatic Hydrocarbons from Soil** — 367

    Zdeněk Košnář, Johanka Wernerová, Petr Frühbauer, and Pavel Tlustoš

    12.1 Introduction — 368

		12.1.1	General Description of Polycyclic Aromatic Hydrocarbons (PAHs)	368
		12.1.2	Basic Description of 16 Individual US EPA PAHs	371
		12.1.3	Sources of PAHs in the Environment	375
		12.1.4	Emissions of PAHs in the Environment	377
		12.1.5	Soil Contamination by PAHs	378
		12.1.6	Impact of PAHs on Animal and Human Health	379
	12.2	Conventional Remediation of Soils Contaminated by PAHs		381
	12.3	Bioremediation of Soil Contaminated by PAHs		382
		12.3.1	Phytoremediation of Soil Contaminated by PAHs	384
		12.3.2	Bacterial Remediation of Soil Contaminated by PAHs	391
		12.3.3	Mycoremediation of Soil Contaminated by PAHs	395
	12.4	Conclusions		403

Part VII Biochemical Conversion

13. Enzymatic Saccharification of Lignocellulosic Biomass — 413

Madhavi Latha Gandla, Chaojun Tang, Carlos Martín, and Leif J. Jönsson

	13.1	Introduction		414
	13.2	Lignocellulosic Biomass		415
	13.3	Biodegradation of Lignocellulose in Nature		420
	13.4	Fungal Enzymes		422
		13.4.1	Glycoside Hydrolases	422
		13.4.2	Polysaccharide Lyases	431
		13.4.3	Carbohydrate Esterases	434
		13.4.4	Auxiliary Activities	436
		13.4.5	Associated Modules	439
	13.5	Bacterial Enzymes		441
	13.6	Determination of Cellulolytic Activity		443
	13.7	Biorefining of Lignocellulosic Feedstocks		445
	13.8	Pretreatment to Facilitate Enzymatic Saccharification		448

13.9	Inhibition of Enzymatic Saccharification	454
13.10	Process Configurations	455
13.11	Future Outlook	459

14. Biological Biorefineries Based on Orange Peel Wastes — 471

Alberto García-Martín, Itziar A. Escanciano, V. Martin-Domínguez, Álvaro Lorente-Arévalo, Jorge García-Montalvo, Jesús Esteban, Juan M. Bolívar, Victoria E. Santos, and Miguel Ladero

14.1	Introduction	472
14.2	Upstream Processes in Biological Biorefineries from OPW	476
	14.2.1 Pretreatment of OPWs	476
	14.2.2 Enzymatic Saccharification of OPWs	481
14.3	Biological Processes to Platform Chemicals and Materials	484
	14.3.1 Bioethanol and Superior Alcohols	484
	14.3.2 Gas Energy and Material Vectors from OPW	487
	14.3.3 Monomers and Other Organic Compounds	496
	14.3.4 Production of Enzymes from OPWs	499
	14.3.5 Biopolymers, Exopolysaccharides, and High Molecular Weight Active Ingredients	502
14.4	Techno-Economic and Environmental Impact Studies	504
14.5	Conclusions	506

Index — 515

Preface

The use of new enzymes is of enormous importance in agricultural and industrial areas for environmentally friendly processes because selected agricultural enzymes (lipases and esterases) support reactions that do not occur naturally, such as the bioprocessing of fibers. Although agricultural enzymes are derived from animal or plant tissues and microbes, they often lack optimal features for practical applications. Therefore, metagenomics-based techniques were successfully used in the identification of genes that encode new and highly active agricultural lipases (LipC12, LipG9, and LipMF3) with the required characteristics. Of importance in recent years are also the plant pectin methyl esterase (PME) gene family and the defensive roles of these novel bifunctional isozymes associated with laccase activity as exemplified in chickpea.

This book, the ninth volume of Jenny Stanford Series on Biocatalysis, addresses the important question of why plants have multiple APases as compared to animals. A deep insight into their roles paves the way for its phosphate ion (Pi) provision through either rhizosphere engineering or genetic manipulation. It gives a brief overview of the reactive species and antioxidant functions as well as the evolution and diversity of superoxide dismutase (SOD) metalloenzymes, which are integral components of the cellular antioxidant defense system in plants. It also discusses the enormous relevance of peroxisomes in plants in more detail.

Herbicide tolerance traits can employ enzymes that act on selected herbicides to enable the application of these agrochemicals during the cropping season. In this context, oxygenase enzymes have been proven to be useful in developing several herbicide tolerance traits. A follow-up systematic investigation of P1 proteinase diversity and evolution is predicted to develop not only new antiviral strategies but also innovative biotechnology and synthetic biology devices.

Soil enzymes are often used in agriculture as reliable indicators of soil health, fertility, and productivity as affected by differentiated natural and anthropogenic factors. They are sensitive to alteration in soil ecosystem and, in turn, to plant-soil-enzyme interactions.

By using sustainable soil management practices, the crop and soil productivity of an ecosystem can be advantageously influenced. Plant-assisted mycoremediation treatment significantly enhances the removal of polycyclic aromatic hydrocarbons (PAHs). Therefore, the cultivation of maize plants in association with *Pleurotus ostreatus* grown on wood substrate seems to be a promising *in situ* bioremediation strategy for PAH-contaminated agricultural soils.

Research and technological development of enzymatic lignin biodegradation has made great progress during recent decades and will likely continue to develop rapidly over the coming years. This also has an influence on biological biorefineries based on orange peel wastes (OTWs).

We are sure the readers will enjoy the 14 chapters of this volume and find them to be useful literature sources on the topic of enzymes in agriculture and industry.

Peter Jeschke
Evgeni B. Starikov
July 2022

PART I
AGRICULTURAL ENZYMES MARKET

Chapter 1

Metagenomics as a Tool to Isolate New Enzymes for Application in Hydrolysis and Synthesis Reactions: The Case of Lipolytic Enzymes

Rocío Cuaspa Ropaín,[a] Robson Carlos Alnoch,[a,b] Patrícia Gruening de Mattos,[a] Janaína Marques de Almeida,[a] David Alexander Mitchell,[a,c] and Nadia Krieger[a,d,e]

[a]*Postgraduate Program in Science-Biochemistry, Federal University of Paraná, PO Box 19046, Central Polytechnic, Curitiba 81531-980, Paraná, Brazil*
[b]*Department of Biology, Faculty of Philosophy, Sciences and Letters of Ribeirão Preto, University of São Paulo, Ribeirão Preto, São Paulo, 14040-901, Brazil*
[c]*Department of Biochemistry and Molecular Biology, Federal University of Paraná, PO Box 19046, Central Polytechnic, Curitiba 81531-980, Paraná, Brazil*
[d]*Graduate Program in Chemistry, Federal University of Paraná, PO Box 19061, Central Polytechnic, Curitiba 81531-980, Paraná, Brazil*
[e]*Department of Chemistry, Federal University of Paraná, PO Box 19061, Central Polytechnic, Curitiba 81531-980, Paraná, Brazil*
nkrieger@ufpr.br

The search for new enzymes for industrial application has increased with the demand for environmentally friendly industrial processes.

Agricultural Biocatalysis: Enzymes in Agriculture and Industry
Edited by Peter Jeschke and Evgeni B. Starikov
Copyright © 2023 Jenny Stanford Publishing Pte. Ltd.
ISBN 978-981-4968-47-8 (Hardcover), 978-1-003-31310-6 (eBook)
www.jennystanford.com

This is particularly true for lipolytic enzymes (lipases and esterases), which are among the most used enzymes in biocatalytic processes. However, current enzymes often do not have optimal characteristics for applications. The use of metagenomic-based techniques has been successful in finding genes that encode for new enzymes, particularly lipases, that present high activity, stability in organic solvents, thermostability, and selectivity. Here we present the basic concepts of metagenomics and a case study of a metagenomic library that was constructed from a fat-contaminated soil sample and led to the isolation and characterization of new lipases, LipC12, LipG9, and LipMF3, which are highly active, stable, and potentially useful enzymes.

1.1 Introduction

The demand for enzyme-catalyzed processes has been increasing for the last 30 years. This is due to the fact that these processes are more environmentally friendly than chemical processes: enzymes work in conditions that are milder than those used in chemical processes, such as lower temperatures and intermediate pH values. Due to these properties, many efforts have been made to improve the economic viability of enzymatic processes, since the high cost is one of the main bottlenecks limiting the implantation of enzymatic processes in the industry.

To render enzymatic processes viable, enzymes need to be more stable and active in the reaction media used in industrial processes. In many cases aqueous media are used, but in several other cases, water-restricted media are used, such as organic solvents, in which the performance of enzymes is frequently not as good as in aqueous media. Beyond this, the range of commercially available enzymes with high performance in water-restricted media is still limited. Thus, there is a demand for new enzymes with the required activity and stability.

One way of achieving stable and active enzymes is to immobilize them on solid supports: immobilization allows the recovery and reuse of enzymes, thereby reducing process costs. Another approach, which can be used in tandem with immobilization, is to find new enzymes that are naturally more active and stable in harsh conditions, such as high temperatures and organic solvents.

New enzymes can be found in nature using the classical methods of isolation and cultivation of the microorganisms that produce them, in so-called "biodiversity hotspots," such as rainforests, and extreme environments, such as saline and volcanic environments. However, classical techniques for obtaining pure cultures are often time-consuming, difficult, and challenging, since microorganisms have complex metabolic requirements (Yarza *et al.*, 2014). It is estimated that less than 0.1% of the microorganisms present in environmental samples like soil are susceptible to isolation and laboratory cultivation (Torsvik *et al.*, 1996), due to the lack of knowledge of the appropriate culture conditions and due to the fact that many microorganisms grow in symbiosis with others. Thus, methods that do not require isolation and cultivation of microorganisms become an important tool for the prospection of new enzymes. Such is the case of metagenomics, which is the object of this chapter.

Hydrolases are by far the most important group of enzymes used in bioprocesses. Among them, lipolytic enzymes are of particular interest. Due to their activity and stability in organic solvents and high selectivity, they have been used to produce chiral compounds, which are of great interest for the chemical and pharmaceutical industries.

This chapter focuses on new lipolytic enzymes found using the metagenomic approach. It is important to state clearly what is meant by "lipolytic enzymes." According to Kovacic *et al.* (2019), lipolytic enzymes compose a large group of versatile enzymes (over 5000, considering only bacterial lipolytic enzymes) that include lipases (EC 3.1.1.3) and esterases (EC 3.1.1.1), which have diverse amino acid sequences but have related tridimensional structure. However, an important point about the identification and classification of novel lipolytic enzymes is the lack of clarity regarding the distinction between lipases and esterases. According to Jaeger *et al.* (1994) and Arpigny and Jaeger (1999), lipases can hydrolyze long-chain triacylglycerols, which are water-insoluble substrates, whereas esterases can only hydrolyze small esters that are partially soluble in water. However, some authors do not provide sufficient information for correct classification, and, in any case, there is no simple way of distinguishing lipases from other esterases. Various enzymes that have previously been classified as "lipases" do not have activity or have not been evaluated against triacylglycerols containing long-chain fatty acids, such as vegetable oils or animal fat, which are natural substrates for lipases. Likewise, other enzymes have been classified as "esterases" due to high activities against p-nitrophenol (p-NP) esters with fatty acids shorter than 10 carbons, but have not even been tested against triacylglycerols of long-chain fatty acids. In other words, some enzymes that have been classified as esterases might be capable of attacking substrates containing long-chain fatty acids. This means that many so-called "esterases" might present lipolytic activity against triacylglycerols containing long-chain fatty acids and might, therefore, be reclassified as "lipases." However, in this chapter, we simply use the term, either lipase or esterase, that was used by the author of the original article.

We present metagenomics as a tool for the isolation of new lipolytic enzymes, identifying the advantages and discussing the challenges of the technique. Additionally, we relate the experience of our research group in prospecting for new lipases through the metagenomic approach.

1.2 Metagenomics as an Enzyme Prospecting Tool

The term metagenomics was proposed in 1998 by Handelsman and collaborators. It represents a new approach to obtaining access to biodiversity. The metagenome is defined as the collection of genomes and genes from the members of a microbiota, which, in turn, is defined as the assemblage of microorganisms present in a given environment (Marchesi and Ravel, 2015). Metagenomics has aided in the understanding of the relationships among microbiota (bacteria, archaea, fungi, protists, and algae), microbial metabolites, environmental conditions, and microbial structural elements (Berg et al., 2020). Moreover, metagenomics maximizes the chances of isolating DNA sequences encoding enzymes and pathways for the production of bioactive molecules from microorganisms that are not cultivable in the laboratory, since the technique involves the direct cloning of fragments of DNA from environmental samples without the need for isolation and cultivation of microorganisms.

Microbial communities of a wide variety of natural and unnatural environments have been explored in order to obtain novel lipolytic enzymes (Table 1.1). Land-based habitats that have been explored include forest soil, which has provided the most industrially important enzymes (Castilla et al., 2018), plant rhizosphere soil, compost, and desert and Antarctic soils. Aquatic habitats that have been explored include surface and deep-sea water, hydrothermal vents, mangroves, tidal and coastal sediments, wastewater, and saline and alkaline lakes. Eukaryote-associated microbiomes have also been explored from humans, rumens, the guts of termites and earthworms, marine sponges, and shrimp gills (López-López et al., 2014; Verma et al., 2021). However, global resources remain unexplored in terms of sampling of habitats and the isolation of new enzymes (Ferrer et al., 2016).

The metagenomic approach for prospecting for new enzymes in a selected habitat involves five major steps (Fig. 1.1): (a) environmental sampling and DNA extraction; (b) construction of the metagenomic library; (c) transformation of recombinant clones into a cell host; (d) screening the clones for the desired function; and (e) expression and biochemical characterization of the enzyme.

After the environmental sampling, step (a) in Fig. 1.1, the DNA in the environmental sample can be extracted either by a direct method, in which the cells in the sample are lysed and the whole sample is used for the extraction of the DNA, or by an indirect method, in which the cells are separated from the matrix before the collection of DNA (Almeida and De Martinis, 2019). The extracted DNA is then evaluated for quantity, purity, and integrity by spectrophotometric, fluorometric, and electrophoretic methods, respectively. Cells can be lysed by physical (vortex, silica beads, heating, freezing), enzymatic (lysozyme, proteinase K, pronase) or chemical (detergents) methods, or a combination of different methods (Lombard et al., 2011). If a faithful picture of the microbiota present in the sample is to be obtained, this step must generate a substantial amount of high-quality DNA.

Table 1.1 Representative lipolytic enzymes isolated from metagenomic libraries, selected properties, and suggested applications

Lipolytic Enzyme	Library Source	Screening Method*	Activity (Substrate)/Relevant Features	Suggested Applications	References
LipC12	Fat-contaminated soil from a wastewater treatment plant (Brazil)	SBS and FS	1722 U·mg^{-1} (olive oil), 1767 U·mg^{-1} (pig fat) Stable from pH 6 to 11 and activity from pH 4.5–10 Stable in organic solvents at 15% and 30% (v/v)	Regioselective deacetylation of sugar-type molecules Synthesis of ethyl oleate (biodiesel) Butyl caprylate synthesis (flavor ester) Synthesis of structured lipids	Glogauer et al. (2011) Alnoch et al. (2016) Madalozzo et al. (2016)
LipMF3	Fat-contaminated soil from a wastewater treatment plant (Brazil)	FS	1650 U·mg^{-1} (tributyrin), 862 U·mg^{-1} (olive oil) Stable in hydrophilic organic solvents (25%, v/v in water)	Synthesis of ethyl oleate (biodiesel) Kinetic resolution of secondary alcohols (organic synthesis)	Almeida et al. (2019)
LipG9	Fat-contaminated soil from a wastewater treatment plant (Brazil)	SBS and FS	1200 U·mg^{-1} (olive oil)	Synthesis of ethyl esters (biodiesel) Kinetic resolution of aliphatic secondary alcohols (organic synthesis)	Alnoch et al. (2015) Bandeira et al. (2016)

Lipolytic Enzyme	Library Source	Screening Method*	Activity (Substrate)/Relevant Features	Suggested Applications	References
JkP01	Hot spring soil (India)	SBS and FS	2022 U·mg^{-1} (p-NP laurate) Stable in n-hexane and acetone (30%)	Detergent formulations	Sharma et al. (2012)
h1Lip1	Baltic Sea sediment bacteria (Sweden)	FS	160 U·mg^{-1} (p-NP butyrate), 150 U·mg^{-1} (p-NP caprylate)	Detergent formulations Bioremediation of soil and water at low temperature	Hårdeman et al. (2007)
OSTL28	Topsoil of Jiang Han oilfield of Hubei (China)	FS	236 U·mg^{-1} (p-NP laurate) High tolerance to glycerol and methanol, broad pH range, and thermostability	Biodiesel production	Fan et al. (2011)
Lip1 and Lip2	Pitcher fluid of *Nepenthes hybrida* in laboratory (Japan)	FS	Lipolytic activity at acidic pH values	Dairy and food industries	Morohoshi et al. (2011)
BDlipA	Water of Baek-du mountain (Korea)	SBS	3.2 U·mg^{-1} (p-NP caprate) Cold-adapted enzyme. Activated by Ca^{2+}, Mg^{2+}, and Mn^{2+}. Inhibited by Zn^{2+} and Cu^{2+}	Detergent formulations (low and high temperatures)	Park et al. (2009)

(Continued)

Table 1.1 (Continued)

Lipolytic Enzyme	Library Source	Screening Method*	Activity (Substrate)/Relevant Features	Suggested Applications	References
KM1	Refrigerators of a meat factory (China)	FS and SBS	1093 U·mg^{-1} (p-NP butyrate) Activated by Ca^{2+} and low concentration (10%) of ethanol, dimethyl sulfoxide, methanol acetonitrile	Detergent formulations (low temperature)	Ji et al. (2015)
PWTSC and PWTSB	Soil from Taishan (China)	FS and SBS	PWTSB 150 U·mg^{-1}, PWTSC 166 U mg^{-1} (p-NP palmitate) Lower sensitivity to metal ions	Detergent formulations (low temperature)	Wei et al. (2009)
EM3L4	Deep-sea sediment (near Papua New Guinea)	FS	5.3 U·mg^{-1} (p-NP caproate), Salt-resistant	Biocatalysis in pharmaceutical and fine chemical industries	Jeon et al. (2011)
Lip906	Mangrove soil (China)	FS	220 U·mg^{-1} (p-NP myristate) Activated by Hg^{2+}, inhibited by Fe^{2+}, Ca^{2+}, Co^{2+} and Mg^{2+}	Detergent formulations	Tang et al. (2017)
LipZ01	Oil-contaminated soil (China)	FS	Activity 42 U·mL^{-1} (olive oil) Stable in the range 35–60 °C and under alkaline conditions (pH 7–10) Activated by Ca^{2+} and Mn^{2+}	Biodiesel production	Zheng et al. (2013).

Lipolytic Enzyme	Library Source	Screening Method*	Activity (Substrate)/Relevant Features	Suggested Applications	References
LipCE	Oil-contaminated soil (Germany)	FS	2021 U·mg^{-1} (p-NP caprylate)	Kinetic resolution of ibuprofen derivatives	Elend et al. (2006)
LipS	Garden soil (Germany)	FS	12 U·mg^{-1} (p-NP caprylate) Hydrolysis and esterification at 70 °C	Kinetic resolution of ibuprofen derivatives at high temperatures	Chow et al. (2012)
LipR1	Soil from hot spring (India)	FS	8756 U·mg^{-1} (p-NP laurate)	Transesterification of secondary alcohols (organic synthesis)	Kumar et al. (2017)
LipZ03	Oil-contaminated soil (China)	FS and SBS	44 U·mL^{-1} (olive oil)	Biodiesel production	Zheng et al. (2013)
Lip479	Hot spring sediment (India)	SBS	597 U·mg^{-1} (p-NP laurate)	Biodiesel production	Sahoo et al. (2017)
Lip-1	Hot spring water (China)	FS	High tolerance to methanol and other organic solvents	Biodiesel production	Yan et al. (2017)
Lipase#8	Commercial supplier (USA)	NI	0.76 U·mg^{-1} (tributyrin)	Synthesis of structured lipids	Bertram et al. (2008)

(Continued)

Table 1.1 (Continued)

Lipolytic Enzyme	Library Source	Screening Method*	Activity (Substrate)/Relevant Features	Suggested Applications	References
LipIAF5-2	Batch reactor enriched biomass	FS	5.46 U·mg^{-1} (p-NP octanoate) Whole-cell biocatalysis Transesterification of glyceryl triacetate into isoamyl acetate in presence of isoamyl alcohol	Synthesis of short-chain fatty acids for aroma production	Brault et al. (2014)
Lip479	Hot spring sediment (India)	FS	Absolute activity not informed. Higher relative activity against p-NP myristate Stability in temperature and organic solvents	Biodiesel production	Sahoo et al. (2020)
Est25	Environmental soil pool (Korea)	FS	103 U·mg^{-1} (p-NP acetate)	Kinetic resolution of ibuprofen derivatives	Kim et al. (2006)
EstAT1 EstAT11	Arctic coastal sediments (Norway)	FS	ESTAT1—200 U·mg^{-1} (p-NP butyrate) ESTAT11—60 U·mg^{-1} (p-NP caproate)	Kinetic resolution of (RS)-ofloxacin ester	Jeon et al. (2009)

Lipolytic Enzyme	Library Source	Screening Method*	Activity (Substrate)/Relevant Features	Suggested Applications	References
EstCS2	Compost soil	FS	Absolute activity not informed. Higher relative activity against p-NP caproate. High stability in organic solvents	Kinetic resolution of ibuprofen derivatives. Polyurethane degradation	Kang et al. (2011)
EstEH112	Intertidal sediments (Korea)	FS	Absolute activity not informed. Higher relative activity against p-NP butyrate	Synthesis of tertiary alcohols for fragrance and flavor chemicals and pharmaceuticals	Oh et al. (2012)
Est22	Aqueous acidic leachate from landfill site (South Africa)	FS	60 U·mg^{-1} (p-NP butyrate)	Synthesis and modification of cephalosporin-based molecules	Mokoena et al. (2013)
EstP2K and EstF4K	Mixed soil (EstP2K) and contaminated river water (EstF4K) (China)	FS	EstF4K 700 U·mg^{-1} (p-NP butyrate), EstP2K 40 U·mg^{-1} (p-NP caprylate). Organic synthesis in the presence of DMSO and methanol	Synthesis of Taxol®	Ouyang et al. (2013)

(Continued)

Table 1.1 (Continued)

Lipolytic Enzyme	Library Source	Screening Method*	Activity (Substrate)/Relevant Features	Suggested Applications	References
Est3–14	Marine mud (China)	FS	292 U·mg^{-1} (p-NP butyrate)	Production of free all-*trans*-astaxanthin	Lu *et al.* (2018)
EST4	Marine mud (China)	FS	292 U·mg^{-1} (p-NP butyrate)	Production of short-chain flavor esters	Gao *et al.* (2016)
MLC3 and SLC5	Filamentous microbial mat from hot spring (MLC3) and sediment from the coastal region (SL5) (India)	FS and SBS	MLC3 0.51 U·mg^{-1}, SLC5 0.34 U·mg^{-1} (pNP butyrate)	Organic synthesis	Ranjan *et al.* (2018)
Est_p6	Marine sediments (China)	FS	2500 U·mg^{-1} (p-NP butyrate) Salt tolerant	Hydrolysis of milkfat for dairy products	Peng *et al.* (2014)

Lipolytic Enzyme	Library Source	Screening Method*	Activity (Substrate)/Relevant Features	Suggested Applications	References
EstB3 EstC7	Communities associated with the moss *Sphagnum magellanicum* (Austria)	FS	EstB3 85 U·mg^{-1}, EstC7 95 U·mg^{-1} (*p*-NP caproate)	Biodegradation (hydrolysis of polyesters)	Müller et al. (2017)
EstQ7	Cornfield soil (China)	FS	1190 U mg^{-1} (*p*-NP butyrate) Moderate tolerance in organic solvents Acyltransferase activity	Various industrial applications for food, pharmaceutical, and biotechnological products	Yan et al. (2021)
Tan410	Cottonfield soil (China)	FS	Absolute activity not informed. Optimal activity against *p*-NP acetate Stable from pH 4.5 to 10.0	Degradation of phenolic compounds	Yao et al. (2021)
PtEst1	Wastewater treatment plant (Germany)	FS	k_{cat} of 3574 min^{-1} (ethyl 3-oxohexanoate) Broad substrate specificity Active in organic solvents	Biodegradation of cyclic molecules like cyclohexanone or dioxane and a broad variety of esters	Höppner et al. (2021)

(Continued)

Table 1.1 (Continued)

Lipolytic Enzyme	Library Source	Screening Method*	Activity (Substrate)/Relevant Features	Suggested Applications	References
XtjR8	Lotus pond sludge (China)	FS	1079 U·mg^{-1} (p-NP acetate), 56 U·mg^{-1} (p-NP caprylate) Phthalate-hydrolyzing activity	Biodegradation of phthalate plasticizer	Qiu et al. (2020)
EST5	Microbial consortium specialized for diesel oil degradation (Brazil)	SBS	Esterification activity 127 U·mg^{-1} (butyric acid/methanol) Cold active. Stable in Triton X-100 and Tween 20 and in organic solvents	Synthesis of flavor esters	Maester et al. (2020), Maester et al. (2016)
EstM2	Municipal waste-contaminated soil	FS	641 U·mg^{-1} (p-NP butyrate) Temperature range: 16 to 55 °C	Biodegradation of phthalate plasticizers	Sakar et al. (2020)
Est1 and Est2	Thermophilic compost soil (Germany)	FS	Est1 23.3 U·mg^{-1} (p-NP butyrate), Est2 10.7 U·mg^{-1} (p-NP valerate) Thermostable (80 and 70 °C) and stable in hydrophilic organic solvents	Detergent formulations (high temperatures, alkaline) Organic synthesis and biodiesel production Bioremediation of environmental waste	Lu et al. (2019)

FS: functional screening, SBS: sequence-based screening, p-NP: p-nitrophenyl esters. The list was created by searching the Web of Science database (accessed June 23rd, 2021) with the following keywords: (lipase OR esterase) AND (metagenom*) AND (applicat* OR synthe*) in topic, date of publication from 2000 to 2021.

Metagenomics as an Enzyme Prospecting Tool | **17**

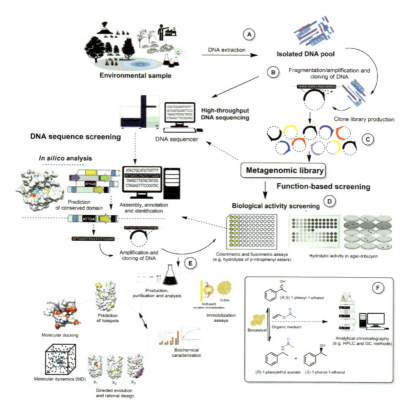

Figure 1.1 Steps of the metagenomic approach for isolating new enzymes. (a) Environmental sampling and DNA extraction, (b) construction of the metagenomic library by either DNA sequencing through high-throughput platforms and further *in silico* analysis for DNA sequence screening, or cloning of the DNA into appropriate vectors for function-based screening, (c) transformation of recombinant clones into a cell host, (d) screening of the clones of the metagenomic library, (e) purification, biochemical characterization, improvement of desired properties and immobilization assays, (f) application of the biocatalyst, for example, in the kinetic resolution of secondary alcohols.

The next step, (b) in Fig. 1.1, is the construction of the metagenomic library, which might be done either by DNA sequencing through high-throughput platforms and further *in silico* analysis for DNA sequence screening (detailed in Section 1.4) or by cloning of DNA in fragments into appropriate vectors and transformation of recombinant clones into a cell host for function-based screening. This step requires the selection of appropriate vectors and hosts. When selecting a vector, one needs to consider the size of insert fragments, which may target one product or complex metabolic pathways, the quality of the extracted DNA, the number of copies, which may be limited to one or more copies inside the host, the selected host, and the screening method (Xing et al., 2012). Frequently used vectors include plasmids (5–10 kb), which are adequate for short inserts, cosmids and fosmids (23–45 kb), which are appropriate for larger clusters of genes and operons (López-López et al., 2014), or even bacterial artificial chromosomes (BAC, about 100 kb), which allow complex gene clusters that encode for numerous enzymatic activities and metabolites (Chu et al., 2008). Fosmid-type vectors have been used most frequently since the sizes of genes that encode for the majority of enzymes are within the fosmid size range (Barzkar et al., 2021).

In the third step, (c) in Fig. 1.1, host selection should consider the efficiency of hosting one or more vectors per cell, the capability of cell machinery for effective protein expression, the stability of the vector inside the cells, and the characteristics for screening, such as expression inside the cells or exporting to the cultivation broth. The most widely used host is *Escherichia coli*, but microorganisms from other genera, such as *Bacillus*, *Pseudomonas*, and *Staphylococcus*, have also been used. Among the yeasts and fungi, *Pichia pastoris* has a major role due to its ability to execute correct posttranslational modifications, such as correct protein folding, phosphorylation and glycosylation, and correct formation of disulfide bridges (Borrelli and Trono, 2015).

The fourth step, (d) in Fig. 1.1, is the screening of the clones for enzyme activity. The screening step is one of the challenges of the metagenomic approach, given that, together with the genetic diversity of the sample collected, the reliability of the screening method determines the success in finding new enzymes (Xing et al., 2012). There are basically two approaches for selecting clones in a metagenomic library: functional screening and sequence-based screening, both having advantages and disadvantages, as detailed in Sections 1.3 and 1.4.

In the last step, (e) in Fig. 1.1, if the screening step is successful, the enzyme is then expressed and recovered from the fermentation broth. This requires several procedures: with the most common host,

E. coli, the enzyme is intracellular, and its recovery will require the breakage of the cell, which can be done using enzymes or physical methods, such as ultrasonic processing, followed by the removal of the cell debris by centrifugation. Finally, the enzyme is purified, generally using affinity chromatography in a nickel column, which is made possible by the insertion of an affinity tag in the vector that was used for enzyme cloning. The most used affinity tag is the His-tag, which corresponds to a string of six histidine residues inserted either at the amino terminus or at the carboxyl terminus of the enzyme. The enzyme purity is then evaluated by electrophoresis (SDS-PAGE) and the enzyme activity is determined by an appropriate method.

The purified enzyme is then ready to be characterized and further processed according to its application. In general, biochemical characterization is done, which includes the determination of kinetic parameters, such as the effects of pH, temperature, organic solvents, salts, and other components of interest, on the activity and stability of the enzyme. If the enzyme is interesting, then it can be crystallized, and its structure determined.

1.3 Functional Screening in a Metagenomic Library

Functional screening is the most used and effective method for enzyme discovery and is based on the expression of functional enzymes and detection of their activity by simple methods, mainly by developing color resulting from the cleavage of appropriate substrates (Guazzaroni *et al.*, 2015; Robinson *et al.*, 2021). As there is no need to know the gene sequence of enzymes *a priori* (Alma'abadi *et al.*, 2015; Madhavan *et al.*, 2017), functional screening is cheaper than sequence-based screening.

Lipolytic enzymes are readily found in metagenomic libraries due to the ease of performing the functional screening. In this case, the screening can be done by cultivating the clones in Petri dishes with a solid medium enriched with appropriate substrates, with the hydrolysis halo formed around the colonies being a qualitative measure of lipolytic activity (Kennedy *et al.*, 2011; Simon and Daniel,

2011). Colorimetric methods can be done in microplates with appropriate substrates (Hosokawa *et al.*, 2015), and clones can also be screened for enantioselectivity (Qian *et al.*, 2007; Liu *et al.*, 2010; Löfgren *et al.*, 2019; Tang *et al.*, 2012; Wahab *et al.*, 2016).

Despite its relative simplicity, screening is potentially a labor-intensive task, given that metagenomic libraries are often very large, containing many thousands of DNA sequences (Choi *et al.*, 2014). Beyond this, it is estimated that simple screening protocols detect less than 0.1% of the potentially positive clones of a metagenomic library (Ferrer *et al.*, 2016), with the ratio of positive hits (based on the total number of clones screened) ranging from 1:11 to 1:193–200 (Peña-Garcia *et al.*, 2016).

High-throughput screening methods have been developed to enable the screening of large metagenomic libraries. These methods are generally based on automation of traditional screening processes and allow the screening of thousands of clones per day (Xiao *et al.*, 2015; Ngara *et al.*, 2018). For example, Ma *et al.* (2021) explored the potential of droplet flow cytometry, an ultrahigh-throughput method. Among one million clones with a 2.5-kb average insert size, they found 180 positive clones, one of which was a novel esterase, EstWY.

Functional screening can lead to failure of gene expression, depending on the heterologous organism used (Madhavan *et al.*, 2017). Low levels of expression occur due to incompatibility of the gene with the heterologous expression system that is used (Choi *et al.*, 2014). This incompatibility is mainly due to difficulties in recognizing the promoter, inefficient translation of the protein, and lack of posttranslational modifications necessary to obtain the active enzyme. Strategies that improve the retrieval of new genes in metagenomics include the use of different host organisms in tandem with the screening, the improvement of heterologous expression in each host, and the development of ever more sensitive screening assays for enzymatic functions of interest (Liebl *et al.*, 2014).

For a more comprehensive description of screening methods, other references may be consulted (Jaeger *et al.*, 1999; Wang *et al.*, 2012; Jacques *et at.*, 2017; Fulton *et al.*, 2018; Markel *et al.*, 2020 Albayati *et al.*, 2020; Qu *et al.*, 2020).

1.4 Sequence-Based Screening in a Metagenomic Library

Sequence-based screening bypasses the limitations of expression that can occur in functional screening because the search for the desired enzyme is done *in silico*, not requiring the expression of the cloned genes in a heterologous host.

The consolidation of New Generation Sequencing (NGS) techniques for screening DNA has facilitated the use of sequence-based screening in metagenomic libraries. These techniques include second-generation platforms (Roche/454, Illumina and Ion Torrent) and third-generation platforms (PacBio and Oxford Nanopore), which use long-read sequencing. These platforms allow the analysis of a huge volume of data from metagenomic libraries with high efficiency, low running costs, and easy forms to analyze results (Prayogo *et al.*, 2020; Kchouk *et al.*, 2017). As such, they have allowed a significant expansion of databases of genes coding for hypothetical functional proteins (Ambardar *et al.*, 2016; Kusnezowa and Leichert, 2017; Madhavan *et al.*, 2017).

The *in silico* screening for new enzymes in metagenomic libraries uses approaches based on homology, sequence analysis of essential motifs, characterization of certain lipolytic enzymes into families, and predictions of enzyme localization to distinguish enzymes based on their functional roles (Vorapreeda *et al.*, 2016). This homology-based prospection uses different algorithms, such as BLAST (https://blast.ncbi.nlm.nih.gov/Blast.cgi) and EMBL-EBI (https://www.ebi.ac.uk/Tools/sss/). Moreover, homology-based approaches can use databases for specific enzymes to guide searches for these enzymes within the sequences of the metagenomic library. For lipolytic enzymes, there are the ESTHER database (Lenfant *et al.*, 2013), the Lipase Engineering Database (LED) (Buchholz *et al.*, 2016), MELDB (Kang *et al.*, 2006), and Lipabase (Messaoudi *et al.*, 2011).

There are essentially two strategies for performing sequence-based or *in silico* screening. In the first strategy, which is based on gene amplification, the genes are identified by PCR (polymerase chain reaction), or by hybridization using degenerated primers and probes derived from conserved regions of known genes (Handelsman, 2004). Since this technique targets internal regions of genes, such as conserved domains and motifs, the regions that flank these motifs need to be cloned or synthesized to obtain the entire gene (Uria and Zilda, 2016). In the second strategy, which is called shotgun metagenome sequencing, the total genetic material is sequenced, and genes are identified by comparison with the information contained in biological databases.

After sequencing the DNA of the metagenomic sample by NGS techniques, the analysis of the sequences includes several steps. The first step is pre-processing, which consists of computational quality control, which minimizes sequence biases or artifacts, and removes sequencing duplicates. The second step is sequence analysis, which can be done either by the "read-based" approach, in which the reads are directly mapped, or by the "assembly-based" approach, in which reads are assembled into contigs and annotated to attribute a given classification and to generate taxonomic and functional categories. The third step is post-processing, which uses multivariate statistical techniques to interpret the data (Quince *et al.*, 2017). All these steps are based on computational algorithms that need to be preselected and adjusted by users and are critical for obtaining successful results.

However, sequence-based screening can have disadvantages. Only new variants of the same functional classes of enzymes can be found, as the method is based on sequence homology (Lee *et al.*, 2010; Simon and Daniel, 2011). Sequencing pipelines are computationally intensive (Robinson *et al.*, 2021) and analysis may require knowledge of programming languages.

Furthermore, sequence-based screening does not dispense the experimental characterization of protein function (Kusnezowa and Leichert, 2017). In fact, as the speed of generation of new sequences is very high, it is necessary to combine the two types of screening, functional and sequential screening, in a coordinated manner.

Effective future exploration of lipolytic enzymes in metagenomic libraries will require integrated analysis through different computational approaches, such as transcriptomics, proteomics, three-dimensional structure determination, and molecular dynamics, in order to gain a better understanding of protein structure and to allow the selection of enzymes based on affinity toward substrates (Vorapreeda *et al.*, 2016). Integrating several types of data, including marker gene sequencing, metagenomics, metaproteomics, and metabolomics, is crucial to understanding the composition and function of microbial communities (Knight *et al.*, 2018). This multi-omics approach would allow exploration of microbial community shifts, phenotypic response to different environment disturbances, and the future engineering of niches within mixed-culture biotechnological processes (Herold *et al.*, 2020). The development of computational tools, even the use of artificial intelligence, will provide better selection tools for identifying suitable biocatalysts from the rich sequence information already accessible in databanks (Bell *et al.*, 2021).

1.5 Lipolytic Enzymes Isolated from Metagenomic Libraries

Lipolytic enzymes are the most representative enzymes of metagenomic libraries. Ferrer *et al.* (2015) surveyed data regarding 6038 clones, enzymes, or coding sequences that were isolated from 256 environments by metagenomic prospecting: 68% of these enzymes were lipolytic enzymes. Likewise, Berini *et al.* (2017) evaluated 332 metagenomic enzymes isolated from January 2014 to March 2017 and, of this total, 161 (48%) were either lipases or esterases.

Many lipolytic enzymes isolated from metagenomic libraries (Table 1.1) present characteristics of industrial relevance, such as stability at low temperatures, halotolerance, tolerance to organic solvents and ions such as calcium, high transesterification activity, and high enantioselectivity. These characteristics are useful in applications involving the resolution of pharmaceutical compounds, the production of biofuels, and the use of lipases in detergents and as bioremediation agents. The most frequently found characteristics are the transesterification of long-chain substrates and resistance to low temperatures; characteristics related to applications in the biofuel industry for the production of biodiesel and in the detergent industry. Most of the esterases listed in Table 1.1 were selected based on their hydrolytic activity and enantioselectivity for application in the resolution of compounds in the pharmaceutical industry. However, most of the articles that have reported the isolation of lipolytic enzymes from metagenomic libraries have focused on biochemical characterization of these enzymes, few studies have been carried out with the aim of applying these enzymes in biocatalytic reactions. In the analysis undertaken by Ferrer *et al.* (2016), among the 288 lipases and esterases studied, only five were tested in synthesis reactions.

Metagenomics has proven to be an important tool for obtaining new lipases with desired characteristics as an alternative to commercially available enzymes: the 14 metagenomic lipases that have been already used for biocatalysis have desirable characteristics, such as stability in organic solvents and activity at low or high temperatures, which are important for applications in the kinetic resolution of optically pure compounds and biodiesel synthesis and for the use of lipases in detergent formulations (Almeida *et al.*, 2020).

It is clear that recent developments in the field of metagenomics are enabling us to access lipases from deeply divergent lineages, including lipases with new characteristics that are classified into novel families (Hitch and Clavel, 2019). However, there are still challenges to be overcome: Although metagenomics has opened the possibility of isolating enzymes from non-culturable microorganisms, there are probably microorganisms from which it is difficult to obtain usable DNA fragments (Quince *et al.*, 2017). Some limitations of heterologous expression of lipases have been circumvented with the co-expression of foldases or chaperones (Martini *et al.*, 2014), removal of signal sequences, and low-temperature induction (Nagarajan, 2012).

1.6 The Lipases LipC12, LipG9, and LipMF3: A Case Study

The lipases LipC12, LipG9, and LipMF3 (Table 1.1) were isolated from the SCGA metagenomic library, which was built by Glogauer *et al.* (2011) from fat-contaminated soil collected from the banks of lagoons of the effluent treatment plant of a meat and dairy processing industry, in the city of Carambeí of the state of Paraná, Brazil. This library was built with DNA fragments of about 36 kb, cloned using a fosmid vector (pCC2FOS), generating a metagenomic library with approximately 500,000 clones, using *E. coli* EPI300 as the host. The library is deposited at the Department of Biochemistry and Molecular Biology of the Federal University of Paraná, Brazil.

The SCGA metagenomic library was screened by culturing the clones in petri dishes with LB (Luria Bertani) agar enriched with different triacylglycerols to identify hydrolysis halos. This selection was performed in three steps with the substrates tributyrin, tricaprylin, and triolein. In the first step, with tributyrin, 2661 clones were identified; of these, 127 clones showed a halo of hydrolysis against tricaprylin, and, finally, only 32 showed a halo of hydrolysis against triolein. Clones were then selected for further characterization according to the size of the hydrolysis halo. From three of the 32 triolein-hydrolyzing clones, the lipases LipC12, LipG9, and LipMF3 were isolated and characterized.

Of the three lipases, LipC12 is so far the most studied. LipC12 has a molecular mass of 33 kDa and 72% identity with the putative lipase from *Yersinia enterocolitica* subsp. palearctica Y11 (Glogauer *et al.*, 2011). Phylogenetic analysis classified LipC12 as belonging to the I.1 subfamily. In addition, the three-dimensional structure of LipC12 was determined by crystallography (Fig. 1.2) (Martini *et al.*, 2012; Martini *et al.*, 2019). Another key feature is that LipC12 folds into its native shape without the need for a foldase, facilitating its expression. LipC12 has high expression levels in *E. coli*, reaching 20% of the total expressed proteins, and is easy to purify by affinity chromatography using a nickel column, since it has a His-tag (>95% purity).

In an aqueous medium, free LipC12 had high specific activity for long-chain triacylglycerols, ranging from 800 to 1800 U mg^{-1}. These specific activities are comparable to those of the commercial lipases of *Rhizopus oryzae*, *Rhizomucor miehei*, and *Thermomyces lanuginosus*. LipC12 is active and stable over a wide range of pH (6.5–11) and temperature (30–60 °C). It is also stable in aqueous solutions of several polar organic solvents (methanol, ethanol, propanol, acetone, and DMSO) after incubation for 48 h, at concentrations of up to 30% (v/v) of the solvents, maintaining 100% of residual activity in all solutions (Glogauer *et al.*, 2011).

LipC12 was immobilized covalently on the support Immobead 150 (Immo-LipC12). Immo-LipC12 was stable in pure organic solvents, maintaining residual activities of 60% in polar solvents (ethanol and isopropanol) and of more than 90% in non-polar solvents after 12 h at 30 °C (Madalozzo et al., 2015). Immo-LipC12 was used to synthesize ethyl oleate in n-hexane (Fig. 1.3a); 99% of conversion was achieved in 60 min. Moreover, the same preparation was used for 10 reaction cycles, maintaining more than 95% of residual activity. Immo-LipC12 was also used to synthesize ethyl oleate in a solvent-free system, where the best result was a conversion of 85% in 48 h, achieved with stepwise addition of the ethanol (Madalozzo et al., 2015).

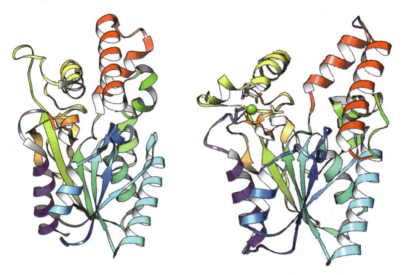

Figure 1.2 Three-dimensional structure of the metagenomic lipase LipC12 (PDB:6CL4). LipC12 with the structure in the "closed" (left-hand side) and "open" (right-hand side) forms. The calcium ion is indicated as a green sphere and the lid domain is indicated in red.

Immo-LipC12 also catalyzes ester synthesis with various saturated and unsaturated fatty acids, giving conversions of over 90% in 1 h. It is also regioselective, being sn-1,3-specific. These features allowed the use of Immo-LipC12 to produce an MLM-type structured lipid from olive oil and caprylic acid, in a solvent-free system (Fig. 1.3b). The product was a modified olive oil containing 23% caprylic acid in the sn-1 and sn-3 positions, a promising result that demonstrates the potential of LipC12 for applications in the food industry (Madalozzo et al., 2016). Based on its regioselectivity, LipC12, immobilized on alkyl-aldehyde support, was evaluated in the regioselective deacetylation of 3,4,6-tri-*O*-acetyl-D-glucal (Fig. 1.3c). The highest yield (69%) was obtained for the C-3 monoacetylated product (4,6-di-*O*-acetyl-D-glucal) at pH 5.0 and 4 °C (Alnoch et al., 2016). These results indicate that the regioselectivity of LipC12 is similar to that of the immobilized lipase B from *Candida antarctica* (CALB) in the same reaction conditions and demonstrate the potential of LipC12 in the regioselective deacetylation of glucose derivatives.

The results presented above show that LipC12 has a great potential in organic synthesis, mainly due to its versatility in catalyzing different reactions. However, although LipC12 remains active and stable in organic solvents at mild temperatures, it is not as stable as commercial immobilized lipases like CALB under more aggressive conditions, such as solvent-free systems or temperatures above 60 °C. Furthermore, studies in kinetic resolution using LipC12 have not been promising. For example, in the transesterification of (*R*,*S*)-1-phenylethanol, LipC12 had low activity (conversion <10% in 24 h), with a low enantiomeric ratio (E = 46). Commercial lipases, such as CALB, or enzymes with high enantioselectivity (e.g., LipG9 isolated from the same metagenomic library, as described below), give enantiomeric ratios above 200.

The second lipase characterized from the SCGA library, LipG9, needs a foldase (Lif) in order to fold correctly. Sequence analyses showed that LipG9 and LifG9 have 96% and 77% of identity, respectively, with the lipase and the foldase of *Aeromonas veronii* B565. Through phylogenetic analysis, LipG9 was classified in the subfamily I.1 of bacterial lipases. Martini et al. (2014) co-expressed the *lipG9* and *lifG9* genes and purified the crude extract using a nickel column. SDS-PAGE analysis of the fractions eluted from the nickel column showed that LipG9 remains complexed with its foldase during the purification. The complex Lip-LifG9 (hereafter referred to simply as LipG9) was characterized. LipG9 has high specific activities against long-chain triacylglycerols 820 U mg^{-1} against triolein). Free LipG9 is active and stable over a wide range of pH (6.0 to 9.0) and temperature (10 to 50 °C).

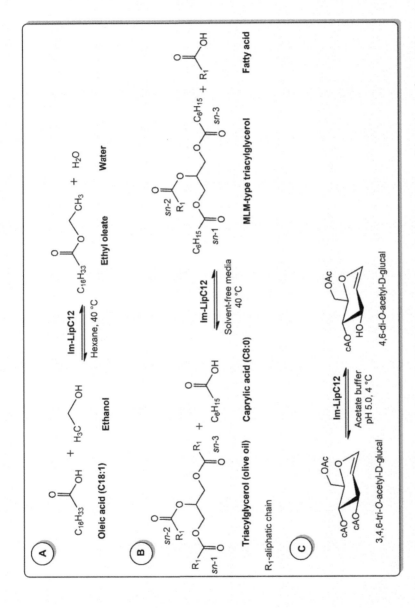

Figure 1.3 Applications of the metagenomic lipase LipC12. (a) Ethyl oleate synthesis in *n*-hexane, (b) synthesis of an MLM-type structured lipid from olive oil and caprylic acid in a solvent-free system, and (c) regioselective deacetylation of 4,6-di-*O*-acetyl-D-glucal.

LipG9 was immobilized on a hydrophobic support (Accurel MP1000) and the immobilized preparation (Acc-LipG9) was characterized in an organic medium. Acc-LipG9 showed high stability (>80%) in pure polar and non-polar organic solvents, such as acetone, ethanol, *n*-heptane, and toluene (Alnoch *et al.*, 2015). Acc-LipG9 was evaluated in the synthesis of ethyl esters of fatty acids of different chain lengths in *n*-heptane. The highest conversions (90% in 3 h) were obtained for medium- and long-chain saturated fatty acids (C8, C14, and C16). Like LipC12, free LipG9 and Acc-LipG9 were regioselective, being *sn*-1,3-specific.

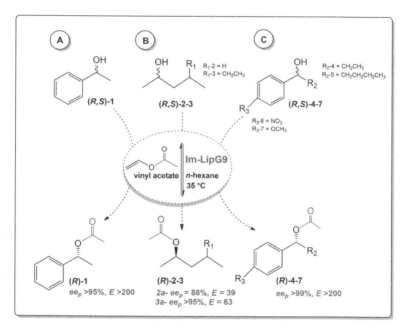

Figure 1.4 Applications of the metagenomic lipase LipG9 in the kinetic resolution of secondary alcohols. (A) Aromatic secondary alcohols, (B) Aliphatic secondary alcohols, and (C) Kinetic resolution of secondary benzylic alcohols. (*R,S*)-**1**: 1-phenyl-1-ethanol; (*R,S*)-**2**: pentan-2-ol; (*R,S*)-**3**: 4-methyl-pentan-2-ol; (*R,S*)-**4**: 1-phenylpropan-1-ol; (*R,S*)-**5**: 1-phenylpentan-1-ol; (*R,S*)-**6**: 1-(4-nitrophenyl)ethan-1-ol; (*R,S*)-**7**: 1-(4-methoxyphenyl)ethan-1-ol.

In the transesterification of (*R,S*)-1-phenylethanol (Fig. 1.4a), Acc-LipG9 was highly enantioselective, giving an enantiomeric excess of the product (ee_p) for (*R*)-1-phenylethyl acetate higher than

99% and an enantiomeric ratio (E) greater than 200 (Alnoch et al., 2015). Later, LipG9 was immobilized covalently onto Immobead (Im-LipG9) and was used in the kinetic resolution of aliphatic sec-alcohols with different carbon chain lengths (Bandeira et al., 2016). Im-LipG9 gave conversions ranging from 19% to 59%, and enantiomeric excesses of substrate (ee_s) from 26 to 88% for alcohols, with high enantioselectivity for (R,S)-pentan-2-ol ($E = 39$) and (R,S)-4-methyl-pentan-2-ol ($E = 63$) (Fig. 1.4b).

More recently, Im-LipG9 was used in the kinetic resolution of different secondary benzylic alcohols (Thomas et al., 2019). Im-LipG9 showed high enantioselectivity for this class of compounds, with enantiomeric excesses of the product (ee_p) above 95%, and $E > 200$ for all alcohols (Fig. 1.4c). The performance of Im-LipG9 was similar to that of CALB and superior to that of *Candida rugosa* lipase in the same kinetic resolution reactions. These results show that Im-LipG9 is highly enantioselective and highlights the potential for further improvement and application of LipG9 for the resolution of chiral compounds.

The third lipase characterized from the SCGA library is LipMF3. Notably, the clone containing this enzyme gave hydrolysis halos against tributyrin and tricaprylin but not triolein, suggesting that LipMF3 was an esterase; however, the enzyme was later shown to be a lipase. LipMF3, similarly to LipG9, was co-expressed with its foldase and remain complexed with the foldase after purification using a nickel column. LipMF3 has a molecular mass of 32.4 kDa and 68% sequence identity with the lipase from *Chromobacterium violaceum*. Phylogenetic analysis classified LipMF3 as belonging to the subfamily I.1 of bacterial lipases. LipMF3 also showed high specific activity for the hydrolysis of long-chain triacylglycerols in aqueous media (862 U mg^{-1} against olive oil), with maximum activity at 40 °C and pH 6.5. It was stable in aqueous solutions of polar organic solvents (25% v/v of DMSO, isopropanol, methanol, ethanol, propanol, and butanol) (Almeida et al., 2019).

LipMF3 was immobilized onto a hydrophobic support (Sepabeads FP-BU). The immobilized preparation (Im-LipMF3) was used to synthesize ethyl oleate in *n*-hexane, giving 94% conversion in 5 h, at 40 °C. It was also used in the kinetic resolution of (R,S)-1-phenyl-1-ethanol in *n*-hexane, with vinyl acetate as the acyl donor.

The conversion of (R)-1-phenylethanol was 40% after 24 h, with an enantiomeric excess of the product (ee_p) of 90% and $E = 33$. Similar to LipC12 and LipG9, LipMF3 also has good catalytic properties and good potential to be used in biocatalysis.

To date, the SCGA metagenomic library has produced three new lipases, which have high activities against long-chain triacylglycerols, activities that are similar to those of commercial lipases. LipC12, LipG9, and LipMF3 were immobilized and successfully used in different reactions in organic media. This success suggests that it would be fruitful to search for other new lipolytic enzymes within this library.

1.7 Conclusions

Metagenomic libraries have been an important source of new lipolytic enzymes over the last 10 years. These metagenomic enzymes have proven to be selective, stable, and active in organic solvents, at low and high temperatures, and over a wide range of pH values. These properties are promising for application in the pharmaceutical, fuel, food, and fine chemistry industries. However, despite much research in the area, there is still an enormous potential to be explored in nature. One of the bottlenecks is the screening of the huge number of clones that are generated through the metagenomic approach. The finding of new lipolytic enzymes can be accelerated by combining high-throughput screening methods with advanced DNA sequencing techniques and new analytical platforms. Future trends will involve the use of computational methods, such as artificial intelligence, molecular dynamics, and molecular docking, to improve the new lipolytic enzymes found in metagenomic libraries; this improvement is necessary to make the new enzymes fully competitive with the available commercial enzymes.

Acknowledgments

We wish to thank CNPq (Conselho Nacional de Desenvolvimento Científico e Tecnológico), a Brazilian government agency for the advancement of science and technology. Research scholarships were granted to Rocío P.C. Ropaín by CAPES (Coordenação de

Aperfeiçoamento de Pessoal de Nível Superior), a Brazilian government agency for the development of personnel in higher education, and to David A. Mitchell, Janaína M. de Almeida and Nadia Krieger by CNPq. Robson C. Alnoch received a postdoctoral fellowship (Grant No: 2020/00081-4) from FAPESP (Fundação de Amparo à Pesquisa do Estado de São Paulo) and Patrícia Gruening received a scientific initiation scholarship (PIBIC) funded by CNPq. The Postgraduate Programs in Science-Biochemistry and in Chemistry of the Federal University of Paraná are financed, in part, by CAPES (Finance Code 001).

References

Albayati S.H., Masomian M., Ishak S.N.H., Mohamad Ali M.S.B., Thean A.L., Mohd Shariff F.B., Muhd Noor N.D.B., and Raja Abd Rahman R.N.Z., *Catalysts*, **10**(7) (2020), 747.

Alma'abadi A.D., Gojobori T., and Mineta K., *Genom Proteom Bioinform*, **13**(5) (2015), 290–295.

Almeida J.M., Martini V.P., Iulek J., Alnoch R.C., Moure V.R., Muller-Santos M., Souza E.M., Mitchell D.A., and Krieger N., *Int J Biol Macromol*, **137** (2019), 442–454.

Almeida J.M., Alnoch R.C., Souza E.M., Mitchell D.A., and Krieger N., *Biochim Biophys Acta Proteins Proteom*, **1868**(2) (2020), 140320.

Almeida O.G.G., and De Martinis E.C.P., *Appl Microbiol Biotechnol*, **103**(1) (2019), 69–82.

Alnoch R., Rodrigues de Melo R., Palomo J., Maltempi de Souza E., Krieger N., and Mateo C., *Catalysts*, **6**(12) (2016), 191.

Alnoch R.C., Martini V.P., Glogauer A., Costa A.C., Piovan L., Muller-Santos M., de Souza E.M., de Oliveira Pedrosa F., Mitchell D.A., and Krieger N., *PLoS One*, **10**(2) (2015), e0114945.

Ambardar S., Gupta R., Trakroo D., Lal R., and Vakhlu J., *Indian J Microbiol*, **56**(4) (2016), 394–404.

Arpigny J.L., and Jaeger K.-E., *Biochem J*, **343**(1) (1999), 177–183.

Bandeira P.T., Alnoch R.C., de Oliveira A.R.M., de Souza E.M., de Pedrosa F.O., Krieger N., and Piovan L., *J Mol Catal B Enzym*, **125** (2016), 58–63.

Barzkar N., Sohail M., Tamadoni Jahromi S., Gozari M., Poormozaffar S., Nahavandi R., and Hafezieh M., *Appl Biochem Biotechnol*, **193**(4) (2021), 1187–1214.

Bell E.L., Finnigan W., France S.P., Green A.P., Hayes M.A., Hepworth L.J., Lovelock S.L., Niikura H., Osuna S., Romero E., Ryan K.S., Turner N.J., and Flitsch S.L., *Nat Rev Methods Primers*, **1**(1) (2021), 46.

Berg G., Rybakova D., Fischer D., Cernava T., Verges M.C., Charles T., Chen X., Cocolin L., Eversole K., Corral G.H., Kazou M., Kinkel L., Lange L., Lima N., Loy A., Macklin J.A., Maguin E., Mauchline T., McClure R., Mitter B., Ryan M., Sarand I., Smidt H., Schelkle B., Roume H., Kiran G.S., Selvin J., Souza R.S.C., van Overbeek L., Singh B.K., Wagner M., Walsh A., Sessitsch A., and Schloter M., *Microbiome*, **8**(1) (2020), 103.

Berini F., Casciello C., Marcone G.L., and Marinelli F., *FEMS Microbiol Lett*, **364**(21) (2017).

Bertram M., Hildebrandt P., Weiner D.P., Patel J.S., Bartnek F., Hitchman T.S., and Bornscheuer U.T., *J Am Oil Chem Soc*, **85**(1) (2008), 47–53.

Borrelli G.M., and Trono D., *Int J Mol Sci*, **16**(9) (2015), 20774–20840.

Brault G., Shareck F., Hurtubise Y., Lépine F., and Doucet N., *PLoS One*, **9**(3) (2014), e91872.

Buchholz P.C., Vogel C., Reusch W., Pohl M., Rother D., Spiess A.C., and Pleiss J., *Chembiochem*, **17**(21) (2016), 2093–2098.

Castilla I.A., Woods D.F., Reen F.J., and O'Gara F., *Marine Drugs*, **16**(7) (2018), 227.

Choi S.-L., Rha E., Lee S.J., Kim H., Kwon K., Jeong Y.-S., Rhee Y.H., Song J.J., Kim H.-S., and Lee S.-G., *ACS Synth Biol*, **3**(3) (2014), 163–171.

Chow J., Kovacic F., Dall Antonia Y., Krauss U., Fersini F., Schmeisser C., Lauinger B., Bongen P., Pietruszka J., Schmidt M., Menyes I., Bornscheuer U.T., Eckstein M., Thum O., Liese A., Mueller-Dieckmann J., Jaeger K.-E., and Streit W.R., *PLoS One*, **7**(10) (2012), e47665.

Elend C., Schmeisser C., Hoebenreich H., Steele H.L., and Streit W.R., *J Biotechnol*, **130**(4) (2007), 370–377.

Fan X., Liu X., Wang K., Wang S., Huang R., and Liu Y., *J Mol Catal B Enzym*, **72**(3) (2011), 319–326.

Ferrer M., Martínez-Martínez M., Bargiela R., Streit W.R., Golyshina O.V., and Golyshin P.N., *Microb Biotechnol*, **9** (2016), 22–34.

Fulton A., Hayes M.R., Schwaneberg U., Pietruszka J., and Jaeger K.-E., *Protein Engineering: Methods and Protocols* (Bornscheuer U.T., and Höhne M., eds), 2018, Humana Press.

Gao W., Wu K., Chen L., Fan H., Zhao Z., Gao B., Wang H., and Wei D., *Microb Cell Fact*, **15**(1) (2016), 41.

Glogauer A., Martini V.P., Faoro H., Couto G.H., Muller-Santos M., Monteiro R.A., Mitchell D.A., de Souza E.M., Pedrosa F.O., and Krieger N., *Microb Cell Fact*, **10** (2011), 54.

Guazzaroni M.E., Silva-Rocha R., and Ward R.J., *Microb Biotechnol*, **8**(1) (2015), 52–64.

Handelsman J., Rondon M.R., Brady S.F., Clardy J., and Goodman R.M., *Chem Biol*, **5**(10) (1998), R245–R249.

Handelsman J., *Microbiol Mol Biol Rev*, **68**(4) (2004), 669–685.

Hårdeman F., and Sjöling S., *FEMS Microbiol Ecol*, **59**(2) (2007), 524–534.

Herold M., Martinez Arbas S., Narayanasamy S., Sheik A.R., Kleine-Borgmann L.A.K., Lebrun L.A., Kunath B.J., Roume H., Bessarab I., Williams R.B.H., Gillece J.D., Schupp J.M., Keim P.S., Jager C., Hoopmann M.R., Moritz R.L., Ye Y., Li S., Tang H., Heintz-Buschart A., May P., Muller E.E.L., Laczny C.C., and Wilmes P., *Nat Commun*, **11**(1) (2020), 5281.

Hitch T.C.A., and Clavel T., *PeerJ*, **7** (2019), e7249.

Höppner A., Bollinger A., Kobus S., Thies S., Coscolín C., Ferrer M., Jaeger K.-E., and Smits S.H.J., *FEBS J*, **288**(11) (2021), 3570–3584.

Hosokawa M., Hoshino Y., Nishikawa Y., Hirose T., Yoon D.H., Mori T., Sekiguchi T., Shoji S., and Takeyama H., *Biosens Bioelectron*, **67** (2015), 379–385.

Jacques P., Béchet M., Bigan M., Caly D., Chataigné G., Coutte F., Flahaut C., Heuson E., Leclère V., Lecouturier D., Phalip V., Ravallec R., Dhulster P., and Froidevaux R., *Bioprocess Biosyst Eng*, **40**(2) (2017), 161–180.

Jaeger K.E., Ransac S., Dijkstra B.W., Colson C., van Heuvel M., and Misset O., *FEMS Microbiol Rev*, **15**(1) (1994), 29–63.

Jaeger K.E., Dijkstra B.W., and Reetz M.T., *Annu Rev Microbiol*, **53**(1) (1999), 315–351.

Jeon J.H., Kim J.-T., Kang S.G., Lee J.-H., and Kim S.-J., *Mar Biotechnol*, **11**(3) (2009), 307–316.

Jeon J.H., Kim J.T., Lee H.S., Kim S.-J., Kang S.G., Choi S.H., and Lee J.-H., *Evid Based Complementary Altern Med*, **2011** (2011), 271419.

Ji X., Chen G., Zhang Q., Lin L., and Wei Y., *J Basic Microbiol*, **55**(6) (2015), 718–728.

Kang C.-H., Oh K.-H., Lee M.-H., Oh T.-K., Kim B.H., and Yoon J.-H., *Microb Cell Fact*, **10**(1) (2011), 41.

Kang H.Y., Kim J.F., Kim M.H., Park S.H., Oh T.K., and Hur C.G., *FEBS Lett*, **580**(11) (2006), 2736–2740.

Kchouk M., Gibrat J.F., and Elloumi M., *Biol Med*, **09**(03) (2017).

Kennedy J., O'Leary N.D., Kiran G.S., Morrissey J.P., O'Gara F., Selvin J., and Dobson A.D.W., *J Appl Microbiol*, **111**(4) (2011), 787–799.

Kim Y.-J., Choi G.-S., Kim S.-B., Yoon G.-S., Kim Y.-S., and Ryu Y.-W., *Protein Expr Purif*, **45**(2) (2006), 315–323.

Knight R., Vrbanac A., Taylor B.C., Aksenov A., Callewaert C., Debelius J., Gonzalez A., Kosciolek T., McCall L.I., McDonald D., Melnik A.V., Morton J.T., Navas J., Quinn R.A., Sanders J.G., Swafford A.D., Thompson L.R., Tripathi A., Xu Z.Z., Zaneveld J.R., Zhu Q., Caporaso J.G., and Dorrestein P.C., *Nat Rev Microbiol*, **16**(7) (2018), 410–422.

Kovacic F., Babic N., Krauss U., and Jaeger K.-E., *Handbook of Hydrocarbon and Lipid Microbiology*, 2019, Springer, pp. 1–35.

Kumar R., Banoth L., Banerjee U.C., and Kaur J., *Int J Biol Macromol*, **95** (2017), 995–1003.

Kusnezowa A., and Leichert L.I., *BMC Bioinformatics*, **18**(1) (2017), 267.

Lee H.S., Kwon K.K., Kang S.G., Cha S.S., Kim S.J., and Lee J.H., *Curr Opin Biotechnol*, **21**(3) (2010), 353–357.

Lenfant N., Hotelier T., Velluet E., Bourne Y., Marchot P., and Chatonnet A., *Nucleic Acids Res*, **41**(Database issue) (2013), D423–D429.

Liebl W., Angelov A., Juergensen J., Chow J., Loeschcke A., Drepper T., Classen T., Pietruszka J., Ehrenreich A., Streit W.R., and Jaeger K.E., *Appl Microbiol Biotechnol*, **98**(19) (2014), 8099–8109.

Liu D., Trodler P., Eiben S., Koschorreck K., Müller M., Pleiss J., Maurer S.C., Branneby C., Schmid R.D., and Hauer B., *ChemBioChem*, **11**(6) (2010), 789–795.

Löfgren J., Görbe T., Oschmann M., Svedendahl Humble M., and Bäckvall J.-E., *ChemBioChem*, **20**(11) (2019), 1438–1443.

Lombard N., Prestat E., van Elsas J.D., and Simonet P., *FEMS Microbiol Ecol*, **78**(1) (2011), 31–49.

Lopez-Lopez O., Cerdan M.E., and Gonzalez Siso M.I., *Curr Protein Pept Sci*, **15**(5) (2014), 445–455.

Lu M., Dukunde A., and Daniel R., *Appl Microbiol Biotechnol*, **103**(8) (2019), 3421–3437.

Lu P., Gao X., Dong H., Liu Z., Secundo F., Xue C., and Mao X., *J Agric Food Chem*, **66**(11) (2018), 2812–2821.

Ma F., Guo T., Zhang Y., Bai X., Li C., Lu Z., Deng X., Li D., Kurabayashi K., and Yang G.-y., *Environ Microbiol*, **23**(2) (2021), 996–1008.

Madalozzo A.D., Martini V.P., Kuniyoshi K.K., de Souza E.M., Pedrosa F.O., Glogauer A., Zanin G.M., Mitchell D.A., and Krieger N., *J Mol Catal B Enzym*, **116** (2015), 45–51.

Madalozzo A.D., Martini V.P., Kuniyoshi K.K., Souza E.M., Pedrosa F.O., Zanin G.M., Mitchell D.A., and Krieger N., *Biocatal Agric Biotechnol*, **8** (2016), 294–300.

Madhavan A., Sindhu R., Parameswaran B., Sukumaran R.K., and Pandey A., *Appl Biochem Biotechnol*, **183**(2) (2017), 636–651.

Maester T.C., Pereira M.R., Machado Sierra E.G., Balan A., and de Macedo Lemos E.G., *Appl Microbiol Biotechnol*, **100**(13) (2016), 5815–5827.

Maester T.C., Pereira M.R., Malaman A.M.G., Borges J.P., Pereira P.A.M., and Lemos E.G.M., *Catalysts*, **10**(10) (2020), 1100.

Marchesi J.R., and Ravel J., *Microbiome*, **3** (2015), 31.

Markel U., Essani K.D., Besirlioglu V., Schiffels J., Streit W.R., and Schwaneberg U., *Chem Soc Rev*, **49**(1) (2020), 233–262.

Martini V.P., Glogauer A., Iulek J., Souza E.M., Pedrosa F.O., and Krieger N., *Acta Crystallogr Sect F Struct Biol Cryst Commun*, **68**(Pt 2) (2012), 175–177.

Martini V.P., Glogauer A., Müller-Santos M., Iulek J., de Souza E.M., Mitchell D.A., Pedrosa F.O., and Krieger N., *Microb Cell Fact*, **13**(1) (2014), 171.

Martini V.P., Krieger N., Glogauer A., Souza E.M., and Iulek J., *N Biotechnol*, **53** (2019), 65–72.

Messaoudi A., Belguith H., Ghram I., and Hamida J.B., *Int J Bioinform Res Appl*, **7**(4) (2011), 390–401.

Mokoena N., Mathiba K., Tsekoa T., Steenkamp P., and Rashamuse K., *Biochem Biophys Res Commun*, **437**(3) (2013), 342–348.

Morohoshi T., Oikawa M., Sato S., Kikuchi N., Kato N., and Ikeda T., *J Biosci Bioeng*, **112**(4) (2011), 315–320.

Muller C.A., Perz V., Provasnek C., Quartinello F., Guebitz G.M., and Berg G., *Appl Environ Microbiol*, **83**(4) (2017), e02641–e02616.

Nagarajan S., *Biotechnol Appl Biochem*, **168**(5) (2012), 1163–1196.

Ngara T.R., and Zhang H., *Genomics, Genomics Proteomics Bioinformatics*, **16**(6) (2018), 405–415.

Oh K.-H., Nguyen G.-S., Kim E.-Y., Kourist R., Bornscheuer U., Oh T.-K., and Yoon J.-H., *J Mol Catal B Enzym*, **80** (2012), 67–73.

Ouyang L.-M., Liu J.-Y., Qiao M., and Xu J.-H., *Biotechnol Appl Biochem*, **169**(1) (2013), 15–28.

Park I.H., Kim S.H., Lee Y.S., Lee S.C., Zhou Y., Kim C.M., Ahn S.C., and Choi Y.L., *J Microbiol Biotechnol*, **19**(2) (2009), 128–135.

Peña-Garcia C., Martinez-Martinez M., Reyes-Duarte D., and Ferrer M., *Comb Chem High Throughput Screen*, **19**(8) (2016), 605–615.

Peng Q., Wang X., Shang M., Huang J., Guan G., Li Y., and Shi B., *Microbial Cell Factories*, **13**(1) (2014), 1.

Prayogo F.A., Budiharjo A., Kusumaningrum H.P., Wijanarka W., Suprihadi A., and Nurhayati N., *J Genet Eng Biotechnol*, **18**(1) (2020), 39.

Qian Z., Fields C.J., and Lutz S., *ChemBioChem*, **8**(16) (2007), 1989–1996.

Qiu J., Yang H., Yan Z., Shi Y., Zou D., Ding L., Shao Y., Li L., Khan U., Sun S., and Xin Z., *Int J Biol Macromol*, **164** (2020), 1510–1518.

Qu G., Li A., Acevedo-Rocha C.G., Sun Z., and Reetz M.T., *Angew Chem Int Ed*, **59**(32) (2020), 13204–13231.

Quince C., Walker A.W., Simpson J.T., Loman N.J., and Segata N., *Nat Biotechnol*, **35**(9) (2017), 833–844.

Ranjan R., Yadav M.K., Suneja G., and Sharma R., *Int J Biol Macromol*, **119** (2018), 572–581.

Robinson S.L., Piel J., and Sunagawa S., *Nat Prod Rep*, **38** (2021), 1994–2023.

Sahoo R.K., Kumar M., Sukla L.B., and Subudhi E., *Environ Sci Pollut Res Int*, **24**(4) (2017), 3802–3809.

Sahoo R.K., Das A., Sahoo K., Sahu A., and Subudhi E., *Int Microbiol*, **23**(2) (2020), 233–240.

Sarkar J., Dutta A., Pal Chowdhury P., Chakraborty J., and Dutta T.K., *Microb Cell Fact*, **19**(1) (2020), 77.

Sharma P.K., Singh K., Singh R., Capalash N., Ali A., Mohammad O., and Kaur J., *Mol Biol Rep*, **39**(3) (2012), 2795–2804.

Simon C., and Daniel R., *Appl Environ Microbiol*, **77**(4) (2011), 1153–1161.

Tang L., Xia Y., Wu X., Chen X., Zhang X., and Li H., *Gene*, **625** (2017), 64–71.

Tang M., Zhang J., Zhuang S., and Liu W., *TrAC Trends Analyt Chem*, **39** (2012), 180–194.

Thomas J.C., Alnoch R.C., Costa A.C.d.S., Bandeira P.T., Burich M.D., Campos S.K., de Oliveira A.R.M., de Souza E.M., Pedrosa F.d.O., Krieger N., and Piovan L., *Mol Catal*, **473** (2019), 110402.

Torsvik V., Sørheim R., and Goksøyr J., *J Ind Microbiol Biotechnol*, **17**(3–4) (1996), 170–178.

Uria A.R., and Zilda D.S., *Adv Food Nutr Res* (Kim S.K., and Toldrá F., eds), 2016, Academic Press, pp. 1–26.

Verma S., Meghwanshi G.K., and Kumar R., *Biochimie*, **182** (2021), 23–36.

Vorapreeda T., Thammarongtham C., and Laoteng K., *World J Microbiol Biotechnol*, **32**(7) (2016), 122.

Wahab R.A., Basri M., Raja Abdul Rahman R.N.Z., Salleh A.B., Abdul Rahman M.B., and Leow T.C., *Enzyme Microb Technol*, **93–94** (2016), 174–181.

Wang M., Si T., and Zhao H., *Bioresour Technol*, **115** (2012), 117–125.

Wei P., Bai L., Song W., and Hao G., *Arch Microbiol*, **191**(3) (2009), 233–240.

Xiao H., Bao Z., and Zhao H., *Ind Eng Chem Res*, **54**(16) (2015), 4011–4020.

Xing M.-N., Zhang X.-Z., and Huang H., *Biotechnol Adv*, **30**(4) (2012), 920–929.

Yan W., Li F., Wang L., Zhu Y., Dong Z., and Bai L., *Biotechnol Rep*, **14** (2017), 27–33.

Yan Z., Ding L., Zou D., Wang L., Tan Y., Guo S., Zhang Y., and Xin Z., *Arch Microbiol*, **203**(7) (2021), 4113–4125.

Yao J., Gui L., and Yin S., *AMB Express*, **11**(1), (2021), 38.

Yarza P., Yilmaz P., Pruesse E., Glöckner F.O., Ludwig W., Schleifer K.-H., Whitman W.B., Euzéby J., Amann R., and Rosselló-Móra R., *Nat Rev Microbiol*, **12**(9) (2014), 635–645.

Zheng J., Liu C., Liu L., and Jin Q., *Syst Appl Microbiol*, **36**(3) (2013), 197–204.

Chapter 2

Plant Pectin Methylesterase: An Insight into Agricultural and Industrial Applications

Zeba Khan, Rakesh Srivastava, Sumit K. Bag, and Praveen C. Verma

Molecular Biology & Biotechnology Division, Council of Scientific and Industrial Research, National Botanical Research Institute (CSIR-NBRI), Lucknow, Uttar Pradesh, India
raakeshshrivastav@yahoo.com

Pectin methylesterase (PME) is one of the ubiquitous enzymes, being a major component of the plant cell wall, and catalyzes the demethoxylation of pectin. PMEs protein structures are highly conserved among isoforms and classified into two groups, Type I and Type II. In plants, *PMEs* correspond to multigene families, which are regulated in an extremely dynamic way. PMEs are involved in many important plants; developmental processes, including wood and pollen formation, cellular adhesion, stem elongation, and others; stress responses such as cold and wounding as well as plant-pathogen interactions. This chapter highlights useful information

---

Agricultural Biocatalysis: Enzymes in Agriculture and Industry
Edited by Peter Jeschke and Evgeni B. Starikov
Copyright © 2023 Jenny Stanford Publishing Pte. Ltd.
ISBN 978-981-4968-47-8 (Hardcover), 978-1-003-31310-6 (eBook)
www.jennystanford.com

for application in agricultural and industrial uses of the plant *PME* gene family.

2.1 Introduction

The plant cell wall is an exceedingly complex and dynamic structure, comprising different polysaccharides and structural proteins, associated with the determination of the cell shape and size, provides mechanical strength and rigidity, development and growth, as well as facilitates intercellular communication and interaction with the various environmental cues. Plant cell walls are organized into three different layers; a primary wall, that is made during cell cycle division and accumulated during the process of cell elongation; a secondary wall, which is deposited inside the primary cell wall of particular cell types; and the middle lamella, which is present between the two layers of the primary cell wall and formed after cell division. The primary cell wall predominantly consists of polysaccharides, structural proteins, enzymes, hemicelluloses, and pectins (Cosgrove, 2005; Anderson and Kieber, 2020). Polysaccharides are present up to 90–95% of the cell wall mass, while structural and polysaccharide-modifying proteins account for 5 to 10% (Cassab and Varner, 1988; Silva *et al.*, 2020). Interestingly, about 15% of *Arabidopsis thaliana* genes participate in the modification, production, and turnover of the cell wall (Wang *et al.*, 2012; Silva *et al.*, 2020).

Pectins are polysaccharides and the key components of the primary plant cell walls and the middle lamellae in the dicotyledonous plant, accounting for approximately 30–35% of the dry weight of the cell wall. (Pelloux *et al.*, 2007; Koziel *et al.*, 2021; Zhang *et al.*, 2021). Mainly, four pectic polysaccharides in the primary cell wall have been recognized; homogalacturonan, rhamnogalacturonan I, rhamnogalacturonan II, and xylogalacturonan (Pelloux *et al.*, 2007; Gigli-Bisceglia *et al.*, 2020). Homogalacturonan is particularly the main pectic component and is found in a higher than 60% methyl esterified state in the cell wall (Pelloux *et al.*, 2007; Caffall and Mohnen, 2009). Pectins with a high level of complexity are dynamically modified by pectin methylesterases (PMEs). PMEs are ubiquitous enzymes and present in fruits, leaves, flowers, stems, and roots in all higher plants and are also reported in fungi and phytopathogenic bacteria (Jolie *et al.*, 2010). Additionally, it is also produced by symbiotic microorganisms during their communications with plants (Lievens *et al.*, 2002). Several PME isoforms have been identified in numerous plants, both at the expression and genetic levels, that differ in isoelectric pH or metabolic activity (Jolie *et al.*, 2010). Furthermore, dicotyledonous plants have a greater diversity of PME isoforms than monocotyledonous plants (Louvet *et al.*, 2006; Jolie *et al.*, 2010; Yang *et al.*, 2013). The PME isoforms are encoded by large multigene families in all plants examined, which evidently question their biochemical and molecular specificity as well as the rationale behind their abundance. (Louvet *et al.*, 2006; Pelloux *et al.*, 2007; Jolie *et al.*, 2010; Levesque-Tremblay *et al.*, 2015; Wu *et al.*, 2017).

2.2 Pectin Methylesterases Classification

In the Carbohydrate Active Enzymes database (CAZy), the *PME* gene family is categorized as class 8 of carbohydrate esterases (EC 3.1.1.11), which catalyze the particular hydrolysis of the methyl ester link at the C-6 carboxy of homogalacturonan to release methanol and protons. PMEs are classified into two types of classes on the basis of whether or not the PRO-domain is present: Group-I PMEs, which are without PRO-domain, and Group-II PMEs, which comprise a PRO-domain, which is a domain similar to the PME inhibitor (PME-I) (Fig. 2.1, Table 2.1). The PME domain is found in both sets of *PME* genes. The PRO-domain is found at the protein *N*-terminus. The PME domain and the PRO-domain are both translated simultaneously in Group-II PMEs; however, the PRO-domain is separated from the PME domain by a subtilisin-like protease in the Golgi body as a prerequisite for emission to the cell wall (Pelloux *et al.*, 2007; Wang *et al.*, 2013). The PRO-domain is similar to a PME-I domain which has a function to inhibit the premature demethoxylation, suggesting auto-inhibitory activity of this PRO-domain (Wang *et al.*, 2013). The PME domain of *A. thaliana* is expected to have a basic isoelectric point, but the PRO domain could have a neutral to acidic isoelectric point (Bosch *et al.*, 2005; Bosch and Hepler, 2005). PME proteins of fungi and bacteria do not contain any PRO domain (Markovic and Janecek, 2004). The three-dimensional structure from the carrot and tomato PMEs suggests a high similarity in the structure, superimposibility, and high similarity in the overall folding topology (Johansson et al., 2002; D'Avino et al., 2003; Jolie et al., 2010). Both Group-I and -II PMEs contain a signal peptide (SP) and transmembrane (TM or signal anchor) domain, which are processed to form the mature active PMEs (Pelloux et al., 2007).

Table 2.1 Comparison of the number of PME and PME-I domains in different plants

Class	Species	Type I PME	Type II PME + PME-I	Total	Reference
Dicotyledonous	Arabidopsis thaliana	23	43	66	(Pelloux et al., 2007)
	Solanum lycopersicum	21	36	57	(Wen et al., 2020)
	Populus euphratica	28	21	49	(Li et al., 2021)
	Solanum tuberosum	26	28	54	(Li et al., 2021)
	Prunus persica	35	36	71	(Zhu et al., 2017)
	Linum usitatissimum	45	60	105	(Pinzón-Latorre and Deyholos, 2013)
	Fragaria vesca	25	29	54	(Xue et al., 2020)
	Asian cotton	33	47	80	(Li et al., 2021)
Monocotyledonous	Oryza sativa	23	20	43	(Jeong et al., 2015)
	Sorghum bicolor	23	19	42	(Ren et al., 2019)
	Zea mays	23	20	43	(Zhang et al., 2019)

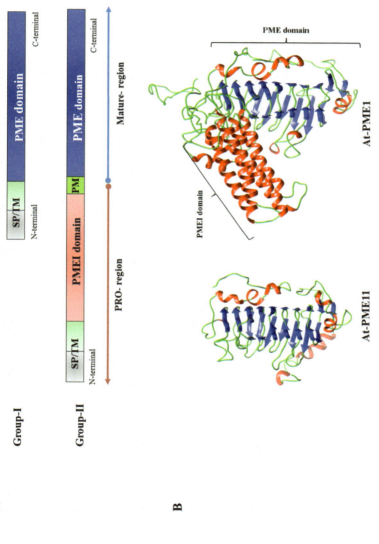

Figure 2.1 The classification and structure of pectin methylesterase (PME): (A) Group-I and Group-II PMEs encompass a conserved PME domain. Both Group-I and -II PMEs proteins comprise a SP and transmembrane (TM) domain; (B) an example for Group-I PME secondary structure: A. thaliana PME-11 (NCBI GenBank accession numbers for protein sequences NP_179755, AT2G21610). An example for Group-II PME secondary structure: PME-1 (NCBI GenBank accession numbers for protein sequences NP_175787, AT1G53840). The secondary structure predicted from PME1 and PME11 was generated using the Phyre2 web portal for protein modeling (Kelley et al., 2015).

Table 2.2 *A. thaliana* Group-I and Group-II PMEs

A. thaliana PME Group-I	*A. thaliana* PME + PME-I Group-II	
AT1G05310	**AT1G02810**	AT3G60730
AT1G11370	AT1G11580	AT3G62170
AT1G44980	AT1G11590	AT4G00190
AT1G69940	AT1G23200	AT4G02300
AT2G19150	AT1G53830	AT4G02320
AT2G21610	AT1G53840	AT4G02330
AT2G36700	AT2G26440	AT4G03930
AT2G36710	AT2G26450	AT4G15980
AT2G47280	AT2G43050	AT4G33220
AT3G17060	AT2G45220	AT4G33230
AT3G24130	AT2G47030	AT5G04960
AT3G27980	AT2G47040	AT5G04970
AT3G29090	AT2G47550	AT5G09760
AT3G42160	AT3G05610	AT5G20860
AT5G07410	AT3G05620	AT5G27870
AT5G07420	AT3G06830	AT5G49180
AT5G07430	AT3G10710	AT5G51490
AT5G18990	AT3G14300	AT5G51500
AT5G19730	AT3G14310	AT5G53370
AT5G26810	AT3G43270	AT5G64640
AT5G47500	AT3G47400	
AT5G55590	AT3G49220	
AT5G61680	AT3G59010	

In *A. thaliana*, there are 66 PME proteins, in which 23 proteins comprise the PME domain and 43 possess both PRO-domain and

PME domain (Table 2.2), however, the majority of these genes' functions are yet unknown (Wang et al., 2013). In contrast, the monocotyledonous rice plant has fewer *PME* genes (43 putative ORFs) than the dicotyledonous plant (Table 2.1), which might be attributed to differences in the cell wall structure, such as grass species having less methyl esterified homogalacturonan (HGA) (Vogel, 2008; Burton et al., 2010; Jeong et al., 2015). In an analysis involving comparison of the amino acid sequence of the PME gene, Markovic and Janecek (2004) revealed five conserved structural motifs: Motif I (Gx Yx E), Motif II (QAVAL), Motif III (QDTL), Motif IV (DFIFG), and Motif V (LGRPWK). Even though the conservation of these five conserved structural areas varies between plants, Motif I (Gx Yx E), is preserved in all *PME* genes (Markovic and Janecek, 2004). The *PME* gene has the same three-dimensional (3D) crystal structure in bacteria as it does in plants, showing that the PME protein structure is greatly conserved and that PME gene function is comparable across species (Jenkins et al., 2001). As a result, accumulating evidence revealed the structure, classification, and different functions of plant PMEs, however, many challenges remain to be examined and need to be determined to further advance our knowledge and thoughtful progressive role of these proteins. Further, work should examine how these different PMEs isoforms are regulated by these developments and environmental stress conditions (Srivastava et al., 2014; Srivastava et al., 2018; Pandey et al., 2019).

2.3   Pectin Methylesterases: An Insight into Their Functions

The gene expression and regulation are very complex and dynamic cellular processes, which are controlled by multistep process and depends on different types of cellular and environmental signaling perceived by cells (Srivastava et al., 2014; Srivastava et al., 2018). The plant *PMEs* expressions are to be tissue or cell-specific and regulated by various developmental and environmental cues. *PMEs* are also engaged in plant defense and are regulated by various stress conditions.

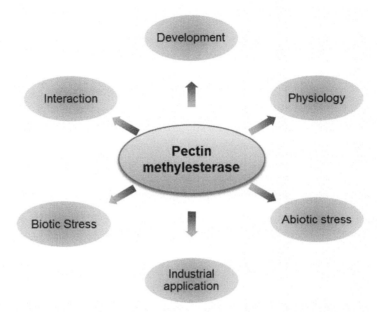

Figure 2.2 Different functions of plant PMEs in different aspects of plant development, growth, and stress conditions as well as agricultural and industrial applications.

2.3.1 Role of PMEs in Different Aspects of Plant Development

The diversity of roles of PMEs in plants has been demonstrated in plant development by accumulating evidence. It is represented by various expression patterns as well as physiological or developmental processes (Figs. 2.2 and 2.3). Several reports have revealed that PMEs have been found to have a role in various vegetative and reproductive plant growth, either directly or indirectly. PMEs are important for cell wall expansion and thickening (Al-Qsous et al., 2004). PMEs promote numerous physiological and/or biochemical processes in plants by mediating the de-esterification of cell wall pectins, which modulates the features of cell walls and hence enables a variety of physiological and biochemical activities. The role of PME has been demonstrated in the dormancy termination and germination of yellow cedar seeds (Ren and Kermode, 2000). During moist cooling, germination, and early post-germinative development, the PME enzyme is

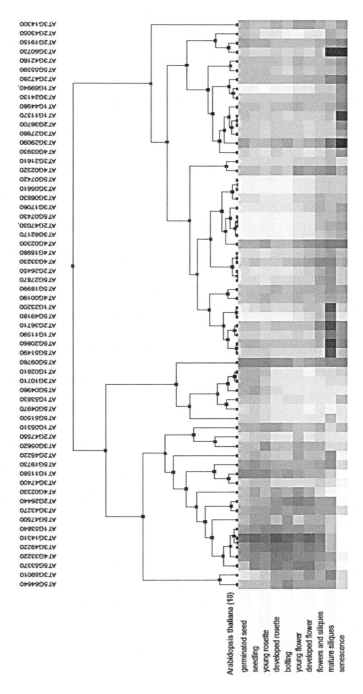

Figure 2.3 Gene expression of 66 *PMEs* in the different development parts of *A. thaliana* plant. This analysis was done by the GENEVESTIGATOR® software (Zimmermann *et al.*, 2008).

generated in various seed portions and seeds at different times. PME appears to play a role in the megagametophyte's weakening, allowing radicle development and the completion of germination, suggesting PME activity is associated with seed germination (Ren and Kermode, 2000). Similarly, hypocotyl elongation has been associated with the activities of the PME isoforms. (Bordenave and Goldberg, 1993). PMEs are also aided in microsporogenesis, pollen tube growth, and cambial cell differentiation (Wakeley *et al.*, 1998; Micheli *et al.*, 2000). For example, AtPPME1, an *A. thaliana* pollen-specific PME, is involved in determining the form of the pollen tube and the pace at which it elongates (Tian *et al.*, 2006). PME's involvement in fruit ripening has been extensively researched, and it has been discovered that variations in PME activity enable changes in the pericarp's cell wall structure (Brummell and Harpster, 2001; Eriksson *et al.*, 2004; Arancibia and Motsenbocker, 2006; Verma *et al.*, 2015). PME causes cell wall solubilization in the root cap, which aids in the parting of root border cells from the root tip. An increase in root cap *PME* transcript, and therefore enzyme activity, led to an increase in soluble, de-esterified pectin levels in the root tip, as well as a decrease in cell wall pH (Stephenson and Hawes, 1994; Weraduwage *et al.*, 2016). PME activity is higher in the leaves and tubers but low in the apical portions of transgenic lines' stems, according to the transformation of *Petunia inflate*–derived cDNA expressing a *PME* under a constitutive 35S promoter in transgenic potato plants. Surprisingly, stems of the transgenic plant extended faster than wild-type plants during the early phases of the growth, displaying that PME also promotes stem elongation (Pilling *et al.*, 2000). PME participation in wood development is one of the emerging functions for PMEs in vegetative growth. The primary constituents of wood are cellulose, lignin, and non-cellulosic polysaccharides (containing neutral and pectic polysaccharides). Accumulating evidence suggests that *PME* also participated in influencing solid wood characteristics. For example, two *PME* genes influence many wood properties of *Eucalyptus pilularis* (blackbutt). *PME7* is largely linked to cellulose, pulp yield, and lignin, whereas *PME6* is mostly linked to contraction and collapse, suggesting that the connections between *PME6* and *PME7* and various wood properties are compatible with our knowledge of the wood formation and *PME* biochemical activity (Sexton *et al.*, 2012). In *A.*

thaliana, five different *PME* encoding genes *At1g11580, At3g59010, At5g53370, At5g09760, and At3g29090* are highly expressed in the xylem (Pelloux *et al.*, 2007). Similarly, transcripts encoding *PME* encoding genes in *Populus trichocarpa* wood-forming tissues have been discovered and demonstrated to be strongly controlled inside the cambial meristem and during xylogenesis (Geisler-Lee *et al.*, 2006). In *A. thaliana*, PMEs are also involved in embryo development and seed germination. In *A. thaliana*, seven *PMEs* are expressed in a regulated manner during development in the seed coat and embryo (Louvet *et al.*, 2006; Muller *et al.*, 2013; Levesque-Tremblay *et al.*, 2015). However, due to functional redundancy within the *PMEs* gene family, the knockout process for the majority of these genes did not disclose any distinct phenotype changes in the seeds. Nonetheless, a *PME* gene [also called highly methyl esterified seeds (HMS)] was recently discovered, which is highly expressed in the embryo and seed coat during the development of seed (Levesque-Tremblay *et al.*, 2015).

2.4 Role of PMEs in Plant Defense-Related Mechanism

To counteract the impacts of biotic and abiotic stressors, plants employ a variety of morphological, biochemical, and molecular strategies (Lodhi *et al.*, 2008; Srivastava *et al.*, 2014; Srivastava *et al.*, 2018; Agarwal *et al.*, 2020; Dixit *et al.*, 2020; Mishra *et al.*, 2020; Kaur *et al.*, 2021). The biochemical and molecular mechanisms of plant defense against the biotic and abiotic stresses are extensive, dynamic, and are facilitated both by direct and indirect processes. The different defense chemicals are created either naturally or constitutively or as a result of plant damage. Interestingly, since PMEs are found in the cell wall, which can act as a physical barrier between the environment and the contents of plant cells' inner organelles. As a result, cell wall changes are commonly linked to plant defense mechanisms responses. Expression analyses of *A. thaliana* suggest changes in the expression levels of around 75% of the projected PME, which fluctuate in response to biotic and abiotic stresses. For instance, some *PME* transcripts are regulated by the cold (such as *A. thaliana PME5* and *At2g47030*), wounding, ethylene, oligogalacturonides, and phloem-feeding insects (Jung et al., 2003; Thompson and Goggin, 2006; Pelloux et al., 2007). Interestingly, early reports suggest PME is thought to be a host-cell receptor for the Tobacco Mosaic Virus (TMV) movement protein, according to early findings. TMV cell-to-cell migration was inactivated when the PME-binding area was removed, indicating that PME is also important in plant intercellular connections during pathogenesis. (Chen et al., 2000).

PMEs activities from plants and pathogens and the degree, as well as patterns of pectin methyl esterification, are important for the consequence of plant-pathogen interaction. In *A. thaliana*, wheat, pepper, and tobacco, inhibitors of *PME* overexpression reduce sensitivity to fungal, bacterial, and viral diseases (Lionetti et al., 2007; Raiola et al., 2011; Lionetti et al., 2014; Lionetti et al., 2015). Since these plants have greater level of methyl esterification, pectin becomes less sensitive to hydrolysis by microbial pectinases, and consequently, limits microbial development. During the pathogen infestation process, plants regulate pectin methyl esterification due to the recruitment of specific plant PME. For example, *A. thaliana PME3* is required for necrotrophic pathogen infection and is triggered by pathogen infection with *Pectobacterium carotovorum* and *Botrytis cinerea* (Raiola et al., 2004). Another report also suggests that plant PME activity is augmented due to pattern-triggered immunity, and after inoculation with either the bacterial hemibiotroph *Pseudomonas syringae* pv *maculicola* ES4326 or necrotrophic fungus *Alternaria brassicicola* (Bethke et al., 2014; Bethke and Glazebrook, 2019).

The PME activity produces different types of substances or chemical products that are contributed to plant defenses directly or indirectly, such as methanol, carboxylic groups, or pectin-derived compounds. In plants, methanol released during PME activity plays important functions such as, protecting photosynthetic machinery against photo-inhibition or encouraging the C3 plant growth (Nonomura and Benson, 1992; Dixit et al., 2013). Due to wounding and in the presence of caterpillar larval oral secretions, PMEs activity and expression are upregulated, thereby, an increase in methanol production has been observed in the tobacco plant, suggesting that PME-induced methanol emissions are significant for plant defenses to protect against-herbivore (von Dahl et al., 2006). The negative charge of carboxylic groups produced by PME facilitates cation binding, which affects plant growth and activity. Interestingly, metals in soils, such as aluminum, calcium, or magnesium, can enhance PME activity *in vivo* (Pelloux *et al.*, 2007). Calcium divalent ion forms a calcium–pectate gel model structure when it interacts with negatively charged carboxylic groups, providing cell wall resistance (Kieffer *et al.*, 2000).

2.5 Agriculture and Industrial Applications of PMEs

PMEs with a wide range of actions are subject to be beneficial in developing bioengineered pectins to fulfill new agricultural and industrial demands. Interestingly, the quality of plant-based food items is modulated by pectin alteration through PMEs.

Methanol released by plants was formerly thought to be a metabolic by-product. During growth and development, methanol is involved in metabolic biochemical activities. Cell wall pectins, which are dimethyl esterified by PMEs, are the major source of plant-derived methanol. Methanol emissions rise in reaction to mechanical wounding or other stressors because damaging in the cell wall, which is the primary source of methanol production. PME activity and levels of plant bio-methanol in the fruit tissues from wild-type tomato and antisense mutant of a *PME* gene were initially suggested that *PME* is involved in the major biochemical route for methanol generation in tomato fruit (Frenkel *et al.*, 1998). PME and pectin methyl esterification have previously been shown to play key roles in plant resistance to insects, fungi, and bacteria (Dixit *et al.*, 2013; Bethke *et al.*, 2014; Lionetti *et al.*, 2017). The wounded plant triggers the gaseous bio-methanol production, which leads to the defense signaling within the plant as well as to adjacent plants. The plant-induced bio-methanol production initiates methanol-inducible genes that control plant tolerance to abiotic and biotic stresses (Dorokhov *et al.*, 2018). Mechanical damage and pathogen infestation enhance tobacco PME production, speed up de-esterification processes, and significantly increase methanol emission (von Dahl *et al.*, 2006; Korner *et al.*, 2009; Dorokhov *et al.*,

2012; Lionetti *et al.*, 2012; Komarova *et al.*, 2014; Dorokhov *et al.*, 2015). It was demonstrated that the overexpression of pectin methyl esterases from *Aspergillus niger* (*AnPME*) and *A. thaliana* (*AtPME*) confers resistance against chewing as well as sucking insects and high PME activity was enriched by the overexpression of *AnPME* and *AtPME* in transgenic tobacco plants. Transgenic plants have up to 16-folds high methanol content and 12-folds high methanol emissions in comparison to control plants (Dixit *et al.*, 2013). Plant PME activity augmented during pattern-triggered immunity after inoculation with the bacterial hemibiotroph *P. syringae* pv maculicola ES4326 and the necrotrophic fungus *A. brassicicola* (Bethke *et al.*, 2014).

The structural integrity of the major cell walls and middle lamella is strongly connected to the texture which is an essential quality feature of fresh and processed fruits and vegetables. Most industrial methods are used to preserve fruits and vegetables, such as bleaching, drying, freezing, sterilization, and pasteurization, which cause irreversible physical damage to biological structures and tissues. However, various procedures including the usage of the PME enzyme can be used to counteract the detrimental effects of processing on texture. Therefore, the PME enzyme can be significantly used to enhance the texture of fruits and vegetables by reducing the negative effects of processing. The solutions of PME and calcium chloride, for instance, are used to firmness fruits such as apples, strawberries, and raspberries by vacuum impregnation or traditional infusion, implying that PME-mediated vacuum pretreatment reduced fruit hardness loss (Degraeve *et al.*, 2003). When vegetables and fruits are treated with PME and calcium infusion, the structural loss induced by freezing can be mitigated. The demethylation of naturally existing pectin in plant tissues by PME and the chelation of extra or natural calcium with the free carboxyl groups generated in pectin molecules are the mechanisms of firming in this technique.

As, PME is used in the agriculture industry to promote the formation of gel in pectin solutions in a variety of ways, depending on the nature of the pectin. Due to different regions with varying compositions, therefore, pectin is not a totally homogeneous molecule. The methylated form of pectin is favored in the agricultural food sector for gelling in high-sugar systems similar to jellies and jams. The low water activity in this situation reduces the hydration of the pectins, resulting in the development of a gel. On a dry matter basis, PMEs were isolated from potato tubers and enhanced 23 times relative to the original potato tubers (Spelbrink and Giuseppin, 2014). This potato PME is used for gel formation with calcium pectate over a wide pH range, which will be highly appropriate for application in the food and agricultural industry. Three PME isoforms have been identified in the tomato, named PE1, PE2, and PE3 (Simons and Tucker, 1999). The role of PME in tomato fruit ripening was investigated using transgenic tomatoes with a 10-fold decrease in PME activity. Reduced PME activity resulted in approximately complete tissue loss during fruit senescence, but had only a minor impact on fruit firmness during ripening (Gaffe *et al.*, 1994; Wen *et al.*, 2013).

PME is used to make clear fruit juices, which is an important industrial use. In particular, the cloudiness in fruit juices is caused by pectic compounds. To break down pectin, the PME enzyme can be employed alone or in conjunction with other pectinases (Wicker *et al.*, 2002). Pectin degradation not only lowers the viscosity of fruit liquids but also makes filtering and concentration easier. For example, *Datura stramonium* PME, when combined with polygalacturonase, improves the clarity of apple, orange, pineapple, and pomegranate juice (Dixit *et al.*, 2013). Orange, apple, pomegranate, and pineapple juices were improved by 2.9, 2.6, 2.3, and 3.6 folds, respectively, when pectin methylesterase from *Datura stramonium* was combined with polygalacturonase (Dixit *et al.*, 2013).

2.6 Conclusion

Advances in high-throughput technology in genomics and proteomics have presented several PME isoforms in different plants, which indicate the complication of their functions in plant growth and stress conditions. Defining the roles of different plant PME isoforms in a distinct set of favorable and unfavorable conditions can be facilitated by new strategies for agricultural and industrial transnational applications.

Acknowledgments

Authors are thankful to CSIR, New Delhi for financial support in the form of "FBR project MLP0037." Institute's Manuscript Number is CSIR-NBRI_MS/2022/05/12.

References

Agarwal N, Srivastava R, Verma A, Mohan Rai K, Singh B, Chandra Verma P, *Plants* **9** (2020), 999.

Al-Qsous S, Carpentier E, Klein-Eude D, Burel C, Mareck A, Dauchel H, Gomord V, Balange AP, *Planta* **219** (2004), 369–378.

Anderson CT, Kieber JJ, *Annu. Rev. Plant Biol.* **71** (2020), 39–69.

Arancibia RA, Motsenbocker CE, *J. Plant Physiol.* **163** (2006), 488–496.

Bethke G, Glazebrook J, *Methods Mol. Biol.* **1991** (2019), 55–60.

Bethke G, Grundman RE, Sreekanta S, Truman W, Katagiri F, Glazebrook J, *Plant Physiol.* **164** (2014), 1093–1107.

Bordenave M, Goldberg R, *Phytochemistry* **33** (1993), 999–1003.

Bosch M, Cheung AY, Hepler PK, *Plant Physiol.* **138** (2005), 1334–1346.

Bosch M, Hepler PK, *Plant Cell* **17** (2005), 3219–3226.

Brummell DA, Harpster MH, *Plant Mol. Biol.* **47** (2001), 311–340.

Burton RA, Gidley MJ, Fincher GB, *Nat. Chem. Biol.* **6** (2010), 724–732.

Caffall KH, Mohnen D, *Carbohydr. Res.* **344** (2009), 1879–1900.

Cassab GI, Varner JE, *Annu. Rev. Plant Physiol. and Plant Molecul. Biol.* **39** (1988), 321–353.

Chen MH, Sheng J, Hind G, Handa AK, Citovsky V, *EMBO J.* **19** (2000), 913–920.

Cosgrove DJ, *Nat. Rev. Mol. Cell Biol.* **6** (2005), 850–861.

D'Avino R, Camardella L, Christensen TM, Giovane A, Servillo L, *Proteins* **53** (2003), 830–839.

Degraeve P, Saurel R, Coutel Y, *J. Food Sci.* **68** (2003), 716–721.

Dixit G, Srivastava A, Rai KM, Dubey RS, Srivastava R, Verma PC, *Plant Signal. Behav.* **15** (2020), e1747689–e1747610.

Dixit S, Upadhyay S, Singh H, Pandey B, Chandrashekar K, Verma P, *Plant Signal. Behav.* **8** (2013), e25681.

Dixit S, Upadhyay SK, Singh H, Pandey B, Chandrashekar K, Verma PC, *Plant Signal. Behav.* **8** (2013), doi: 10.4161/psb.25681.

Dixit S, Upadhyay SK, Singh H, Sidhu OP, Verma PC, *PLoS One* **8** (2013), e79664.

Dorokhov YL, Komarova TV, Petrunia IV, Frolova OY, Pozdyshev DV, Gleba YY, *PLoS Pathog* **8** (2012), e1002640.

Dorokhov YL, Sheshukova EV, Komarova TV, *Front Plant Sci.* **9** (2018), 1623.

Dorokhov YL, Shindyapina AV, Sheshukova EV, Komarova TV, *Physiol. Rev.* **95** (2015), 603–644.

Eriksson EM, Bovy A, Manning K, Harrison L, Andrews J, De Silva J, Tucker GA, Seymour GB, *Plant Physiol.* **136** (2004), 4184–4197.

Frenkel C, Peters JS, Tieman DM, Tiznado ME, Handa AK, *J. Biol. Chem.* **273** (1998), 4293–4295.

Gaffe J, Tieman DM, Handa AK, *Plant Physiol.* **105** (1994), 199–203.

Geisler-Lee J, Geisler M, Coutinho PM, Segerman B, Nishikubo N, Takahashi J, Aspeborg H, Djerbi S, Master E, Andersson-Gunneras S, Sundberg B, Karpinski S, Teeri TT, Kleczkowski LA, Henrissat B, Mellerowicz EJ, *Plant Physiol.* **140** (2006), 946–962.

Gigli-Bisceglia N, Engelsdorf T, Hamann T, *Cell Mol. Life Sci.* **77** (2020), 2049–2077.

Jenkins J, Mayans O, Smith D, Worboys K, Pickersgill RW, *J. Mol. Biol.* **305** (2001), 951–960.

Jeong HY, Nguyen HP, Lee C, *J. Plant. Physiol.* **183** (2015), 23–29.

Johansson K, El-Ahmad M, Friemann R, Jornvall H, Markovic O, Eklund H, *FEBS Lett.* **514** (2002), 243–249.

Jolie RP, Duvetter T, Van Loey AM, Hendrickx ME, *Carbohydr. Res.* **345** (2010), 2583–2595.

Jolie RP, Duvetter T, Vandevenne E, Van Buggenhout S, Van Loey AM, Hendrickx ME, *J. Agric. Food Chem.* **58** (2010), 5449–5456.

Jung SH, Lee JY, Lee DH, *Plant Mol. Biol.* **52** (2003), 553–567.

Kaur G, Prakash P, Srivastava R, Verma PC, Enhanced secondary metabolite production in hairy root cultures through biotic and abiotic elicitors, in *Plant Cell and Tissue Differentiation and Secondary Metabolites, Reference Series in Phytochemistry* (Ramawat K.G., et al. eds); *Reference Series in Phytochemistry* (Ramawat K.G., et. al. eds), 2021, https://doi.org/10.1007/978-3-030-30185-9_38. Springer, Cham; Springer Nature, Switzerland AG 2020; 978-3-030-11253-0, pp. 625–660.

Kelley LA, Mezulis S, Yates CM, Wass MN, Sternberg MJE, *Nat. Protoc.* **10** (2015), 845–858.

Kieffer F, Lherminier J, Simon-Plas F, Nicole M, Paynot M, Elmayan T, Blein JP, *J. Exp. Bot.* **51** (2000), 1799–1811.

Komarova TV, Pozdyshev DV, Petrunia IV, Sheshukova EV, Dorokhov YL, *Biochemistry (Mosc)* **79** (2014), 102–110.

Korner E, von Dahl CC, Bonaventure G, Baldwin IT, *J. Exp. Bot.* **60** (2009), 2631–2640.

Koziel E, Otulak-Koziel K, Bujarski JJ, *Front. Microbiol.* **12** (2021), 656809.

Levesque-Tremblay G, Müller K, Mansfield SD, Haughn GW, *Plant Physiol.* **167** (2015), 725–737.

Levesque-Tremblay G, Pelloux J, Braybrook SA, Muller K, *Planta* **242** (2015), 791–811.

Li Y, He H, He L-F, *Potato Res.* **64** (2012), 1–19.

Lievens S, Goormachtig S, Herman S, Holsters M, *Mol. Plant Microbe Interact.* **15** (2002), 164–168.

Lionetti V, Cervone F, Bellincampi D, *J. Plant Physiol.* **169** (2012), 1623–1630.

Lionetti V, Fabri E, De Caroli M, Hansen AR, Willats WG, Piro G, Bellincampi D, *Plant Physiol.* **173** (2017), 1844–1863.

Lionetti V, Giancaspro A, Fabri E, Giove SL, Reem N, Zabotina OA, Blanco A, Gadaleta A, Bellincampi D, *BMC Plant Biol.* **15** (2015), 6.

Lionetti V, Raiola A, Camardella L, Giovane A, Obel N, Pauly M, Favaron F, Cervone F, Bellincampi D, *Plant Physiol.* **143** (2007), 1871–1880.

Lionetti V, Raiola A, Cervone F, Bellincampi D, *Mol. Plant Pathol.* **15** (2014), 265–274.

Lodhi N, Ranjan A, Singh M, Srivastava R, Singh SP, Chaturvedi CP, Ansari SA, Sawant SV, Tuli R, *Biochimica et Biophysica Acta (BBA)* **1779** (2008), 634–644.

Louvet R, Cavel E, Gutierrez L, Guenin S, Roger D, Gillet F, Guerineau F, Pelloux J, *Planta* **224** (2006), 782–791.

Markovic O, Janecek S, *Carbohydr. Res.* **339** (2004), 2281–2295.

Micheli F, Sundberg B, Goldberg R, Richard L, *Plant Physiol.* **124** (2000), 191–199.

Mishra J, Srivastava R, Trivedi PK, Verma PC, *3 Biotech* **10** (2020), 547.

Muller K, Levesque-Tremblay G, Bartels S, Weitbrecht K, Wormit A, Usadel B, Haughn G, Kermode AR, *Plant Physiol.* **161** (2013), 305–316.

Nonomura AM, Benson AA, *Proc. Natl. Acad. Sci. U.S.A.* **89** (1992), 9794–9798.

Pandey B, Prakash P, Verma PC, Srivastava R, Regulated gene expression by synthetic modulation of the promoter architecture in plants, in *Current Developments in Biotechnology and Bioengineering: Synthetic Biology, Cell Engineering and Bioprocessing Technologies*, 2019, Elsevier, 2018, 9780444640857, https://doi.org/10.1016/B978-0-444-64085-7..., pp. 235–255.

Pelloux J, Rustérucci C, Mellerowicz EJ, *Trends in Plant Sci.* **12** (2007), 267–277.

Pilling J, Willmitzer L, Fisahn J, *Planta* **210** (2000), 391–399.

Pinzón-Latorre D, Deyholos MK, *BMC Genomics* **14** (2013), 742.

Raiola A, Camardella L, Giovane A, Mattei B, De Lorenzo G, Cervone F, Bellincampi D, *FEBS Lett.* **557** (2004), 199–203.

Raiola A, Lionetti V, Elmaghraby I, Immerzeel P, Mellerowicz EJ, Salvi G, Cervone F, Bellincampi D, *Mol. Plant-Microbe Interact.* **24** (2011), 432–440.

Ren A, Ahmed RI, Chen H, Han L, Sun J, Ding A, Guo Y, Kong Y, *Genes (Basel)* **10** (2019), E755.

Ren CW, Kermode AR, *Plant Physiol.* **124** (2000), 231–242.

Sexton TR, Henry RJ, Harwood CE, Thomas DS, McManus LJ, Raymond C, Henson M, Shepherd M, *Plant Physiol.* **158** (2012), 531–541.

Silva J, Ferraz R, Dupree P, Showalter AM, Coimbra S, *Fron Plant Sci.* **11** (2020).

Simons H, Tucker GA, *Phytochemistry* **52** (1999), 1017–1022.

Spelbrink RE, Giuseppin ML, *Appl. Biochem. Biotechnol.* **174** (2014), 1998–2006.

Srivastava R, Rai KM, Srivastava M, Kumar V, Pandey B, Singh SP, Bag SK, Singh BD, Tuli R, Sawant SV, *Molecular Plant* **7** (2014), 626–641.

Srivastava R, Rai KM, Srivastava R, Plant biosynthetic engineering through transcription regulation: an insight into molecular mechanisms during environmental stress, in *Biosynthetic Technology and Environmental Challenges*, 2018, Springer Nature Singapore Pte Ltd, doi: 10.1007/978-981-10-7434-9; , pp. 51–72.

Srivastava R, Srivastava R, Singh UM, Understanding the patterns of gene expression during climate change, in *Climate Change Effect on Crop Productivity*, 2014, CRC Press, Taylor & Francis Group, pp. 279–328.

Stephenson MB, Hawes MC, *Plant Physiol.* **106** (1994), 739–745.

Thompson GA, Goggin FL, *J. Exp. Bot.* **57** (2006), 755–766.

Tian GW, Chen MH, Zaltsman A, Citovsky V, *Dev. Biol.* **294** (2006), 83–91.

Verma C, Singh RK, Singh RB, Mishra S, *Open Biochem. J.* **9** (2015), 15–23.

Vogel J, *Curr. Opin. Plant Biol.* **11** (2008), 301–307.

von Dahl CC, Havecker M, Schlogl R, Baldwin IT, *Plant J.* **46** (2006), 948–960.

Wakeley PR, Rogers HJ, Rozycka M, Greenland AJ, Hussey PJ, *Plant Mol. Biol.* **37** (1998), 187–192.

Wang M, Yuan D, Gao W, Li Y, Tan J, Zhang X, *PLoS One* **8** (2013), e72082.

Wang S, Yin Y, Ma Q, Tang X, Hao D, Xu Y, *BMC Plant Biol.* **12** (2012), 138.

Wen B, Strom A, Tasker A, West G, Tucker GA, *Plant Biol.* **15** (2013), 1025–1032.

Wen B, Zhang F, Wu X, Li H, *Front. Plant Sci.* **11** (2020), 238.

Weraduwage SM, Kim SJ, Renna L, Anozie FC, Sharkey TD, Brandizzi F, *Plant Physiol.* **171** (2016), 833–848.

Wicker L, Ackerley JL, Corredig M, *J. Agricul. Food Chem.* **50** (2002), 4091–4095.

Wu HC, Huang YC, Stracovsky L, Jinn TL, *Plant Signal. Behav.* **12** (2017), e1338227.

Xue C, Guan S-C, Chen J-Q, Wen C-J, Cai J-F, Chen X, *BMC Plant Biol.* **20** (2020), 13.

Yang XY, Zeng ZH, Yan JY, Fan W, Bian HW, Zhu MY, Yang JL, Zheng SJ, *Physiol. Plant* **148** (2013), 502–511.

Zhang B, Gao Y, Zhang L, Zhou Y, *J. Integr. Plant Biol.* **63** (2012), 251–272.

Zhang P, Wang H, Qin X, Chen K, Zhao J, Zhao Y, Yue B, *Sci. Rep.* **9** (2019), 19918.

Zhu Y, Zeng W, Wang X, Pan L, Niu L, Lu Z, Cui G, Wang Z, *J. Amer. Soc. Hort. Sci.* **142** (2017), 246.

Zimmermann P, Laule O, Schmitz J, Hruz T, Bleuler S, Gruissem W, *Mol. Plant* **1** (2008), 851–857.

Chapter 3

Induced Polyphenol Oxidases Are Associated with Laccase Activity in Different Genotypes of Resistant Chickpea Cultivars Infected by *Fusarium oxysporm* f.sp. *ciceris* and Salicylic Acid

Shivashankar Gayatridevi,[a] Kuruba Sreeramulu,[a] and Senigala K. Jayalakshmi[b]

[a]*Department of Biochemistry, Gulbarga University, Kalaburagi 585-106, India*
[b]*Department of Plant Pathology, College of Agriculture (University of Agricultural Sciences, Raichur), Kalaburagi 585-103, India*
skjl64@rediffmail.com

Differential expression of polyphenol oxidase (PPO) and laccase isozymes in different cultivars of chickpea, resistant genotypes - A1, JG-315, WR-315, R1-315, Vijaya, GBS-963, GBS-2; susceptible genotypes - MNK, GCP-107, GBS-6, KW-104; and moderately susceptible genotypes GBS-11 and GCP-100 for wilt disease caused by Foc (*Fusarium oxysporum* f.sp. *ciceris*) was analyzed. PPOs

---

Agricultural Biocatalysis: Enzymes in Agriculture and Industry
Edited by Peter Jeschke and Evgeni B. Starikov
Copyright © 2023 Jenny Stanford Publishing Pte. Ltd.
ISBN 978-981-4968-47-8 (Hardcover), 978-1-003-31310-6 (eBook)
www.jennystanford.com

and laccase activities were increased by 30–70% and 12–20%, respectively, in all the resistant genotypes, whereas no increased activities of PPOs and laccases were observed in all the susceptible genotypes upon treatments with the Foc or salicylic acid (SA). Polyphenol oxidase and laccase isozyme activities were detected in the gel and it was found that the induction of new polyphenol oxidases in all the resistant genotypes. The induced polyphenol oxidase isozymes were associated with the laccase activity; whereas, no induction of polyphenol oxidase isozymes was observed in all the susceptible and moderately susceptible genotypes upon treatments with Foc or SA. The defensive roles of these novel bifunctional isozymes associated with laccase activity are discussed for chickpeas.

3.1 Introduction

Polyphenol oxidase (PPO) (EC 1.14.18.1 or EC 1.10.3.2) is a nuclear-encoded enzyme distributed universally in all plants (Mayer and Harel, 1979; Mayer, 1987; Boeckx et al., 2015). PPOs oxidizes the phenols to quinones; they are highly reactive molecules, which can covalently modify and cross-link a variety of cellular nucleophiles via a 1, 4-addition mechanism, resulting in the biosynthesis of toxic condensed polymers which exerts an anti-nutritional effect against pests, plant pathogens, and herbivores by the covalent modification and cross-linking of nucleophilic substituents of amino acids and proteins. Hence PPOs are involved in plant defense mechanisms (Duffey and Felton, 1991; Thipyapong et al., 1995; Thipyapong and Steffens, 1997; Raj et al., 2006; Taranto et al., 2017) It is known that PPOs are induced by wounding, plant hormones like systemin (Constabel et al., 1995), SA, and jasmonic acid (Flurkey and Inlow, 2008) and also by plant pathogens (incompatible), wilt caused by *Fusarium* and potato bacteria, wheat head blight, potato late blight (Thipyapong et al., 2007; Poiatti et al., 2009) as well as compatible interactions with potato soft rot, bacterial spot of citrus in potato, indicating that the induction of PPO genes is part of the plant defense mechanism. A direct link has been established between herbivore growth and PPOs overexpressing and antisense genotypes of tomato, to the decreased or increased PPO activities, respectively, related to the susceptibility of the diseases (Thipyapong et al., 2007). Thus, the induction of PPOs by different plant pathogens and the increased

PPO activities during the diseases and herbivory suggest that they were involved in plant defense-related processes.

PPOs have been studied in relation to the commercial significance of browning. However, their role is less understood in plants. There are few reports on the relationship between the levels of PPOs and resistance under biotic or abiotic stress. For example, potato varieties exhibit higher PPO activities when infected by *Pectobacterium atrosepticum, Pectobacterium carotovorum* subsp. *brasiliensis* and *Dickeya* spp. (Ngadze *et al.*, 2012) causing soft rot disease. Similarly, the expression of PPO isoforms can be used as markers to assess the results between various genotypes of tomato and pathogens, such as *Ralstonia solanaceae* and *Xanthomonas axonopodis* PV. *Vesicatoria* causes bacterial wilt and bacterial leaf spot disease, respectively (Kavita *et al.*, 2008; Vanitha *et al.*, 2009). High levels of PPOs were found in the pearl millet resistant to the fungi, *Sclerospora graminicola*, which causes downy mildew, whereas in susceptible genotypes, even after a prolonged time, no PPOs were detected (Niranjan Ray *et al.*, 2006). Hence, resistant genotypes of wheat and chickpea exposed to soil-borne pathogens such as *Fusarium graminearum* and Foc, respectively, elicit an overexpression of multiple isoforms of PPOs (Mohammadi *et al.*, 2002; Raju *et al.*, 2008; Jayalakshmi *et al.*, 2009). High levels of PPOs could be correlated with the high tolerance of potatoes to the Colorado beetle (*Leptinotarsa decemlineata*) (Castañera *et al.*, 1996). Evidence is available to prove that PPOs are involved in plant defense mechanisms. Li and Stefens (2002) reported that potato PPO overexpressed in tomato plants showed increased tolerance to *Pseudomonas syringae* pv. tomato, a causal agent of the bacterial speck disease. On the contrary, plants overexpressing antisense PPO cDNA, remained highly susceptible for disease as there was a significant decrease in the levels of PPOs (Thipyapong *et al.*, 2004). Similarly, in transgenic poplar, overexpression of PPOs increased tolerance to herbivory, and caterpillar (*Malacosoma disstria*) (Wang *et al.*, 2004; Constabel, 2008).

F. oxysporum f.sp. *ciceris* is a serious wilt-causing agent in chickpea cultivar (cv) (*Cicer arietinum* L.). Our earlier studies indicated that chickpea cv. ICCV-10 treated with Foc or SA, strengthened cell wall structures and accumulation of phenolic substances, chitinase, and *PR* proteins, thereby preventing the entry of *Fusarium* wilt pathogen. Several factors responsible for the induction of systemic acquired resistance (SAR) in the resistant and susceptible cultivars of chickpea by exogenously added SA or infected with Foc were reported (Raju et al., 2007; 2008; 2009). Chickpea cultivar ICCV-10, resistant to wilt pathogen was shown to establish SAR whereas, susceptible cultivar L-550 did not. Resistant genotype ICCV-10 exerted localized, elevated concentrations of several isoforms of PPOs induced upon treatment with Foc or SA, whereas the susceptible cv. L-550 failed to induce PPO even after a considerable time (Raju et al., 2008). SA is a signal molecule and its physiological effects are well known including induction of SAR against a range of pathogens (Volts et al., 2009; Hayat et al., 2010). Earlier we have reported that the chickpea plant infected with Foc was shown to contain 3.47 ± 0.52 µM g^{-1} of fresh weight of SA (Gayatridevi et al., 2012). Changes in isozyme pattern of PPOs by VAM (vesicular-arbuscular mycorrhizal) fungi in the root of *Ziziphus* species have been reported (Mathur, 1995).

This prompted us to investigate the distinctive properties of native and induced PPOs and their significance in different genotypes of chickpea infected by Foc or exogenously applied SA. However, the native and elicited PPOs have different activities, substrate specificities, and typical inhibitors and have their own biochemical roles to play in the plant. The fundamental question to be addressed in this study is how the induced PPOs differ from native PPOs and their role under pathological conditions. Hence, this study reports the screening of PPO and laccase activities in different genotypes of chickpea treated with SA or Foc. Further, their possible role in plant defense is discussed.

3.2   PPO and Laccase Activity

The PPO activity in the roots of the resistant genotype JG-315 increased significantly by 40% when treated with SA (0.8 mM) or Foc. The PPO activities were increased by 70% and 30% in roots and shoots of WR-315 treated with SA and Foc. Similarly, PPO activities were found to be increased by 30% in the shoot of R1-315, and 40 to 50% in root and shoot extract of Vijaya, treated with SA or Foc, respectively. On the other hand, PPO activities of susceptible genotype KW-104 and MNK remained the same in both SA or Foc treated root and shoot compared to the control root and shoot extract (Fig. 3.1). Laccase activity was observed in all the resistant cv. of roots and shoots, viz. JG-315 (12% and 10%), WR-315 (13% and 18%) and R1-

315 (19% and 20%), respectively, upon treatment with the SA or Foc (Fig. 3.2), when compared with their respective controls, whereas no laccase activity was detected in all the susceptible genotypes.

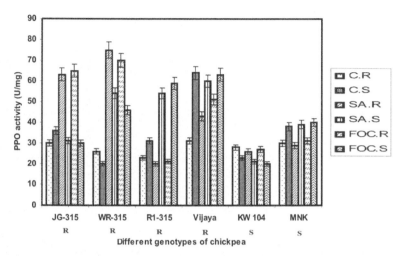

Figure 3.1 PPO activity in chickpea of different genotypes: control root (C.R), control shoot (C.S), SA (0.8 mM) treated root (SAR) and shoot (SAS), and Foc-infected root (FOC.R) and shoot (FOC.S). The conidia were adjusted to 3000 conidial mL^{-1}. Then, the 10-day-old seedlings (shoot length: 10 cm) were sprayed with a spore suspension. The shoots and roots of the genotypes were collected after 10 days of treatment for the isolation of PPO and laccase. Each bar represents the mean ± S.E. of three independent experiments.

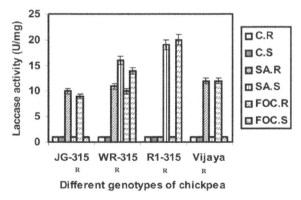

Figure 3.2 Laccase activity in different genotypes of chickpea: control root (C.R), control shoot (C.S), SA treated root (SA.R) and shoot (SA.S), and Foc-infected root (FOC.R) and shoot (FOC.S). Each bar represents the mean ± S.E. of three independent experiments.

3.3 Detection of PPO and Laccase Isozymes in Native PAGE

In plant cells, PPO enzymes exhibit multiple isoforms and their compositions were analyzed by native PAGE. PPO activity in the stained gels of control shoots and roots of resistant genotypes revealed single isoforms, whereas, upon treatments with SA or Foc, elicitation of new PPOs was observed. However, no induction of new PPOs was observed in all the susceptible genotypes either in control or in treated plants. For example, in the JG-315 genotype, induction of newly synthesized PPO has been observed upon treatment with SA and Foc. Similar induction was also observed in other resistant cvs. WR-315, R1-315, GBS-963, GBS-2, A-1, and Vijaya (Table 3.1).

PPO (Figs. 3.3a, 3.4a, 3.5a, and 3.6a) and laccase activities of chickpea (Figs. 3.3b, 3.4b, 3.5b, and 3.6b) were detected in the native gels and are shown for some of the resistant genotypes of chickpea. The chickpea genotype JG-315 showed a single isoform in control root (Fig. 3.3, a-A) and control shoot (Fig. 3.3, a-B) extract, whereas upon treatments with SA or Foc, induction of new PPO isoforms has been observed in root extract (Fig. 3.3, a-C and a-E) but not in the shoot extract (Fig. 3.3, a-D and a-F), respectively. The induced PPO was found to be associated with laccase activity (Fig. 3.3, b-C and b-E). Similarly, in all the resistant genotypes, WR-315, R1-315, and Vijaya, the induced PPOs were screened and found to be associated with the laccase activity (Figs. 3.4–3.6).

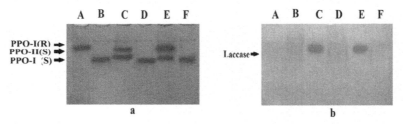

Figure 3.3 Native gel stained for polyphenol oxidase (a) and laccase (b) activity from the root and shoot extract of JG-315 (resistant) varieties of chickpea. (A) control root; (B) control shoot; (C) SA treated root; (D) SA treated shoot; (E) pathogen-infected root; (F) pathogen-infected shoot. Equal amount of protein was loaded on gels (20 µg).

Table 3.1 PPO isoforms of chickpea in different genotypes treated with SA and Foc

Sl. No.	Cultivar	Genotype	No. of PPO isoforms*						No. of Laccase isoforms*					
			Control		SA treated		Foc treated		Control		SA treated		Foc treated	
			Root	Shoot	Root	Shoot	Root	Shoot	Root	Shoot	Root	Shoot	Root	Shoot
1	JG-315	R	1	1	2	1	2	1	0	0	1	0	1	0
2	WR-315	R	1	1	3	1	3	1	0	0	1	1	1	1
3	R1-315	R	1	1	1	2	1	2	0	0	0	1	0	1
4	Vijaya	R	1	2	2	1	2	2	0	0	1	0	1	0
5	GBS-963	R	1	1	3	1	3	1	0	0	2	0	2	0
6	GBS-2	R	1	1	2	1	2	1	0	0	1	0	1	0
7	A-1	R	1	1	2	1	2	1	0	0	1	0	1	0
8	KW-104	S	1	1	1	1	1	1	0	0	0	0	0	0
9	MNK	S	1	1	1	1	1	1	0	0	0	0	0	0
10	GBS-6	S	1	1	1	1	1	1	0	0	0	0	0	0
11	GCP-107	S	1	1	1	1	1	1	0	0	0	0	0	0
12	GBS-11	M	1	1	2	1	1	2	0	0	1	0	1	0
13	GCP-100	M	1	2	1	2	1	2	0	0	0	0	0	0

*PPO and laccase isoforms were identified by native PAGE. S: susceptible, R: resistant, M: moderately resistant.

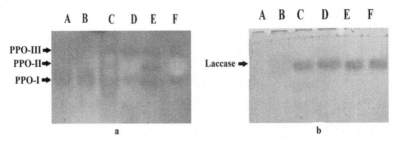

Figure 3.4 Native gel stained for polyphenol oxidase (a) and laccase (b) activity from the root and shoot extract of WR-315 (resistant) varieties of chickpea. (A) control root; (B) control shoot; (C) SA treated root; (D) SA treated shoot; (E) pathogen-infected root; (F) pathogen-infected shoot. Equal amount of protein was loaded on gels (20 μg).

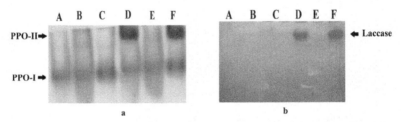

Figure 3.5 Native gel stained for polyphenol oxidase (a) and laccase (b) activity from the root and shoot extract of R1-315 (resistant) varieties of chickpea. (A) control root; (B) control shoot; (C) SA treated root; (D) SA treated shoot; (E) pathogen-infected root; (F) pathogen-infected shoot. Equal amount of protein was loaded on gels (20 μg).

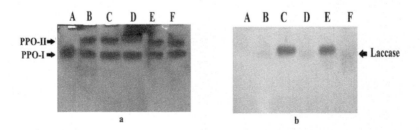

Figure 3.6 Native gel stained for polyphenol oxidase (a) and laccase (b) activity from the root and shoot extract of Vijaya (resistant) varieties of chickpea. (A) control root; (B) control shoot; (C) SA treated root; (D) SA treated shoot; (E) pathogen-infected root; (F) pathogen-infected shoot; Equal amount of protein was loaded on gels (20 μg).

On the other side, the susceptible genotype KW-104 and MNK were shown to contain a single isoform of PPO in both the control root and shoot extract (Fig. 3.7a and 3.8a). However, upon treatments with SA or Foc, no induction of new isoforms of PPO or laccase activity was observed in shoots as well as in roots extracts (Figs. 3.7b and 3.8b).

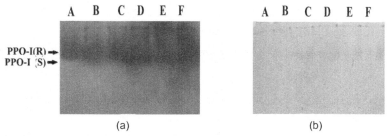

Figure 3.7 Native gel stained for polyphenol oxidase (a) and laccase (b) activity from root and shoot extract of KW-104 (susceptible) varieties of chickpea. (A) control root; (B) control shoot; (C) SA treated root; (D) SA treated shoot; (E) pathogen-infected root; (F) pathogen-infected shoot. Equal amount of protein was loaded on gels (20 µg).

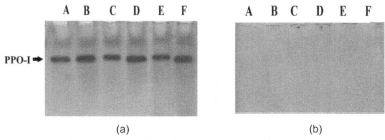

Figure 3.8 Native gel stained for polyphenol oxidase (a) and laccase (b) activity from root and shoot extract of MNK (susceptible) varieties of chickpea. (A) control root; (B) control shoot; (C) SA treated root; (D) SA treated shoot; (E) pathogen-infected root; (F) pathogen-infected shoot. Equal amount of protein was loaded on gels (20 µg).

The majority of research work on PPO has been focused on the characterization of its potential role as a defense mechanism in plants. It is now common practice to examine the expression of isozymes of PPO when exposed to herbivore or injury or pathogenic attack or various biological or abiotic stressors. Plants have developed various defense mechanisms, such as being able to synthesize large amounts of SA and pathogen-related proteins. In the present study, constitutional and induced PPOs were distinguished on the basis of enzymatic activity in the gel.

In this study different genotypes of chickpea plants infected with the Foc or treated with SA, were screened for PPOs. It was observed that the resistant genotype plants infected with the Foc or treated SA were found to induce new PPOs along with constitutive PPOs whereas susceptible genotypes did not induce new PPO. Further, native and induced PPOs were screened for other enzymes such as cresolase, tyrosinase, DOPA oxidase (data not shown), and laccase activities. Significantly to note that, in all the resistant genotypes, the induced PPOs were associated with the laccase activity, whereas no such laccase activity was observed in all the susceptible genotypes.

Laccase was found to be an important virulence factor in many fungal infections of plants. Among other functions, laccase protects against fungal pathogens in the host environment from toxic phytoalexins and tannins (Pezet *et al.*, 1992). For example, in the root pathogen, the aggression of the *Heterobacidian anosum* is related to the presence of laccase (Johansson *et al.*, 1999). Dutch elm disease has also been linked to laccase secretion by causative agents (Binz and Kenevsky. 1996).

It was observed from the substrate specificities that newly induced PPOs were associated with laccase activity. Laccases (EC 1.10.3.2.) belong to the group of phenol oxidases and have been found to be widespread in higher plants, both in monocotyledonous and dicotyledonous (O'Malley *et al.*, 1993; Mayer and Staples, 2002; Mayer, 2006). The high laccase activity is related to the cell wall lignification (Markle, 1998) and can oxidize monoliognols, with high lignifications for stem tissue of *Zinnia elegans* (Liu *et al.*, 1994), xylem of *P. taeda* (Bao *et al.*, 1993), and tobacco (Richardson and McDougall, 1997). These data show that laccase activity is present in different plant tissues which undergo lignification. Lignification of the cell walls by laccases was detected by the immunolocalization method (Driouich *et al.*, 1992). The purified laccases from different plants were shown to synthesize lignin precursors, monolignol alcohols in *in vitro* (Sterjiades *et al.*, 1992; Bao *et al.*, 1993; Ranocha *et al.*, 1999). Further, laccases genes have either been overexpressed (Dean *et al.*, 1998; Sato *et al.*, 2001) or down-regulated and proved their involvement in the lignification process. It is now clear that the phenolic compounds undergo polymerization by PPOs and laccase helps the plants to protect against biotic stress (Lavid *et al.*, 2001).

SA is a natural phenolic compound present in many plants. In infected tissues, SA levels can approach 100 µM, a concentration enough to trigger some physiological changes in the plant. In chickpea, accumulation of SA was reported (Gayatridevi *et al.*, 2012) upon infection with Foc. Exogenous application of SA mimic response of plants infected with Foc. Since PPOs are sensitive to SA, they are more likely to be activated at the physiological concentration of SA. As a result, the increased PPOs and laccase activities are associated with the synthesis of lignin.

This is further supported by our earlier report (Raju *et al.*, 2008) on histochemical analysis pertaining to the invasion of Foc in root tissues of the chickpea resistant cv. ICCV10 and the susceptible cv. L550. In the resistant cv ICCV10, they observed that the fungal mycelium could not enter the tissue as the root cell walls were highly lignified, which could prevent intracellular invasion. In contrast, susceptible genotype showed profuse invasion of mycelia even inside the cells.

3.4 Conclusion

Based on the previous and present results, we conclude that the native PPOs are responsible for the oxidation of endogenous phenols to quinones thereby providing natural immunity while the bifunctional PPOs/laccase must be involved in the phenolic oxidation as well as lignin biosynthesis during the Foc infection. On combining, the enzymes may provide the additional line of defense resistance in the chickpea plant against Foc.

References

Bao W., O'Malley D. M., Whetten R., Sederoff R. R., *Science,* **260** (1993), 672–674.

Binz T., Canevascini G., *Mycol. Res.,* **100** (1996), 1060–1064.

Boeckx T., Winters A. L., Webb K. J., Kingston-Smith A. H., J., *Expt. Bot.,* **66** (2015), 3571–3579.

Castañera P., Steffens J. C., Tingey W. M., *J. Chem. Ecol.*, **22** (1996), 91–101.

Constabel C. P., Bergey D. R., Ryan C. A., *Proc. Natl. Acad. Sci.* USA, **92** (1995), 407–411

Constabel C. P., Barbehenn R. Defensive roles of polyphenol oxidase in plants, in *Induced Plant Resistance to Herbivory* (Schaller A., ed), 2008, Springer Science and Business Media B.V., Dordrecht, pp. 253–269.

Dean J. F. D., Lafayette P. R., Rugh C., Tristram A. M., Hoopes J. T., Eriksson K. E. L., Driouich A., Laine A. C., Vian B., Faye L., *Plant. J.*, **2** (1992), 13–24.

Driouich A., Laine A. C., Vian B., Faye L., *Plant J.*, **2** (1992), 13–24.

Duffey S. S, Felton G. W. Enzymatic antinutritive defenses of the tomato plant against insects, in *Naturally Occurring Pest Bioregulators* (Hedin P. A., ed), 1991, ACS Press, Washington, DC, pp.167–197.

Flurkey W. H., Inlow J. K., *J. Inorg. Biochem.*, **102** (2008), 2160–2170.

Gayatridevi S., Jayalakshmi S. K., Sreeramulu K., *Plant Physiol. Biochem.*, **52** (2012), 154–161.

Hayat Q., Hayat S., Irfan M., Ahmad A., *Environ. Exp. Bot.*, **68** (2010), 14–25.

Johansson M., Denekamp M., Asiegbu F. O., *Mycol. Res.*, **10** (1999), 365–371.

Jayalakshmi S. K., Raju S., Rani S. U., Benagi, V. I., Sreeramulu K., *Aust. J. Crop Sci.*, **3** (2009), 44–52.

Kavitha R., Umesha S., *Phytoparasitica*, **36** (2008), 144–159.

Lavid N., Schwartz A., Lewinsohn E., Tel-Or E., *Planta.*, **214** (2001), 189–195.

Li L., Steffens J. C., *Planta.*, **2** (2002), 239–247.

Liu L., Dean J. F. D., Friedman W. E., Eriksson K. E., *Plant J.*, **6** (1994), 213–224.

Mathur N., Vyas A., *J. Plant Physiol.*, **14** (1995), 498–500.

Mayer A. M., Harel E., *Phytochemistry*, **18** (1979), 193–215.

Mayer A. M., *Phytochemistry*, **26** (1987), 11–20.

Mayer A. M., Staples R. C., *Phytochemistry*, **60** (2002), 551–565.

Mayer, A. M., *Phytochemistry*, **67** (2006), 2318–2331.

Markle S. A. Laccase associated with lignifying vascular tissues, in *Lignin and Lignan Biosynthesis* (Lewis N. G., and Sarkanen S., eds), 1998, Washington DC, *J. Am. Chem. Soc.*, **44** (1998), 96–108.

Mohammadi M., Kazemi H., *Plant Sci.*, **162** (2002), 491–498.

Ngadze E., Icishahayo D., Coutinho T. A., Van der Waals J. E., *Plant Dis.*, **96** (2012), 186–192.

Niranjan Ray S., Sarosh B. R., Shetty H. S., *Funct. Plant Biol.*, **33** (2006), 563–571.

O'Malley D. M., Whetten R., Bao W., Chen C. L, Sederoff R. R., *Plant J.,* **4** (1993), 751–757.

Pezet R., Pont V., Hoang-Van K., Enzymatic detoxication of stilbenes by Botrytis cinerea and inhibition by grape berries proanthrocyanidins, in *Recent Advances in Botrytis Research* (Verhoeff K., Malathrakis N. E., Williamson B., eds), 1992, Pudoc Scientific, Wageningen, pp. 87–92.

Poiatti V. A. D., Dalmas F. R., Astarita L. V., *Biol. Res.,* **42** (2009), 205–215.

Raj S., Sarosh B. R., Shetty H., *Funct. Plant Biol.,* **33** (2006), 563–571.

Raju S., Jayalakshmi S. K., Sreeramulu K., *Physiol Mol Biol Plant.,* **13** (2007), 27–36.

Raju S., Jayalakshmi S. K., Sreeramulu K., *Aust. J. Crop Sci.,* **2**(3), (2008), 121–140.

Raju S., Jayalakshmi S. K., Sreeramulu K., *J. Plant Physiol.,* **166** (2009), 1015–1022.

Ranocha P., McDougall G., Hawkins S., Sterjiades R., Borderies G., Stewart D., Cabanes-Macheteau M., Boudet A. M., Goffner D., *Eur. J. Biochem.,* **259** (1999), 485–495.

Richardson A., McDougall G. J., *Phytochemistry,* **44** (1997), 229–235.

Sato Y., Wuli B., Sederoff R., Whetten R., *J. Plant Res.,* **114** (2001), 147–155.

Sterjiades R., Dean J. F. D., Eriksson K. E., *Plant Physiol,* **99** (1992), 1162–1168.

Taranto F., Pasqualone A., Mangini G., Tripodi P., Miazzi M. M., Pavan S., Montemurro C., *Int. J. Mol. Sci.,* **18**(2), (2017), 377–393.

Thipyapong P., Hunt M. D., Steffens J. C., *Phytochemistry,* **40** (1995), 673–676.

Thipyapong P., Stiffens J. C., *Plant Physiol.,* **115** (1997), 409–418.

Thipyapong P., Melkonian J., Wolfe D. W., Steffens J. C., *Plant Sci.,* **167** (2004), 693–703.

Thipyapong, P., Stout M. J., Attajarusit J., *Molecules,* **12** (2007), 1569–1595.

Volts A. C., Dempsey M. A., Klessig D. F., *Annu. Rev. Phhyto. Pathol.,* **47** (2009), 177–206.

Vanitha S. C., Niranjana S. R., Umesha S., *J. Phytopathol.,* **157** (2009), 552–557.

Wang J., Constabel C. P., *Planta,* **220** (2004), 87–96.

PART II
PLANT ENZYMES

Chapter 4

Classification and Evolutionary Landscape of Acid Phosphatase–Encoding Gene Families in Plants

Amir Feizi,[a,b] Mohammad Ali Malboobi,[a] Javad Zamani,[a] Tahmineh Lohrasebi,[a] and Shahrokh Kazempour-Osaloo[c]

[a]*Department of Plant Molecular Biotechnology, National Institute of Genetic Engineering and Biotechnology, P.O. Box 14965/161, Tehran, Iran*
[b]*OMass Therapeutics, The Oxford Science Park, The Schrödinger Building, Heatley Rd, Oxford OX4 4GE*
[c]*Department of Plant Biology, Faculty of Biological Sciences, Tarbiat Modares University, Tehran 14415-154, Iran*
malboobi@nigeb.ac.ir

Monosteric phosphatases, commonly known as acid phosphatase (APase) enzymes, catalyze the hydrolysis of phosphoric ester bonds of various substrate types including, phosphorylated sugars, lipids, proteins, and nucleic acids. These enzymes play a key role in the absorption, recycling, and scavenging of phosphate ion (Pi) from internal and external resources, particularly in plants as sessile organisms. Having exhaustive reiterated sequence searches in protein

---

Agricultural Biocatalysis: Enzymes in Agriculture and Industry
Edited by Peter Jeschke and Evgeni B. Starikov
Copyright © 2023 Jenny Stanford Publishing Pte. Ltd.
ISBN 978-981-4968-47-8 (Hardcover), 978-1-003-31310-6 (eBook)
www.jennystanford.com

databases, we retrieved an inventory of plant APases, particularly those from *Arabidopsis thaliana* and *Oryza sativa* as representatives of dicotyledonous and monocotyledonous plants, respectively. Discrepancies in the protein sequences length, conserved motifs, number of exons, structural features, and active site residues are all indicative of remarkable levels of diversity among functionally similar APases. A comprehensive sequence-based clustering analysis anchored on the *Arabidopsis thaliana* and rice annotated genomes led to the classification of the plant APases into five discrete groups with distinct family-specific signatures. Based on the inference of orthologous and paralogous relationships among the members of each family, divergence from common ancestors and lineage-specific expansions within the protein families were discriminated. As the classified plant APase families do not show any ortholog relationships in sequence and structural level, we proposed that these families are the products of convergent evolution from distinct ancestral proteins toward gaining the function of Pi-bond hydrolysis from a wide range of substrates. Subsequent divergent evolution has expanded each APase family to further broaden the substrate ranges and, thus, ensure the Pi homeostasis in plants.

4.1 Introduction

Phosphorus (P), in the form of phosphate ion (Pi), uptake, mobilization, and redistribution are essential for cell survival as it contributes to virtually all developmental, metabolic, and physiological processes in plants (Vance *et al.*, 2003; Raghothama and Karthikeyan, 2005; Crombez *et al.*, 2019). Pi is not only a basic constituent of essential biological molecules, such as ATP, phosphoproteins, phospholipids, sugar phosphates, and nucleotides, but also it is a vital regulator in many biochemical processes such as photosynthesis, respiration, energy transfer, and signal transduction (Vance *et al.*, 2003). Therefore, it is important to maintain Pi homeostasis in the cell, particularly in chloroplasts as the organelles responsible for the photosynthesis (Raghothama and Karthikeyan, 2005; Fabiańska *et al.*, 2019).

Despite the high abundance of P in the soil, in the form of mineral and organic compounds, plants can only absorb free Pi (Vance *et al.*,

2003; Deng *et al.*, 2017). Consequently, a range of adaptive strategies has been evolved in plants to salvage Pi from both internal and external resources, including the involvement of phosphatases that play a central role in Pi metabolism (Raghothama and Karthikeyan, 2005). As sessile organisms, plants rely on these enzymes for the absorption, recycling, and scavenging of Pi from internal and external resources (Wang and Liu, 2018).

Monoesteric phosphatases (EC 3.1.3) catalyze the hydrolysis of phosphoric ester bonds of various substrate types including, inorganic compounds, phosphorylated sugars, lipids, proteins, and nucleic acids (Malhotra *et al.*, 2018). Depending on their optimum pH for their catalysis, phosphatases are classified into two distinct categories: alkaline phosphatase (EC 3.1.3.1) and acid phosphatase (APase; EC 3.1.3.2) (Dick *et al.*, 2011). The APases are grouped based on substrate specificity by the International Union of Biochemistry and Molecular Biology (IUBMB) nomenclature, however, grouping the subsets of these enzymes is of limited use as it is now clear that most of the known APases display a broad range of substrate specificity, although at different levels. Other classifications of APases were based on the biochemical properties of these enzymes such as molecular size (high and low molecular weights), interacting residues (histidine, serine, and cysteine APases) and to some extent, amino acid sequence similarities (Schenk *et al.*, 2013). For instance, three distantly related families of bacterial APases were proposed by Thaller and colleagues (1998) as molecular classes A, B, and C on the basis of shared conserved motifs that are mostly placed in the catalytic activities (Thaller *et al.*, 1998). Despite these attempts, the relationship and, thus, the classification of plant APases remain rather vague and limited.

APases are widely present in microorganisms (Schenk *et al.*, 2013; Chu *et al.*, 2019), animals, and plants (Tagad and Sabharwal, 2018). This wide distribution in various living organisms reflects the pivotal roles that APases play in many morphological, physiological, and biochemical processes. In plants, APases are engaged in several developmental stages including seed germination, root growth, flowering, fruit ripening, and senescence (Chafik *et al.*, 2020). In particular, the induced level of their expression in shoot and root is a hallmark for plant response to Pi starvation (Zhang *et al.*, 2014; Mission *et al.*, 2010).

The analysis of substantial genomic data has revealed that plant cells are equipped with several distinct APases. Yet, due to the high diversity of the APases at the sequence level, the previous efforts for the classifications of plant APases have been limited to purple acid phosphatase (PAP) family as a subset of these enzymes (Del Pozo et al., 1999; Hegeman and Grabau, 2001; Li et al., 2002a; Olczak and Olczak, 2002; Olczak and Wątorek, 2003). One of the inclusive works was conducted on 29 predicted *Arabidopsis thaliana* PAP protein sequences demonstrating the complex biology of PAPs in plants compared to animal carrying only a single PAP enzyme (Li et al., 2002).

Despite the vast amount of knowledge on genetics and biochemistry of prokaryotes and eukaryotes APases, their functions and roles in Pi homeostasis in plants are less understood. This is mainly due to the high sequence and structure diversities among these enzymes, and the complexity of the Pi metabolism in plants. Besides these biological sides of the problem, understanding the precise mechanism of Pi homeostasis is critical for agricultural biotechnology as the demand for absorbable Pi in the soil will be peaking over the coming decades (Cordell et al., 2009), and usage of Pi fertilizers will increase the unsustainable environmental effects. Therefore, it is crucial to develop phosphorous-use-efficient crops in near future, which requires a better understanding of the mechanisms that plants developed through the evolution to adapt to the Pi limitation.

In this chapter, we have examined plant APases with focusing on *A. thaliana* and rice as representatives of the monocotyledonous and dicotyledonous plants both with relatively small genomes. It must be noted that a comparison of chloroplast DNA of several flowering plants has shown the occurrence of the divergence of monocotyledons and dicotyledons 140–150 million years ago (Chaw et al., 2004). A comparative analysis between *A. thaliana* and rice showed that despite a three-fold difference between their genome sizes and little micro-collinearity, the distribution of total gene copy numbers is quite similar (Itoh et al., 2007). In addition, exon and intron structures were also found to be comparable, indicating a stable gene structure between these two species despite their long period of evolutionary divergence. Although a majority of the genes and functional motifs are shared, there are 5663 and 3402 species-specific genes in rice and *A. thaliana*, respectively (Itoh *et al.*, 2007). Furthermore, it has already been recognized that *the A. thaliana* genome has undergone several rounds of duplications (Blanc *et al.*, 2000), resulting in multigene families through both gene duplications and segmental chromosome doubling (Cannon *et al.*, 2004). Gene multiplications increase the complexity of the puzzling nature of the highly diversified APases in plants. We have collected and performed an additional integrative analysis of multiple data sets including protein sequences, conserved motifs, domain architectures, three-dimensional (3D) structures, and experimental evidence to adopt a better classification for APases. This coherent classification is required to portray how plants have invented a multitude of phosphatase enzymes as a critical toolbox to ensure access for adequate levels of Pi from endogenous and exogenous resources. Untangling the complexity of APases can pave the way to understand how their expansion in number and diversification in sequence have contributed to the evolution of Pi homeostasis in plants.

4.2 Plant APase Sequences Retrieval and Comparison

Plant APase sequences were initially retrieved by searching the "acid phosphatase" term in relevant DNA and protein databases. Then, experimentally well-studied and dissimilar plant APases sequences including GenBank Accession P80366 (Pierrugues *et al.*, 2001; Zhu *et al.*, 2005; Sun *et al.*, 2012; Del Vecchio *et al.*, 2014), GenBank Accession AAG40473 (Bladwin *et al.*, 2001; Baldwin *et al.*, 2001), GenBank Accession NP_193986 (Carman and Han, 2006), GenBank Accession NP_560374 (Mura *et al.*, 2003), and GenBank Accession AAA00007 (Ostanin *et al.*, 1992) were used as seeds in BLASTP and subsequent PSI-BLAST searches against non-redundant (nr) version of protein sequence databases (Schäffer *et al.*, 2001).

Because of the high level of diversity among the APase protein sequences, we used the weight matrix BLOSUM 45 (E-value < 0.005) in sequence searches or multiple alignments. We also performed additional BLASTP searches in the Arabidopsis Information Resource (TAIR, http://www.Arabidopsis.org/) to identify additional encoding loci. Similarly, we retrieved APase sequences for rice by BLASTP searches in International Rice Genome Research Program (IRGSP, http://rgp.dna.affrc.go.jp/IRGSP). To ensure no locus encoding APases was missed, the retrieved data were cross-checked with annotated Arabidopsis APases and rice APases in relevant divisions of Map Viewer (**http://rgp.dna.affrc.go.jp/IRGSP/**). Additionally, InterPro (**http://www.ebi.ac.uk/interpro/**) was used to retrieve additional sequences having the presence of previously known APase motifs in protein domains for both *A. thaliana* and rice.

This exhaustive search led to a collection of plant APases that catalyze the breakdown of abundant Pi compounds. We excluded protein phosphatases that are coupled with protein kinases in reversible phosphorylation reactions (e.g., in signal transduction pathways or regulation of gene expression). To avoid any redundancy, we removed sequences with 95% or higher identities or enzymes with the same locus number, if available. As a result, a total of 192 annotated plant APase protein sequences were obtained including 58 proteins belonging to *A. thaliana* and 47 belonging to *O. sativa* (Table 4.1). We also included APases from other plants in the phylogenetics analysis to delineate their ancestral and orthologs/paralogs relationships. These sequences varied in their lengths, ranging from 200 to 1062 amino acids, and in their number of exons, ranging from 1 to 31.

Table 4.1 Classifications and annotations of plant APases

Proposed name	Old names	Locus no.[1]	Accession no.[2]	Protein length[3]	No. of exons[3]
***Arabidopsis thaliana* (At)**					
HRP1		At1g04040	NP_563698	271	3
HAP1		At1g09870	NP_563856	487	11
PAP1		At1g13750	NP_172830	613	10
PAP2		At1G13900	NP_172843	656	2
PAP3		At1g14700	NP_172923	366	7
PLP1	ATPAP2	At1g15080	NP_172961	290	7
HRP3		At1g17710	NP_173213	279	4
PAP4		At1g25230	NP_173894	339	7

Proposed name	Old names	Locus no.[1]	Accession no.[2]	Protein length[3]	No. of exons[3]
PAP5		At1g52940	NP_564619	396	7
PAP6		At1g56360	NP_176033	466	7
SAP2		At1g72880	NP_177431	385	10, 11
HRP2		At1g73010	NP_565052	293	4
PLP2	ATPAP1	At2g01180	NP_565255	327	1, 2
PAP7		At2g01880	NP_178297	328	7
PAP8		At2g01890	NP_178298	335	7
PAP9		At2G03450	NP_178444	651	2
PAP10		At2G16430	NP_179235	468	8, 7
PAP11		AT2G18130	NP_179405	441	7
PAP12	Psr12	At2g27190	NP_180287	469	7
PAP13		At2G32770	NP_973585	454	5, 6
HRP4		At2g38600	NP_181394	251	3
HRP5		At2g39920	NP_565918	283	5
PAP14		At2g46880	NP_973704	327	4, 6
HAP2		At3g01310	NP_186780	1056	31
PLP3		At3g02600	NP_566177	364	9
PAP15		At3g07130	NP_187369	532	6
PAP16		At3g10150	NP_187626	367	4
PLP4		At3g15820	NP_566527	301	3
PLP5		At3g15830	NP_188204	296	3
PAP17	AtACP5	At3g17790	NP_566587	338	3
PLP6		At3g18220	NP_566602	308	7
PAP18		At3g20500	NP_188686	437	5
PAP19		AT3G46120	NP_190198	388	6
PLP7		At3g50920	NP_001030835	279	4, 5
PAP20		At3G52780	NP_190846	427	6
PAP21		At3g52810	NP_190849	437	6
PAP22		At3g52820	NP_190850	434	6
PLP8		At3g54020	NP_190970	305	11
PLP9		At3g58490	NP_001078308	416	8

(Continued)

Table 4.1 (Continued)

Proposed name	Old names	Locus no.[1]	Accession no.[2]	Protein length[3]	No. of exons[3]
PAP23		At4g13700	NP_193106	474	6
SAP1		At4g14930	NP_567449	315	9
PLP10		At4g22550	NP_193986	213	1
PAP24		At4g24890	NP_194219	615	12
HRP6		**At4g25150**	NP_194245	260	3
HRP7		At4g29260	NP_194655	256	3
HRP8		At4g29270	NP_194656	256	3
PAP25		At4g36350	NP_195353	446	7
PLP11		At5g03080	NP_195928	226	2
HAP3		At5g15070	NP_568308	1049	31
HRP10	VSP2	At5g24770	NP_568454	265	2, 3
HRP9	VSP1	At5g24780	NP_568455	270	3
PAP26		At5g34850	NP_198334	475	9
HRP11		At5g44020	NP_199215	272	3
PAP27		At5G50400	NP_199851	611	10
HRP12		At5g51260	NP_199939	257	3
PAP28		At5g57140	NP_200524	397	4
PAP29		At5g63140	NP_201119	389	3
PLP12		At5g66450	NP_001078807	286	4
Oryza sativa (Os)					
		Os01g0139600	NP_001041977	313	1
		Os01g0191200	NP_001042269	303	2
		Os01g0600500	NP_001043492	284	4
		Os01g0666000	NP_001043798	295	7
		Os01g0693300	NP_001043945	322	7
		Os01g0709400	NP_001044033	418	10
		Os01g0720400	NP_001044089	274	1
		Os01g0776600	NP_001044416	465	8
		Os01g0777500	NP_001044423	347	7
		Os01g0777700	NP_001044424	1062	26

Proposed name	Old names	Locus no.[1]	Accession no.[2]	Protein length[3]	No. of exons[3]
		Os01g0800500	NP_001044534	630	13
		Os01g0941800	NP_001045361	382	5
		Os02g0226200	NP_001046344	296	2
		Os02g0661800	NP_001047648	205	1
		Os02g0704500	NP_001047860	275	4
		Os03g0332500	NP_001050017	532	7
		Os03g0568900	NP_001050513	458	5
		Os03g0689100	NP_001050945	1044	26
		Os03g0805400	NP_001051628	415	8
		Os03g0818100	NP_001051705	519	11
		Os04g0410600	NP_001052730	452	4
		Os05g0189300	NP_001054846	251	2
		Os05g0189900	NP_001054847	243	2
		Os05g0190500	NP_001054848	265	2
		Os05g0191500	NP_001054849	209	1
		Os05g0192100	NP_001054851	204	2
		Os05g0549900	NP_001056238	369	7
		Os06g0607100	NP_001058029	307	2
		Os06g0139800	NP_001056747	293	3
	ossap1	Os06g0643900	NP_001058182	476	9
		Os07g0681200	NP_001060651	244	3
		Os07g0204500	NP_001059144	305	10
		Os07g0111600	NP_001058738	653	2
		Os08g0359100	NP_001061628	310	7
		Os08g0359200	NP_001061629	310	7
		Os09g0308900	NP_001062829	307	7
		Os11g0151800	NP_001065770	439	5
		Os12g0150700	NP_001066168	390	3
		Os12g0151000	NP_001066169	443	2
		Os12g0576600	NP_001067109	607	12
		Os12g0576700	NP_001067110	611	12
		Os12g0637000	NP_001067368	460	3

(Continued)

Table 4.1 (Continued)

Proposed name	Old names	Locus no.[1]	Accession no.[2]	Protein length[3]	No. of exons[3]
		Os12g0637100	NP_001067369	463	1
		Os12g0637200	NP_001067370	337	5
		NA	ABA99053	564	
		NA	ABA94167	294	
		NA	BAD53728	264	3
		NA	ABA99980	337	
Glycine max (Gm)					
	PAP		AAF60316	332	
			1609232A	257	
			AAK49438	547	
	VSPA		P15490	254	
	VSP25		CAA11075	264	
			P10742	291	
			BAB86895	234	
	GmPAP3		AAN85417	512	
			AAF19820	464	
			AAN85416	512	
Phaseolus vulgaris (Pv)					
			AAF60317	331	
	KBPAP		P80366	432	
			BAA19152	225	
			AAL17638	264	
			BAD05167	457	7
			CAA04644	459	
			ABP52095	271	
Hordeum vulgare (Hv)					
			CAB71336	272	
			ABJ98329	517	

Proposed name	Old names	Locus no.[1]	Accession no.[2]	Protein length[3]	No. of exons[3]
Ipomoea batatas (Ib)					
	IbPAP2		AAF19822	465	
	IbPAP3		CAA07280	427	
			AAF60315	312	
			CAA06921	465	
	IbPAP1		AAF19821	473	
Ipomoea nil (In)					
			AAG49895	209	
Lupinus albus (La)					
	lasap2		BAA82130	638	
			BAA97745	462	
	AP1		AAK51700	460	
Nicotiana tabacum (Nt)					
	NtPAP4		BAC55154	461	
	NtPAP12		BAC55155	470	
	NtPAP19		BAC55156	468	
	NtPAP21		BAC55157	470	
			ABP96799	551	
Solanum tuberosum (St)					
	PAP2		AAT37527	447	
	PAP3		AAT37528	477	
	PAP1		AAT37529	328	
Spirodela punctata (Sp)					
			BAA92365	455	
Tagetes patula (Tp)					
	TPAP1		BAA97038	466	

(*Continued*)

Table 4.1 (Continued)

Proposed name	Old names	Locus no.[1]	Accession no.[2]	Protein length[3]	No. of exons[3]
*Glycine falcata*n (Gf)					
	VSPa		AAS07026	253	
Brachypodium sylvaticum (Bs)					
		57h21.11	ABL85037	248	
Musa acuminate (Ma)					
			ABC60344	180	
Medicago truncatula (Mt)					
	MtPAP1		AAX20028	465	7
		AC149269g8v2	ABE84853	252	
		AC147434g32v2	ABE88130	297	
		AC151524g43v2	ABN07938	1058	
		AC136955g15v1	ABE81309	389	
		AC145222g31v2	ABE91728	307	
		AC155880g17v2	ABN08118	272	
Lupinus luteus (Ll)					
	acpase2*		CAD44185	463	
	PPD2		CAD12837	612	
	acPase1*		CAD30328	477	
			CAD12839	629	
			CAD12836	615	
Ostreococcus tauri (Ot)					
		Ot03g02120	CAL52864	291	

Proposed name	Old names	Locus no.[1]	Accession no.[2]	Protein length[3]	No. of exons[3]
Solanum lycopersicum (Sl)					
	APSAA2		CAA39369	120	
	ASP1		P27061	255	
	Apase1		AAC60539	174	
			AAG40473	269	
Pinus pinaster (Pp)					
			CAC84485		
Vitis vinifera (Vv)					
			CAN67288	256	
			CAO68115	320	
			CAO42204	343	
			CAO42205	321	
			CAO49375	313	
			CAO22812	224	
			CAO70346	214	
			CAO18122	222	
			CAO62718	242	
Vigna unguiculata (Vu)					
			AAF89579	374	
			AAF89745	322	
Thellungiella halophila (Th)					
			ABB45850	296	
Brachypodium sylvaticum (Bs)					
			ABL85037	248	

(*Continued*)

Table 4.1 (Continued)

Proposed name	Old names	Locus no.[1]	Accession no.[2]	Protein length[3]	No. of exons[3]
Populus trichocarpa (Ps)					
			ABK92516	285	
Picea sitchensis (Ps)					
			ABK25074	338	
			ABK25679	297	
			ABK21060	226	
			ABK93524	223	
Physcomitrella patens (Pp)					
			XP_001772861	218	
			XP_001778706	301	
			XP_001752483	231	
			XP_001755528	221	
			XP_001758316	321	
			XP_001781090	234	
			XP_001759893	304	
			XP_001769023	388	
			XP_001779824	266	
			XP_001763589	245	
			XP_001773743	254	
			XP_001753925	420	
			XP_001756514	427	
			XP_001754917	241	
Ostreococcus lucimarinus (Ol)					
			XP_001416918	264	
			XP_001420094	229	

[1]Locus no. are based on MapViewer Built 7.0 and 3.0 of *Arabidopsis thaliana* and rice genome, respectively.
[2]Accession no. are from GenBank database (*www.ncbi.nlm.nih.gov/Genbank/GenbankSearch.html*).
[3]The number of amino acids.

4.3 Sequence Alignments, Clustering, and Phylogenetic Analysis

To analyze the diversity of APases, we first performed multiple alignments of the protein sequences using the Clustal W algorithm of the MEGA X software package (Kumar *et al.*, 2018). The outputs of the alignments were used for the phylogenetic tree constructions by the phylogeny package of MEGA X. Initially, 58 *A. thaliana* APases and 47 *O. sativa* APases sequences (Table 4.1) were aligned to assess the overall clustering patterns, using the neighbor-joining method (with pairwise deletion of gaps and missing residues and bootstrapping for 1000 replications). As a result, the internal nodes were not statistically supported (bootstrap values <50), and the constructed tree did not provide a reliable basis for the phylogenetic relationship among the major clades (data not shown). This reflects remarkable sequence diversities among the APase groups as noted earlier by other researchers (Stukey and Carman, 1997; Raghothama, 1999; Li *et al.*, 2002a; Olczak and Wątorek, 2003). Gerlt and Babbitt, (2001) have defined a protein superfamily as "a group of homologous enzymes that catalyze the same chemical reaction with different substrate specificities." Based on the phylogenetic tree of *A. thaliana* APases and the multiple alignments results, it is quite conceivable that the so-called APases do not form a superfamily by definition and instead they cluster into five distinct protein families with possibly independent evolutionary paths. Therefore, we proceeded to explore each of these families separately.

For each family, the conserved motifs were primarily recognized through multiple alignments as well as searches in InterPro (http://www.ebi.ac.uk/interpro/) and Pfam databases (Bateman *et al.*, 2004) (http://www.sanger.ac.uk/Software/Pfam/). In some cases, APase sequences from organisms other than plants were incorporated in the alignments to resolve the conserved sequences. Furthermore, we defined conserved motifs for each protein family by carefully scanning the alignments manually looking for consensus sequences in MEGA. In addition, the motif search tools of the MEGA alignment builder module (Kumar *et al.*, 2018) were used to detect the known conserved motifs in misaligned regions.

4.4 PAP Family

As the best studied and the largest group, the PAP family include 29 *A. thaliana* PAPs (AtPAPs) and 19 *O. sativa* PAPs (OsPAPs) as well as several known ones identified in other plant species (Bhadouria et al., 2017; Kong et al., 2018; 2014; Srivastava et al., 2020) (Table 4.1; Figs. 4.1 and 4.2). Transcripts for all *A. thaliana* PAP genes as well as splicing variants have been detected in various tissues (Li et al., 2002; Zhu et al., 2005; Lohrasebi and Malboobi, unpublished data). The reconstructed phylogenetic tree showed that this family could be clustered into five subfamilies I to V (Fig. 4.1). Sequence identities among the members of subfamilies are high enough so that phylogenetic trees based on whole sequences and the conserved motifs resembled each other (data not shown). All five PAP motifs and seven conserved residues described by (Schenk et al., 2013) were found in most of the plant PAP family members. Data compiled by Koonin and Tatusov (1994) showed that APase enzymes carrying GD/GNH motifs catalyze the dephosphorylation of a wide range of phosphoproteins and phospho-nucleotide and polynucleotides. Here, by the addition of some conserved residues, we redefined the plant PAP family signature as **GD**lg, **GD**lsYadXy, **GNH**eXdf, livlX**H**, and G**H**v**H**Xy (X is any amino acid, upper-case and bold letters are well-conserved residues and metal-ligating residues, respectively; Fig. 4.2). The binuclear metal center of these enzymes in its active form consists of either Fe (III)-Me (II) (Me stands for iron, zinc, or manganese and Fe (II) in mammalian PAPs) (Schenk et al., 2005). The characteristic pink or purple color of purified PAP proteins is related to charge transitions between a tyrosine residue and chromophoric ferric ion in the binuclear center (Tran et al., 2010; Plaxton and Tran, 2011; Feder et al., 2020).

Structurally, plant PAP proteins are categorized into high molecular weight (HMW) and low molecular weight (LMW) phosphatases. The HMW PAPs are functional in homodimeric form while the LMW PAPs are typically monomeric carrying only metallophoesterase motifs (Schenk et al., 2000). Multiple PAP genes were identified in Arabidopsis (Li et al., 2002a), rice (Zhang et al., 2011), chickpea (Bhadouria et al., 2017), tomato (González-Muñoz et al., 2015; Srivastava et al., 2020), *Moso bamboo* (Zhou et al., 2021), *Jatropha curcas* (Venkidasamy et al., 2019), tea (Yin et al.,

PAP Family | 91

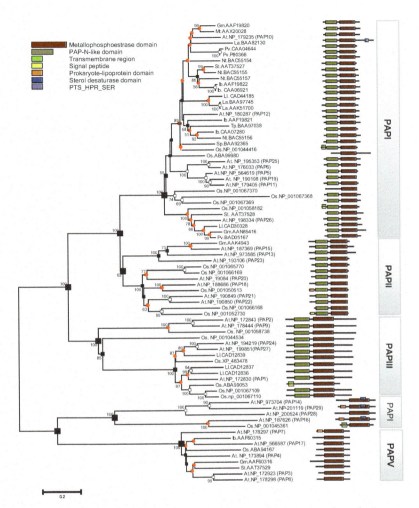

Figure 4.1 Phylogenetic clustering, domain architecture and evolutionary scenario of retrieved plant PAP proteins. Retrieved sequences were clustered into five major groups, PAP I to V. Orthologous, out-paralogous and in-paralogous relationships are depicted by filled circle, filled square, and open square, respectively, at the nodes. Schematic domain architectures were drawn using InterPro data. Each patterned box represents a specific domain as indicated at the left-hand side of the tree. The uprooted tree was constructed by MEGA X package (Kumar *et al.*, 2018) using minimum evolution method with Poisson correction and pairwise deletion options. The numbers besides the nodes are bootstrap values ≥50 percent based on 1000 replication. Abbreviated genus and species names (the first two letters), and GenBank Accession Numbers are shown at the right side.

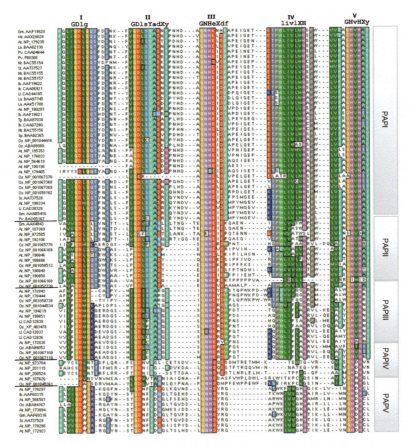

Figure 4.2 Multiple alignments of PAP family conserved amino acid sequences. Plant PAP sequences were aligned by ClustalW program integrated in MEGA X package (Kumar et al., 2018). Decorated report was prepared by BioEdit software (Hall, 1999). The identical residues and biochemically equivalent residues were decorated by the same gray scales. Motifs are organized according to the order of occurrence in the alignment and separated by dashes. Family signatures are shown on the top. Residues conserved in almost all sequences are illustrated with upper letter and the other highly conserved residues that are only substituted by equivalent amino acid residues are in lower case.

2019), and soybean (Zhu et al., 2020) based on conserved structural features. Respectfully, we have used the same nomenclatures for PAP proteins as annotated by Li et al. (2002) that are based on chromosomal locations (Table 4.1).

While subfamily PAPI and PAPII include PAPs with small to medium size proteins, subfamily PAPIII encompasses larger PAPs. Subfamilies PAPIV and PAPV include smaller PAPs with the least sequence similarities- sharing only GD/GNH/GHXH motif- with other PAP subfamilies (Fig. 4.1). (Schenk *et al.*, 1999) showed that small and large PAPs isolated from plants and animals align with their cognates better than those within the same kingdom suggesting the divergence of small and large PAPs predate the divergence of plant and animal. Later, two consequent duplication events have occurred leading to the emergence of PAPIII in the first round and to PAPI and II in the second one. PAPIV and V are likely to be the outcomes of a single duplication event (Fig. 4.1). The time of such events remains obscure since the presence of both large and small PAPs are shown in all kingdoms (Flanagan *et al.*, 2006), though the number of encoding genes is quite different (e.g., 1 in humans *vs.* 29 in *A. thaliana*). Most of the knowledge about the PAP structure and function has been extracted from various studies performed on the red kidney bean PAP. The 3D structure of kidney bean PAP showed that it is functional as a 110-kDa homodimer (Beck *et al.*, 1986). Recent structural studies on plant PAPs in complex with Pi or other analogous anions have shed light on the possible roles of the metal ions in the formation of pre-catalytic complex and the subsequent nucleophilic attack (Schenk *et al.*, 2008).

4.4.1 PAP I Subfamily

Members of the Arabidopsis PAPI genes subfamily are distributed over various chromosomes. In this subfamily, AtPAP10 and AtPAP26 show one-to-one orthologous relationships with their rice counterparts (Fig. 4.1). Many other known monocotyledonous (1 sequence) and dicotyledonous (23 sequences) PAPs are orthologs of these two proteins (Fig. 4.1). Three Arabidopsis PAPs, AtPAP10 to 12, located close to chromosome 2 are collinear with their three OsPAPI orthologs, Os12g0637000, Os12g0637100, and Os12g0637200 (GenBank Accession NP_001067368 to 70) that are positioned in tandem on chromosome 12 in rice. High sequence similarities among these enzymes indicate the occurrence of a series of gene duplications before and after monocots and dicots divergence. For instance, Arabidopsis PAP11 is clustered with four others AtPAPs resulting from a recent lineage-specific expansion (LSE) of the encoding genes in dicots while Os.NP_001058182 is clustered with other encoding genes from dictos (including AtPAP26) indicating an old LSE (Fig. 4.1). However, for example, such an expansion was not observed for AtPAP26 and its orthologs.

According to the InterPro searches, all PAPI subfamily members carry a couple of domains known as metallophosphoesterase and PAP-N-like, except for two OsPAPIs, ABA99980 and Os12g0637200 (GenBank Accessions NP_001067370), in which the latter domain is missing. Interestingly two other OsPAPI members Os01g0776600 and Os06g0643900 (GenBank Accessions NP_001044416 and NP_001058182), acquired transmembrane region and signal peptide as well.

Several experimental examples, support the PAPI subfamily members' involvement in Pi metabolism. KbPAP (GenBank Accession P80366) isolated from *Phaseolus vulgaris* was one of the first PAPs for which the catalytic and structural properties had been studied in detail (Beck et al., 1986; Flanagan et al., 2006; Klabunde et al., 1994; Schenk et al., 2008; Strater et al., 1995). Three PAPI-encoding genes isolated from *Ipomoea batatas*, IbPAP1 (GenBank Accession AAF19821) IbPAP2 (GenBank Accession AAF19822,) and IbPAP3 (GenBank Accession CAA07280) were highly similar to each other and KbPAP and are expressed in response to Pi deprivation (Durmus et al., 1999; Hegeman and Grabau, 2001). However, the core metals of the IbPAP1 are Fe(III)–Mn(II) in comparison to those of KbPAP, which are Fe(III)–Zn(II) (Schenk et al., 2004). In addition, four members of the PAPI subfamily were isolated from a cDNA library prepared from tobacco cultured cells and designated as NtPAP4 (GenBank Accession BAC55154), NtPAP12 (GenBank Accession BAC55155), NtPAP19 (GenBank Accession BAC55156), and NtPAP21 (GenBank Accession BAC55157). The transcript levels of both NtPAP12 and NtPAP21 were increased in the protoplasts immediately after transferring into a medium that induced cell wall regeneration (Kaida et al., 2003). MtPHY1 (GenBank Accession AAX71115), as an extracellular phytase in *Medicago truncatula*, belong to the PAPI subfamily and is shown to be induced in leaves and roots when grown in low Pi condition (Xiao et al., 2006). *P. vulgaris* PAPI member, KhACP (GenBank Accession BAD05167), is a colorless APase purified from embryonic axes that exhibited vanadate-dependent chloroperoxidase activity (Yoneyama *et al.*, 2004 &2007). This protein clustered with another characterized PAPI protein, GmPAP3 (GenBank Accession AAN85416), from *Glycine max* carries a putative mitochondrial targeting transit peptide and is induced by salt and oxidative stress (Liao *et al.*, 2003). AtPAP26 (GenBank Accession NP_198334), a vacuolar enzyme, and two PAPI members isolated from *Solanum tuberosum*, *StPAP2* (GenBank Accession AAT37527) and *StPAP3* (GenBank Accession AAT37528), was shown to be induced in Pi starvation (Bozzo *et al.*, 2002; Zimmermann *et al.*, 2004; Veljanovski *et al.*, 2006; Zhang *et al.*, 2014). Altogether, these data suggest that PAPI members are mostly responsive to the Pi stress and are targeted to subcellular or extracellular locations where they catalyze the hydrolysis of certain substrates.

4.4.2 PAP II Subfamily

With the exception of AtPAP13 and 23, all other genes encoding AtPAPII members are located on chromosome 3. Like PAPI, all PAPII subfamily members carry metallophosphoesterase and PAP-N-like domains. Two OsPAPIIs, Os03g0568900 and Os04g0410600 (GenBank Accessions NP_001050513 and NP_001052730), possess a prokaryotic lipoprotein domain and a signal peptide, respectively (Fig. 4.1). Apart from AtPAP18 and its ortholog, Os.NP_001050513, all other enzymes in this subfamily comprise members with paralogous and co-orthologs relationships (Fig. 4.1). As no orthologs for AtPAP13, 15, and 23 exist in rice, the encoding genes could be solely expanded in dicots. The only reported ortholog for these three AtPAPII in other plants is *Glycine max* APase, GmPhy (GenBank Accession AAK49438) which shows phytase activity in cotyledons of germinated seeds (Hegeman and Grabau, 2001). This protein is unrelated to previously characterized microbial or maize phytases, which are classified as histidine APases. The work of (Zhu *et al.*, 2005) revealed that the level of AtPAP23 transcription was high in flower apical meristem cells and is restricted to petals and anther filaments in fully developed flowers. The available data show a probable key role for the members of this subfamily in germination and flower development by mobilizing Pi from stocked-up molecules such as phytate.

4.4.3 PAP III Subfamily

The third clade includes large PAPs which are clustered together as the members of the PAPIII subfamily (Fig. 4.1). As shown, PAPIII orthologs between Arabidopsis and rice has been expanded in each species for extra paralogous enzymes. It is noteworthy that no orthologs for Os.NP_001044534 is known in dicots. Similarly, all PAPIII subfamily members carry metallophosphoesterase and PAP-N-like domains, except for one OsPAPIII, ABA99053, which lacks the latter. Instead, this protein possesses signal peptide and the transmembrane region at N-terminal which suggest it most probably sits in cell membrane than being secreted to the extracellular space. Furthermore, motifs I and IV in the metallophosphatase domain of PAPIII are slightly modified (Fig. 4.2). Functionally, PAPIII members are known to have diphosphonucleotide phosphatase activity as demonstrated for the purified enzymes isolated from *O. sativa* (Choisne *et al.*, 2005) and *Lupinus leteus* (Olczak and Olczak, 2002).

4.4.4 PAP IV Subfamily

The fourth clade includes four known members of AtPAPIV and only one ortholog from rice (Fig. 4.1). These PAPs are grouped with small-size enzymes detected in mammalians (Li *et al.*, 2002a; Schenk *et al.*, 2000) which only carry the metallophosphoesterase domain, therefore, parts of motif I and II and the whole motif IV of this domain are missing in this subfamily (Fig. 4.2). AtPAP16 and 29 and their rice ortholog gained additional trans-membrane domain that could place them on the cell membrane.

4.4.5 PAP V Subfamily

The last clade is the PAPV subfamily which encompassed five AtPAPV and one OsPAPV ortholog containing only the metallophosphoesterase domain (Fig. 4.1). Experimental analyses show that several members of this subfamily possess exo-nuclease or phosphodiesterase activities (Imamura *et al.*, 1996). AtPAP17 (GenBank Accession NP_566587) also known as AtACP5, is a 35 kDa monomeric enzyme induced during Pi stress (Wasaki *et al.*, 1997; 1999; Li *et al.*, 2002b), however, *StPAP1* (GenBank Accession

AAT37529), isolated from *S. tuberosum* was not responsive to Pi supply (Zimmermann *et al.*, 2004).

4.5 Halo Acid Dehalogenases (HAD)-Related APase Family

In the initial reconstructed phylogenetic tree, two APases groups sharing a Rossmann-like structure and motifs typical of HAD superfamily were clustered separately (Fig. 4.3) due to highly diverse primary sequences. Both sequences carry two characteristic motifs: (*i*) DXD motif found at the end of the first β-strand in the Rossmann-like structures; and (*ii*) DXXXD motif shown to occur at the strand adjacent to the first β-strand in a 3D-structural model (Burroughs *et al.*, 2006). The conservation of these sequences, known as motif, I and IV, have possible mechanistic similarities with HAD proteins. The HADs superfamily, include enzymes that catalyze the cleavage of C-Cl, P-C, and P-O-P bonds via the nucleophilic substitution reaction (Lahiri *et al.*, 2004; Lu *et al.*, 2005). Similar to the HAD catalytic domains, it is assumed that the first aspartic acid (Asp) residue in the DXD motif coordinates a magnesium ion (Mg^{2+}) along with the backbone carbonyl (C=O) of the second Asp residue. The fourth motif, GDXXXD, of HAD family also coordinates the Mg^{2+} ion and interacts with negatively charged Pi, preparing it for nucleophilic attack by the first Asp in DXD motif through the formation of aspartyl-intermediate (Burroughs *et al.*, 2006). Therefore, we named these groups as HAD-related phosphatase (HRP) family and divided them into subfamilies I and II with their own specific motifs (Fig. 4.3). It is noteworthy that several other HAD-like proteins have been shown to display phosphoprotein phosphatase activity (Kerk *et al.*, 2008). However, the *A. thaliana* and rice HAD-like phosphoprotein phosphatase sequences did not align with the ones in this study.

4.5.1 HRP I Subfamily

This subfamily included 10 sequences found in both *A. thaliana* and rice (Fig. 4.3). Retrieved homologs from other plants and additional representative sequences from other organisms assisted the accuracy of phylogenetic relationships and motifs recognitions. According to the constructed tree, five OsHRPI sequences, Os05g0189300, Os05g0189900, Os05g0190500, Os05g0191500, Os05g0192100 and Os01g0191200 (GenBank Accession NP_001054846-49, NP_001054851, and NP_001042269) and one protein from barley, CAB71336, clustered together. Interestingly, this sub-cluster shares an ancestor node with a sub-cluster including only HRP from dicots. This suggests the ancestral gene of these sequences has undergone LSE right after the monocot and dicot speciation. This is supported by the tandem locations of Os.NP001054846-49 on chromosome 5. Similarly, a pair of AtHRPI-encoding genes, AtHRP9 (GenBank Accession NP_568455) and AtHRP10 (GenBank Accession NP_568454), are collocated on chromosome 5. Another pair of gene encoding for AtHRPI, AtHRP7 (GenBank Accession NP_194655) and AtHRP8 (GenBank Accession NP_194656), are collocated on chromosome 4. In addition, two genes belonging to the OsHRPI subfamily, Os06g0139800, and BAD53728 (GenBank Accession NP_001056747) are collocated together on chromosome 6. High levels of sequence identities and the colocalization of the genes are indicative of recent gene duplications.

Pfam and InterPro motif searches for the members of this group indicated that these sequences have regions that were conserved in bacterial class IIIB subfamily of APase and plant vegetative storage proteins, known as VSPs (Calderone *et al.*, 2004; Liu *et al.*, 2005). A close examination of multiple alignments for this group (Fig. 4.3) revealed six blocks of conserved motifs including **CX**sw**R**XX**v**EXX**N**, d**XW**v**FDXDXTXLS**XX**PY**, **G**X**KXXXLTXR**, **NL**XXX**GY**XX**W**, **G**nX**GDQWSDLXG**, and **RXFKLPNP**X**YYV** (X is any amino acid, residues involved in the catalytic activity are bold) (Burroughs *et al.*, 2006). Five invariable residues Asp44, Asp48, Asp167, Ser168, and Asp171, in the active site coordinates the metal-ion binding (Lahiri *et al.*, 2004; Lu *et al.*, 2005; Burroughs *et al.*, 2006). Interestingly, Ser168 is replaced by glutamine (Gln) in all HRPI subfamily members (Fig. 4.3). Furthermore, the first Asp in some HRPI homologs isolated from *G. max* and *P. vulgaris* have been replaced by Ser, Gly, and Asn (Fig. 4.3). It has been shown that the expressions of the genes in this subfamily are restricted to vegetative and floral organs (Berger *et al.*, 1995; Utsugi *et al.*, 1998; Sun *et al.*, 2018). In addition, Liu *et al.* (2005) showed that the expressions of genes coding for AtHRP7 and 8 were induced by Pi starvation and methyl jasmonate.

Halo Acid Dehalogenases (HAD)-Related APase Family | 99

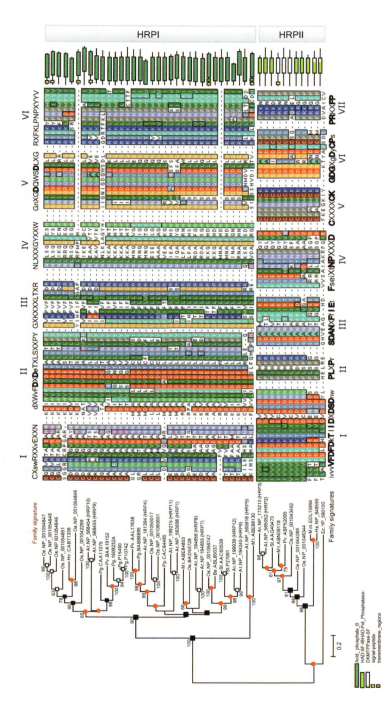

Figure 4.3 Minimum evolution tree, multiple alignments of conserved sequences and domain architecture of plant HRP family members. These sequences were classified to two major subfamilies, HRPI and HRPII.

4.5.2 HRP II Subfamily

HRPII subfamily includes two genes from *A. thaliana* and three genes from rice that encode putative APases as appeared in the literature (Fig. 4.3). In contrast to the HRPI subfamily, HRPII proteins have low sequence diversity in plants. Phylogenetically, AtHRP2 and 3 (GenBank Accession NP_173213 and NP_565052) are the only predicted in-paralogous in this subfamily distantly located on chromosome 1. Multiple sequence alignment of animal and plant homologs revealed seven well-conserved motifs, ivvv**VFDFD**k**TIIDXDSD**nw, **PLXPr**, **SDANXFfiEt**, **FseiXtNPXXXD**, **CXXXXCK**, **GDGXgDyCPs**, **PRKXFP** (X is any amino acid, residues involved in the catalytic activity are bold; Fig. 4.3). One HRPII member, LePS2 phosphatase, has already been cloned from *Lycopersicon esculentum*. The expression of LePS2 was rapidly induced in the Pi-starved plant roots and shoots (Baldwin *et al.*, 2001). Moreover, recombinant LEPS2 exhibited limited APase activity in the presence of *p*-nitrophenyl phosphate substrate (Baldwin *et al.*, 2001).

4.6 Phospholipid Phosphatase (PLP) Family

Ten AtAPase and four OsAPase annotated as phosphatidic APase or PAP2 families were clustered together (Fig. 4.4). We preferred to designate these as phospholipid phosphatase or PLP family to avoid confusion with the PAP family and subfamilies. The PLP family includes several phospholipid phosphatases, such as type 2 phosphatidic APase (EC: 3.1.3.4), phosphatidylglycerol phosphatase phosphatase B (EC: 3.1.3.27) as well as glucose-6-phosphatase (EC: 3.1.3.9), and a group of bacterial-like APase (EC: 3.1.3.2) (Ishikawa *et al.*, 2000; Carman *et al.*, 2006). To construct the phylogenetic relationships of the PLP family, we performed further BLASTP searches using primarily detected PLPs in rice and *A. thaliana*. As a result, we retrieved two additional sequences in *A. thaliana* and seven for rice. We also added a collection of all known PLP homologs in other lineages from chlorophyte to flowering plants as well as representative sequences from other kingdoms. The multiple sequence alignments of the retrieved sequences were used for phylogenetic analysis (Fig. 4.4). Based on the constructed tree, PLP family members were divided into six groups (PLP I to VI subfamilies) supported by high bootstrap values (Fig. 4.4).

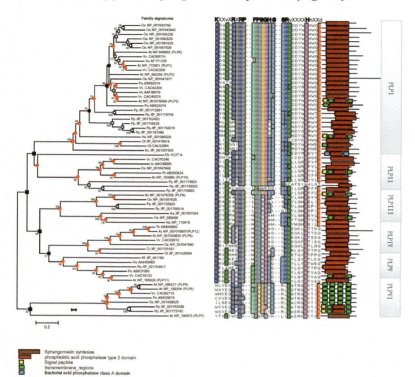

Figure 4.4 Minimum evolution tree, multiple alignments of conserved sequences and domain architecture of plant PLP family members. These sequences were classified to six subfamilies, PLPI and PLPVI.

Based on the multiple alignments, we identified three conserved motifs for this family including **KXXvXRXRP**, **FPSGHtS**, and **iSRvXXXXHhXXDVd** (X is any amino acid, residues involved in the catalytic activity are indicated in bold; Fig. 4.4) with some modification to the previously reported motifs (Carman and Han, 2006; Stukey and Carman, 1997). The conserved arginine residues in motif 1, and the conserved histidine (His) residues in motifs 2 and 3, are essential for the catalytic activity of PLP enzymes (Stukey and Carman, 1997; Toke *et al.*, 1999; ZHANG *et al.*, 2000). Although such conserved motifs exist in almost all examined *A. thaliana* and *O. sativa* sequences, there are members of this family in both plants that display a high degree of variations within these motifs (Fig. 4.4). The PLP family includes several phospholipid phosphatases, such as type 2 phosphatidic APase (EC: 3.1.3.4), phosphatidylglycerol phosphatase phosphatase B (EC: 3.1.3.27) as well as glucose-6-phosphatase (EC: 3.1.3.9), and a group of bacterial APase (EC: 3.1.3.2) (Ishikawa *et al.*, 2000; Carman *et al.*, 2006). Three of the PLP-like proteins, At3g15820, At3g50920, At5g66450 (GenBank Accession NP_566527, NP_001030835 and NP_001078807) were proposed to be chloroplastic-like and one mitochondrial-like, At5g03080 (GenBank Accession NP_195928; unpublished data). It is postulated that PLPs are involved in the replacement of phosphorylated metabolites, such as phospholipids and phosphosugars with functionally equivalent molecules in subcellular organelles in plants subjected to severe Pi starvation (van der Rest *et al.*, 2002). The role of PLPs in lipid signaling has been proposed as well (Carman and Han, 2006).

4.7 Histidine Acid Phosphatase Family

We identified three genes in *A. thaliana* and four genes in rice encoding proteins like the histidine acid phosphatase (HAP) proteins. Aligning with all other known HAP sequences from prokaryotes and eukaryotes, this group was clearly divided into two clusters, named HMW and LMW subfamilies (Fig. 4.5). We observed low sequence similarities between HMW and LMW HAPs. The HWM HAPs carry a highly conserved region named RimK located at the *N*-terminal. The RimK motif was also found in glutathione synthase or glutaminyl transferase (Galperin and Koonin, 1997). Interestingly, no significantly similar sequence to HMW HAPs was found in prokaryotes despite having many sequences containing the RimK motif. Given the striking sequence divergence between the two subfamilies, it is difficult to determine if the HMW HAPs are the product of domain exchange between genes encoding the RimK-containing proteins and LMW HAPs. We noticed a short OsHAPs, Os01g0777500 (GenBank Accession NP_001044423), with no RimK region, that aligned with HMW HAPs. Based on separate multiple sequence alignments, motifs for this subfamily were defined as **RHGXRXPT** for the LMW HAPs and **ELRcVIAviRHGDRTPKQKvK**

Histidine Acid Phosphatase Family | 103

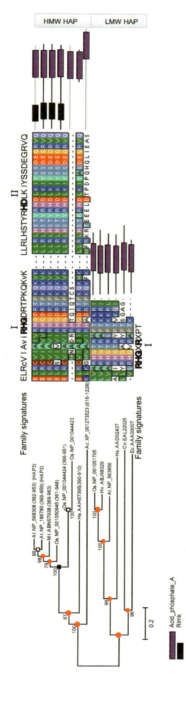

Figure 4.5 Minimum evolution tree, multiple alignments of conserved sequences and domain architecture of plant HRP family members. These sequences were classified to two subfamilies, LMW HAP and HMW HAP.

and **LIRHDLKIY**X**S**dE**g**R**V**q for the HMW HAPs (X is any amino acid, residues involved in the catalytic activity are bold; Fig. 4.5). Similar motifs have been detected in some prokaryotic APases with phytase and glucose-1-phosphatase activities (Vats and Banerjee, 2004). The majority of the known phytases carry two conserved motifs, **RHGXRXP** and **XHDX**. The histidine residue in the RHGXRXP motif and Asp in the XHDX motif, located in the catalytic site of the enzyme serves as a nucleophile and serves as a proton donor, respectively (Oh et al., 2004). As shown in Fig. 4.5, the former motif is shared in both subfamilies, while the latter is missing within the LMW HAPs. It is worth noting that the phytase term refers to at least three structurally different enzyme families, HAP, PAP, and a prokaryotic enzyme named β-propeller phytase or BPP (Lung et al., 2008; Mullaney and Ullah, 2003). We have also isolated a phytase from *Psudomomase putida* strain P13 with strong phytase activity (Sarikhani et al., 2019). For instance, phytase activities were reported for some PAP proteins, such as AtPAP15 (GenBank Accession NP_187369) (Kuang et al., 2009; p. 15), GmPhy (GenBank AccessionAAK43438) (Hegeman and Grabau, 2001). Xiao et al. (2006) found a PAPI member in *M. truncatula*, named MtPHY1 (GenBank Accession AAX20028) that is expressed in the roots during growth under low Pi condition and when introduced in the transgenic Arabidopsis plants expressing MtPHY1 exhibits significantly increased capacity for Pi acquisition from phytate and, thus, higher plant growth (Xiao et al., 2005).

4.8 Protein E (SurE)-Related Acid Phosphatase Family

This group includes only two sequences in each model plant species (Fig. 4.6) that share similarities with the well-known prokaryotic survival protein E (SurE) with reported APase activities (Lee et al., 2001; Mura et al., 2003). Therefore, we designated this family as SurE acid phosphatase (SAP). We conducted further searches for the related sequences in other organisms and utilized a few of them to portray the clustering of the SAPs. Apparently, this family has not been expanded as much and only one pair of SAPs exist in every plant species (Fig. 4.6). In other words, each cluster encompasses a set of orthologous sequences resulting from their common ancestor

Protein E (SurE)-Related Acid Phosphatase Family | 105

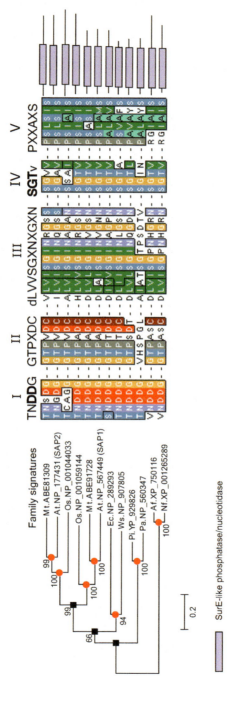

Figure 4.6 Minimum evolution tree, multiple alignments of conserved sequences and domain architecture of plant SAP family members.

with a duplication time preceding the divergence of monocots and dicots. Plant SAPs are moderately similar to each other and we detected four well-conserved motifs for this family including **TNDDG, GTPXDC, LVVSGXNXGXN,** and **SGTXXAXEAXXXGXPXXAXS** (X is any amino acid, residues involved in the catalytic activity are bold; Fig. 4.6). These motifs are well-conserved in prokaryotes and fungi while none was found in mammalians. We also noticed plant SAPs are phylogenetically closer to bacterial SAPs indicating possible endosymbiosis, and subsequent gene transfer from organelle to nucleolus and might be a plausible scenario for the origin of plant SAPs. There is no experimental evidence for plant SAPs function, however, based on the comprehensive structural and functional works conducted by Mura *et al.* (2003), prokaryotic SAP enzymes displayed substrate specificity toward purine nucleotides.

4.9 Structural Comparisons of APase Families

Analyzing the diversity of plants APase at the sequence level, we also explored their variations in 3D structures. We used the ConSurf program (Landau *et al.*, 2005) to map the conservation scores from multiple alignments of the family members on the selected structures for each family available in PDB (https://www.rcsb.org/). These representing structures include chain A of kidney bean purple APase (PDB ID:1KBP) for PAP family, chain A of *Escherichia coli* APase (PDB ID: 1N9K) for HRP family, chain A of *E. Blattae* APase (PDB ID: 1EOI) for PLP family, chain A of *Francisella tularensis* (PDB ID: 2GLC) for HAP family, and chain A of *Thermotoga maritime* APase (PDB ID: 1ILV) for SAP family. After mapping the conservation scores by ConSurf, the output was imported into the PyMol program (http://www.pymol.org) to visualize the 3D structures in ribbon format with the color-coded scale of the conservation. As shown in Fig. 4.7, despite variations in details, four of the five APase families share the general Rossmannoid structure composed of repeating α/β units that are arrayed as β-strands in the core covered by α-helices on the surface of proteins. Exceptionally, the 1EOI structure from the PLP family is only composed of α-helices. In the Rossmann-like structures, the conserved residues mostly occur in the turns and loops, as well as in the β-strands, while residues in the α-helices are highly variable. In other words, there is a tendency for conservation toward the cores of proteins where the active sites are positioned.

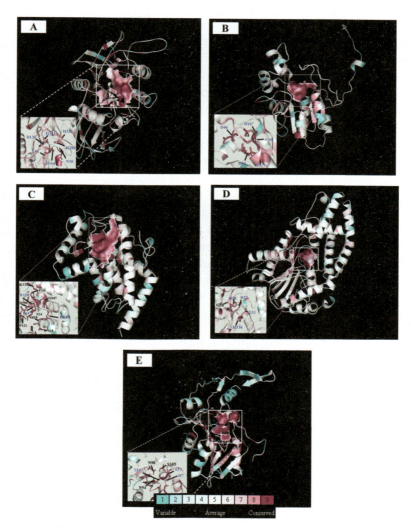

Figure 4.7 Structural comparisons of plant APs. Representative 3D structures for each family of plant APases were exploited for ConSurf analysis (Landau et al., 2005) using multiple alignment data imported from ClustalW data sets. The computed scores for each position were used to infer conservation level and illustrated by gray scales (by colored scales in supplementary Fig. X.8) on the ribbon structures drawn by PyMol software (DeLano, 2002). Small boxes are magnifications of proposed catalytic regions in which the active residues directly involve in Pi hydrolysis are shown in blue. (a) Chain A of kidney bean purple acid phosphatase (PDB ID: 1KBP) representing PAP family. (b) Chain A of *Escherichia coli* APase (PDB ID: 1N9K) representing HRP family. (c) Chain A of E. Blattae APase (PDB ID: 1EOI) representing PLP family. (d) Chain A of *Francisella tularensis* (PDB ID: 2GLC) representing HAP family. (e) Chain A of *Thermotoga maritime* APase (PDB ID: 1ILV) representing SAP family.

Active sites were also magnified based on available information in the literature with the use of the mesh option (Fig. 4.7). Except for the SAPs, all catalytic sites are composed of distantly located individual residues on turns or loops and are organized closely in the 3D structures. These include one or more residues that are believed to coordinate the Mg^{2+} which is key for nucleophile catalysis (Burroughs et al., 2006). The common feature of these residues is being charged amino acids fulfilling the need for nucleophilic attacks. It is worth noticing that while all of the enzymes catalyze similar reactions, the residues that are directly interacting with Pi bonds are not completely conserved, for example His residues in PAPs (Schenk et al., 2008), Asp residues in HRPs (Burroughs et al., 2006; Burroughs et al., 2006) and SAPs (Lee et al., 2001) or Arg and His residues in PLP (Stukey and Carman, 1997; Toke et al., 1999; Zhang et al., 2000) and HAP (Ostanin et al., 1992). The overall shape of the active site also shows an open shape which allows these APase with non-specific binding for boarding the substrate space of Pi bonds.

4.10 Concluding Remarks

Phosphate is a key for cellular processes such as signal perception and transduction, regulation of gene expression, and regulation of enzymatic activities. Furthermore, it is an essential component of biomolecules such as DNA, RNA, phospholipids, phosphosugars, and phosphoproteins. Unlike animals as the consuming section in the upper level of the energy conversion pyramid, plants are producers and are in the first level of the energy pyramid. Therefore, plants are the primary gate for integrating inorganic Pi into the building blocks of life. APases can be seen as molecular machines that are invented and engineered by evolution to provide plants with the capability of converting the trapped Pi in the soil compounds into an absorbable form by the roots.

In this chapter, we have tried to address an important and not previously explored question of why plants have multiple APases in comparison to animals. We further investigated types of evolutionary forces in shaping these heterogeneous groups of functionally (and probably mechanistically) similar enzymes. To address these questions, we have comprehensively re-examined the evolutionary landscape of all known APase protein sequences in *A. thaliana* and *O. sativa* representing monocotyledonous and dicotyledonous plants that are diverged 140 to 200 million years ago (Chaw *et al.*, 2004). As discussed above, the pairwise identity-based clustering of the retrieved APase sequences grouped them into five distinct families. Consequently, the phylogenetic analysis and defining the conserved motifs enabled us to identify family-specific signatures. Indeed, the conserved sequences are characteristic tools to discrete APase families from each other as none is shared among them.

The high level of diversity in the primary sequence, structure, and conserved active sites; in the protein length; and in the number of exons among APase families suggests that likely these enzymes did not diverge from a common ancestor. Here, we propose a convergent evolutionary scenario for APases in plants involving multiple ancestral genes. In other words, the ancestral genes have originated from other superfamilies and have undergone independent evolutionary processes (e.g., duplications, mutations, recombinations, and rearrangements) to ensure that plants sustain the Pi homeostasis (Fig. 4.8). As a result, five distinct families of plant APases are evolved and share mechanistic characteristics in hydrolyzing Pi phosphoric ester bonds.

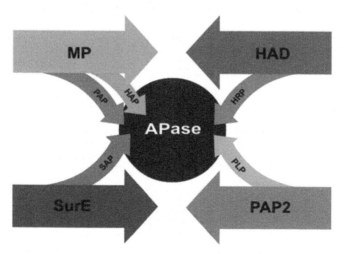

Figure 4.8 Schematic representation of APase families converging relationships with other superfamilies. As shown, PAP and HAP families have been deviated from metallophosphatase superfamily: HRP family from HAD superfamily, PLP family from PAP2 superfamily, and SAP family from Surival E superfamily.

A similar phenomenon has already been reported for morphological characters such as wings in insects and birds as well as molecular entities such as anhydrases in mammals and plants (Breton, 2001), transcriptional regulators (Conant *et al.*, 2003; Conant and Wagner, 2003) and plant disease resistance genes (Ashfield *et al.*, 2004). All of these examples show the emergence of biological structures that exhibit similar functions that evolved through widely discrete evolutionary tracks allowing adaptation to ecological niches or physical constraints. Therefore, like the analogies between morphological characters, we do expect analogies between structural and/or functional features of plant APases rather than sequence homologies among them. Here, we speculate having similar functions (APase activity) and, possibly, roles in Pi acquisition as well as resemblance at 3D structures, the use of charged amino acids in the catalytic residues, and utilizing metal ions (Table 4.2) are instances of analogies among APase protein families. It is noteworthy that the PLP subfamily differs from other families for not having a Rassmonidal structure and lacking metal ions in the active site.

Table 4.2 Protein families and the number of known APase encoding genes in *A. thaliana*, *O. sativa*, and other plant genomes

Acid Phosphatase Families	Catalysis Residues	Interacting Anions	A. thaliana	O. sativa	Other plants
PAP	His	Fe & Mn/Zn	29	19	30
HRP	Asp	Mg	12	13	17
PLP	Arg & His	-	12	11	34
HAP	His & Asp	Ca	3	4	2
SAP	Asp	Ca/Mg	2	2	2
Total			58	49	85

Despite having distinct last common ancestral genes, it is quite possible that each APase family has undergone gene multiplications and diversifications independently afterward. This is supported by out-paralogous relationships between several ancestral genes within the APase families conforming to the duplications to predate the divergence of the monocot and dicots. For example, in Arabidopsis,

PAP5, 6, 25, 19, and *11* form clear in-paralog relationships and are the result of gene duplication after speciation, while *PAP10* and *PAP12* are out-paralogs and are the result of gene duplication before mono and dicot speciation (Fig. 4.1). Therefore, APase genes expansions in plants and multiple LSEs could be explained by divergence from the common ancestors within each family. The gene expansions along with subtle variations were particularly essential for plants to be able to retrieve Pi from as many mineral or organic compounds as possible. Consequently, the large numbers of APase enzymes have possibly been favored by natural selection as plants carrying numerous APase-encoding genes were able to withstand and propagate in suboptimal concentrations of Pi by hydrolyzing various compounds in the soil. Considering the non-mycorrhizal nature of *Arabidopsis*, it is not unexpected that this plant possesses 23% more APase-encoding genes (mostly PAPs) than rice despite having a smaller genome size. To be able to sustain its potential for retrieving Pi from various substrates, Arabidopsis has been under the evolutionary force of inventing more APases in comparison to rice which relies on mycorrhiza symbiosis.

To conclude, it is conceivable that the necessity for Pi homeostasis for cellular survival was the main selective force to favor sequence and structural adaptations of various superfamily members toward APase activity to target as many alternative Pi substrate types as possible. Then, divergent evolution within the families allowed the broadening of substrate subtypes. This is more pronounced for plants as sessile organisms, particularly for those with no mycorrhizal symbiosis.

Acknowledgments

We are grateful to the National Institute of Genetics Engineering and Biotechnology for providing services and support. We would also like to acknowledge Dr. Mehdi Sadeghi for his technical advice. Also, we greatly acknowledge Dr. William Plaxton for his deep comments.

References

Baldwin, J.C., Karthikeyan, A.S., Raghothama, K.G., *Plant Physiology* **125** (2001), 728–737.

Beck, J.L., McConachie, L.A., Summors, A.C., Arnold, W.N., De Jersey, J., Zerner, B., *Biochimica et Biophysica Acta (BBA): Protein Structure and Molecular Enzymology* **869** (1986), 61–68.

Berger, S., Bell, E., Sadka, A., Mullet, J.E., *Plant Molecular Biology* **27** (1995), 933–942.

Bhadouria, J., Singh, A.P., Mehra, P., Verma, L., Srivastawa, R., Parida, S.K., Giri, J., *Scientific Reports* **7** (2017), 1–12.

Blanc, G., Barakat, A., Guyot, R., Cooke, R., Delseny, M., *The Plant Cell* **12** (2000), 1093–1101.

Bozzo, G.G., Raghothama, K.G., Plaxton, W.C., *European Journal of Biochemistry* **269** (2002), 6278–6286.

Breton, S., *JOP: Journal of the Pancreas* **2** (2001), 159–164.

Burroughs, A.M., Allen, K.N., Dunaway-Mariano, D., Aravind, L., *Journal of Molecular Biology* **361** (2006), 1003–1034.

Calderone, V., Forleo, C., Benvenuti, M., Thaller, M.C., Rossolini, G.M., Mangani, S., *Journal of Molecular Biology* **335** (2004), 761–773.

Cannon, S.B., Mitra, A., Baumgarten, A., Young, N.D., May, G., 2004. *BMC Plant Biology* **4** (2004), 1–21.

Carman, G.M., Han, G.-S., *Trends in Biochemical Sciences* **31** (2006), 694–699.

Chafik, A., Essamadi, A., Çelik, S.Y., Mavi, A., *International Journal of Biological Macromolecules* **160** (2020), 991–999.

Chaw, S.-M., Chang, C.-C., Chen, H.-L., Li, W.-H., *Journal of Molecular Evolution* **58** (2004), 424–441.

Choisne, N., Perchat Demange, N., Orjeda, G., Samain, S., D'Hont, A., Cattolico, L., Pelletier, E., Couloux, A., Segurens, B., Wincker, P., Scarpelli, C., Weissenbach, J., Salanoubat, M., Quetier, F., Singh, N., Mohapatra, T., Sharma, T., Gaikwad, K., Singh, A., et al. *BMC Biology* **3** (2005), 18.

Chu, Y.-H., Yu, X.-X., Jin, X., Wang, Y.-T., Zhao, D.-J., Zhang, P., Sun, G.-M., Zhang, Y.-H., *RSC Advances* **9** (2019), 354–360.

Conant, G.C., Wagner, A., *Nature Genetics* **34** (2003), 264–266.

Cordell, D., Drangert, J.-O., White, S., *Global Environmental Change, Traditional Peoples and Climate Change* **19** (2009), 292–305.

Crombez, H., Motte, H., Beeckman, T., *Developmental Cell* **48** (2019), 599–615.

Del Pozo, J.C., Allona, I., Rubio, V., Leyva, A., De La Peña, A., Aragoncillo, C., Paz-Ares, J., *The Plant Journal* **19** (1999), 579–589.

Del Vecchio, H.A., Ying, S., Park, J., Knowles, V.L., Kanno, S., Tanoi, K., She, Y.-M., Plaxton, W.C., *Plant Journal* **80** (2014), 569–581.

DeLano, W.L., *The PyMOL Molecular Graphics System*, Delano Scientific, San, 2002.

Deng, M.-J., Wang, F., Mao, C.-Z., *Plant Physiology Journal* **53** (2017), 377–387.

Dick, C.F., Dos-Santos, A.L.A., Meyer-Fernandes, J.R., *Enzyme Research* **2011** (2011), 1–7.

Durmus, A., Eicken, C., Sift, B.H., Kratel, A., Kappl, R., Hüttermann, J., Krebs, B., *European Journal Biochem*stry **260** (1999), 709–716.

Fabiańska, I., Bucher, M., Häusler, R.E., *Plant Science* **286** (2019), 57–67.

Feder, D., McGeary, R.P., Mitić, N., Lonhienne, T., Furtado, A., Schulz, B.L., Henry, R.J., Schmidt, S., Guddat, L.W., Schenk, G., *Plant Science* **294** (2020), 110445.

Flanagan, J., Cassady, A., Schenk, G., Guddat, L., Hume, D., *Gene* **377** (2006), 12–20.

Galperin, M.Y., Koonin, E.V., *Protein Science* **6** (1997), 2639–2643.

Gerlt, J.A., Babbitt, P.C., *Annual Review of Biochemistry* **70** (2001), 209–246.

González-Muñoz, E., Avendaño-Vázquez, A.-O., Montes, R.A.C., de Folter, S., Andrés-Hernández, L., Abreu-Goodger, C., Sawers, R.J., *Frontiers in Plant Science* **6** (2015), 341.

Hegeman, C.E., Grabau, E.A., *Plant Physiology* **126** (2001), 1598–1608.

Imamura, R., Yamanaka, K., Ogura, T., Hiraga, S., Fujita, N., Ishihama, A., Niki, H., *Journal of Biological Chemistry* **271** (1996), 25423–25429.

Itoh, T., Tanaka, T., Barrero, R.A., Yamasaki, C., Fujii, Y., Hilton, P.B., Antonio, B.A., Aono, H., Apweiler, R., Bruskiewich, R., *Genome Research* **17** (2007), 175–183.

Kaida, R., Sage-Ono, K., Kamada, H., Okuyama, H., Syono, K., Kaneko, T.S., *Biochimica et Biophysica Acta (BBA)-Gene Structure and Expression* **1625** (2003), 134–140.

Kerk, D., Templeton, G., Moorhead, G.B., *Plant Physiology* **146** (2008), 351–367.

Klabunde, T., Stahl, B., Suerbaum, H., Hahner, S., Karas, M., Hillenkamp, F., Krebs, B., Witzel, H., *European Journal of Biochemistry* **226** (1994), 369–375.

Kong, Y., Li, X., Ma, J., Li, W., Yan, G., Zhang, C., *Plant Cell Rep*ort **33** (2014), 655–667.

Kong, Y., Li, X., Wang, B., Li, W., Du, H., Zhang, C., *Frontiers in Plant Science* **9** (2018), 292.

Koonin, E.V., Tatusov, R.L., *Journal of Molecular Biology* **244** (1994), 125–132.

Kuang, R., Chan, K.-H., Yeung, E., Lim, B.L., *Plant Physiology* **151** (2009), 199–209.

Kumar, S., Stecher, G., Li, M., Knyaz, C., Tamura, K., *Molecular Biology and Evolution* **35** (2018), 1547.

Lahiri, S.D., Zhang, G., Dai, J., Dunaway-Mariano, D., Allen, K.N., *Biochemistry* **43** (2004), 2812–2820.

Landau, M., Mayrose, I., Rosenberg, Y., Glaser, F., Martz, E., Pupko, T., Ben-Tal, N., *Nucleic Acids Research* **33** (2005), W299–W302.

Lee, J.Y., Kwak, J.E., Moon, J., Eom, S.H., Liong, E.C., Pedelacq, J.-D., Berendzen, J., Suh, S.W., *Nature Structural Biology* **8** (2001), 789–794.

Li, D., Zhu, H., Liu, K., Liu, X., Leggewie, G., Udvardi, M., Wang, D., *Journal of Biological Chemistry* **277** (2002b), 27772–27781.

Liao, H., Wong, F.-L., Phang, T.-H., Cheung, M.-Y., Li, W.-Y.F., Shao, G., Yan, X., Lam, H.-M., *Gene* **318** (2003), 103–111.

Liu, Y., Ahn, J.-E., Datta, S., Salzman, R.A., Moon, J., Huyghues-Despointes, B., Pittendrigh, B., Murdock, L.L., Koiwa, H., Zhu-Salzman, K., *Plant Physiology* **139** (2005), 1545–1556.

Lu, Z., Dunaway-Mariano, D., Allen, K.N., *Biochemistry* **44** (2005), 8684–8696.

Lung, S.-C., Leung, A., Kuang, R., Wang, Y., Leung, P., Lim, B.-L., *Phytochemistry* **69** (2008), 365–373.

Malhotra, H., Sharma, S., Pandey, R., *et al.* Phosphorus nutrition: plant growth in response to deficiency and excess, in *Plant Nutrients and Abiotic Stress Tolerance*, 2018, Springer, pp. 171–190.

Misson, J., Raghothama, K. G., Jain, A., Jouhet, J., Block, M. A., Bligny, R., Thibaud, M. C., *Proceedings of the National Academy of Sciences* **102**(33), (2005), 11934–11939.

Mullaney, E.J., Ullah, A.H., *Biochemical and Biophysical Research Communications* **312** (2003), 179–184.

Mura, C., Katz, J.E., Clarke, S.G., Eisenberg, D., *Journal of Molecular Biology* **326** (2003), 1559–1575.

Oh, B.-C., Choi, W.-C., Park, S., Kim, Y.-O., Oh, T.-K., *Applied Microbiology and Biotechnology* **63** (2004), 362–372.

Olczak, M., Olczak, T., *FEBS Letters* **519** (2002), 159–163.

Olczak, M., Wątorek, W., *Physiologia Plantarum* **118** (2003), 491–498.

Ostanin, K., Harms, E.H., Stevis, P.E., Kuciel, R., Zhou, M.-M., Van Etten, R., *Journal of Biological Chemistry* **267**(1992), 22830–22836.

Pierrugues, O., Brutesco, C., Oshiro, J., Gouy, M., Deveaux, Y., Carman, G.M., Thuriaux, P., Kazmaier, M., *Journal of Biological Chemistry* **276** (2001), 20300–20308.

Plaxton, W.C., Tran, H.T., *Plant Physiology*, **156** (2011), 1006–1015.

Raghothama, K., *Annual Review of Plant Biology* **50** (1999), 665–693.

Raghothama, K., Karthikeyan, A., *Plant and Soil* **274** (2005), 37–49.

van der Rest, B., Boisson, A.-M., Gout, E., Bligny, R., Douce, R., *Plant Physiology* **130** (2002), 244–255.

Sarikhani, M.R., Malboobi, M.A., Aliasgharzad, N., Greiner, R., 2019. *Journal of Applied Microbiology* **127** (2002), 1113–1124.

Schäffer, A.A., Aravind, L., Madden, T.L., Shavirin, S., Spouge, J.L., Wolf, Y.I., Koonin, E.V., Altschul, S.F., *Nucleic Acids Research* **29** (2001), 2994–3005.

Schenk, G., Elliott, T.W., Leung, E., Carrington, L.E., Mitić, N., Gahan, L.R., Guddat, L.W., *BMC Structural Biology* **8** (2008), 1–13.

Schenk, G., Gahan, L.R., Carrington, L.E., Mitić, N., Valizadeh, M., Hamilton, S.E., de Jersey, J., Guddat, L.W., *Proceedings of the National Academy of Sciences* **102** (2005), 273–278.

Schenk, G., Ge, Y., Carrington, L.E., Wynne, C.J., Searle, I.R., Carroll, B.J., Hamilton, S., de Jersey, J., *Archives of Biochemistry and Biophysics* **370** (1999), 183–189.

Schenk, G., Korsinczky, M.L., Hume, D.A., Hamilton, S., DeJersey, J., *Gene* **255** (2000), 419–424.

Schenk, G., Mitić, N., Hanson, G.R., Comba, P., *Coordination Chemistry Reviews* **257** (2013), 473–482.

Srivastava, R., Parida, A.P., Chauhan, P.K., Kumar, R., et al. *International Journal of Biological Macromolecules* **165** (2020), 2253–2266.

Strater, N., Klabunde, T., Tucker, P., Witzel, H., Krebs, B., *Science* **268** (1995), 1489–1492.

Stukey, J., Carman, G.M., *Protein Science* **6** (1997), 469–472.

Sun, F., Carrie, C., Law, S., Murcha, M.W., Zhang, R., Law, Y.S., Suen, P.K., Whelan, J., Lim, B.L., *Plant Signal Behavior* **7** (2012), 927–932.

Sun, L., Wang, L., Zheng, Z., Liu, D., *Plant Science* **277** (2018), 278–284.

Tagad, C.K., Sabharwal, S.G., *Journal of Food Science and Technology* **55** (2018), 313–320.

Thaller, M.C., Schippa, S., Rossolini, G.M., *Protein Science* **7** (1998), 1647–1652.

Toke, D.A., McClintick, M.L., Carman, G.M., *Biochemistry* **38** (1999), 14606–14613.

Tran, H., Hurley, B., Plaxton, W., *Plant Science* **179** (2010), 14–27.

Utsugi, S., Sakamoto, W., Murata, M., Motoyoshi, F., *Plant Molecular Biology* **38** (1998), 565–576.

Vance, C.P., Uhde-Stone, C., Allan, D.L., *New Phytologist* **157** (2003), 423–447.

Vats, P., Banerjee, U.C., *Enzyme and Microbial Technology* **35** (2004), 3–14.

Venkidasamy, B., Selvaraj, D., Ramalingam, S., *International Journal Of Biological Macromolecules* **123** (2019), 648–656.

Wang, L., Liu, D., *Plant Science* **271** (2018), 108–116.

Wasaki, J., Ando, M., Ozawa, K., Omura, M., Osaki, M., Ito, H., Matsui, H., Tadano, T., Properties of secretory acid phosphatase from lupin roots under phosphorus-deficient conditions, in *Plant Nutrition for Sustainable Food Production and Environment,* 1997, Springer, pp. 295–300.

Wasaki, J., Omura, M., Osaki, M., Ito, H., Matsui, H., Shinano, T., Tadano, T., *Soil Science and Plant Nutrition* **45** (1999), 439–449.

Xiao, K., Harrison, M., Wang, Z.-Y., *Journal of Integrative Plant Biology* **48** (2006), 204–211.

Xiao, K., Harrison, M.J., Wang, Z.-Y., *Planta* **222** (2005), 27–36.

Yin, C., Wang, F., Fan, H., Fang, Y., Li, W., *International Journal of Molecular Sciences* **20** (2019), 1954.

Yoneyama, T., Shiozawa, M., Nakamura, M., Suzuki, T., Sagane, Y., Katoh, Y., Watanabe, T., Ohyama, T., *Journal of Biological Chemistry* **279** (2004), 37477–37484.

Yoneyama, T., Taira, M., Suzuki, T., Nakamura, M., Niwa, K., Watanabe, T., Ohyama, T., *Protein Expression and Purification* **53** (2007), 31–39.

Zhang, Q., Wang, C., Tian, J., Li, K., Shou, H., *Plant Biology* **13** (2011), 7–15.

Zhang, Y., Wang, X., Lu, S., Liu, D., *Journal of Experimental Botany,* **65** (2014), 6577–6588.

Zhang, Q.-X., Pilquil, C.S., Dewald, J., Berthiaume, L.G., Brindley, D.N., *Biochemical Journal* **345** (2000), 181–184.

Zhou, M., Chen, W., Zhao, M., Li, Y., Li, M., Hu, X., *Forests* **12** (2021), 326.

Zhu, H., Qian, W., Lu, X., Li, D., Liu, X., Liu, K., Wang, D., *Plant Molecular Biology* **59** (2005), 581–594.

Zhu, S., Chen, M., Liang, C., Xue, Y., Lin, S., Tian, J., *Frontiers in Plant Science* **11** (2020), 661.

Zimmermann, P., Regierer, B., Kossmann, J., Frossard, E., Amrhein, N., Bucher, M., *Plant Biology* **6** (2004), 519–528.

Chapter 5

Acid Phosphatases Roles in Plant Performance

Mohammad Ali Malboobi,[a] Mohammad Sadegh Sabet,[b] Katayoun Zamani,[c] Tahmineh Lohrasebi,[a] Zahra Fathi,[a] and Javad Zamani[a]

[a]*Department of Plant Molecular Biotechnology, National Institute of Genetic Engineering and Biotechnology, P.O. Box 14965/161, Tehran, Iran*
[b]*Department of Plant Genetics and Breeding, Faculty of Agriculture, Tarbiat Modares University, Tehran, Iran*
[c]*Department of Genetic Engineering and Biosafety, Agricultural Biotechnology Research Institute of Iran, Agricultural Research, Education and Extension Organization, Karaj, Iran*
malboobi@nigeb.ac.ir

Phosphorus (P), in the form of its phosphate ion (Pi), plays an essential role in many pathways, including energy transfer, photosynthesis, respiration, metabolic reactions, signaling, and various levels of regulations in plants. It is also a structural component of many biomolecules such as nucleic acids, proteins, sugar-phosphates, and phospholipids. Therefore, it is essential to retain a certain homeostatic level of Pi to keep cellular reactions running and reduce

---

Agricultural Biocatalysis: Enzymes in Agriculture and Industry
Edited by Peter Jeschke and Evgeni B. Starikov
Copyright © 2023 Jenny Stanford Publishing Pte. Ltd.
ISBN 978-981-4968-47-8 (Hardcover), 978-1-003-31310-6 (eBook)
www.jennystanford.com

disturbance in plant performance when subjected to various biotic and abiotic environmental conditions. A collectively named large family of acid phosphatase (APase) enzymes play primary roles in Pi homeostasis by mobilizing, recycling, and scavenging Pi from internal and external resources. Having broad substrates ranges, their expression patterns and activity levels could determine when and where they operate in a perfectly tuned manner depending on which available substrates to target in effective order. Still, multiple APases and interplay networking among them with relevance to cellular Pi complicate the utilization of these enzymes. A deep insight into their roles and concerted operations paves the way for Pi provision through either rhizosphere engineering, genetic manipulation, or agricultural and industrial innovations.

5.1 Introduction

Phosphorus (P) is the most vital element for plants growth and productivity (Vance *et al.*, 2003). In general, soil P usually ranges from 100 to 2000 mg P kg^{-1} soil equivalent to approximately 350 to 7000 kg P ha^{-1} in the top 20–30 cm of surface soil (Grant *et al.*, 2005). Since plants only uptakes P in the form of soluble phosphate ion (Pi), it is limited in over 40% of arable lands (Vance *et al.*, 2003). Besides, Pi solubility and mobility in soil is so low that only a small portion of it (15–25%) is available for crop uptake even after using Pi fertilizer. About 30–65% of P in soil is in organic P compounds (Po) and the remaining can be found as inorganic compounds, aluminum/iron in acidic soil, or as calcium/magnesium in alkaline soil. The production of Pi fertilizers is resource-limited. On the other hand, it is predicted that the world Pi consumption exceeds the production by the year 2033 (Cordell, 2009). Considering the growth rate of the world population while diminishing the supply of Pi fertilizers, the production of human food will face a serious challenge. Therefore, deep insight into aspects of Pi provision to plants is necessary to grow crops with improved efficiency in Pi uptake and usage. Here, we will review the molecular mechanisms that naturally support plants to cope with Pi-deficient condition, mainly fulfilled by taking advantage of APase enzymes.

5.2 Phosphate Ion and Its Significance

P level ranges from 0.05% to 0.5% of total plant dry weight and exists either as free inorganic Pi or as esterified Po form (Vance et al., 2003; Veneklaas et al., 2012). The main pools for esterified P are biomolecules such as nucleic acids ranging from 0.3 to 2.0 mg P g^{-1} dry weight in various crops which carry the genetic information (Elser et al., 2010; Veneklaas et al., 2012). The largest portion of them is ribonucleic acid (RNA) (~80%) which is metabolically active, particularly in the translation process (Dissanayaka et al., 2021). Other structural forms are phospholipids (PLs), sugar-phosphates, and phosphorylated proteins. PLs are the essential constituent of cell membranes that contain up to 30% of the total Po pool in nutrient-sufficient plant cells. Membrane PL degradation in Pi-depleted plants is coupled to the synthesis of sulfo- and galactolipids to maintain membrane integrity (Malhotra et al., 2018; Dissanayaka et al., 2021).

Sugar-phosphates are the Pi esters formed by phosphorylation of mono/polysaccharides produced through photosynthesis, glycolysis, and respiratory reactions. They are mostly the prime intermediate metabolites that integrate with other molecules such as phytic acid, glucose-6-phosphate, and dihydroxyacetone phosphate (Malhotra et al., 2018).

Phosphoproteins are posttranslationally modified by the attachment of one or more Pi group(s) through kinase activities. These amino acids are most often serine, threonine, or tyrosine residues. Indeed, Pi regulates the function of many proteins via covalent attachment to proteins acting as an allosteric activator or inhibitor of key regulatory enzymes of central metabolic or signaling pathways (Bykova et al., 2003; Veneklaas et al., 2012; Plaxton and Shane, 2018).

Pi is also a component of high-energy bonds, including phosphoanhydrides, acyl phosphates, and enol phosphates. It becomes evident as a constituent of essential biomolecules such as ATP, ADP, or NADPH acting as universal cellular energy cofactors (Malboobi et al., 2012; Malhotra et al., 2018).

The main roles of Pi in plant growth and development could be categorized in three different aspects:

(1) Seeds of crops contain large amounts of Pi, mostly in phytate form. Increasing seed Pi content can improve seedling vigor in the early growth stage which is eventually reflected in higher yield. This is thought to be needed for faster initial root growth giving seedlings earlier access to growth-limiting resources, such as water and mineral elements. Seed Pi reserves can sustain maximal growth of cereal seedlings for several weeks after germination until three or more leaves and an intensive root system are established (White and Veneklaas, 2012; Wang et al., 2021).

(2) Pi plays a crucial role in improving vegetative growth and development by increasing the number of leaves and their expansion, the root strength, and the formation of flower and seed (Malhotra et al., 2018). In a Pi-limited condition, plants invest little in sexual reproduction, reduce flowering time, produce fewer seeds, and have conservative leaf economy traits, such as a low leaf area and a high leaf dry-matter content (Fujita et al., 2014). In contrast, when subjected to high soluble Pi concentration in soil, there are increases in the seed number, seed dry-matter, seed yield, and, hence, high harvest index (Prajapati et al., 2017; Taliman et al., 2019; Naomi et al., 2021).

(3) Pi alters the shape of plants from cellular to organ levels. Changes appear in affected plant height, leaf area, leaf number, shoot dry biomass, and root architecture primarily influenced by cell division and cell enlargement (Prajapati et al., 2017; Balzergue et al., 2017; Gutiérrez-Alanís et al., 2018; Malhotra et al., 2018; Naomi et al., 2021). In Pi limitation condition, changes comprise increasing both root hair length and density, thereby expanding the absorptive root surface area (Niu et al., 2013; Crombez et al., 2019).

These are all indicative of the indispensable roles of Pi in many fundamental physiological processes in plants, including photosynthesis, respiration, nutrients absorption, and reproduction. For instance, the requirement for Pi in photophosphorylation and the exchange of triose-Pi between the chloroplast and cytosol demonstrates its central role in photosynthesis. As a result, plant performance relies heavily on the level of Pi and mechanisms for keeping its homeostasis (Veneklaas *et al.*, 2012; Dissanayaka *et al.*, 2021).

5.3 Stepwise Plant Response to Available Pi

An adequate amount of Pi is essential for plant growth and survival in various environmental conditions. When the available Pi level is low, a signaling pathway leads to a change in root system architecture to enhance Pi foraging from topsoil. This involves cessation in primary root growth and initiation of lateral roots appearance (Ham *et al.*, 2018). These are accompanied by the release of Pi from immobilized soil compounds through exudation of organic acids, like malate, citrate and gluconate, as well as secretion of several enzymes including nucleases and APases that work together synergistically in the root rhizosphere (Plaxton and Tran, 2011; Malboobi *et al.*, 2012). Additionally, induced expression of high-affinity Pi transporters helps the efficient Pi acquisition (Amtmann *et al.*, 2005; Morcuende *et al.*, 2007; Peret *et al.*, 2011; Plaxton and Tran, 2011; Lohrasebi *et al.*, 2013; Zhang *et al.*, 2014; Scheible and Rojas-Triana, 2015). Among these, the upregulation of APases is believed to be the primary means for the remobilization, recycling, and scavenging of Pi from both intracellular and extracellular resources.

Within the plant cells, reprogramming of biochemical pathways includes upregulation of Pi- and adenylate-independent 'bypass' enzymes of central metabolism changes in the allocation of Pi between cell compartments facilitated by the transporters, Pi recycling from compounds like rRNA and organellar DNA, replacement of membrane phospholipids with galactolipids and sulfolipids, and Pi remobilization from older leaves to younger organs (Nussaume *et al.*, 2010; Plaxton and Tran, 2011; Siebers *et al.*, 2015; Dissanayaka *et al.*, 2018). It is already shown that Pi scavenging from nucleic acid pools occurs in two steps initiated by RNases, such as the RNase T2 family. RNases T2 catabolizes RNA via a 2′,3′-cyclic nucleotide monophosphate intermediate (cNMP) which is turned into nucleotide monophosphate (NMP) by a cyclic nucleotide phosphodiesterase. Finally, the released nucleotides then act as a substrate for APases (Abel *et al.*, 2000; Hillwig *et al.*, 2011).

Interestingly, we have found that in a long-term, severe Pi-starvation condition, a *trans*-spliced *APase* mRNA is accumulated that presumably releases Pi from DNA directly. This APase is translated via a frameshift at the border of sequences encoding zinc finger and APase catalytic domains (Lohrasebi *et al.*, 2013). Transient expression of an mRNA transcribed from a recombinant DNA sequence carrying these domains triggered apoptosis of leaf tissue up to the petioles of the injected tobacco or lettuce leaves (Malboobi and Samaian, unpublished data). It is assumed that this is the last attempt to remobilize Pi from its genome for extending the survival of plants. However, due to the high risk for cell life, it is accompanied by two stringent controlling checkpoints, *trans*-splicing and frameshifting, allowed only when needed.

5.4 APases Types and Functions

As described above, hydrolysis of Pi esters by APases is indeed a critical process in the energy metabolism and metabolic regulation of plant cells (Duff *et al.*, 1994). The possible substrates include many phosphorylated sugars, lipids, proteins, and nucleic acids. The roles of APases in the release, mobilization, and recycling of Pi are clear now (Tran *et al.*, 2010b; Araujo and Vihko, 2013). By a survey in the *Arabidopsis thaliana* genome, Li and colleagues (2002) identified over 50 putative APases including 10 vegetative storage protein type APases, four phosphatidic APases, 29 purple APase, and one histidine APases. The number has been changed to 58 annotated genes (Feizi *et al.*, Chapter 4) coding for APases which are categorized into five distinct families, purple acid phosphatase (29 genes), haloacid dehalogenase (HAD)-related acid phosphatase (12 genes), phospholipid phosphatase (12 genes), histidine acid phosphatase (3 genes) and survival protein E (SurE) acid phosphatase (2 genes). As described, due to the indispensable roles of Pi in living organisms, some members of unrelated gene families may acquire APases function to broaden the possible substrates. For example, Pi starvation induces the secretion of HAD-related APases in *A. thaliana*, which participate in the utilization of extracellular Po (Du *et al.*, 2021). Five families of APases have been described.

5.4.1 Purple Acid Phosphatase (PAP) Family

Purple acid phosphatase (PAPs; EC 3.1.3.2) are members of the metallo-phosphoesterase family of binuclear metal-containing acid hydrolases, have been identified in animals, plants, and some bacterial species (Schenk et al., 2013; Olczak et al., 2003). This type of APases comprises the largest group of plant APases. Most PAPs catalyze the hydrolysis of a broad range of phosphoric acid mono- or diesters and anhydrides, such as ATP, phosphoenolpyruvate (PEP), and sugar esters, at acidic or neutral pH (Cox et al., 2007). According to the literature, overexpression of PAPs in transgenic plants indicate possible applications for improving crop Pi acquisition efficiency (Tran et al., 2010a; Wang and Liu, 2018; Feder et al., 2020). Furthermore, vacuolar PAPs present a key role in Pi remobilizing and scavenging from dispensable intracellular Pi monoesters and anhydrides.

A common feature of PAPs is their induction by low Pi in plants and their role in Pi scavenging and recycling. For example, *AtPAP12* secreted by Pi-deficient *A. thaliana* suspension cells and seedlings was highly active against several Pi ester substrates over a broad range of pH range, making it ideally suited for scavenging Pi from the Po pools prevalent in many soils (Tran et al., 2010b). Yet, current knowledge suggests other functions for some plant PAPs as well. For example, both *AtPAP17* and *AtPAP26* have alkaline peroxidase activity metabolizing reactive oxygen species (del Pozo et al., 1999; Veljanovski et al., 2006). Increased expressions of PAP genes have also been reported in response to other environmental conditions including heat stress (Reddy et al., 2017), bacterial or fungal infections (Jakobek and Lindgren, 2002; Feng et al., 2003; Ravichandran et al., 2013; Zamani et al., 2014), high NaCl (Liao et al., 2003; Abbasi-vine et al., 2021), oxidative stresses (del Pozo et al., 1999; Li et al., 2008), and senescence (Robinson et al., 2012a, Gao et al., 2017). Several PAPs are predominantly expressed in flowers, suggesting their potential function in reproduction and seed development (Zhu et al., 2005; Bhadouria et al., 2017). Moreover, an extracellular PAP was shown to be involved in the regulation of cell wall biosynthesis by activation of β-glucan synthases (Kaida et al., 2009). *AtPAP9* has a potential role in the plasma membrane and cell wall adhesion for the *N*-terminal domain of a high molecular weight PAP protein (Zamani et al., 2014). Also, the expression of some PAPs is required for nodule formation and nitrogen fixation (Wang et al., 2015; Wang et al., 2020; Maryanto et al., 2021).

5.4.2 Haloacid Dehalogenase (HAD)-Related Acid Phosphatase (HRP) Family

The presence of HAD superfamily is ubiquitous in all eukaryotes (Burroughs et al., 2006). The HAD enzymes catalyze carbon or phosphoryl group transfer reactions on a diverse range of substrates in acidic pH. The majority of HAD proteins are found to show phosphatases activities, such as P-type ATPases, dehalogenases, sugar phosphomutases, phosphonatases, and phosphotransferases so we named them HAD-related phosphatase (HRP) family (Du et al., 2021; Feizi et al., Chapter 4).

All proteins of the HAD superfamily contain an α/β-Rossmannoid core domain (parallel β sheets in $\alpha/\beta/\alpha$ units), with the active site formed by four loops containing three conserved amino acid motifs, DxD, GDxxxD, or GDxxxxD. A smaller domain with a dynamic hinge-like structure linked to the core domain acts as a cap over it. This domain is responsible for substrate diversification within the family. As a result, substrate recognition is associated with the cap residues, while catalytic activity is modulated by the residues located deep inside the core cleft (Zamani Amirzakaria et al., 2020; Du et al., 2021).

Several members of the HRP family are transcriptionally upregulated in response to Pi deficiency. For instance, in the Arabidopsis, the *AtPPsPase1* (*HRP2*) gene is highly activated in Pi starvation and encodes a pyrophosphatase, suggesting that the function *AtPPsPase1* gene is to liberate Pi from pyrophosphate (PPi; May et al., 2012). Recombinant OsHAD1 also removes Pi from phosphorylated serine and sodium phytate (Pandey et al., 2017). By searching genomic sequences, 41 and 40 HAD genes have been identified in rice and *A. thaliana*, respectively. At least, the expression levels of 17 HAD genes are induced by Pi starvation in shoots or roots. Some of these annotated as HRP proteins are predicted to be involved in intracellular or extracellular Po recycling under low Pi in plants (Du et al., 2021). Several studies have indicated their accumulation in response to herbivore or insect attacks during flower development, Pi starvation, jasmonate induction, and glycerol metabolism (Caparrós-Martín *et al.*, 2007). Shewanella-like protein phosphatases 1 and 2 (SLP1 and SLP2) are localized to the chloroplast and mitochondria, respectively. Originally uncovered through bioinformatics, these enzymes have been proven to be *bona fide* protein serine/threonine phosphatases that are initially found in bacteria while displaying limited distribution across eukaryotes. They are remarkably conserved in several plant species suggesting fundamental roles in chloroplasts and mitochondria (Johnson *et al.*, 2020).

Vegetative storage proteins (VSPs) are also classified as APases of the HAD superfamily based on sequence motif analysis (Chen *et al.*, 2012). These proteins have been found in a variety of plant species. Although 10 VSP genes in the *A. thaliana* genome have been annotated based on the existence of common DXDXT motifs, the encoded products of only three of these genes, *AtVSP1* (AT5G24780), *AtVSP2* (AT5G24770), and *AtVSP3* (AT4G29260) have been molecularly and biochemically characterized (Sun *et al.*, 2018). *AtVSP 1* and *2* are differentially induced by methyl jasmonate, wounding, sugars, light, and Pi starvation. *AtVSP2* also has insecticidal activity, but whether it is involved in plant adaptation to Pi deficiency is not known. *AtVSP3* does not function in *A. thaliana* responses to Pi starvation and lacks insecticidal activity (Sun *et al.*, 2018). It must be noted that some vegetative storage proteins, as shown in the case of soybean, can accumulate to 40% of soluble proteins in leaves, yet contribute less than 1% to the extractable APase activity (Leelapon *et al.*, 2004).

5.4.3 Phospholipid Phosphatases (PLP) Family

Lipids are the major constituent of the plasma membrane accounting for over 30% of the cell total Po pool (Nakamura, 2018; Poirier *et al.*, 1991). In Pi-starved plants, membrane lipids scavenging and remobilizing Pi is catalyzed by a group of APases, earlier known as phosphatidic acid phosphatases (EC 3.1.3.4). These enzymes were later renamed phospholipid phosphatase (PLP) to avoid confusion in classification (Feizi *et al.*, Chapter 4). PLPs are evolutionarily conserved enzymes sharing the same motifs. Members of this family dephosphorylate phosphatidic acid to yield diacylglycerol (DAG) and Pi. DAG is a precursor for galactolipids, a primary component of photosynthetic membranes (Nakamura et al., 2007). In plants, phosphatidic acid is both a metabolic precursor for all glycerolipids and a key signaling lipid that regulates numerous reactions involved in developmental and physiological processes, particularly in response to environmental stresses (Dubots et al., 2012). From another point of view, PLP has a major role in lipid homeostasis by controlling the cellular levels of its substrates (Carman and Han, 2019).

A. thaliana has two types of PLPs, a membrane-bound type named lipid-Pi phosphatase with nine members and a soluble type termed phosphatidate phosphohydrolase with two members (Yunus et al., 2015). One of the former types was isolated as a radiation stress-inducible isoform and another one is a negative regulator of ABA signaling (Nakamura and Ohta, 2010). Two mutants of the latter type, *pah1*, and *pah2*, showed flower developmental defects, suggesting the roles of PLPs in flower development (Nakamura et al., 2014).

5.4.4 Histidine Acid Phosphatase (HAP) Family

A commercial enzyme, named "phytase" catalyzes the hydrolysis of phytate carrying six Pi groups, and is widely used as an animal feed additive (Kumar et al., 2012). Most bacterial, fungal, and plant phytases belong to histidine acid phosphatase (HAP; EC 3.1.3.2) enzymes which are further classified as 3-phytase (EC 3.1.3.8) or 6-phytase (EC 3.1.3.26) depending on their high activity for the first specific position to initiate the hydrolysis of phytate.

The HAP family contains α/β Rossmannoid folding which uses a histidine residue as a nucleophile during the process of the sequential Pi group removal from the substrate. At the sequence level, the members of the histidine APase family are characterized by the general signature motif RHGXRXP, C-terminal "HD," and eight cysteine residues in its sequence (Araujo and Vihko, 2013). In plants, HAPs with phytase activity has been known in *A. thaliana* and rice, particularly during Pi limitation (Mullaney and Ullah, 1998; Li et al., 2011; Cangussu et al., 2018).

It is noteworthy that the phytase activity has been observed in PAP members in plants too. Two of them with experimental data are *AtPAP15* (NP_187369) (Zhang *et al.*, 2016) and *G. max GmPhy* (AF272346) (Hegeman and Grabau, 2001). Xiao *et al.* (2006) found a PAPI member in *M. truncatula*, named *MtPHY1* (AAX20028), expressed in the roots during growth under low Pi conditions. They have also shown that the transgenic *A. thaliana* plants expressing *MtPHY1* exhibit significantly increased capacity for Pi acquisition from phytate and, thus, higher plant growth (Xiao *et al.*, 2005).

5.4.5 SurE-Related Acid Phosphatase (SAP) Family

As a small family of plant APases with sequences similar to the well-known prokaryotic SurE family (Mura *et al.*, 2003), it was designated as SurE acid phosphatase (SAP; Feizi *et al.*, Chapter 4). Apparently, this family has not expanded as much in plant evolution such that only a pair of such sequences exist in every plant species.

There is no experimental evidence for plant SAPs function; however, based on the structural and functional analysis, prokaryotic SAP enzymes displayed nucleotidase and exopolyphosphatase and may be involved in the stress response (Mura *et al.*, 2003; Iwasaki and Miki, 2007).

5.5 Multiple Isoforms and Broad Substrates Range of APases

Plants secrete an enormous variety of hydrolytic enzymes to uptake nutrients from different natural environments. The study of these processes reveals a complex network of gene expression regulations that control not only the synthesis but also the activities and secretions of enzymes in response to environmental factors. Experimentally, APases are among the most proficient natural catalysts known to date. Interestingly, a large number of these enzymes are promiscuous catalysts that exhibit phosphatase and sulfatase activities in the same active site (Pabis *et al.*, 2016) Besides, they catalyze the hydrolysis of a wide range of substrates with varying degrees of efficiency rather than a specific substrate like most enzymes (Pabis *et al.*, 2016). The concentration of soluble

Pi in the soil is low (0.1–10 µM) (Secco et al., 2017) in which organic substrates such as phytates, PEP, phospholipids, nucleotides, organic polyphosphate, etc. offer alternative sources of Pi and account for 30–90% of the soil P pool. Phytate serves a range of biological functions in plants, most notably as a seed Pi storage and energy source molecule (Feder et al., 2020). PEP is an essential precursor in plants for the synthesis of chorismate in the shikimate pathway, as a major branch point between central and specialized plant metabolism, particularly for plant glycolysis and respiration. Consequently, plants have evolved several enzymes that hydrolyze Pi ester bonds in phytate and PEP (Feder et al., 2020).

Besides, the biological functions of PAPs are diverse and the assignment of specific roles is complicated by the occurrence of multiple isoforms of these enzymes (Tran et al., 2010a and b; Robinson et al., 2012a and b; Tian and Liao, 2015). Importantly, in the context of the role of plant PAPs in P acquisition, for example, A. thaliana, soybean, chickpea, and tobacco can hydrolyze phytate. rkbPAP a PAP from red kidney bean is the most extensively studied plant PAP with respect to enzymatic properties (Schenk et al., 2013; Feder et al., 2020). AtPAP15 is another phytase which effectively involved during seed and pollen germination by mobilizing Pi from stored phytate.

The emerging pictures indicate that different PAP isoforms may have different functions and preferred substrates. Some PAP isoforms act as phytases as identified in *Nicotiana tabacum* (tobacco), *Oryza sativa* (rice), *Cicer arietnum* (chickpea), *Glycine max* (soybean), and *A. thaliana* (Kaida et al., 2009; Kuang et al., 2009; Bhadouria et al., 2017; Wang et al., 2011). Other PAPs prefer PEP as their substrate, including two PAP isoforms from *A. thaliana*, that is, *AtPAP12* and *AtPAP26* (Tran et al., 2010b; Sabet et al., 2018; Farhadi et al., 2020; Abbasi-Vineh et al., 2021), while others are known to be ATPases, like *AtPAP10*, a PAP from sweet potato (*IbPAP1*) and *rkbPAP* (Beck et al., 1986; Cashikar et al., 1997). Proteins, such as AtPAP15 (Kuang et al., 2009), GmPAP4 (Kong et al., 2014), TapAPhyb1 (Dionisio et al., 2011), and CaPAP7 (Bhadouria et al., 2017) only catalyze the decomposition of phytic acid and possess substrate specificity, whereas most PAP proteins can hydrolyze ATP, PEP, phosphorylated proteins, and other types of Pi monoesters (Table 5.1).

Table 5.1 A summary of Arabidopsis APases with experimentally known substrates and subcellular localizations

Gene/protein name	Subcellular locations in cell	Organ	Substrate and function	Reference
AT1G73010/HRP2	Nucleus	Senescent leaf	Cleavage of pyrophosphate	(May et al., 2012)
AT1G17710/HRP3	Nucleus	Senescent leaf	Phosphoethanolamin	(May et al., 2012)
AT5G24770/HRP10	Chloroplast, cytosolic ribosome, plant-type vacuole	Flower	4-Methylumbelliferyl phosphate	(Chen et al., 2012)
AT2G01180/PLP2	Chloroplast, integral component of plasma membrane, plasma membrane	Senescent leaf	Phosphatidate	(Pierrugues et al., 2001)
AT3G50920/PLP7	Chloroplast/intracellular membrane-bounded organelle	Young leaf	1,2-Diacyl-sn-glycerol-3-phosphate	(Nakamura et al., 2007)
AT3G58490/PLP8	Endoplasmic reticulum membrane	Flower	Sphingosine phosphate	(Nakagawa et al., 2012)
AT5G03080/PLP10	Chloroplast/integral component of endoplasmic reticulum membrane	Flower	Lipid biosynthetic process	(Cantagrel & Lefeber, 2011), and Sequence Homology
AT3G54020/PLP12	Golgi membrane, endoplasmic reticulum membrane, plasma membrane	Flower	Ceramide biosynthetic process	(Mina et al., 2010)

(Continued)

Table 5.1 (Continued)

Gene/protein name	Subcellular locations in cell	Organ	Substrate and function	Reference
AT2G16430/PAP10	Cell wall, extracellular region, plasmodesma	Seed germination	Phosphoserin, ATP, Pi scavenging	(Wang et al., 2011)
AT2G27190/PAP12	Extracellular region	Senescent leaf	PEP complex component	(Tran et al., 2010)
AT4G36350/PAP25	Cell wall, extracellular region	Young flower	Phosphothreonine, phosphoserine, and phosphotyrosine	(Del Vecchio et al., 2014)
AT5G34850/PAP26	Extracellular region, plant-type vacuole, plastid, secretory vesicle, vacuole	Flower	PEP, Phenyl P, Inorganic pyrophosphate, NADP	(Tran et al., 2010; Veljanovski et al., 2006)
AT3G07130/ PAP15	Extracellular region	Flower	Na-pyrophosphate, tetrasodium pyrophosphate, PEP, phytate, modulate ascorbate levels by controlling the input of myoinositol into this branch of ascorbate biosynthesis	(Kuang et al., 2009; Zhang et al., 2015)

Gene/protein name	Subcellular locations in cell	Organ	Substrate and function	Reference
AT4G13700/PAP23	Extracellular region	Flower	dATP, O-phosphothreonine	(Zhu et al., 2005)
AT1G13900/PAP2	Golgi apparatus, chloroplast extracellular region, intracellular mitochondrial	Flower	Sugar phosphate, regulation of plant carbon metabolism, facilitates the import of selected proteins into chloroplasts	(Sun et al., 2012; Zhang et al., 2016)
AT5G50400/PAP27	Chloroplast	Flower	GDP L galus	(Wolucka & Van Montagu, 2007)
AT3G20500/PAP18	Vacuole, apoplast	-	Pi scavenging	Zamani et al., 2012
AT2G03450/PAP9	Plasma membrane and cell wall	Stipule and vascular tissue	A potential role in plasma membrane and cell wall adhesion	Zamani et al., 2014, Arae et al., 2022
AT3G17790/PAP17	Vacuole, extracellular matrix	Leaf, root	Pi scavenging and metabolizing reactive oxygen species, broad APase substrate selectivity	O'Gallagher, 2022 del Pozo et al., 1999

Root-associated PAPs are well known to play a role in the utilization of extracellular Po sources, such as ATP, phytate, and dNTPs (Liang et al., 2010; 2012; Wang et al., 2011; 2014; Robinson et al., 2012b; Liu et al., 2018; Lu et al., 2016; Gao et al., 2017; Mehra et al., 2017; Wu et al., 2018). For example, *AtPAP10/12/26* are suggested to participate in the hydrolysis of extracellular DNA and ADP in *A. thaliana* (Wang et al., 2011; 2014). Similarly, the functions of *PvPAP3* in bean and *OsPAP10a/21b/26/10c* in rice have been suggested to mediate extracellular ATP utilization (Liang et al., 2010; Tian et al., 2012; Lu et al., 2016; Gao et al., 2017; Mehra et al., 2017). In addition to extracellular ATP utilization, plant PAP members have also been suggested to participate in extracellular dNTP hydrolysis, including *PvPAP1/3* from common bean, *SgPAP7/10/26* from Stylo (*Stylosanthes* spp.), and *GmPAP1*-like from soybean (Liang et al., 2012; Liu et al., 2016; Wu et al., 2018). Recently, some PAP members exhibiting phytase activity have been suggested to mediate extracellular phytate utilization, including *SgPAP23* from Stylo, *OsPHY1* from rice, *MtPHY1* from Medicago (*Medicago truncatula*), and *GmPAP4* and *GmPAP14* from soybean (Ma et al., 2009; Li R. J. et al., 2012; Kong et al., 2014; Liu et al., 2018), suggesting diverse functions of PAP members in Pi scavenging and recycling in plants. A pioneering study on PAP function in extracellular ATP utilization has been conducted in common bean (*Phaseolus vulgaris*) hairy roots. A summary of known preferred substrates of *A. thaliana* APases present in subcellular locations is presented in Table 5.1.

5.6 Tissue-Specific Expression of APases

Plant APases have been studied in various tissues of plant species. Several APases were purified and biochemically characterized from seeds (Tagad et al., 2018), roots (Coello et al., 2002), tubers (Durmus et al., 1999), leaves (Huang et al., 2012), bulbs (Guo et al., 1997), and fruits (Turner et al., 2001). As well, two root-associated APase isozymes, GmPAP1-like and GmPAP21, have been found by proteomic analysis of cell wall proteins (Wu et al., 2018) that were shown to be involved in the adaptation of soybean roots to Pi starvation (Li et al., 2017; Wu et al., 2018). Similarly, NtPAP12 and OsPAP21*b* were reported to affect cell wall biosynthesis and root development (Kaida et al., 2009; Mehra et al., 2017).

Most characterized secreted APases belong to the PAP family that carry a signal peptide guiding them through the cell secretory pathways. Interestingly, the signal peptides of secreted PAPs from *A. thaliana*, soybean, onion, and tomato are all processed at the same site, beginning after an invariant arginine residue (Del Vecchio *et al.*, 2014). The alignment of the *N*-terminal amino acid sequences revealed highly conserved amino acid residues at the 6-, 5-, and 3-positions (Tran *et al.*, 2010a).

With the aid of genomic and transcriptomic data availability, annotations and expression patterns of a variety of PAPs have been documented. For example, Pi deficiency leads to upregulation of PAP members in rice (10 out of 26;), maize (11 out of 33), physic nut (20 out of 25), *A. thaliana* (11 out of 29), soybean (23 out of 35), and chickpea (12 out of 25) (Del Pozo *et al.*, 1999; Haran *et al.*, 2000; Zhang *et al.*, 2011; Li *et al.*, 2012; Wang *et al.*, 2014; González-Muñoz *et al.*, 2015; Bhadouria *et al.*, 2017; Venkidasamy *et al.*, 2019). It is assumed that the upregulation of transcription of PAPs reflects increases in intracellular and extracellular APase activities in these species (Zimmermann *et al.*, 2004; Liang *et al.*, 2010; Chiou and Lin, 2011).

To find tissue-specific expression profiles of APases, Zhu *et al.* (2005) compared the transcript levels of 28 *A. thaliana* PAP (*AtPAP*) genes in five *A. thaliana* organs. Although the expression patterns of 28 *AtPAP* members differed in vegetative organs, all of them were transcribed in flower. To find out the roles of *AtPAP* genes in flower development, further expression and functional analyses were conducted using *AtPAP23*. Histochemical staining of transgenic plants carrying *AtPAP23* promoter fused to β-glucuronidase (GUS) gene revealed that its transcription was very high in flower apical meristems, but not in petals and anther filaments in fully developed flowers (Zhu *et al.*, 2005).

To identify the tissue-specific expression of *GmPAP* genes in soybean, the expression patterns of 35 *GmPAP* genes were analyzed in six tissues. Once again the results showed that flowers possessed the largest number of expressed *GmPAP* genes, followed by seeds and roots (six, four, and three genes, respectively) (Li *et al.*, 2012). Similarly, RNAseq analysis in maize plants reveals PAP transcripts accumulation differs in various plant tissues at multiple stages of plant development. In seedlings, there is a trend toward the greater accumulation of *PAP* transcripts in the roots than in the shoot. In older vegetative stages, however, transcripts levels increase in the aerial parts of the plant, with the highest levels in mature leaves (González-Muñoz *et al.*, 2015).

Genome-wide analysis of *APase* gene structure and expression in 10 vegetable species plants including three *Brassicaceae* (*A. thaliana*, *Brassica oleracea*, and *B. rapa*), five Solanaceae (*Solanum lycopersicum*, *S. pennellii*, *S. tuberosum*, *S. melongena*, and *Capsicum annuum*), three *Cucurbitaceae* (*Cucumis sativus*, *C. melo*, and *Citrullus lanatus*), and one basal angiosperm (*Amborella trichopoda*), exhibited tissue-specific expression patterns for PAP genes. In these comparisons, most genes exhibited similar tissue-specific expression patterns among taxonomic categories (Xie and Shang, 2018). However, some PAPs from different taxonomies exhibited more diverse expression patterns. Evolutionary or developmental reasons as well as differences in sampling times and data collection methods must be considered for the cause of the inconsistencies.

With genome-wide analysis of Moso Bamboo (*Phyllostachys edulis*), Zhou *et al.* (2021) identified 17 *PePAP* genes which showed higher expression in roots and stems than that in leaves. Yet, *PePAP1*, *PePAP2*, *PePAP11*, and *PePAP14* were highly expressed in all examined organs (Zhou *et al.*, 2021). These data infer that some APases accumulated like typical housekeeping proteins, consistent with roles in Pi acquisition and utilization in plants. Others are expressed more flexibly during different growth stages and may help to ensure Pi homeostasis in any conditions or any developmental stages (Xie and Shang, 2018).

The isoforms of AtPAP26 are strongly upregulated on root surfaces and in cell walls of Pi-starved seedlings (Farhadi *et al.*, 2020; Abbasi-Vineh *et al.*, 2021). The ortholog of AtPAP26 in rice (OsPAP26) is also upregulated during Pi deprivation and senescence and may thus fulfill similar crucial roles in Pi metabolism. There are several pieces of evidence indicating the regulation occurring at the posttranscriptional and posttranslational levels affect the subcellular and extracellular compartments localization and substrate range (Tian and Liao, 2015). For example, differentially glycosylated forms of AtPAP26-S1 and AtPAP26-S2 make them vacuolar and secreted in Arabidopsis, respectively (Tran et al., 2010b). Furthermore, purified AtPAP26-S1 and AtPAP26-S2 exhibited different substrate specificities which strongly suggests that differential glycosylation influences PAP kinetic properties (Tran et al., 2010b). Additionally, a role for *N*-glycosylation in PAP secretion has been proposed as shown for PAPs from *Lupinus luteus* and KbPAP from beans (Olczak and Olczak, 2007).

Protein phosphorylation is often another critical common regulatory modification (Tian and Liao, 2015). Similarly, 36 out of 38 GmPAP members of soybean were predicted to exhibit more than one glycosylation site. Moreover, it has been suggested that the enzymatic properties of plant PAPs could be affected by their glycosylation (Navazio et al., 2002; Olczak and Olczak, 2007; Tran et al., 2010b). Therefore, it is believable that posttranslational modifications of APases may influence their targeting and/or kinetic properties.

5.7 Responsiveness of APases to Pi Status

As an important mechanism, the increased APase activity has been correlated with induced gene expression of APase in several plant species, including *Brassica nigra* (black mustard), *Lycopersicon esculentum* (tomato), and also *A. thaliana* suspension cells and seedlings as a model plant (Duff et al., 1994.; Tran et al., 2010b). In one study, the expression patterns of 29 *A. thaliana AtPAPs* were revealed together. In Pi deprivation, gene transcription levels of *AtPAP11* and *AtPAP12* were induced and increased, respectively (Li et al., 2002). In Hammond et al. (2003) study, the expression patterns for an array containing 8100 *A. thaliana* genes were analyzed under Pi deprivation (0.01 mM) or provision (1 mM Pi) in hydroponic plant culture. Their results showed that *AtPAP1, AtPAP5, AtPAP6, AtPAP7, AtPAP10, AtPAP12, AtPAP14, AtPAP16, AtPAP17, AtPAP22, AtPAP21*, and *AtPAP23* genes were highly inducible in the leaves Pi starved as compared to the fed *A. thaliana* seedlings. Among them, *AtPAP5, AtPAP14*, and *AtPAP17* genes were reported to be highly inducible (Hammond et al., 2003).

The possible changes in 22,810 *A. thaliana* genes were investigated in medium supplemented with either 500 µM or 5 mM Pi in the short-term (3, 6, and 12 hours), medium-term (1 and 2 days), and long-term 14-day series treatments. Among 42 APase genes in this array, *AtPAP1*, *AtPAP5*, *AtPAP14*, *AtPAP22*, and *AtPAP23* genes were introduced as Pi-inducible genes in leaf tissue during long-term stress while *AtPAP14* and *AtPAP17* genes were also introduced as highly induced genes in the root (Misson et al., 2005). Morcuende et al. (2007) studied the expression of *A. thaliana* genes under 0.2 mM and 3 mM Pi status conditions. They showed that the expression of APases, as well as nucleases, increased under Pi stress conditions. The ATH1 array used by this group carries 47 *APase* genes, 27 of which were PAP family members. They showed the expression of 11 *PAP* genes and *HRP2* (At1g17710) and *HRP3* (At1g73010) increases specifically in response to Pi stress conditions. In another study, global gene expression patterning was demonstrated by *A. thaliana* microarrays comprising 21,500 genes in which the influence of sucrose and Pi concentrations individually and together on gene regulation was investigated. Consequently, 40 Pi-inducible genes with twice or higher expression levels, including *PAP17* and *HRP2* genes, were identified (Muller et al., 2007).

To examine the link between transcriptional regulation of maize *ZmPAP* genes and the Pi deprivation response, González-Muñoz et al. (2015) generated root and leaf transcriptomes of young maize seedlings grown in Pi-sufficient (1 mM) and Pi-limiting (10 µM) conditions and quantified *ZmPAP* transcripts by RNAseq technique. Mapping of sequencing reads to maize PAP gene models revealed a broad trend toward greater transcript accumulation under P limitation. In comparison to the fed plants, 11 *ZmPAP* transcripts accumulated to significantly high levels under Pi deprivation. Similar to *A. thaliana*, transcripts of *ZmPAP26* showed no significant difference in the level of accumulation between the treatments, although its level of expression was relatively high.

Zhang et al. (2011) identified 26 putative *OsPAP* genes by genome-wide analysis of rice out of which 25 possess sets of metal-ligating residues typical of known PAPs. They detected transcripts of 21 *OsPAP* genes in roots or leaves of rice seedlings. The transcripts levels of 10 genes were upregulated by Pi deprivations and increased activities were detected for both intracellular and secretory APases in rice roots.

The effects of Pi deficiency on the APase activity and growth in two wheat cultivars (*Triticum aestivum* L.) were studied by Ciereszko *et al.* (2011a). Pi deficiency increased the activity of extracellular and intracellular APases in comparison to Pi-sufficient plants. As a result, Pi starvation led to reduced shoot and root mass up to 8–11% of the control plants. In addition, the ratio of root/shoot fresh weight increased (2–3 times compared to control), and shoot height decreased to about 50–60% of the control in the starved plants after two to three weeks of culture. Similar data were reported for barley subjected to moderate Pi deficiency (Ciereszko *et al.*, 2011b).

In a recent report, it is shown that the expression levels of *PePAP10*, *PePAP12*, and *PePAP16* in the roots of Moso Bamboo (*Phyllostachys edulis*) plants treated with low Pi were significantly increased, which is consistent with the expression trend of APase activity in other plants (Zhou *et al.*, 2021).

5.8 Roles of APases in Pi Homeostasis

Pi homeostasis is defined as "the maintenance of cytoplasmic Pi levels irrespective of nutritional Pi status" that is between 2.5 to 10 mM (Rebeille *et al.*, 1984; Dissanayaka *et al.*, 2021). Since plants are habitually exposed to the limitation of free Pi in soil, a series of morphological and physiological adaptation mechanisms have evolved to cope with low Pi and other environmental conditions. Briefly, a series of alterations in root architecture, organic acid metabolism enhancement, APase secretion allows promoting efficient Pi acquisition from soil (Wang and Liu, 2018; Zhou *et al.*, 2021). Besides, low Pi induces intracellular APases activity involved in the remobilization and recycling of Pi from internal reservoirs to keep Pi homeostasis in the cytoplasm (Dissanayaka *et al.*, 2021). These adaptive mechanisms are described in detail below.

Soil Po compounds are composed of about 20–50% of phytates, 10% of nucleic acids, 1–5% phospholipids, trace amounts of phosphoproteins, and 30–50% of others. In the past two decades, secreted APases have been purified and biochemically characterized from a variety of plant species including tomato, tobacco, common bean, soybean, and *A. thaliana* (Tian and Liao, 2015) that solubilize Pi-containing soil compounds. Several *A. thaliana* secreted APases, including AtPAP10, AtPAP12, AtPAP25, and AtPAP26, have been characterized in detail (Tian and Liao, 2015; Wang and Liu, 2018). AtPAP12 and AtPAP26 are two predominant isozymes secreted into the culture media or located on shoot cell walls during Pi starvation of *A. thaliana* suspension cells. Knockout of *AtPAP12* or *AtPAP26* resulted in more than 70% reductions of root-secreted and shoot cell wall APase activity assays demonstrated that AtPAP12 and AtPAP26 account for most of the secreted APase activities of *A. thaliana* under Pi-starvation conditions (Tran *et al.*, 2010b; Robinson *et al.*, 2012b; Del Vecchio *et al.*, 2014).

Another secreted APase of *A. thaliana* is AtPAP10 which probably exists in plants as a tetramer. The recombinant AtPAP10 protein has APase activity against a variety of substrates and has an optimal pH of ~5.0. Knockout of *AtPAP10* reduces ~40% of total root-associated APase activity. Rather than being released into the growth medium, AtPAP10 is predominantly associated with the root surface (Wang *et al.*, 2011). AtPAP25 is also a secreted APase and is also closely related to AtPAP10, AtPAP12, and AtPAP26 (Li *et al.*, 2002). AtPAP25 has been purified from the cell walls of *A. thaliana* suspension cells. Unlike AtPAP10, AtPAP12, and AtPAP26, AtPAP25 is exclusively synthesized under Pi-deficient conditions and has a very low Vmax against its known substrates (Del Vecchio *et al.*, 2014).

Within the cells, Pi redistribution between subcellular compartments allows maintenance of cytoplasmic homeostasis as well. For better clarification of the physiological roles of PAPs, it is also important to find out about their subcellular localization of expression. Using a variety of methods, such as immunolocalization, imaging of transformed cells expressing specific PAPs fused with marker proteins, and the purification from various subcellular fractions, the localizations of APases have been recognized to be cytoplasm, vacuole, plasma membrane, nucleus, cell wall, plastid, mitochondria, and apoplast, in addition to secretome (Tian and Liao, 2015). Vacuoles as a major storage pool of Pi in higher plants may contain up to 95% of the total Pi in the fed cells. Vacuolar Pi concentration is estimated to range from micromolar to millimolar depending on the available extracellular Pi concentrations as revealed by the ^{31}P-nuclear magnetic resonance (NMR) study (Foyer and Spencer C, 1986). Plant cells selectively distribute Pi between cytoplasmic (metabolic) and vacuolar (storage) pools;

assuming cytoplasmic Pi is maintained essentially in a certain range at the expense of large fluctuations in vacuolar Pi (Yang *et al.*, 2017; Dissanayaka *et al.*, 2021). In addition, APases of Pi-starved plant cells likely remobilize and recycle Pi from expendable intracellular Pi monoesters and anhydrides. This is accompanied by marked reductions in cytoplasmic Pi metabolites during extended Pi deprivation (Duff *et al.*, 1994). For instance, AtPAP26, a dual-targeted enzyme, remobilizes Pi from the vacuolar and senescent leaves (Robinson *et al.*, 2012a). Pi recycling from endogenous nucleic acid pools makes a crucial contribution to its utilization efficiency in Pi-starved plants. In Arabidopsis and maize, vacuolar rRNA is degraded in autophagy-like pathways by Pi starvation-inducible and senescence-inducible RNases followed by the activity of PAP enzymes (Bassham and MacIntosh, 2017; Yang *et al.*, 2017; Dissanayaka *et al.*, 2021).

A dual-targeted protein, AtPAP2, was documented to be targeted to both plastids and mitochondria via its *C*-terminal hydrophobic motif (Sun *et al.*, 2012). Furthermore, the analysis of several plant genomes has consistently revealed a single PAP gene encoding a protein having a *C*-terminal hydrophobic motif, which suggests a conserved function for the *C*-terminal hydrophobic motif in plants (Sun *et al.*, 2012). Similarly, PvPAP1 and PvPAP5 have each been localized to both the plasma membrane and nucleus (Liang *et al.*, 2012). A recent review by Wu *et al.* (2019) describes the identification of 14 AtPAPs in cell wall proteomes that function in Pi mobilization and even cell wall synthesis. The upregulation of intracellular APase activity is an important biochemical hallmark of plant response to Pi deprivation. Cell wall-associated AtPAP12 and AtPAP26 were hypothesized to recycle Pi from endogenous resources that may leak into the cell wall from the cytoplasm during P-deprivation or senescence (Robinson *et al.*, 2012a; Shane *et al.*, 2014; Wu *et al.*, 2019).

Another source for internal Pi is phospholipids as the most abundant class of lipids in cell membranes. PLPs are involved in phospholipids remodeling with alternative non-Pi lipids, particularly sulfo- and galactolipids in Pi-starved plants (Dissanayaka *et al.*, 2021). Furthermore, HRPs are upregulated under Pi deprivation in order to dephosphorylate cellular Po. Overexpression of *OsHAD1* in rice resulted in enhanced APase activity, biomass, and total and soluble Pi contents in Pi-deficient transgenic seedlings fed with phytate (Pandey *et al.*, 2017).

5.9 APases Responsive to Other Stresses

The expression levels of some APase-encoding genes are also largely influenced by other abiotic and biotic conditions, such as the lack of nutrients, high salt concentration, or pathogenic attacks (Williamson *et al.*, 1991; Beber *et al.*, 2000; Jakobek and Lindgren, 2002; Petters *et al.*, 2002; Stenzel *et al.*, 2003). Based on this concept, when Pi-fed *A. thaliana* plants were subjected to fungal infections, a remarkable reduction was observed for the three indicators related to Pi metabolism, total P level, Pi concentration, and APase activity (Lohrasebi *et al.*, 2013). In line with this, expression profiling of 58 *A. thaliana* APase-encoding genes after inoculation with *Alternaria brassicicola* showed that the rates of transcription of several *APase* genes were affected. As a result, total APases activity increased in the root and shoots of treated seedlings. Whether these are the consequences of competitive nutrient consumption in the hydroponic culture or the pathogenic interaction of fungus with the plant is still a valid question. Experimentally, it was found all fungal-induced genes, except for *AtHRP2* and *AtPLP7*, were affected by the addition of chitin as an elicitor. Also, chitin treatment led to the upregulation of four other genes, *AtPAP5*, *AtPAP8*, *AtHRP1*, and *AtHRP2* (Lohrasebi *et al.*, 2013). These discrepancies could be related to the dosage of applied chitin and/or complicity of fungal infection. Both reverse northern blot and RT-PCR methods revealed almost the same expression patterns for the induced genes (Tamaoki *et al.*, 2008). Genes coding for *AtPAP9*, *AtPAP13*, and *AtPLP7* in the root samples and *AtPAP7*, *AtPAP9*, *AtPAP11*, *AtPAP13*, and *AtPLP7* in the shoots were highly transcribed after fungal inoculation.

Analysis of the expression profiles of 58 *A. thaliana* APase-encoding genes showed that some of these genes respond to salinity, cold, and heat stresses regardless of the Pi content of the plant (Lohrasebi *et al.*, unpublished data; Kuang *et al.*, 2009). Abbasi-Vineh *et al.* (2021) showed the overexpression of *A. thaliana AtPAP17* and *AtPAP26* genes enhanced the expression level *of AtSOS1*, *AtSOS2*, *AtSOS3*, *AtHKT1*, *AtVPV1*, and *AtNHX1* genes, involved in the

K$^+$/Na$^+$ level that led to facilitating intracellular Na$^+$ homeostasis and reducing the ion-specific damages. In addition, they showed lower content of sodium accumulated in the overexpressing *AtPAP17* or *AtPAP26* lines while the activity of the catalase, guaiacol peroxidase, and ascorbate peroxidase increased as well (Abbasi-Vineh *et al.*, 2021).

Transcriptome analyses elucidated that the regulation of four *PAP* genes in the tea plant was also affected by Fe status (Yin *et al.*, 2019), suggesting they might participate in iron homeostasis. Different expression patterns suggest that the transcript levels of APase genes are regulated by distinct pathways. For example, *A. thaliana* vegetative storage proteins (VSPs) with APase activity were rapidly induced by wounding, jasmonate or insect feeding on leaves (Berger *et al.*, 1995; 2002, Stotz *et al.*, 2000; Reymond *et al.*, 2004). Among them, *VSP1* (At5g24780) and *VSP2* (At5g24770) genes exhibited different expression patterns in response to methyl jasmonate and Pi starvation while another VSP gene, At1g04040, responded to Pi starvation only. Taken together, these results illustrate that the expression regulation of APases is more complex than previously described.

5.10 Interplay between APases to Keep Pi Homeostasis

Gene overexpression and mutation phenotyping have provided an exceptional opportunity for understanding the functions and roles of APases in Pi homeostasis. Overexpression of several genes coding for APases have been exploited to generate transgenic crops with enhanced capability in releasing Pi and thus improved growth performance. For example, overexpression of *AtPAP2* accelerates the growth of rape, *Camelina sativa*, potato, *A. thaliana*, and some other plants (Sun *et al.*, 2018). Metabolite analysis shows that *AtPAP2* overexpressing lines contained higher levels of sugar and tricarboxylic acid cycle metabolites indicating that the increased carbon metabolism resulted in faster growth and higher yields (Sun *et al.*, 2018).

Similarly, transgenic *A. thaliana* overexpressing *AtPAP10*, *AtPAP12*, and *AtPAP26* growth rates were improved when plants were supplied with ADP and Fru-6-P (Wang *et al.*, 2011; 2014).

Transgenic rape (*Brassica napus*) expressing AtPAP26 showed a 1.3-fold increase in APase activity, 1.5 fold in free Pi content, and 1.9 fold in dry weight compared to non-transgenic plants at 1.2 mM Pi condition (Sabzalipoor et al., unpublished data). Overexpression of *AtPAP15* and *SgPAP23* (from *Stylosanthes guianensis*), which show high phytase activities, facilitates the utilization of phytate and significantly improves the growth of the transgenic plants (Wang et al., 2009; Liu et al., 2018). Transgenic soybean lines with overexpression of *AtPAP15* exhibit improved yields when grown on acidic soils (Wang et al., 2009). Other studies have also shown that by overexpressing the *AtPAP15* gene into soybean hairy roots, the activity of PAPs in the roots increased by 1.5 times. Consistently, overexpression of *AtPAP15* in soybean exhibits significant PAPs and phytase activity in leaves and root exudates so that the P content and the dry weight of the plants improved significantly (Wang et al., 2009). In rice, overexpression of *OsPAP10a*, *OsPAP10c* and *OsPAP21b* increased APase activity and Po degradation level (Tian et al., 2012; Lu et al., 2016; Mehra et al., 2017). The extracellular utilization of ATP was significantly enhanced in hairy roots of transgenic beans with overexpression of *PvPAP3* or *GmPAP1*-like (Liang et al., 2010; Wu et al., 2018). Transfer of soybean *GmPAP4* into Arabidopsis leads to reduced Pi deficiency symptoms and higher biomass than the wild-type plants (Wang and Liu, 2012). By the overexpression of *MtPAP1* plants in *A. thaliana*, the APase activity in the root rhizosphere significantly increased which caused high Pi and total P content in the plant and thus the higher yield than the control ones (Xiao et al., 2006). Studies have shown that using dNTP as the sole Pi source, the dry weight and total P content of kidney bean plants overexpressing *PvPAP3* are higher than the control ones (Tian et al., 2012). With ATP in the medium, the average fresh weight and P content of soybean hairy roots overexpressing *PvPAP3* were increased significantly higher than the control (Liang et al., 2010). Similarly, when incubating rice in the medium containing ATP as the sole P source, the Pi concentration in the overexpressed *OsPAP10a* plant solution reached to significantly higher level than that in the control plant medium (Tian et al., 2012). If ADP was used, the shoot and root biomass of Arabidopsis overexpressing *AtPAP10*, *AtPAP12*, and *AtPAP26* were improved compared to control plants (Wang et al., 2014). In addition, our recent research shows that heterologous expression of *AtPAP26* and Pi limitation leads to substantial production of chicoric acid in *Echinacea purpurea* transgenic hairy roots (Salmanzadeh *et al.*, 2020).

Besides listing utilized substrates by the plant APases, the above results suggest increased activities of APases through genetic modification could enhance Pi content and dry weight as indicators for Pi metabolism and biomass gain in plants (Deng *et al.*, 2020). However, in some other cases such as the *OsPAP10c* overexpressing plants, the growth rate was reduced both in the pot and in field studies (Lu *et al.*, 2016). Likewise, the overexpressing of *GmPAP1* and *GmPAP21* in soybean roots resulted in lower fresh weight than the control ones under sufficient Pi conditions (Wu *et al.*, 2018; Li *et al.*, 2017). These data imply that there must be a networking relationship among APases such that overexpression of one influences the regulation of the other genes.

The above hypothesis was further supported by the analysis APase knocked-out mutants. The availability of T-DNA insertional mutant (Pan *et al.*, 2003) and gene-specific silenced lines (Hilson *et al.*, 2004) are other means for functional analysis of APases. Three independent *A. thaliana* mutants defective in APases activity have already been characterized. *pho3* with reduced APase activity phenotype was found defective in Pi deficiency responses (Zakhleniuk *et al.*, 2001). Reduced APase activity on the root surface but not in the whole-cell extract of *pup1* indicated restriction of APase activities to certain locations (Trull and Deikman, 1998). Tomscha *et al.* (2004) have introduced an *A. thaliana* mutant, *pup3*, with a 25% to 49% reduction in APase activity, mainly related to PAP26 and PAP12 isozymes. In *A. thaliana*, AtPAP12 and AtPAP26 have been shown to be the predominant PAP isozymes that are secreted into the medium under Pi starvation (Tran *et al.*, 2010b; Ghahremani *et al.*, 2019). In 2010, Hurley and colleagues showed that an *A. thaliana* T-DNA knockout line of *AtPAP26* exhibits impaired growth under Pi deficiency. Mutations of *AtPAP12* and *AtPAP26* result in a significant reduction in the activity of secreted APases and hence in the ability to utilize extracellular Po (Robinson *et al.*, 2012b). In triple-knockout mutant *atpap12/atpap15/atpap26*, the total root-associated APase activity against *p*NPP, as a general substrate, was reduced to about 50% compared to the wild type under both Pi-sufficient and -deficient conditions (Zhang *et al.*, 2014). Despite highly specific expression pattern and the demonstrated biochemical function of the AtPAP23 protein product, RNAi (RNA interference), T-DNA knockout and overexpression lines of *the AtPAP23* gene have been reported indistinguishable from wild-type plants in the development of flower or other organs (Zhu *et al.*, 2005).

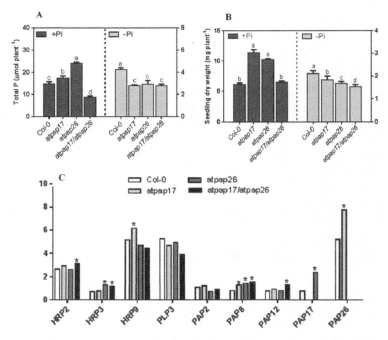

Figure 5.1 Mutational analysis of *A. thaliana* APases. P content (A), seedling dry weight (B) and expression patterns of some APases (C) in *A. thaliana atpap17*, *atpap26*, and *atpap17/atpap26* mutants compared to wild type (Col-O). Seven-day old seedlings were grown for 14 days with Pi (+P) or without it (−Pi). Values are the means ± SE of three biological replicates. Significant differences are indicated by different letters or asterisks ($P < 0.05$). Adapted from Farhadi *et al.*, 2020.

As a well-studied case, the isoforms of AtPAP26 are strongly upregulated on root surfaces and in cell walls of Pi-starved seedlings while its function is compensated by AtPAP17 in the mutant line (Farhadi *et al.*, 2020; Abbasi-Vineh *et al.*, 2021). P content and dry weight of *atpap26* or *atpap17* single-mutant lines were unexpectedly increased in Pi-sufficient conditions while these were reduced significantly in *atpap17/atpap26* double mutant line (Fig. 5.1; Farhadi *et al.*, 2020). Such that, P content of *atpap17/atpap26* double mutant line was 51 and 64% lower than that of either *atpap17* or *atpap26* single-mutant lines fed for Pi. In line with this, the lower expression of the *AtPAP26* gene is accompanied by increased expression of the *AtPAP17* gene under Pi sufficiency in the *atpap26* mutant and vice versa (Farhadi *et al.*, 2020).

A new approach for *APase* gene clustering was proposed by Sobhe Bidari *et al.*, (2008). According to this method, 58 Arabidopsis *APases* genes were clustered based on data from quantitative RT-PCR in different Pi concentrations and growth time courses. The patterns of gene expression were reconstructed by K-means and FCM methods and, then, new features are defined for the genes by calculating Pearson correlation between new vectors for genes with similar expression patterns. As a result, *APase* genes were clustered into five groups in the roots and two groups in the shoots according to their time-series data sets (Sobhe Bidari *et al.*, 2008; Lohrasebi *et al.*, 2012).

Putting together the overexpression and mutant data while considering the expression patterns of APase-encoding genes, it is plausible that the maintenance of Pi homeostasis is governed by complex networking among these genes mainly regulated at the transcriptional level.

5.11 Concluding Remarks

Several APases participate in the maintaining of Pi homeostasis through releasing, remobilizing, and recycling of Pi in the right place and time. Figure 5.2 summarizes the experimental data for *A. thaliana* APases compiled by a survey in current literature. Accordingly, APase enzymes catalyze the hydrolysis of phosphoric ester bonds of various substrate types in different subcellular localizations to be named cytoplasm, vacuole, plasma membrane, nucleus, cell wall, plastid, mitochondria, apoplast, and secretome in various tissues.

As shown in Fig. 5.2A, PAPs are believed to play a major role in plant Pi metabolism in leaves through hydrolysis of intra- and extracellular substrates, especially under Pi deprivation. Among them, secreted or cell wall-associated PAPs, AtPAP12, AtPAP25, and AtPAP26, hydrolyze PEP, PPs, PPi, located in the intracellular or extracellular compartments, or they may recycle Pi from endogenous phosphomonoesters leaked from the cytoplasm across the plasma membrane, for example, AtPAP12 and AtPAP26. HRP family members catalyze the dephosphorylation of PPi and PL substrates. PLP enzymes as a large APase family release Pi from PLs of the plasma membrane of various organelles. PLP2 (AtLPP1) and PLP7 (LPPepsilon1) activated in chloroplast are functioned in the plasma membrane, particularly in senescent leaves. PLP8, PLP10, and PLP12 are active in the endoplasmic reticulum membrane, chloroplast, and Golgi membrane, respectively (Pierrugues *et al.*, 2001; Nakamura *et al.*, 2007; Nishikawa *et al.*, 2008; Mina *et al.*, 2010).

Figure 5.2B demonstrates PAP members hydrolyze phytic acid to free Pi and lower phosphoric esters of myoinositol in flowers and seeds. AtPAP15, as an extracellular APase, is playing an important role in mobilizing Pi from phytate reserves in pollen, seed, and also roots during germination. AtPAP2, hydrolyzing sugar-phosphate substrates, is targeted to both chloroplasts and mitochondria that modulate carbon metabolism. *PLP12* is also expressed in flowers targeting PL substrates there.

Root cells secret organic acid anions, like malate and citrate, especially during Pi starvation that increase the solubility of mineral-bound Pi. Synergistically, in this acidic condition, secreted nucleases, RNases, phosphodiesterases, and PAPs (e.g., AtPAP26, AtPAP10) mobilize Pi from soil DNA and RNA, derived from decaying biomatters (Fig 5.2C).

The importance of APases-encoding genes for the provision of Pi has been clearly shown through transgenesis too. For instance, overexpression of *OsPAP21b* (Mehra *et al.*, 2017), *OsPAP26* (Gao *et al.*, 2017), *MtPAP1* (Ma *et al.*, 2009), *AtPAP26* (Sabet *et al.*, 2018), *AtPAP18* (Zamani *et al.*, 2012), *AtPAP17* (Frahadi *et al.*, 2020), *OsPAP10c* (Deng *et al.*, 2020) improved Pi acquisition, utilization, or remobilization. Therefore, APases have become attractive candidates for developing crops with high potency in Pi acquisition from agricultural soils producing higher yields (Feder *et al.*, 2020). The current knowledge should yield insights into the physiological roles of these important enzyme families and deepen ongoing efforts to exploit the tools of biotechnology to improve Pi acquisition and utilization efficiency to reduce the over-usage of polluting nonrenewable Pi-containing fertilizers.

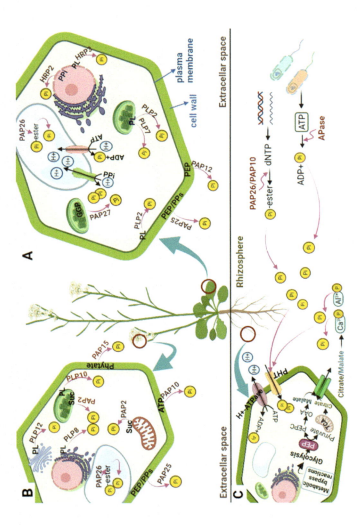

Figure 5.2 A schematic model for the contributions of various acid phosphatases in Pi homeostasis. (A) In leave subcellular localizations, acid phosphatase (APase) enzymes catalyze the hydrolysis of phosphoric ester bonds of various substrate types including inorganic pyrophosphate (PPi), phosphoenolpyruvate (PEP), sugar phosphate (Suc), phosphoproteins (PPs), *para*-Nitrophenyl phosphate (*p*-NPP), GDP-L-galactose phosphorylase (GGP), phospholipid (PL), and ATP; (B) in flowers and seeds, PAP members are functional inside the cells and some are secreted to extracellular space hydrolyzing sugar-Pi, phospholipids and phytic acid (myoinositol hexakisphosphate) as shown; (C) root secreted organic acid anions, nucleases, RNases, phosphodiesterases, and PAPs (AtPAP26, AtPAP10) all contribute in mobilize Pi from soil decaying organic matters in rhizosphere. Drawing was created in Biorender.com.

Yet, the importance of fine-tuning of Pi homeostasis in cell survival and growth complex requires interactions among all genes playing roles in different ways. A deep insight into APases interactions, networking, and their regulation mechanisms is only possible through introducing dynamic biomodel of Pi metabolism to go beyond its static image as presented in Fig. 5.2. In the reconstructed biomodels produced so far, Pi metabolism modules have been neglected or oversimplified. Such as big gap in biomodels necessitates collaborations of researchers to produce quantitative data for the expression and the activities of APases, Pi transporters, kinases, etc. The integration of these data in Pi modules of introduced biomodel facilitates applications from fertilization to harvesting higher yield.

Acknowledgments

The authors would like to appreciate the National Institute of Genetic Engineering and Biotechnology and Tarbiat Modaress University for providing experimental and data processing facilities to fill some gaps in the current knowledge as described in the text.

References

Abbasi-Vineh M. A., Sabet M. S., Karimzadeh G., *Frontiers in Plant Science*, **15** (2021), 11–2326.

Abel S., Nürnberger T., Ahnert V., Krauss G. J., Glund K., *Plant Physiology*, **122** (2000), 543–552.

Amtmann A., Hammond J. P., Armengaud P., White P. J., *Advances in Botanical Research*, **43** (2005), 209–257.

Arae T., Nakakoji M., Noguchi M., Kamon E., Sano R., Demura T., Ohtani M., *Development, Growth & Differentiation* **64** (2022), 5–15.

Araujo C. L., Vihko P. T., *Phosphatase Modulators*, 2013, Humana Press, pp. 155–166

Balzergue C., Dartevelle T., Godon C., Laugier E., Meisrimler C., Teulon J. M., Creff A., Bissler M., Brouchoud C., Hagège A., Müller J., *Nature Communications*, **15** (2017), 1–6.

Bassham D. C., MacIntosh G. C., *Plant Science*, **262** (2017) 169–174.

Beber K., Jarosch B., Langen G., Kogel K. H., *Molecular Plant Pathology*, **1** (2000) 277–289.

Beck J. L., McConachie L. A., Summors A. C., Arnold W. N., De Jersey J., Zerner B., *Biochimica et Biophysica Acta (BBA) – Protein Structure and Molecular Enzymology*, **869** (1986), 61–68.

Berger S., Bell E., Sadka A., Mullet J. E., *Molecular Plant Pathology*, **27** (1995) 933–942.

Berger S., Mitchell-Olds T., Stotz H. U., *Physiologia Plantarum*, **114** (2002), 85–91.

Bhadouria J., Singh A. P., Mehra P., Verma L., Srivastawa R., Parida S. K., Giri J., *Scientific Reports*, **7** (2017), 1–2.

Burroughs A. M., Allen K. N., Dunaway-Mariano D., Aravind L., *Journal of Molecular Biology*, **361** (2006), 1003–1034.

Bykova N. V., Egsgaard H., Møller I. M., *FEBS Letters*, **540** (2003), 141–146.

Cangussu A. S. R., Aires Almeida D., Aguiar R. W. D. S., Bordignon-Junior S. E., Viana K. F., Barbosa L. C. B., Lima, W. J. N., *Enzyme Research*, **2018** (2018), 1–12.

Cantagrel V., Lefeber D. J., *Journal of Inherited Metabolic Disease*, **34** (2011), 859–867.

Caparrós-Martín J. A., Reiland S., Köchert K., Cutanda M. C., Culiáñez-Macià F. A., *Plant Molecular Biology*, **63** (2007), 505–517.

Carman G. M., Han G. S., *Journal of Lipid Research*, **60** (2019), 2–6.

Cashikar A. G., Kumaresan R., Rao N. M., *Plant Physiology*, **114** (1997), 907–915.

Chen Y., Wei J., Wang M., Shi Z., Gong W., Zhang M., *PloS One*, **7** (2012), 1–8, e49421.

Chiou T. J., Lin S. I., *Annual Review of Plant Biology*, **62** (2011), 185–206.

Ciereszko I., Szczygła A., Żebrowska E., *Journal of Plant Nutrition*, **34** (2011a), 815–829.

Ciereszko I., Żebrowska E., Ruminowicz M., *Acta Physiologiae Plantarum* **33** (2011b), 2355–2368.

Coello P., *Physiologia Plantarum*, **116** (2002), 293–298.

Cordell D., Drangert J.-O., White S., *Global Environmental Change, Traditional Peoples and Climate Change*, **19** (2009), 292–305.

Cox R. S., Schenk G., Mitić N., Gahan L. R., Hengge A. C., *Journal of the American Chemical Society*, **129** (2007) 9550–9551.

Crombez H., Motte H., Beeckman T., *Developmental Cell*, **48** (2019), 599–615.

Del Pozo J. C., Allona I., Rubio V., Leyva A., De La Peña A., Aragoncillo C., Paz-Ares J., *The Plant Journal*, **19** (1999), 579–589.

Del Vecchio H. A., Ying S., Park J., Knowles V. L., Kanno S., Tanoi K., She Y.-M., Plaxton W. C., *The Plant Journal* **80** (2014), 569–581.

Deng S., Lu L., Li J., Du Z., Liu T., Li W., Xu F., Shi L., Shou H., Wang C., *Journal of Experimental Botany*, **71** (2020), 4321–4332.

Dionisio G., Madsen C. K., Holm P. B., Welinder K. G., Jørgensen M., Stoger E., Arcalis E., Brinch-Pedersen H., *Plant Physiology*, **156** (2011), 1087–1100.

Dissanayaka D. M. S. B., Plaxton W. C., Lambers H., Siebers M., Marambe B., Wasaki J., *Plant Cell and Environment,* **4** (2018), 1483–1496.

Dissanayaka D. M., Ghahremani M., Siebers M., Wasaki J., Plaxton W. C., *Journal of Experimental Botany,* **72** (2021), 199–223.

Du Z., Deng S., Wu Z., Wang C., *PLoS One* **16** (2021).

Dubots E., Botté C., Boudière L., Yamaryo-Botté Y., Jouhet J., Maréchal E., Block M. A., *Biochimie,* **94** (2012), 86–93.

Duff S. M., Sarath G., Plaxton W. C., *Physiologia Plantarum*, **90** (1994), 791–800.

Durmus A., Eicken C., Horst Sift B., Kratel A., Kappl R., Hüttermann J., Krebs B., *European Journal of Biochemistry*, **260** (1999), 709–716.

Elser J. J., Peace A. L., Kyle M., Wojewodzic M., McCrackin M. L., Andersen T., Hessen, D. O., *Ecology Letters* **13** (2010), 1256–1261.

Farhadi S., Sabet M. S., Malboobi M. A., Moieni A., *Frontiers in Plant Science*, **11** (2020), 1–15.

Feder D., McGeary R. P., Mitić N., Lonhienne T., Furtado A., Schulz B. L., Henry R. J., Schmidt S., Guddat L. W., Schenk G., *Plant Science*, **294** (2020), 1–38.

Feng G., Su Y., Li X., Wang H., Zhang F., Tang C., Rengel Z., *Journal of Plant Nutrition* **25** (2002), 969–980.

Foyer C., Spencer C., *Planta* **167** (1986), 369–375.

Fujita Y., Venterink H. O., Van Bodegom P. M., Douma J. C., Heil G. W., Hölzel N., Jabłońska E., Kotowski W., Okruszko T., Pawlikowski P., De Ruiter P. C., *Nature*, **505** (2014), 82–86.

Gao W., Lu L., Qiu W., Wang C., Shou H., *Plant and Cell Physiology*, **58** (2017), 885–892.

Ghahremani M., Park J., Anderson E. M., Marty-Howard N. J., Mullen R. T., Plaxton W. C., *Plant, Cell & Environment*, **42** (2019), 1158–1166.

González-Muñoz E., Avendaño-Vázquez A. O., Montes R. A., de Folter S., Andrés-Hernández L., Abreu-Goodger C., Sawers R. J., *Frontiers in Plant Science*, **6** (2015), 1–12.

Grant C., Bittman S., Montreal M., Plenchette C., Morel C., *Canadian Journal of Plant Science*, **85** (2005), 3–14.

Guo J., Pesacreta T. C., *Journal of Plant Physiology*, **151** (1997), 520–527.

Gutiérrez-Alanís D., Ojeda-Rivera J. O., Yong-Villalobos L., Cárdenas-Torres L., Herrera-Estrella L., *Trends in Plant Science*, **23** (2018), 721–730.

Ham B. K., Chen J., Yan Y., Lucas W. J., *Current Opinion in Biotechnology*, **49** (2018), 1–9.

Hammond J. P., Bennett M. J., Brown H. C., Broadly J., Eastwood D. C., May S. T., Rahn C., Swarup R., Woolaway K. E., Whlte P. J., *Plant Physiology*, **132** (2003), 578–596.

Haran S., Logendra S., Seskar M., Bratanova M., Raskin I., *Plant Physiology*, **124** (2000), 615–626.

Hegeman C. E., Grabau E. A., *Plant Physiology*, **126** (2001), 1598–1608.

Hillwig M. S., Contento A. L., Meyer A., Ebany D., Bassham D. C., MacIntosh G. C., *Proceedings of the National Academy of Sciences*, **108** (2011), 1093–1098.

Hilson P., Allemeersch J., Altmann T., Aubourg S., Avon A., Beynon J., Bhalerao R. P., Bitton F., Caboche M., Cannoot B., Chardakov V., *Genome Research*, **14 (**2004), 2176–2189.

Huang S., Zhang J., Ma Y., Wei S., Huang L., *Plant Physiology and Biochemistry*, **57** (2012), 114–119.

Iwasaki W., Miki K., *Journal of Molecular Biology*, **371** (2007), 123–136.

Jakobek J. L., Lindgren P. B., *Journal of Experimental Botany*, **53** (2002), 387–389.

Johnson J. J., White-Gloria C., Toth R., Labandera A.-M., Uhrig R. G., Moorhead G. B., *Plants: Functional Genomic Perspective*, 2020, Springer International Publishing, Cham, 2020, pp. 1–9.

Kaida R., Satoh Y., Bulone V., Yamada Y., Kaku T., Hayashi T., Kaneko T. S., *Plant Physiology*, **150** (2009), 1822–1830.

Kong Y., Li X., Ma J., Li W., Yan G., Zhang C., *Plant Cell Reports*, **33** (2014), 655–667.

Kuang R., Chan K. H., Yeung E., Leong L. B., *Plant Physiology*, **151** (2009), 199–209.

Kumar V., Singh G., Verma A. K., Agrawal S., *Enzyme Research*, **2012** (2012), 1–8.

Leelapon O., Sarath G., Staswick P. E., *Planta* **219** (2004), 1071–1079.

Li C., Gui S., Yang T., Walk T., Wang X., Liao H., *Annals of Botany*, **109** (2012), 275–285.

Li C., Li C., Zhang H., Liao H., Wang X., *Physiologia Plantarum*, **159** (2017), 215–227.

Li D., Zhu H., Liu K., Liu X., Leggewie G., Udvardi M., Wang D., *Journal of Biological Chemistry*, **277** (2002), 27772–27781.

Li R., Lu W., Gu J., Li X., Guo C., Xiao K., *African Journal of Biotechnology*, **10** (2011), 11110–11123.

Li W. Y., Shao G., Lam H. M., *New Phytologist*, **178** (2008), 80–91.

Liang C. Y., Tian J., Lam H. M., Lim B. L., Ya X., Liao H., *Plant Physiology*, **152** (2010), 854–865.

Liang C., Sun L., Yao Z., Liao H., Tian J., *PLoS One*, **7** (2012), 1–11, e38106.

Liao H., Wong F. L., Phang T. H., Cheung M. Y., Li W. Y., Shao G., Yan X., Lam H. M., *Gene*, **318** (2003), 103–111.

Liu P., Cai Z., Chen Z., Mo X., Ding X., Liang C., Liu G., Tian J., *Plant, Cell & Environment* **41** (2018), 2821–2834.

Liu P.-D., Xue Y.-B., Chen Z.-J., Liu G.-D., Tian J., *Journal Experimental Botany* **67** (2016), 4141–4154.

Lohrasebi T., Zamani K., Sabet M. S., Malboobi M. A., Yazdanbakhsh P., *Progress in Biological Sciences*, **2** (2013), 42–57.

Lu L., Qiu W., Gao W., Tyerman S. D., Shou H., Wang C., *Plant, Cell & Environment,* **39** (2016), 2247–2259.

Ma X. F., Wright E., Ge Y., Bell J., Xi Y., Bouton J. H., Wang Z. Y., *Plant Science*, **176** (2009), 479–488.

Malboobi M. A., Samaeian A., Sabet M. S., Lohrasebi T., *Plant Science* (Dhal N. K., ed), 2012, InTech Press, Croatia, pp. 1–33

Malhotra H., Sharma S., Pandey R., *Plant Nutrients and Abiotic Stress Tolerance* (Hasanuzzaman M., Fujita M., Oku H., Nahar K., Hawrylak-Nowak B., eds), 2018, Springer, Singapore, pp. 171–190.

Maryanto S. D., Tanjung Z. A., Roberdi R., Sudania W. M., Pujianto P., Hairinsyah H., Utomo C., Liwang T., *Biodiversitas Journal of Biological Diversity*, **22** (2021), 1385–1390.

May A., Spinka M., Köck M., *Biochimica et Biophysica Acta (BBA) – Proteins and Proteomics*, **1824** (2012), 319–325.

Mehra P., Pandey B. K., Giri J., *Plant Biotechnology Journal*, **15** (2017), 1054–1067.

Mina J. G., Okada Y., Wansadhipathi-Kannangara N. K., Pratt S., Shams-Eldin H., Schwarz R. T., Steel P. G., Fawcett T., Denny P. W., *Plant Molecular Biology*, **73** (2010), 399–407.

Misson J., Raghothama K. G., Jain A., Jouhet J., Block M. A., Bligny R., Ortel P., Creff A., Somerville S., Rolland N., *Proceedings of the National Academy of Sciences of the United States of America*, **102** (2005), 11934–11939.

Morcuende R., Gibon Y., Zheng W., Pant B. D., Blasing O., Usadel B., Czechowskit T., Udvardi M. K., Stti M., Scheible W. R., *Plant, Cell & Environment*, **30** (2007), 85–112.

Mullaney E. J., Ullah A. H., *Biochemical and Biophysical Research Communications*, **251** (1998), 252–255.

Muller R., Morant M., Jarmer H., Nilsson L., Nielsen T. H., *Plant Physiology*, **143** (2007), 156–171.

Mura C., Katz J. E., Clarke S. G., Eisenberg D., *Journal Molecular Biology*, **326** (2003), 1559–1575.

Nakagawa N., Kato M., Takahashi Y., Shimazaki K., Tamura K., Tokuji Y., Kihara A., Imai H., *Journal of Plant Research*, **125** (2012), 439–449.

Nakamura Y., Ohta H., Phosphatidic acid phosphatases in seed plants, in *Lipid Signaling in Plants* (Munnik T., ed), Springer, Berlin, Heidelberg, *Plant Cell Monographs*, **16** (2010), pp. 131–141.

Nakamura Y., *Plant and Cell Physiology*, **59** (2018), 441–447.

Nakamura Y., Teo N. Z., Shui G., Chua C. H., Cheong W. F., Parameswaran S., Koizumi R., Ohta H., Wenk M. R., Ito T., *New Phytologist*, **203** (2014), 310–322.

Nakamura Y., Tsuchiya M., Ohta H., *Journal of Biological Chemistry*, **282** (2007), 29013–29021.

Naomi M. R., Nurmalasari I. A., *IOP Conference Series: Earth and Environmental Science*, vol. 637, 2021, IOP Publishing.

Navazio L., Miuzzo M., Royle L., Baldan B., Varotto S., Merry A. H., Harvey D. J., Dwek R. A., Rudd P. M., Mariani P., *Biochemistry*, **41** (2002), 14141–14149.

Nishikawa M., Kenta H., Mai I., Hiroki M., Kentaro T., Ikuko H. N., Yohei T., Kenichiro Sh., Hiroyuki I., *Plant and Cell Physiology*, **49** (2008), 1758–1763.

Niu Y. F., Chai R. S., Jin G. L., Wang H., Tang C. X., Zhang Y. S., *Annals of Botany*, **112** (2013), 391–408.

Nussaume L., Maréchal E., Thibaud M. C., Block M. A., *Plant Cell Monographs*, **19** (2010), 237–251.

O'Gallagher B., Ghahremani M., Stigter K., Walker E. J., Pyc M., Liu A. Y., MacIntosh G. C., Mullen R. T., Plaxton W. C., *Journal of Experimental Botany* **73** (2022), 382–399.

Olczak M., Morawiecka B., Watorek W., *Acta Biochimica Polonica*, **50** (2003), 1245–1256.

Olczak M., Olczak T., *Arch Biochem Biophys* **461** (2007), 247–254.

Pabis A., Duarte F., Kamerlin, S. C. L., *Biochemistry*, **55** (2016), 3061–3081.

Pan X., Liu H., Clark J., Jones J., Bevan M., Stein L., *Nucleic Acids Research*, **31** (2003), 1245–1251.

Pandey B. K., Mehra P., Verma L., Bhadouria J., Giri J., Plant Physiology **174** (2017), 2316–2332.

Peret B., Clément M., Nussaume L., Desnos T., *Trends in Plant Science*, **16** (2011), 442–450.

Petters J., Göbel C., Scheel D., Rosahl S., *Plant Cell Physiology*, **43** (2002), 1049–1053.

Pierrugues O., Brutesco C., Oshiro J., Gouy M., Deveaux Y., Carman G. M., Thuriaux P., Kazmaier M., *Journal of Biological Chemistry*, **276** (2001), 20300–20308.

Plaxton W. C., Shane M. W., *Annual Plant Reviews Online,* **15** (2018), 99–123.

Plaxton W. C., Tran H. T., *Plant Physiology*, **156** (2011), 1006–1015.

Poirier Y., Thoma S., Somerville C., Schiefelbein J., *Plant Physiology,* **97** (1991), 1087–1093.

Prajapati B. J., Gudadhe N. I., Gamit V. R., Chhaganiya H. J., *Farming and Management*, **2** (2017), 36–40.

Ravichandran S., Stone S. L., Benkel B., Prithiviraj B., *BMC Plant Biology*, **13** (2013), 1–2.

Rebeille F., Bligny R., Douce R., *Plant Physiology,* **74** (1984), 355–359.

Reddy C. S., Kim K. M., James D., Varakumar P., Reddy M. K., *Acta Physiologiae Plantarum*, **39** (2017), 1–10.

Reymond P., Bodenhausen N., Van Poecke R. M. P., Krishnamurthy V., Dicke M., Farmer E. E., *Plant Cell*, **16** (2004), 3132–3147.

Robinson W. D., Carson I., Ying S., Ellis K., Plaxton W. C., *New Phytologist*, **196** (2012a), 1024–1029.

Robinson W. D., Park J., Tran H. T., Del Vecchio H. A., Ying S., Zins J. L., Patel K., McKnight T. D., Plaxton W. C., *Journal of Experimental Botany*, **63** (2012b), 6531–6542.

Sabet M. S., Zamani K., Lohrasebi T., Malboobi M. A., Valizadeh M., *Iranian Journal of Biotechnology*, **16** (2018), 31–34.

Salmanzadeh M., Sabet M. S., Moieni A., Homaee M., *Planta*, **251** (2020), 1–14.

Scheible W. R., Rojas-Triana M., *Annual Plant Reviews* (Plaxton W. C., Lambers H., eds), **48** (2015), 23–63, Wiley-Blackwell, Hoboken, New Jersey.

Schenk G., Mitić N., Hanson G. R., Comba P., *Coordination Chemistry Reviews*, **257** (2013), 473–482.

Secco D., Bouain N., Rouached A., Hanin M., Pandey A., *Critical Reviews in Biotechnology* **37** (2017), 898–910.

Shane M. W., Stigter K., Fedosejevs E. T., Plaxton W. C., *Journal of Experimental Botany*, **65** (2014), 6097–6106.

Siebers M., Dörmann P., Hölzl G., *Annual Plant Reviews* (Plaxton W. C., Lambers H., eds), **48** (2015), 237–264, Wiley-Blackwell, Hoboken, New Jersey.

Sobhe Bidari P., Manshaei R., Lohrasebi T., Feizi A., Malboobi M. A., Alirezaie J., *8th IEEE International Conference on Bioinformatics and Bioengineering*, (2008), 10412467, Athens, Greece.

Stenzel I., Ziethe K., Schurath J., Hertel S. C., Bosse D., Köck M., *Physiologiae Plantarum*, **118** (2003), 138–146.

Stotz H. U., Pittendrigh B. R., Kroymann J., Weniger K., Fritsche J., Bauke A., Mitchell-Olds T., *Plant Physiology*, **124** (2000), 1007–1018.

Sun F., Carrie C., Law S., Murcha M. W., Zhang R., Law Y. S., Suen P. K., Whelan J., Lim B. L., *Plant Signaling & Behavior*, **7** (2012), 927–932.

Sun F., Suen P. K., Zhang Y., Liang C., Carrie C., Whelan J., Ward J. L., Hawkins N. D., Jiang L., Lim B. L., *New Phytologist*, **194** (2012), 206–219.

Sun Q. Q., Li J. Y., Cheng W. Z., Guo H. H., Liu X. M., Gao H. B., *Genes*, **9** (2018), 1–18.

Tagad C. K., Sabharwal S. G., *Journal of Food Science and Technology*, **55** (2018), 313–320.

Taliman N. A., Dong Q., Echigo K., Raboy V., *Plants.* **8** (2019), 1–13.

Tamaoki M., Freeman J. L., Pilon-Smits E. A. H., *Plant Physiology*, **146** (2008), 1219–1230.

Tian J., Liao H., *Annual Plant Reviews*, **48** (2015), 265–288.

Tian J., Wang C., Zhang Q., He X., Whelan J., Shou H., *Journal of Integrative Plant Biology*, **54** (2012), 631–639.

Tomscha J. L., Trull M. C., Deikman J., Lynch J. P., Guiltinan M. J., *Plant Physiology*, **135** (2004), 334–345.

Tran H. T., Hurley B. A., Plaxton W. C., *Plant Science*, **179** (2010a), 14–27.

Tran H. T., Qian W., Hurley B. A., She Y. M., Wang D., Plaxton W. C., *Plant, Cell & Environment*, **33** (2010b), 1789–1803.

Trull M. C., Deikman J., *Planta*, **206** (1998), 544–550.

Turner W. L., Plaxton W. C., *Planta*, **214** (2001), 243–249.

Vance C. P., Uhde-Stone C., Allan D. L., *New Phytologist*, **157** (2003), 423–447.

Veljanovski V., Vanderbeld B., Knowles V. L., Snedden W. A., Plaxton W. C., *Plant Physiology*, **142** (2006), 1282–1293.

Veneklaas E. J., Lambers H., Bragg J., Finnegan P. M., Lovelock C. E., Plaxton W. C., Price C. A., Scheible W.-R., Shane M. W., White P. J., Raven J. A., *New Phytology* **195** (2012), 306–320.

Venkidasamy B., Selvaraj D., Ramalingam S., *International Journal of Biological Macromolecules*, **123** (2019), 648–656.

Wang J., Si Z., Li F., Xiong X., Lei L., Xie F., Chen D., Li Y., Li Y., *Plant Molecular Biology*, **88** (2015), 515–529.

Wang L. S., Lu S., Zhang Y., Li Z., Du X., Liu D., *Journal of Integrative Plant Biology*, **56** (2014), 299–314.

Wang L., Li Z., Qian W., Guo W., Gao X., Huang L., Wang H., Zhu H., Wu J.-W., Wang D., Liu D., *Plant Physiology* **157** (2011), 1283–1299.

Wang L., Liu D., *Plant Science*, **271** (2018), 108–116.

Wang L., Liu D., *Plant Signaling & Behavior*, **7** (2012), 306–310.

Wang X., Pang J., Wen Z., Gadot G., de Borda A., Siddique K. H., Lambers H., *Plant and Soil*, **5** (2021), 1–2.

Wang X., Wang Y., Tian J., Lim B. L., Yan X., Liao H., *Plant Physiology*, **151** (2009), 233–240.

Wang Y., Yang Z., Kong Y., Li X., Li W., Du H., Zhang C., *Frontiers in Plant Science*, **11** (2020), 1–12.

White P. J., Veneklaas E. J., *Plant and Soil*, **357** (2012), 1–8.

Williamson V. M., Colwell G., *Plant Physiology*, **97** (1991), 139–146.

Wolucka B. A., Van Montagu M., *Phytochemistry* **68** (2007), 2602–2613.

Wu W. W., Lin Y., Liu P. D., Chen Q. Q., Tian J., Liang C. Y., *Journal of Experimental Botany*, **69** (2018), 603–617.

Wu W., Zhu Sh., Chen Q., Lin Y., Tian J., Liang C., *International Journal of Molecular Sciences*, **20** (2019), 1–13.

Xiao K., Harrison M., Wang Z. Y., *Journal of Integrative Plant Biology*, **48** (2006), 204–211.

Xiao K., Harrison M. J., Wang Z.-Y., *Planta,* **222** (2005), 27–36.

Xie L., Shang Q., *BMC Genomics*, **19** (2018), 1–12.

Yang S. Y., Huang T. K., Kuo H. F., Chiou T. J., *Journal of Experimental Botany*, **68** (2017), 3045–3055.

Yin C., Wang F., Fan H., Fang Y., Li W., *International Journal of Molecular Sciences*, **20** (2019), 1–17.

Yunus I. S., Cazenave-Gassiot A., Liu Y. C., Lin Y. C., Wenk M. R., Nakamura Y., *Plant Signaling & Behavior*, **10** (2015), 1–10, e1049790.

Zakhleniuk O. V., Raines C. A., Lioyd J. C., *Planta*, **212** (2001), 529–534.

Zamani Amirzakaria J., Malboobi M. A., Marashi S. A., Lohrasebi T., *Journal of Biomolecular Structure and Dynamics*, **39** (2020), 1–12.

Zamani K., Lohrasebi T., Sabet M. S., Malboobi M. A., Mousavi A., *Gene Expression Patterns,* **14** (2014), 9–18.

Zamani K., Sabet M. S., Lohrasebi T., Mousavi A., Malboobi M. A., *Biologia*, **67** (2012), 713–720.

Zhang Q., Wang C., Tian J., Li K., Shou H., *Plant Biology*, **13** (2011), 7–15.

Zhang R., Guan X., Law Y.-S., Sun F., Chen S., Wong K. B., Lim B. L., *Plant Signaling & Behavior* **11** (2016), e1239687.

Zhang W., Gruszewski H. A., Chevone B. I., Nessler C. L., *Plant Physiology*, **146** (2008), 431–440.

Zhang Y., Wang X., Lu S., Liu D., *Journal of Experimental Botany,* **65** (2014), 6577–6588.

Zhou M., Chen W., Zhao M., Li Y., Li M., Hu X., *Forests*, **12** (2021), 1–9.

Zhu H., Qian, W., Lu X., Li D., Liu X., Liu K., Wang D., *Plant Molecular Biology* **59** (2005), 581–594.

Zimmermann P., Regierer B., Kossmann J., Frossard E., Amrhein N., Bucher M., *Plant Biology*, **6** (2004), 519–528.

Chapter 6

Superoxide Dismutases in Plants: New Insights into Regulation and Functioning

Ravi Prakash Sanyal,[a] Abiraami T. V.,[a] Sabiha Perween,[b] Satish B. Verulkar,[b] Hari S. Misra,[a,c] and Ajay Saini[a,c]

[a]*Molecular Biology Division, Bhabha Atomic Research Centre, Trombay, Mumbai, Maharashtra, India*
[b]*Department of Plant Molecular Biology and Biotechnology, Indira Gandhi Krishi Vishwavidyalaya (IGKV), Raipur, Chhattisgarh, India*
[c]*Homi Bhabha National Institute, Anushaktinagar, Trombay, Mumbai, Maharashtra, India*
hsmisra@barc.gov.in, ajays@barc.gov.in

Superoxide dismutases (SODs) are ubiquitous metalloenzymes that are an integral component of the cellular antioxidant defense system. The origin and evolution of the SODs was an outcome of the transitions in the atmospheric conditions ~2.4 billion years ago (Bya), due to the 'Great Oxygenation Event' (GOE). This resulted in an increase in atmospheric oxygen, and the subsequent evolution of diverse aerobic life forms. Aerobic metabolism, though more efficient,

---

Agricultural Biocatalysis: Enzymes in Agriculture and Industry
Edited by Peter Jeschke and Evgeni B. Starikov
Copyright © 2023 Jenny Stanford Publishing Pte. Ltd.
ISBN 978-981-4968-47-8 (Hardcover), 978-1-003-31310-6 (eBook)
www.jennystanford.com

was also associated with the generation of reactive oxygen species (ROS), as metabolic byproducts. The SODs evolved to dismutate the harmful superoxide radical ($O_2{}^{\cdot-}$) and confer protection against ROS-mediated oxidative damage. Factors like the availability of soluble metal cofactors for catalysis, endosymbiosis, and genomic events contributed toward the diversity of SODs among simple and complex life forms. Based on the metal cofactors there are four SOD types (Fe, Mn, Ni, and CuZn SOD), which show diversity in distribution among different organisms, as well as cellular localization (cytosol, mitochondria, chloroplast, peroxisome, apoplast, etc.). The functional significance of SODs in diverse physiological processes has increased several folds, due to their contribution in localized antioxidant function, regulation of levels of other reactive species, maintenance of appropriate cellular redox environment, and cellular signaling. The regulation of SODs operates at multiple levels, where different mechanisms play important roles in controlling the expression, transcript/protein levels, and activities of SODs in response to intrinsic and extrinsic factors. This chapter gives an overview of important aspects of reactive species and antioxidant functions, evolution and diversity of SODs, different modes of regulation of expression and function of SODs, and important applications with recent insights.

6.1 Introduction

Environmental factors (biotic and abiotic) are important for all life forms, and any deviation from their optimal levels affects the growth, development, and survival of living organisms. Environmental conditions continuously change over a period of time and may include slow, incremental, or drastic changes, which results in the evolution of adaptive strategies among organisms (Rago *et al.*, 2019). Unlike other organisms, plants being sessile are more prone to environmental stress conditions (heat, low temperature, light, drought, salinity, nutrient deprivation, heavy metal stress, radiation, etc.), which significantly affect their growth, development, and productivity (Boyer, 1982; He *et al.*, 2018). In natural conditions, plants face multiple stresses (individual or in combination) that affect almost all aspects of normal physiology (Mittler, 2006; Zhu, J-K, 2016; Mittler *et al.*, 2017; Pandey *et al.*, 2017). The unfavorable conditions perceived by plants result in a complex, inter-linked reprogramming of cellular machinery to induce a battery of adaptive responses regulated at multiple levels (Mittler, 2006; Haak *et al.*, 2017). Certain types of molecular damage are common to different stresses, albeit to a different extent, resulting in the activation of similar adaptive/protective responses. For example, the generation of reactive species is common to many stress conditions, which results in the activation of antioxidant defense systems for protection against oxidative damage to cellular components (Hasanuzzaman *et al.*, 2020).

This chapter is focused on 'superoxide dismutases (SODs),' an important group of ubiquitous, antioxidant metalloenzymes. SODs, initially identified as a metalloprotein with no known function (McCord and Fridovich, 1969), have come a long way to be regarded as an indispensable group of proteins involved in crucial cellular functions (Perry *et al.*, 2010). Multiple SOD isoforms are an integral component of the cellular antioxidant defense system (Alscher *et al.*, 2002; Del Río *et al.*, 2018). The chapter discusses different aspects of reactive species, the evolution of multiple SOD isoforms, structural and functional differences, localization and functions, modes of regulation, and biotechnological applications, with emphasis on some important and recent insights.

6.2 Impact of Great Oxygenation Event (GOE) on Cellular Metabolism

Atmospheric changes as a result of the 'GOE' (~2.4 Bya) resulted in the evolution of more energy-efficient metabolism in aerobic organisms compared to anaerobes (Miller, 2012). On the negative side, aerobic metabolism was associated with the generation of ROS (metabolic byproducts), with detrimental effects on cellular functions and integrity (Case, 2017). Evolutionary pressure against this oxidative damage resulted in the origin and evolution of SOD enzymes (Miller, 2012). Further course of evolution diversified the SODs into multiple isoforms as a consequence of factors like atmospheric conditions, metal cofactor availability, endosymbiosis, genomic events, etc. These antioxidant enzymes protected the living systems from the detrimental effects of ROS (Alscher *et al.*, 2002). Over time, the diversity of reactive species (and associated biological damage) increased substantially, which resulted in the evolution of a complex, integrated, multi-layered antioxidant defense system that enables living systems to maintain a suitable 'redox environment,' minimize damage, and utilize diverse reactive species for important cellular processes (Case, 2017).

6.3 Reactive Species: Generation, Molecular Targets, and Scavenging

Generation of reactive chemical species (ROS) is a continuous process in different cell compartments, and these species can have different fates/outcomes based on their levels and reactivity. The ROS species are reduced/excited species of molecular oxygen (O_2) that exists in the triplet ground state ($^3O_2$), as a relatively stable, paramagnetic biradical (Apel and Hirt, 2004). However, activation of O_2 by either energy transfer or sequential reduction can cause a change in the electron spins leading to the formation of species such as singlet oxygen ($^1O_2$), superoxide ($O_2^{·-}$), hydrogen peroxide (H_2O_2), and hydroxyl ($^·OH$) radicals that are more reactive than molecular oxygen (Sharma *et al.*, 2012). There are additional categories of reactive species *viz.* reactive nitrogen species or RNS (e.g., nitric oxide, ·NO; peroxynitrite, ONOO⁻; nitrogen dioxide, ·NO_2), reactive sulfur species or RSS (e.g., thiyl radical, RS·; sulfenic acid, RSOH, etc.) and reactive carbonyl species (RCS) (Hasanuzzaman *et al.*, 2020). The relative levels of these reactive species including RSS, RNS, and RCS are influenced by levels of different antioxidants in the cell (Biswas *et al.*, 2019; Kaur, *et al.*, 2019; Hasanuzzaman *et al.*, 2020; Cejudo *et al.*, 2021). A lot of information is still needed to delineate the precise roles of these reactive species in cellular processes. A brief account of the characteristics of some important reactive species is described below and also listed in Table 6.1.

Table 6.1 Overview of characteristics of some important reactive chemical species (ROS, RNS, RCS, and RSS) in plants

Reactive Species Types	Molecules	Major Cellular Location	Metabolic Reactions/Sites Involved	Reactions/Biological Damage	Antioxidant/Scavenging System Involved	
					Nonenzymatic	Enzymatic
ROS	Superoxide ($O_2^{\cdot-}$)	Cytosol, Chloroplast, Mitochondria, Peroxisome, Apoplast, Membranes	Photosynthesis (PSI and PSII), Mitochondrial electron transport chain (ETC) Complex I and III, NADPH oxidase, Xanthine oxidase (XOD), Aldehyde oxidase (AO), Xanthine dehydrogenase (XDH)	Moderately reactive, Damages proteins (Fe-S center), participates in the generation of other reactive species	Ascorbic acid, Flavonoids, Phenolic acids, Alkaloids, and Amino acids	Multiple Superoxide dismutase (SODs) isoforms in different cellular compartments and cytosol
	Hydroxyl radical ($^{\cdot}OH$)	Chloroplast, Mitochondria, Membranes, Peroxisome,	Fenton reaction and Haber–Weiss reaction	Highly reactive, reacts with all biomolecules	Ascorbic acid, Tocopherol, Phenolic acids, Alkaloids, Glutathione	No enzyme-based system for direct scavenging

(Continued)

Table 6.1 (Continued)

Reactive Species		Major Cellular Location	Metabolic Reactions/Sites Involved	Reactions/Biological Damage	Antioxidant/Scavenging System Involved	
Types	Molecules				Nonenzymatic	Enzymatic
	Hydrogen peroxide (H_2O_2)	Peroxisomes, Chloroplasts, Mitochondria, Apoplast, Cell wall	Dismutation of $O_2^{\cdot -}$ in different, organelles, Glycolate oxidase (GOX), Polyamine oxidase (PAO), Copper amine oxidase (CuAO), Sulfite oxidase (SO)	Protein damage via modifications (Cys residues, aromatic amino acids) and indirectly by $\cdot OH$ radical generation via Fenton reaction	Ascorbic acid, Glutathione, Flavonoids, Amino acids	Catalases (CAT), Peroxidases (POX), Ascorbate peroxidases (APX), Glutathione peroxidase (GPX), Peroxiredoxins (PRX)
	Singlet oxygen ($^1O_2$)	Chloroplast, Mitochondria, Membranes	Photosystem II (PSII), Cytochrome-b6f complex	DNA damage, PSII damage, Protein damage (Trp, Met, His, Tyr, and Cys residues), Protein carbonylation, Lipid peroxidation	Ascorbic acid, Glutathione, Tocopherol, Carotenoids, Alkaloids	No dedicated enzyme for direct scavenging
RNS	Nitric Oxide (NO)	Cytoplasm, Chloroplast, Plasma membrane, Apoplast, Mitochondria, Peroxisome	Nitric oxide-forming nitrite reductase, Nitrate reductase (NR), Nonenzymatic reduction, Xanthine oxidoreductase (XOR)	Posttranslational modifications (S-nitrosylation, tyrosine nitration), interacts with heme center of metalloproteins	Superoxide radical, thiols, and Fe-containing molecules	NAD(P)H- and non-symbiotic hemoglobin-dependent NO-scavenging system S-nitrosoglutathione reductase (GSNOR),

Reactive Species Types	Molecules	Major Cellular Location	Metabolic Reactions/Sites Involved	Reactions/Biological Damage	Antioxidant/Scavenging System Involved	
					Nonenzymatic	Enzymatic
	Peroxynitrite (ONOO⁻)	Peroxisomes, Chloroplast	Rapid nonenzymatic reaction between NO and $O_2^{\cdot -}$	Tyrosine nitration, lipid modification, protein damage, DNA damage	Ascorbic acid, Glutathione, γ-Tocopherol, Carotenoids, Flavonoids	Thiol-dependent peroxidases, Peroxiredoxins (PRX), Glutathione peroxidase (GPX)
RCS	Reactive molecules with carbonyl-conjugated C–C double bonds	Chloroplast Membrane, Mitochondrial membrane	Nonenzymatic lipid peroxidation and action of redox catalyst, enzymatic lipid oxidation (lipoxygenase, LOX), and oxylipin metabolism	Carbonylation of proteins (Trp, His, Tyr, Met, and Cys residues), modification/inactivation	Cysteine, Glutathione NADH/NADPH mediated reduction	Alkenal/one oxidoreductase (AER), Glutathione S-transferase (GST), Aldo-keto reductase (AKR) Aldehyde dehydrogenase (ADH), Aldehyde oxidase (AO)
RSS	Thiyl radicals (RS·)	Peroxisomes	Multiple reactions generate different types of RS· radicals, reactions involving H_2S, oxidation of thiols, etc.	Alters redox status of thiols/disulfides, S-nitrosation, protein modifications	Phenolic acids, β-Carotene,	Glutaredoxin (GRx, thioltransferase), Thioredoxin (TRX)

6.3.1 Superoxide Radical ($O_2^{\cdot-}$)

It is an important ROS generated by single electron transfer to molecular O_2, at multiple locations in the plant cell *viz.* chloroplast, mitochondria, peroxisomes, cytosol, apoplast (Alscher *et al.*, 2002; Gill and Tuteja, 2010; Das and Roychoudhury, 2014). The $O_2^{\cdot-}$ is moderately reactive ($t_{1/2}$: 2–4 µs) and less damaging compared to $\cdot$OH and H_2O_2 (Halliwell, 2006). In general, $O_2^{\cdot-}$ is the first free radical to be generated, serves as reductant or oxidant, and also participates in reactions to generate other ROS (e.g., $\cdot$OH, H_2O_2) and RNS ($ONOO^-$) (Halliwell, 2006; Satomi *et al.*, 2008; Gill and Tuteja, 2010). As the $O_2^{\cdot-}$ is unable to cross membranes, it needs to be scavenged at the site of generation to minimize the direct and indirect damage, and here predominantly multiple SOD isoforms are involved (Alscher *et al.*, 2002).

6.3.2 Hydrogen Peroxide (H_2O_2)

It is produced at multiple cellular locations (peroxisome, chloroplast, mitochondria, endoplasmic reticulum, etc.) due to both nonenzymatic and enzymatic reactions (Mishra and Sharma, 2019), in both normal and unfavorable conditions (Sharma *et al.*, 2012). Superoxide dismutase catalyzed dismutation of $O_2^{\cdot-}$ is an important source of H_2O_2 (Janků *et al.*, 2019). Hydrogen peroxide is neutral, relatively stable at physiological conditions ($t_{1/2}$: 1 ms), highly diffusible (migration distance: 1 µm), and traverse across membranes (Das and Roychoudhury, 2014). These characteristics are important for H_2O_2-mediated oxidative damage at multiple cellular locations, as well its role in physiological processes, cellular signaling and plant-pathogen interactions (Torres *et al.*, 2002; Sharma *et al.*, 2012). It causes oxidative damage (sulfhydryl groups and aromatic amino acids)-mediated inactivation of enzymes/proteins, generates highly reactive $\cdot$OH radical, and is also involved in programmed cell death (PCD) (Halliwell, 2006; Dat *et al.*, 2000).

6.3.3 Hydroxyl Radical ($\cdot$OH)

It is the most reactive ($t_{1/2}$: 1 µs), toxic, and a strong oxidizing ROS (redox potential: +2.40 V) (Halliwell and Gutteridge, 1999; Das and Roychoudhury, 2014). It is generated in transition-metal catalyzed reactions, from H_2O_2 and $O_2^{·-}$ (Haber–Weiss reaction) or directly from H_2O_2 (Fenton reaction). It is also generated in reactions catalyzed by heme oxygenases, cytochrome P450s and class III peroxidases (Demidchik, 2015; Podgórska *et al.*, 2017). The ˙OH radical reacts and causes extensive oxidative damage to proteins, nucleic acids, lipids, which may lead to cell death (Pinto *et al.*, 2003). Antioxidant molecules (flavonoids, proline, etc.), reduction in levels of metal ions, as well as the ROS involved in generation (H_2O_2 and $O_2^{·-}$), can reduce the cellular ˙OH levels and associated damage (Das and Roychoudhury, 2014).

6.3.4 Singlet Oxygen ($^1O_2$)

Its generation does not involve the transfer of electrons to molecular oxygen (O_2). In fact, the interaction of chlorophyll triplet state (^{3}Chl) and the molecular oxygen at triplet ground state ($^3O_2$,) leads to the formation of reactive $^1O_2$ species (Gill and Tuteja, 2010). Conditions such as abiotic stresses (salinity, drought, etc.), which cause stomatal closure and affect CO_2 availability also result in the generation of $^1O_2$. Singlet oxygen is highly reactive (half-life: 1–4 μs), and can diffuse to several hundred nanometers (Das and Roychoudhury, 2014). Singlet oxygen reacts with several biological molecules causing oxidative damage to proteins, nucleic acids, DNA, unsaturated fatty acids. It is quenched by the antioxidant molecules, β-carotene and α-tocopherol (Krieger-Liszkay and Fufezan, 2008). The $^1O_2$ is also suggested to play beneficial roles in the activation of several stress-responsive pathways (Op den *et al.*, 2003).

6.3.5 Other Reactive Species (RNS, RCS, RSS)

These are also present in different cellular compartments. Different RNS vary in their reactivity and decay kinetics, which is responsible for their roles in different pathways (Arnao and Hernández-Ruiz, 2019). For example, the NO (important RNS) is a lipophilic molecule, is highly diffusible, and can form several reactive intermediates (Hasanuzzaman *et al.*, 2020). The reaction between NO and $O_2^{·-}$ generates $OONO^-$, which can decompose to ·NO_2 and ˙OH radicals. It is relatively a stronger oxidant than $O_2^{·-}$ or NO and causes damage to lipids, proteins, and DNA (Del Río, 2015). The reaction of NO with peroxy radical generates ·NO_2 (strong oxidant) which can cause lipid peroxidation, oxidization of ascorbic acid, and reacts with tyrosine to form 3-nitrotyrosine (Del Río, 2015). RCS are generated by enzymatic as well as nonenzymatic reactions and can cause modifications by forming covalent bonds. These species modulate the protein function in different organelles and play important roles in signaling related to several physiological mechanisms (Mano et al., 2019). The reactive species (ROS, RNS, RSS, RCS) have both detrimental as well as beneficial effects.

6.4 Reactive Species and Important Sites of Generation in Plants

The cellular metabolic environment is highly complex and contains thousands of enzymes/regulators working in a coordinated manner, for dynamic inter-conversion of a large number of metabolites for diverse fates in different compartments (Elia and Alain, 2020). The formation of even detrimental metabolic byproducts cannot be stopped completely, however they can be scavenged for minimum impact on cellular integrity and metabolism. One such intriguing category comprises highly reactive metabolic byproducts including ROS ($O_2^{\cdot-}$, $\cdot OH$, $HO_2^{\cdot}$, H_2O_2, $^1O_2$, etc.) and RNS ($\cdot NO$, $\cdot NO_2$, HNO_2, N_2O_4, $ONOO^-$) (Halliwell, 2006; Halliwell and Gutteridge, 2007; Del Río, 2015). Initially, these reactive species were considered detrimental as they damage important cellular macromolecules, leading to metabolic dysfunction (Das and Roychoudhury, 2014). However, advancements in this field showed their involvement in diverse physiological processes, cellular signaling, growth, development, abiotic/biotic stress responses, and PCD (Apel and Hirt, 2004; Gill and Tuteja, 2010; Dietz et al., 2016; Mittler, 2017; Del Río, 2015). These reactive species are the direct and inevitable outcome of aerobic metabolism in different cellular compartments in plant cells viz. chloroplast, mitochondria, peroxisomes, cytosol, endoplasmic reticulum, cell membrane, cell wall, and apoplast (Kar, 2011; Das and Roychoudhury, 2014; Mittler et al., 2017). Some of the prominent sites/reactions generating reactive species in plants are also listed in Table 6.1.

In plants, chloroplasts are major sites of ROS generation (during photosynthesis), particularly due to reactions at electron transport chains (ETCs) associated with photosystem I (PS I) and photosystem

(PS II) (Gill and Tuteja, 2010). ROS such as $^1O_2$, $O_2^{·-}$, $·OH$, and H_2O_2 are generated in chloroplasts (Sharma et al., 2010; Hasanuzzaman et al., 2020). ROS generated in chloroplasts are important for organellar signaling, however, their excess accumulation causes damage to thylakoid membranes harboring photosystems, leading to photoinhibition (Takagi et al., 2016).

Mitochondria (the powerhouse of a cell) are metabolically active and generate ROS at multiple sites of the ETC, complex I, NADH ubiquinone oxidoreductase, and complex III, cytochrome bc_1 complex (Turrens, 2003; Rasmusson et al., 2008). Certain enzymes present in the mitochondrial matrix (e.g., aconitase, 1-galactono-γ lactone dehydrogenase, GAL) also contributes to the mitochondrial ROS pool (Andreyev et al., 2005; Rasmusson et al., 2008). The primary ROS generated in the mitochondria is $O_2^{·-}$, however it is dismutated to H_2O_2 spontaneously or enzymatically (Mn SOD-catalyzed), which can further generate $·OH$ by Fenton reaction (Møller, 2001). These ROS are important for intracellular signaling, however, their elevated levels cause oxidative damage within the mitochondria, affecting the bioenergetics of the cell (Mittler et al., 2011; Janků et al., 2019).

Peroxisomes, involved in lipid metabolism and photorespiration, are major sites of H_2O_2 production, particularly the glycolate oxidase, superoxide dismutase, flavin oxidase catalyzed reactions, and β-oxidation of fatty acids (Del Río et al., 2002; Del Río et al., 2006). Enzymatic reactions in peroxisomal lumen (xanthine oxidase, XOD) and membrane (contains a NAD(P)H dependent ETC) also contribute to $O_2^{·-}$ production (Del Río et al., 2002). Peroxisomes also generate RNS ($·NO$ and $ONOO^-$) that are involved in inter-organellar signaling, and pathogen-induced PCD (McDowell and Dangl, 2000; Corpas et al., 2001; Corpas et al., 2019; Corpas et al., 2020).

Reactive species are also generated at some secondary sites in plant cells like cytosol, cell wall, cell membrane, and apoplast (Kar, 2011). Plant cytosol is metabolically active and certain reactions result in the generation of ROS. For example, xanthine oxidase (XO, converts xanthine into uric acid) and AO (in aldehyde oxidation) comprise two major sources of $O_2^{·-}$ in the cytosol (Jajic et al., 2015). The cytosolic pool also contains ROS generated in different organelles (e.g., H_2O_2) that have traversed through membranes or via aquaporin-like channels (Bienert et al., 2007). A cell wall-associated peroxidase generates H_2O_2 for pathogen defense (Martinez et al., 1998), whereas plasma membrane-bound RBOH (respiratory burst oxidases homolog) generates $O_2^{\cdot-}$ in the apoplast, which is converted to H_2O_2 by apoplastic SOD and oxalate oxidase (OX) (Shapiguzov et al., 2012). Apoplast-localized class III peroxidases (POXs) are involved in the generation of $O_2^{\cdot-}$, H_2O_2, and $\cdot OH$ radicals (Podgórska et al., 2017). Endoplasmic reticulum (ER)-bound NADPH dependent cytochrome P450 system is also involved in the generation of $O_2^{\cdot-}$ in the ER lumen, which is spontaneously converted to H_2O_2, and results in the generation of $\cdot OH$ radical via Fenton reaction (Das and Roychoudhury, 2014; Janků et al., 2019). Generation of RNS ($\cdot NO$, $\cdot NO_2$, HNO_2, N_2O_4, $ONOO^-$, etc.) at multiple cellular locations by both enzymatic and nonenzymatic reactions also involve other reactive species/metabolites; however, some pathways are still not completely characterized (Del Río et al., 2015). Among these, $\cdot NO$ and $ONOO^-$ are the most important RNS, produced in multiple compartments (mitochondria, peroxisomes, chloroplast, plasma membrane) by different mechanisms (Corpas et al., 2004; Corpas and Barroso, 2014; Del Río et al., 2015).

6.5 Reactive Species: Detrimental and Beneficial Effects

The reactive species were initially considered detrimental, due to their highly reactive nature, however, their involvement in diverse cellular functions is now well established (Dickinson and Chang, 2011). Antioxidant systems maintain cellular 'ROS homeostasis,' and any disturbance in it also affects the cellular redox environment important for normal physiological functions (Mittler, 2017; Hasanuzzaman et al., 2020). The beneficial/detrimental effects of reactive species depend upon their cellular levels, reactivity, ability to traverse across membranes, and scavenging systems.

Reactive species can damage all important components including nucleic acids, proteins, and membranes causing damage to cellular functions and integrity (Table 6.1). Elevated ROS levels damage the DNA in multiple ways, and both nuclear and organellar (mitochondria, chloroplast) are prone to oxidative damage viz. oxidation of deoxyribose sugar, damage to nucleotides, strand breaks, base modifications, and cross-links, with both short-term and long-term effects (Evans et al., 2004; Sharma et al., 2012). The $\cdot OH$ radical causes extensive damage to DNA particularly, oxidation of nucleotide bases and sugars, strand breaks, DNA-protein cross-links, and base modifications (Oleinick *et al.*, 1987; Tsuboi *et al.*, 1998; Halliwell and Gutteridge, 1999). The compartmentalization of certain antioxidant enzymes (e.g., SODs) is important for the protection of organellar DNA, as they lack protection mediated by histones/other proteins, and are present in the vicinity of ROS-generation sites (Richter *et al.*, 1992; Sharma *et al.*, 2012). The reactive species also enhance the lipid peroxidation reaction, which causes extensive damage to membranes leading to loss of integrity of both cell and organelles. The double bonds in unsaturated fatty acids and ester linkage in the lipid molecules are prone to ROS-mediated oxidative damage (Mishra and Sharma, 2019). Both $O_2^{\cdot-}$ and $\cdot OH$ are capable of initiating the lipid peroxidation reaction, which can lead to the generation of additional lipid-derived radicals, thereby aggravating the oxidative stress, and associated damage (Gill *et al.*, 2010; Sharma *et al.*, 2012). Proteins, important structural/functional components of the cell, are damaged by reactive species in multiple ways, direct as well as indirect. Nitrosylation, carbonylation, and glutathionylation are direct modifications and can modulate the function of proteins (Banks and Andersen, 2019). Certain modifications are reversible while many others are irreversible, and may lead to fragmentation, aggregation, and proteolysis of modified protein molecules (Gill *et al.*, 2010). Sulfur-containing amino acids/thiol groups in proteins are more prone to ROS-mediated damage, and damage to Fe-S centers may result in the release of iron that can lead to the generation of $\cdot OH$, by Fenton reaction (Das and Roychoudhury, 2014). Among the RNS, $\cdot NO$ reacts with $O_2^{\cdot-}$ to form $ONOO^-$, a powerful oxidant/nitrating species, which causes nitration of prone residues in proteins (Radi, 2013).

All categories of reactive chemical species (ROS, RNS, RSS, RCS) produced in the cell are equally important for diverse physiological processes *viz.* growth and development, signaling, abiotic/biotic stress responses, protein modifications (Giles *et al.*, 2017; Mano *et al.*, 2019; Saddhe *et al.*, 2019; Hasanuzzaman *et al.*, 2020; Cejudo *et al.*, 2021). Phytohormones (e.g., ethylene and abscisic acid) crosstalk via ROS during stress responses (Kar, 2011) and regulate metabolic flux under stress conditions (Mittler, 2017). Certain ROS also divert the electrons away from the site of generation *viz.* chloroplast and mitochondria, to minimize local damage (Choudhury *et al.*, 2017;

Mittler, 2017). Among different ROS, the role of H_2O_2 as a signaling molecule is crucial for a diverse array of cellular functions related to growth and development, photosynthetic reactions, and in conferring tolerance to different biotic and abiotic stresses (Neill and Desikan, 2002; Niu and Liao, 2016; Hasanuzzaman et al., 2020). Similarly, among the RNS, ·NO functions as a key signaling molecule in several abiotic (UV, high light, high/low temperature, drought, salinity, etc.) and biotic stress responses (Yu et al., 2014; Del Río et al., 2015; Palma et al., 2019). For certain functions, ROS also interacts with other reactive species (RNS, RSS, and RCS) that work at different levels of signal transduction in different stress conditions (Hasanuzzaman et al., 2020). While RSS affects the generation and perception of ROS/RNS-mediated signaling (Kaur et al., 2019), RCS acts at downstream levels and mediates under different stress conditions (Biswas et al., 2019). The precise functional significance of many RNS, RSS, and RCS candidates is still not completely understood, which is also difficult due to their cross talks with each other (Del Río et al., 2015; Astier et al., 2018).

6.6 Cellular Antioxidant Defense Systems

The generation of different types of ROS, RNS, RSS, and RCS in the cell is a continuous, and inevitable process, with beneficial as well as detrimental effects. While the higher levels of reactive species can cause extensive damage to cellular components, extremely low levels can also have a negative impact (Mittler, 2017). Hence, physiological relevant levels of reactive species, important for several functions, are maintained by a complex, and well-coordinated network of antioxidant systems, comprising both nonenzymatic and enzymatic components (Gill and Tuteja, 2010; Hasanuzzaman et al., 2020). The cellular antioxidant defense system is responsible for an intricate balance of generation and scavenging of reactive species (cellular ROS homeostasis), which is important for an appropriate redox environment, and several processes crucial for normal growth and development (Mittler, 2017). Under adverse conditions, the cellular homeostasis of reactive species is disturbed and the antioxidant systems are modulated for protection against oxidative damage (Sharma et al., 2010). The two arms (nonenzymatic and enzymatic) of the antioxidant system include several important components that are briefly described below.

6.6.1 Nonenzymatic Antioxidants

Some of the important nonenzymatic components of the antioxidant system include ascorbic acid (AsA), glutathione (GSH), α-tocopherols, carotenoids, flavonoids, phenolic acids, alkaloids, amino acids (e.g. proline) that are involved in scavenging of reactive species in multiple cellular compartments (Gill and Tuteja, 2010; Hasanuzzaman et al., 2012; Hasanuzzaman et al., 2020). AsA (vitamin C) is highly abundant and one of the most powerful cellular antioxidant molecules, present in all the plant tissues for protection against oxidative damage (Smirnoff, 2005). It is highly abundant in the chloroplast, (~30–40% cellular concentration) while mitochondria play an important role in the synthesis, and continuous regeneration of the reduced ascorbate (ASH) (Foyer and Noctor, 2005; Szarka et al., 2007). ASH is a powerful ROS scavenger, protects cellular membranes from $O_2^{·-}$ and $·OH$ radical-mediated damage, is a component of important ASH-GSH cycle, and protects enzymes containing metal cofactors (Gill and Tuteja, 2010). Glutathione (GSH), actually a tripeptide (γGlu-Cys-Gly) is another important antioxidant molecule for protection against ROS-mediated damage. It is present in almost all cellular compartments and is crucial for diverse physiological processes including growth and development, and stress responses (Jimenez et al., 1998; Mullineaux and Rausch, 2005). Cellular balance of reduced (GSH) and oxidized (GSSG) forms of glutathione play a central role in the maintenance of redox environment, scavenging of ROS (e.g., $^1O_2$, H_2O_2, $·OH$), expression of stress-responsive genes, regeneration of AsA via AsA-GSH cycle, and protection of photosynthetic machinery from oxidative damage (Foyer and Halliwell, 1976; Larson, 1988; Foyer and Noctor, 2005; Gill and Tuteja, 2010). Another important metabolite is proline, a well-known stress-responsive compatible solute (Kavi Kishor et al., 2005), which is important for diverse cellular functions (Szabados and Savouré, 2005). It is an important nonenzymatic antioxidant against lipid peroxidation, damage due to $^1O_2$ and $·OH$ radicals, and therefore plays role in the mitigation of stress-induced ROS-mediated damage and ROS signaling (Alia and Saradhi, 1991; Chen and Dickman, 2005; Trovato et al., 2008). In addition, to the water-soluble metabolites discussed above, lipid-soluble molecules also play important antioxidant roles. Tocopherols (α, β, γ, and δ types) comprise a group of lipid-soluble molecules involved in scavenging of ROS (e.g., $^1O_2$), lipid-free radicals (prevents the chain propagation during oxidative damage), and minimizing membrane damage under stress conditions (Hollander-Czytko et al., 2005; Munné-Bosch, 2005; Liu et al., 2008). Another group of lipophilic antioxidants in plants is carotenoids (e.g., β-carotene), which transfer the absorbed light energy to the chlorophyll, and also serve as important ROS scavengers to protect photosynthetic machinery, signaling molecules in diverse mechanisms, and stress responses (Zigmantas et al., 2002; Li et al., 2008). One more category of antioxidants includes phenolic compounds including flavonoids (includes flavonols, flavones, isoflavones, and anthocyanin) that are involved in a diverse array of mechanisms including protection against UV light, pathogens, insects, and stress conditions (Winkel-Shirley, 2002; Gill and Tuteja, 2010; Sharma et al., 2012; Panche et al., 2016). Certain nonenzymatic antioxidants (e.g., melatonin) are capable of scavenging both ROS and RNS (Reiter et al., 2001).

6.6.2 Enzymatic Antioxidant Defense System

The other arm of the cellular antioxidant defense system comprises a battery of enzymes working in a coordinated manner to scavenge specific reactive species and reduce the levels of other secondary free radicals. The antioxidant enzymes maintain the cellular redox environment, play a crucial role in signaling and processes important for growth, physiology, and stress responses (Hasanuzzaman et al., 2020; Rajput et al., 2021). Some of the prominent antioxidant enzymes include SODs, CAT, POX, GR, APX, etc. (Fig. 6.1). SODs (EC: 1.15.1.1), which exists as multiple isoforms (based on catalytic metal cofactors, Fe, Mn, and CuZn), are responsible for dismutation of $O_2^{·-}$ radical in multiple cellular compartments as well as for reduction of $^·OH$ and H_2O_2 levels, indirectly (Gill et al., 2015). Catalases (CAT, EC: 1.11.1.6), tetrameric enzymes (heme-containing) and the first antioxidant enzyme to be discovered are responsible for the decomposition of H_2O_2. The catalases are present in peroxisomes as well as in a few other compartments and do not require cellular reductant for their catalytic function (Scandalios et al., 1997).

Ascorbate peroxidases (APX, EC: 1.1.11.1) are present in multiple cellular compartments, comprise the central component of the AsA-GSH cycle, and are essential for the maintenance of cellular ROS levels (Caverzan *et al.*, 2012). Guaiacol peroxidases (GOPX; EC: 1.11.1.7) are also heme-containing peroxidases (exists as multiple isoforms) present in multiple cellular compartments and associated with several biosynthetic processes as well as abiotic/biotic stress responses (Gill and Tuteja, 2010). Glutathione reductase (GR, EC: 1.6.4.2) is a flavoprotein oxidoreductase enzyme that catalyzes NAD(P)H dependent reduction of GSSG to GSH, maintains a high cellular GSH/GSSG ratio, and is important for the AsA-GSH cycle (Schulz *et al.*, 1978). Monodehydroascorbate reductase (MDHAR, EC: 1.6.5.4) is also a FAD (Flavin adenine dinucleotide) enzyme that uses NAD(P)H as the electron to catalyze the regeneration of AsA (Eltayeb *et al.*, 2007). Dehydroascorbate reductase (DHAR, EC: 1.8.5.1) catalyzes the reduction of DHA to AsA, in a reaction that uses reduced glutathione (GSH) and generates oxidized glutathione (GSSG) (Ushimaru *et al.*, 1997). Glutathione *S*-transferases (GST, EC: 2.5.1.18), involved in catalytic conjugation of glutathione to electrophilic substrates, are multi-functional enzymes involved in several metabolic processes and abiotic/biotic stress responses (Dixon *et al.*, 2010). Polyphenol oxidases (PPO, EC: 1.14.18.1) are copper-containing enzymes present in the chloroplast (thylakoid membranes) and are involved in the oxidation of mono- or diphenols to quinone, and defense responses (Araji *et al.*, 2014). Additionally, a few other enzymes like peroxiredoxins (PRX, EC 1.11.1.15) and thioredoxins (TRX, EC: 1.8.1.9) also play important role in the scavenging of reactive species (Hasanuzzaman *et al.*, 2020). An overview of coordination among some antioxidant systems is shown in Fig. 6.1.

The ROS and other reactive species (RNS, RSS, RCS) damage cellular components, and disrupts important cellular functions; however, they also play important roles in several physiological processes (Hasanuzzaman *et al.*, 2020). The antioxidant enzymes present in different cellular compartments are specific toward scavenging of a particular type of reactive species (e.g., SODs for $O_2^{\cdot-}$, CAT for H_2O_2), however, this indirectly affects levels of other reactive species also. For example, enzymatic scavenging of $O_2^{\cdot-}$ (by SODs) or H_2O_2 (by CAT) also reduces the generation of $\cdot OH$, as well as other reactive species (Janků et al., 2019). The coordinated action of antioxidant enzymes in different compartments is also important for intra-organellar ROS signaling for various molecular responses. For example, SOD isoforms present in different compartments are responsible for cellular ROS homeostasis, oxidative stress protection, generation of H_2O_2, and maintenance of its gradient, for signaling and different cellular processes (Janků et al., 2019; Rajput et al., 2021).

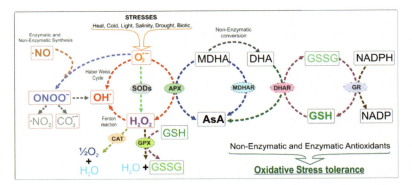

Figure 6.1 Schematic representation of interplay of some important antioxidant systems for ROS management in biological systems. SODs, superoxide dismutases; APX, ascorbate peroxidase; CAT: catalase; GPX, glutathione peroxidase; MDHAR, monodehydroascorbate reductase; DHAR, dehydroascorbate reductase; GR, glutathione reductase; $O_2^{·-}$, superoxide radical, ·OH, hydroxyl radical; H_2O_2, hydrogen peroxide; MDHA, monodehydroascorbate; DHA, dehydroascorbate; AsA, ascorbic acid; GSSG, oxidized glutathione, GSH, reduced glutathione; NADPH, nicotinamide adenine dinucleotide phosphate (reduced); NADP, nicotinamide adenine dinucleotide phosphate; ·NO, nitric oxide; ONOO⁻, peroxynitrite; ·NO₂, nitrogen dioxide; $CO_3^{·-}$, carbonate radical.

6.7 Multiple SOD Isoforms and Their Need in Biological Systems

The discovery of SODs in living systems lead to the theory that ROS are important mediators of oxygen toxicity, and are also important biological products (McCord et al., 1971; Fridovich, 1978; Foyer and Noctor, 2005). The basic reaction of the SODs is the 'metal cofactor catalyzed' dismutation of $O_2^{·-}$ into H_2O_2 and O_2. The SOD isoforms contain different types of metal cofactor for catalysis viz. Ni, Fe, Mn or Cu (Sheng et al., 2014). The SOD-catalyzed dismutation reaction is important for ROS homeostasis in organelles involved in aerobic metabolism, and equally important for the generation of other ROS (e.g., H_2O_2, $^{\cdot}OH$) and RNS (e.g., $OONO^-$) species involved in signaling (Hasanuzzaman et al., 2020).

The SODs have evolved to protect cellular components against ROS-mediated oxidative damage (Alscher, 2002). Plants cells harbor multiple SOD isoforms, localized to different cellular compartments, which play crucial roles in diverse physiological processes, cellular signaling, and oxidative stress tolerance (Alscher et al., 2002 and Gill et al., 2015). Based on the metal cofactor(s) present, plants harbor three types of SODs (Fe, Mn, and CuZn SODs) to maintain the ROS homeostasis in the compartments, active in oxidative metabolic reactions and to scavenge excess ROS generated in different conditions, including environmental perturbations (Alscher, 2002). The Fe SODs use iron as a catalytic cofactor and are localized in the chloroplasts (site of photosynthesis) while Mn SODs are present in mitochondria and are important for ROS scavenging during respiration. In addition, Mn SODs are present in peroxisomes that are metabolically linked to other organelles, and involved in diverse physiological processes, metabolic reactions, development, and abiotic/biotic stress responses (Pan et al., 2019). Plant cells also contain multiple types of CuZn SODs localized to different compartments such as chloroplasts, peroxisomes, cytosol, and apoplast (Alscher, 2002; Dreyer and Schippers, 2019). Multiple SODs are immensely useful in view of the compartmentalization of metabolic reactions in plant cells, and the inability of the $O_2^{\cdot-}$ to membrane barrier (Takahashi and Asada, 1983).

6.8 Nickel Superoxide Dismutase (Ni SOD)

Ni SOD is a special type of SOD that contains Ni metal ion as the catalytic co-actor for dismutation of $O_2^{\cdot-}$ into H_2O_2 and O_2, in diffusion-limiting conditions (Getzoff et al., 1983). The Ni SOD is not ubiquitous like other SOD isoforms, and has been discovered relatively recently in *Streptomyces* and cyanobacteria (Youn et al., 1996; Eitinger, 2004; Schmidt et al., 2009). The Ni SODs are localized in the cytosol, exist as homohexamer, and their presence in certain marine organisms is likely to be an outcome of convergent evolution

(Sheng, et al., 2014). Unlike other SOD isoforms, the active-site geometry of Ni SOD is quite unusual and comprises square planner Ni^{2+} coordinated to one histidine (His-1) and two cysteines (Cys-2, Cys-6) residues present at the N-terminal region of the enzyme (Wuerges et al., 2004). Nickel SOD is the only SOD isoform that contains S-donor ligands in the catalytic site (Ryan et al., 2010). The catalytic mechanism of Ni SOD is similar to the Fe- or Mn SODs, where dismutation of $O_2^{•-}$ occurs by cycling between M(III) and M(II) oxidation states of the metal ion (Ryan et al., 2010). The three-dimensional (3D) structure of the Ni SOD shares no homology with Fe-, Mn-, and CuZn SOD enzymes. Each subunit of the native Ni SOD (homohexamer) comprises a four α-helix bundle fold (up-down-up-down topology), and a hook-like structure at N-terminal for chelating a Ni ion, present at catalytic site (Barondeau et al., 2004). Ni SOD predominantly contains helical regions compared to other isoforms that also contain β-sheet secondary elements. Although the evolution of Nickel SOD is independent of the other three SOD isoforms, it uses similar strategies for restricting access to the catalytic site, and electrostatic steering (Perry et al., 2009; Barondeau et al., 2004). The Ni SOD is limited to only a few organisms, and not present in higher animals and plants (Miller, 2012).

6.9 Cambialistic Superoxide Dismutase (Fe/Mn SOD)

The superoxide dismutases are generally specific for one metal-cofactor type at the catalytic site, viz. Ni (Ni SOD), Fe (Fe SOD), and Mn (MnSOD). The CuZn SOD is a bimetallic SOD containing both the Cu and Zn metal cofactors per subunit, however, only Cu is involved in catalysis, and Zn is involved in stability and subunit interaction (Pelmenschikov and Siegbahn, 2005; Li et al., 2010). Certain types of SODs that are capable of accommodating either Fe or Mn cofactor at the active sites are referred to as 'cambialistic SODs' (Alscher et al., 2002). This special type of SODs belongs to the Fe/Mn SOD family, and share high similarity in primary sequence, secondary and tertiary structural elements, as well as electrical properties, and hence are able to catalyze the dismutation of $O_2^{•-}$ with either metal cofactor (Alscher et al., 2002; Schmidt et al., 1996). The cambialistic SODs are capable of using either cofactor as per the availability of metals in the medium (Gabbianelli *et al.*, 1995). The presence of cambialistic SODs in a certain group of microbes suggests that these might be beneficial under unfavorable conditions (Mandelli, 2013; Garcia *et al.*, 2017). The cambialistic SODs are present in relatively primitive organisms (Miller, 2012), and like Ni SOD this isoform is not present in higher animals and plants.

SOD isoforms in higher organisms use Fe, Mn, and CuZn as metal cofactors, and localize to different cellular compartments. The first and foremost factor important for this diversity of SODs was the preferential availability of certain metal ions due to atmospheric conditions, which was responsible for their integration in different catalytic proteins.

6.10 Iron Superoxide Dismutase (Fe SOD)

In the primitive anaerobic conditions, the major metal element in the soluble form was iron (as Fe^{2+}), which resulted in the evolution of Fe-containing proteins, including Fe SOD, the first SOD isoform to evolve (Bannister and Parker, 1985; Yamano *et al.*, 1999). Hence, Fe SOD (or FSD) with iron as catalytic cofactor are predominantly present in prokaryotic life forms, and it is presumed to have been acquired in the eukaryotic lineage by either endosymbiosis or lateral gene transfer, subsequently (Kanematsu and Asada, 1979; Grace, 1990; Martin *et al.*, 2003; Wolfe *et al.*, 2005). The dismutation of $O_2^{\cdot -}$ by Fe SODs involves the cycling of Fe ion from Fe (III) to Fe (II) and back to Fe (III) state (Miller, 2013). The plant Fe SOD isoforms are generally specific to chloroplasts and contain a chloroplastic targeting signal sequence (Alscher *et al.*, 2002; Fink and Scandalios, 2002). Evidence from the comparative analysis of Fe SODs in plants and cyanobacteria has suggested its origin in the chloroplasts and subsequent transfer to the nuclear genome during evolution (Bowler *et al.*, 1994; Alscher *et al.*, 2002). Fe SODs are sensitive to inactivation by H_2O_2 and are tolerant to KCN (Gill and Tuteja, 2010; Sheng *et al.*, 2014). Among different organisms, both homo-dimeric and homo-tetrameric forms of Fe SODs have been reported (Alscher *et al.*, 2002). In general, plants harbor multiple genomic loci coding for Fe SOD isoforms (Tyagi *et al.*, 2019). For instance, *A. thaliana* contains three chloroplastic Fe SODs, AtFSD1 (AT4G25100), AtFSD2 (AT5G51100), and AtFSD3 (AT5G23310), whereas *O. sativa* contains two, OsFSD1 (LOC_Os06g05110) and OsFSD2 (LOC_Os06g02500) (Kliebenstein *et al.*, 1998; Yadav *et al.*, 2019). However, the multiple Fe SODs show high conservation of catalytic site residues that include three histidines, and one aspartate (Pilon *et al.*, 2011; Fig. 6.2).

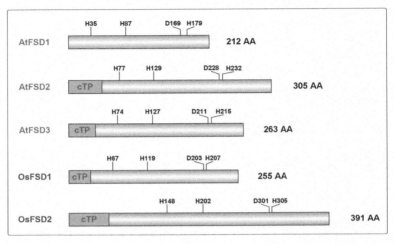

Figure 6.2 Schematic representation of important features of Fe SODs (FSDs) of *A. thaliana* (AtFSD1, AT4G25100; AtFSD2, AT5G51100; AtFSD3, AT5G23310) and *O. sativa* (OsFSD1, LOC_Os06g05110; OsFSD2, LOC_Os06g02500). Length of the different Fe SODs, location of chloroplastic targeting signal peptide (cTP), and positions of conserved active-site residues are indicated.

The plant Fe SODs are localized in chloroplasts, along with other SODs (e.g., Cu Zn SODs), and are responsible for the scavenging of $O_2^{·-}$ generated during photosynthesis (Pilon *et al.*, 2011). The Fe SODs, with relatively high α-helical and low β-sheet content, are structurally different than Cu Zn SODs and more similar to Mn SODs (Bowler *et al.*, 1994). The homology model of three *A. thaliana* Fe SODs and two *O. sativa* Fe SODs showed very similar folds and overall 3D structures (Fig. 6.3). The *N*-terminal contains the α-helical region while the C-terminal contains the α/β-domain (Perry *et al.*, 2011).

Besides chloroplasts, the plant Fe SODs have also been reported in other cellular compartments *viz.* cytoplasm (*V. unguiculata* and *A. thaliana*), nucleus (*A. thaliana*), as well as peroxisomes (*D. caryophyllus*) (Bowler *et al.*, 1994; Droillard and Paulin, 1990; Muñoz *et al.*, 2005; Priya *et al.*, 20007). Recent studies on multiple Fe SODs from *A. thaliana* have shown that these enzymes are also present at multiple locations *viz.* chloroplast, nucleus, and cytoplasm, and in particular AtFSD1 is also localized to the plasma membrane in response to salt stress (DvoEitiřák *et al.*, 2021). The three Fe SODs, AtFSD1, AtFSD2, and AtFSD3, in addition to the basic antioxidant function in chloroplastic, also participate in additional cellular functions (Gallie and Chen, 2019). The difference in the spatial distribution of FSDs also exists within the chloroplast, with AtFSD2 dispersed in stroma and AtFSD3 localized to the nucleoid region (Pilon *et al.*, 2011).

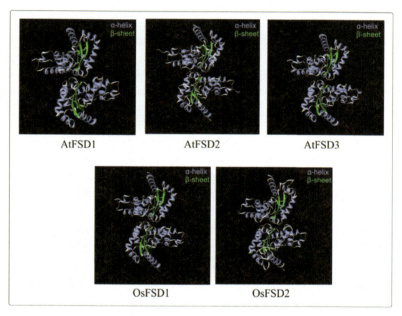

Figure 6.3 Homology models of Fe SODs (FSDs) of *A. thaliana* (AtFSD1, AT4G25100; AtFSD2, AT5G51100; AtFSD3, AT5G23310) and *O. sativa* (OsFSD1, LOC_Os06g05110; OsFSD2, LOC_Os06g02500) generated at SWISS-MODEL workspace homology modeling web server (https://swissmodel.expasy.org). Secondary elements (α-helix, β-sheet) in the two subunits of Fe SODs are shown in different colors.

The multiple Fe SODs also interact with each other and contribute toward additional functions in the chloroplast (Myouga *et al.*, 2008). Of the three *A. thaliana* Fe SODs, AtFSD1 and AtFSD2 are the outcome of an inter-chromosomal block duplication event, involving chromosomes 4 and 5 (https://bioinformatics.psb.ugent.be/plaza_

v4_5_dicots), and seems to have diverged subsequently. Heteromeric interaction between AtFSD2 (duplicate copy of AtFSD1) and AtFSD3 contributes toward chloroplast development and protection from oxidative damage (Myouga et al., 2008).

On the contrary, the rice genome contains only two non-duplicated FSDs (OsFSD1 and OsFSD2) and lacks the third gene corresponding to the *A. thaliana* homolog (AtFSD1). Similarly, the chloroplastic AtFSDs were also found to interact with plastid-encoded RNA polymerase (PEP) associated proteins (PAPs) complex as AtFSD2(PAP9) and AtFSD3(PAP4) that are crucial for activation of genes involved in photosynthesis and chloroplast development (Favier et al., 2021; Lee et al., 2019). Association of AtFSDs with PEP may also be important for the protection of transcription machinery from oxidative damage. Activation of Fe SODs also requires interaction with chaperonin 20 (CPN20), involved in the delivery of iron (Kuo et al., 2013).

Plant Fe SODs are also important for growth and development as *fsd* gene expression is modulated in a tissue- and stage-specific manner (Yadav et al., 2019). The Fe SODs are highly expressed in the early stage of development compared to other stages, which seems to be directed toward the protection of developing photosynthetically active tissues (Pilon et al., 2011; Yadav et al., 2019). The *fsd* genes are responsive to most of the abiotic stress conditions (salinity, heat, drought, cold, etc.), and are upregulated to minimize ROS-mediated mediated oxidative damage (Pilon et al., 2011; Yadav et al., 2019; Y. Zhou et al., 2017). Studies on transgenic *A. thaliana* plants lacking *fsd1* showed minor impact on plant phenotype, compared to plants lacking stromal *fsd* (*fsd2*) gene that showed severe developmental defects (retarded growth, pale yellow leaves), reduced chlorophyll content, and photosynthetic efficiency, while mutant plants lacking nucleoid *fsd* (*fsd3*) gene failed to survive beyond seedling stage (Gallie and Chen, 2019). Further, *fsd* double mutant (lacking *fsd2fsd3*) plants showed severe albino phenotype and high sensitivity to oxidative stress (Myouga et al., 2008). The complementation studies in mutant *fsd* plants showed distinct physiological functions of AtFSD2/AtFSD3. While AtFSD3 overexpression (in *fsd2* mutant) partially restored the AtFSD2 function and displayed improved growth and development, the AtFSD2 overexpression (in *fsd3* mutant) failed to rescue the plants beyond the seedling stage, indicating important and unique functions of stromal and nucleoid FSDs (Gallie and Chen,

2019). Overall the studies on plant Fe SODs show their importance in both stress responses and physiological processes crucial for normal growth and development.

6.11 Manganese Superoxide Dismutase (Mn SOD)

The Mn SOD is considered a primitive isoform like Fe SOD that evolved due to the increase in the concentration of oxygen in the atmosphere, leading to higher availability of soluble Mn (III) compared to iron (Alscher *et al.*, 2002). It is also presumed that the Mn SOD (or MSD) might have evolved from the Fe SODs via cambialistic type Fe/Mn SOD isoform (Alscher *et al.*, 2002; Sheng *et al.*, 2014). The prokaryotic and eukaryotic Mn SODs show high similarity (Bowler *et al.*, 1994). The Mn SODs are present in the mitochondrial compartment to scavenge $O_2^{\cdot-}$ radicals generated from the ETC and other oxidative reactions, which otherwise can damage mitochondrial enzymes containing Fe-S centers (e.g., aconitase) (Morgan *et al.*, 2008). Mn SOD maintains the mitochondrial redox environment by efficient dismutation of $O_2^{\cdot-}$ into H_2O_2, which is subsequently degraded (Morgan *et al.*, 2008). Some reports have also shown the presence of Mn SODs in peroxisomes of some plants (Sandalio and Del Río, 1987; Del Río *et al.*, 1992; Miller *et al.*, 2012). Mn SODs are resistant to either potassium cyanide (KCN) or H_2O_2 but inhibited by sodium azide (NaN_3), and exhibit peroxidase activity (Sheng *et al.*, 2014). Like Fe SOD, the Mn cofactor in the Mn SODs also alternates between (II) and (III) oxidation states for the dismutation of $O_2^{\cdot-}$ radical (Miller, 2012). The structural similarity between the Mn SODs and Fe SODs is also evident in the secondary structure element composition (Marques *et al.*, 2010). Like Fe SODs, the Mn SOD display high α-helical content compared to the β-sheets (Fig. 6.4). It contains one Mn atom per subunit at the catalytic sites and exists as homodimers or homotetramers.

However, despite high structural similarity with Fe SODs, the Mn SODs cannot utilize Fe as a catalytic cofactor for dismutation of $O_2^{\cdot-}$ (like cambialistic Fe/Zn SODs), which is indicative of its substantial divergence (Fridovich, 1986). The catalytic site residues (three histidines and one aspartate) are conserved in different Mn SODs as seen in *A. thaliana* and *O. sativa* (Fig. 6.5) and is similar to Fe SODs (Pilon *et al.*, 2011).

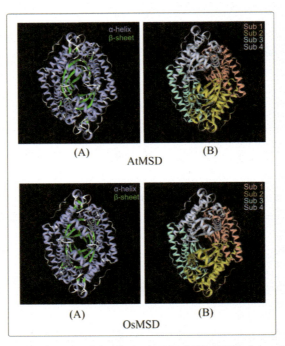

Figure 6.4 Homology models of single Mn SOD (MSD) from *A. thaliana* (AtMSD, AT3G10920, top panel) and *O. sativa* (OsMSD, LOC_Os05g25850, bottom panel) generated at SWISS-MODEL workspace homology modeling web server (https://swissmodel.expasy.org). (A) Secondary elements (α-helix and β-sheet) are indicated by different colors. (B) Arrangement of four monomeric subunits (Sub 1-4, indicated by different colors) to form homo-tetrameric Mn SODs.

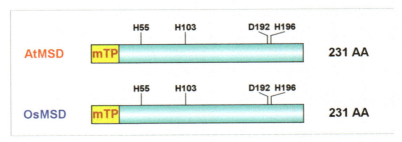

Figure 6.5 Schematic representation of important features of Mn SOD (MSD) of *A. thaliana* (AtMSD, AT3G10920) and *O. sativa* (OsMSD, LOC_Os05g25850). Length of the Mn SODs, location of mitochondrial targeting signal peptide (mTP), and positions of conserved active-site residues are indicated.

Mn SOD analysis in *A. thaliana* has shown that it is expressed to similar extent, in most tissues (Yadav *et al.*, 2019). Mn SOD is a crucial antioxidant enzyme that is responsive to diverse stress conditions such as heat, drought, salinity, low temperature, heavy metals, etc., and is important for the alleviation of stress-associated ROS toxicity (Gill *et al.*, 2015; Li *et al.*, 2017; Tyagi *et al.*, 2019; Saini *et al.*, 2021). It is also important for plant growth, maintenance of ROS homeostasis during embryo-sac development (Martin *et al.*, 2013). A recent study in *A. thaliana* has shown the involvement of 'Mn trafficking transporters for mitochondrial Mn SOD (AtMTM1 and AtMTM2)' in the functioning of Mn SOD, and Mn homeostasis (Hu *et al.*, 2021). Analysis of single (*Atmtm1*, *Atmtm2*) and double mutant (*Atmtm1* and *Atmtm2*) *A. thaliana* plants showed that both the MTM proteins interact with AtMnSOD, responds to oxidative stress, and also play important role in root growth, flowering-time (Hu *et al.*, 2021).

6.12 Copper Zinc Superoxide Dismutases (CuZn SODs)

The evolution of the third category of superoxide dismutase, CuZn SOD, was quite late compared to the Fe and Mn SODs (Saito *et al.*, 2003). The complete transition of atmosphere into oxidizing type (completely replenished with oxygen) resulted in the higher availability of the soluble Cu(II) compared to Fe(II) (Alscher *et al.*, 2002). This resulted in the initiation of incorporation of Cu(II) into cellular metalloproteins including SODs, however, due to differences in characteristics of Cu-metal (w.r.t. Fe or Mn), major structural changes were also incorporated in the protein (Bannister *et al.*, 1991). Hence, the Fe and Mn SODs share substantial structural homology compared to the third isoform or CuZn SODs (Alscher *et al.*, 2002). The CuZn SODs are present in both prokaryotes and eukaryotes, however, the diversity of many isoforms localized in multiple cellular compartments is much higher. In plants, the CuZn SOD isoforms appear to have evolved after the evolution of *M. polymorpha* (common liverwort or umbrella liverwort) (Dreyer, and Schippers, 2019). The major isoforms of plant CuZn SODs are localized in different compartments, cytosol (CSD1), chloroplast (CSD2), and peroxisomes (CSD3) and apoplast (Huang *et al.*, 2012). The different CuZn SOD isoforms show sequence heterogeneity ranging from 10–32% (Alscher *et al.*, 2002); however, the active-site residues are highly conserved. Different CuZn SODs exist as dimers (cytosolic, peroxisomal) or homotetramers (chloroplast, apoplast), where each subunit is capable of full catalytic activity (Bordo *et al.*, 1994; Fridovich, 1986).

The CuZn SOD isoforms show conserved secondary elements (higher β-sheet content and low α-helical content) and a similar overall 3D structure, which is very different from the structure of Fe and Mn SODs (Fig. 6.6). Each subunit of CuZn SOD (in dimeric/tetrameric forms) folds as an eight-stranded, Greek-key β-barrel, with eight β-strands and seven connecting loops, of which Greek-key loop, LIV (contains Zn sub-loop and disulfide sub-loop), and LVII/electrostatic loop are important. Loop LVII acts as an active-site lid to limit solvent access to the metal-binding sites (Yogavel *et al.*, 2008; Perry *et al.*, 2010). The Cu/Zn SOD has an intra-subunit disulfide bond that is important for the stability of the enzyme (Bouldin, 2012).

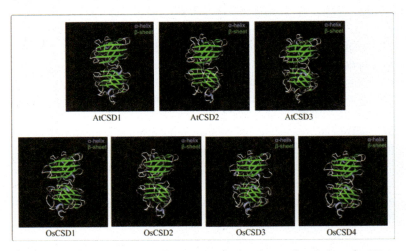

Figure 6.6 Homology model of CuZn SOD (CSD) isoforms of *A. thaliana* (AtCSD1, AT1G08830; AtCSD2, AT2G28190; AtCSD3, AT5G18100) and *O. sativa* (OsCSD1, LOC_Os03g22810; OsCSD2, LOC_Os08g44770; OsCSD3, LOC_Os03g11960; OsCSD4, LOC_Os07g46990) generated at SWISS-MODEL workspace homology modeling web server (https://swissmodel.expasy.org). Secondary elements (α-helix and β-sheet) are indicated by different color.

The CuZn SODs are sensitive to KCN as well as H_2O_2 treatment (Sheng et al., 2014). The conservation of secondary elements and overall structure is evident in the 3D-homology models of CuZn SOD isoforms of *A. thaliana* (cytosolic: AtCSD1, chloroplastic: AtCSD2, peroxisomal: AtCSD3) and *O. sativa* (cytosolic: OsCSD1, LOC_Os03g22810 and OsCSD4, LOC_Os07g46990; chloroplastic: OsCSD2, LOC_Os08g44770; peroxisomal: OsCSD3, LOC_Os03g11960). The two *O. sativa* cytosolic isoforms (OsCSD1 and OsCSD4) have evolved due to a block duplication event in the genome (https://bioinformatics.psb.ugent.be/plaza_v4.5_monocots).

Different CuZn SODs are responsible for scavenging of $O_2^{\cdot-}$ radical generated in different cellular compartments *viz.* chloroplast, peroxisomes, cytosol, and apoplast (Gill and Tuteja, 2015). The cytosolic CuZn SODs (AtCSD1, OsCSD1, and OsCSD4) are responsible for scavenging of $O_2^{\cdot-}$ generated in reactions catalyzed by cytosolic enzymes (e.g., XO and AO) (Janků et al., 2019). The cytosolic CSDs are also known to localize to the nucleus (Xu et al., 2010). The chloroplasts are major sites of ROS production, which is substantially higher than metabolically active mitochondria (Hasanuzzaman et al., 2020), hence multiple SODs (e.g., Arabidopsis: AtCSD2, AtFSD1, AtFSD2, and AtFSD3; Rice: OsCSD2, OsFSD1, and OsFSD2) are present in these organelles for scavenging of $O_2^{\cdot-}$ generated in reactions at both the photosystems (PS I and PS II). The chloroplastic CuZn SODs also contain a chloroplastic targeting signal at *N*-terminal, as seen in the corresponding Fe SODs.

The peroxisomal Cu Zn SODs (AtCSD3 and OsCSD3) are responsible for scavenging of the $O_2^{\cdot-}$ generated due to the enzymatic reactions in the peroxisomes, including photorespiration (Corpas et al., 2001; Del Río et al., 2016). These groups of Cu Zn SODs contain PTS1 (C-terminal tripeptide) or PTS2 (close to *N*-terminal) type signal sequence for targeting the enzyme to the peroxisomes (Huang et al., 2012). The multiple CuZn SODs present in different cellular compartments are not only important for localized $O_2^{\cdot-}$ scavenging but also for regulation of ROS-mediated signaling in a spatio-temporal manner (Janků et al., 2019). A recent study has shown that a chloroplast-localized protein EGY3 helps in chloroplastic

ROS homeostasis and also stabilizes chloroplastic CuZn SOD in *A. thaliana* by inhibiting its degradation (Zhuang *et al.*, 2021).

6.13 Dynamics of Regulation and Functioning of SODs

The expression of genes in prokaryotes and eukaryotes is regulated at multiple levels. Unlike the genes involved in a single reaction/pathway, those involved in multiple pathways/conditions are regulated by complex mechanisms, which may also crosstalk for a more dynamic response, as per cellular needs. As SODs play crucial roles in diverse conditions including growth, development, and abiotic/biotic stress responses (Gill *et al.*, 2015; Janků *et al.*, 2019), the cellular levels of the enzymes need to the dynamically, and precisely regulated in response to different intrinsic and extrinsic factors with involvement of multiple mechanisms.

6.13.1 *cis* Elements–Mediated Regulation of SODs

The expression of a gene is affected by multiple factors including both *cis* and *trans* components. Regulatory regions present upstream to the coding region include general promoter elements such as the TATA box, CAAT box, GC box that are required for the basic transcription machinery (e.g., RNA polymerase, transcription factors) to initiate the transcription (Joshi *et al.*, 2016). Several other condition-specific regulatory elements referred to as '*cis*-regulatory elements' are also present, and are responsible for the expression of the gene in diverse conditions (Singh, 1998; Kaufmann *et al.*, 2010; Bilas *et al.*, 2016; Ng *et al.*, 2018). As the plant SOD genes respond to a variety of conditions (cellular requirements, phytohormone signaling, biotic/abiotic stress responses), they harbor diverse types of *cis*-elements in the vicinity of the coding regions (Mishra *et al.*, 2019).

Some of the common categories of *cis*-regulatory elements present in plant SOD isoforms include motifs responsive to light (3-AF1 binding site, ACE, G-box, Gap-box, I-box, GT-1), ultraviolet light (AP-1), heat stress (heat shock I, II), cold stress (LTR, Y-box), wound response (WUN-motif), defense and stress response (TC-rich repeats), anaerobic induction (ARE/GC-motif), drought inducibility (MBS), GTAC-motif (SPL7), CORE motif, H_2O_2 (AP-1), abscisic acid response (ABRE), auxin response (TGA-element, AuX RR core), gibberellin response (P-box, GARE-motif, TATC-box), jasmonic acid response (TGACG/CGTCA-motif), salicylic acid response (TCA-element), ethylene response (ERE), meristem specific activation (CAT-box), pathogen defense and elicitor (W-box), factor binding (ACGT, leucine zipper; bHLH, helix-loop-helix proteins; bZIP, leucine zipper), circadian rhythm (circadian), etc. (Tsukamoto *et al.*, 2005; Yamasaki *et al.*, 2009; Wang *et al.*, 2018; Tounsi *et al.*, 2019; Zhou *et al.*, 2019).

The expression of multiple *A. thaliana* Fe SODs is regulated by *cis*-acting regulatory elements, which show diversity in copy number and specificity to conditions (Verma *et al.*, 2019; Zhou *et al.*, 2019). *In silico* studies have shown the presence of several *cis*-elements associated with light, phytohormones, defense, and stress responses in both monocots and dicots (Jiang *et al.*, 2019; Verma *et al.*, 2019; Yadav *et al.*, 2019). In addition, several *trans*-acting transcription factors affect the Fe SOD expression in specific conditions. For example, AtMEKK1 mediates activation of AtMKK5-AtMPK6/3 signaling cascade under salinity as well high light to enhance expression *fsds* and *csds* and is important for ROS-induced oxidative stress management (Xing *et al.*, 2013; 2015) (Fig. 6.7, left panel). Similarly, SPL7 (Squamosa promoter-binding-like protein 7) induces multiple genes including miR398 (down-regulates CSDs) for induction of chloroplastic *fsds* under Cu-deprivation (Pilon *et al.*, 2011) (Fig. 6.7, right panel). An overview of the complexity of mechanisms involved in stress perception, signal transduction, and activation of SOD-mediated adaptive responses for salinity, high light, and low copper conditions is shown in Fig. 6.7.

The diversity of *cis*-elements in different SOD isoforms indicates their involvement in response to different intrinsic and extrinsic stimuli, however, many other regulatory mechanisms operating on SODs, or affecting the cross-talking/interacting partners, and upstream/downstream candidates in the response pathways, are also instrumental in the overall expression profiles of the SODs.

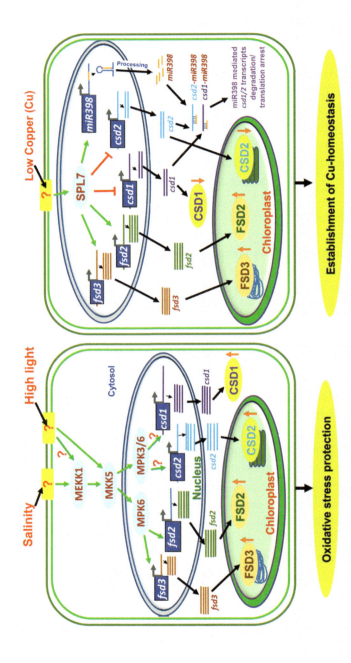

Figure 6.7 Schematic representation of mechanisms involved in stress perception, signal transduction, and activation of expression of SODs in plants, mediated by AtMEKK1 in response to high light and salinity (left panel) and SPL7 under low copper condition (right panel). Green arrows indicate activation, red lines indicate inhibition, orange-colored arrows indicate upward/down-regulation at the protein level.

6.13.2 MicroRNA miR398–Mediated Regulation of CuZn SODs

Regulation of gene expression in higher plants and animals is not as straightforward as in prokaryotes. In addition to transcription and translation level controls, regulatory mechanisms also operate at posttranscription and posttranslation levels (Haak *et al.*, 2017). Recently identified non-coding RNAs (as ncRNAs) operate at multiple levels to make the overall process more dynamic and highly complex (Patil *et al.*, 2014). MicroRNAs (miRNAs), small 21–25 nt ncRNAs, regulate the expression of plant genes in diverse processes (growth, development, phase transitions, circadian rhythm, biotic/abiotic stress responses, etc.) by guiding the cleavage of target transcripts or translation repression (Sunkar *et al.*, 2012; Waititu *et al.*, 2020). Reports have established that miR398 regulates the expression of CuZn SODs in plants (Sunkar *et al.*, 2006; Jagadeeswaran *et al.*, 2009). Regulation of CuZn SODs by multiple miR398 members (e.g., Arabidopsis: *AtmiR398a, AtmiR398b, AtmiR398c*; rice: *OsmiR398a, OsmiR398b*) is affected by several factors. The miR398 members differ in *cis*-regulatory elements resulting in their differential expression under various conditions (Li *et al.*, 2017). Sequence variations also affect the secondary structures of the precursor transcripts resulting in differential cleavage efficiency to generate mature microRNAs (Belén *et al.*, 2018). The sequence differences among mature miR398 members can also affect the recognition/cleavage efficiency of the target CuZn SODs (Li *et al.*, 2010; Saini *et al.*, 2021).

MicroRNA miR398 modulates the RNA and/or protein levels of plant cytosolic as well as chloroplastic CuZn SODs in a dynamic manner for diverse functions (Zhu *et al.*, 2011; Saini *et al.*, 2012). The down-regulation of CuZn SODs under certain conditions (e.g., copper deficiency, sucrose; heat stress) is mediated by up-regulation of miR398 (Yamasaki *et al.*, 2005; Abdel-Ghany and Pilon, 2008; Dugas and Bartels, 2008; Guan *et al.*, 2013), and for up-regulation of CuZn SODs (high light, high Cu^{2+}, Fe^{3+}, methyl viologen/paraquat) miR398 itself is down-regulated (Sunkar *et al.*, 2006). Under Cu limiting conditions, the miR398 down-regulates the CuZn SOD isoform levels and helps to channelize Cu to other proteins important for photosynthesis (Yamasaki *et al.*, 2007; Abdel-Ghany and Pilon, 2008; Shahbaz and Pilon, 2019). Transgenic plant experiments have shown that controlling the levels of *miR398* (or modification of target site complementarity) modulates the levels of CuZn SODs (Dugas and Bartels, 2008), leading to enhanced stress tolerance (Sunkar *et al.*, 2006). In addition to its direct impact, miR398 also affects the folding and maturation of CuZn SODs, indirectly. It targets the copper chaperone for SODs (CCS), which play a crucial role in the delivery of Cu cofactor to the active sites of the different CuZn SODs, and affects their maturation and activity in the cell (Beauclair *et al.*, 2010). The miR398-mediated posttranscriptional regulation can rapidly regulate the CuZn SODs levels in multiple ways, in response to different conditions (Lu *et al.*, 2010), including copper limiting conditions (Fig. 6.7). MicroRNA *miR398* also plays a central role in the regulation of thermotolerance in *A. thaliana* (Guan *et al.*, 2013). The role of miR398-mediated regulation in different conditions is becoming more complex. A recent report has shown that *cis*-natural antisense transcripts (NATs) of *miR398* genes also interfere with the biogenesis of the *miR398*, which has been shown to attenuate the associated thermotolerance (Li *et al.*, 2020). Such *cis*-NAT:miR398 interactions may also have important implications in other regulatory functions associated with *miR398*, and advocates further investigations on such functional dynamics.

6.13.3 Alternative Splicing in Regulation and Functioning of SODs

The genes structure of prokaryotes is simple, whereas in higher organisms including plants the non-coding regions (introns) disrupt the continuity of the coding region in most genes, and this was first reported in 1977 (Reddy, 2007). A posttranscriptional mechanism, known as 'splicing or constitutive splicing (CS),' excises introns and joins exons to generate mature transcripts in eukaryotes (Reddy, 2007). Interestingly, under certain conditions, one precursor transcript may also generate multiple alternative mature transcripts by the 'alternative splicing (AS)' process (Reddy, 2007; Chaudhary *et al.*, 2019) (Fig. 6.8). In recent years, several high-throughput genomics/transcriptomics studies have shown that multiple AS-events (intron retention, IR; exon skipping, ES; mutually exclusive exons, MEE; 5´ alternative splice site, 5´ ASS; 3´ alternative splice site, 3´ ASS) affects a majority of the intron-containing genes in both plants and animals (Barbazuk *et al.*, 2008; Marquez *et al.*, 2012;

Chaudhary *et al.*, 2019). AS enhances the transcriptome/proteome diversity, regulates transcripts and/or protein levels, channelizes transcripts/protein isoforms to different fates, and play important roles in a diverse array of cellular processes in plants including stress responses, and stress-memory (Reddy *et al.*, 2013; Gracz, 2016; Ling *et al.*, 2018; Laloum *et al.*, 2018; Ganie and Reddy, 2021).

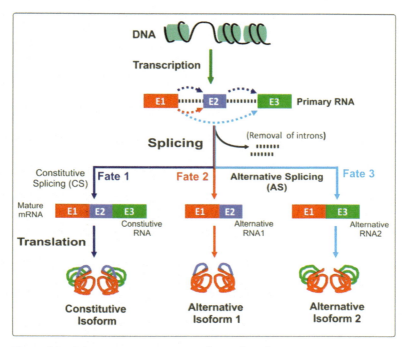

Figure 6.8 Schematic representation of CS and AS of an intron-containing plant gene, leading to the formation of multiple transcripts and protein isoforms. E1–E3 indicates different exons (coding regions), horizontal dashed lines indicate introns and differently colored curved arrows (dashed) indicate various splicing events. Alternative fates of the primary transcript by AS-events are also shown at both RNA and protein levels.

SODs, being important antioxidant enzymes, are regulated at multiple levels, and several studies have indicated the involvement of alternative splicing of certain SODs in different plants including *O. sativa* (Feng *et al.*, 2006; Saini *et al.*, 2021), *P. trichocarpa* (Srivastava *et al.*, 2009), *G. max* (Sagasti *et al.*, 2014) and *A. thaliana* (Lee *et al.*, 2019). The analysis based on RNA-Seq data and *in silico* splicing junction predictions has shown the existence of multiple alternatively spliced transcripts of Fe, Mn, and CuZn SOD isoforms in both *A. thaliana* (https://www.arabidopsis.org) and *O. sativa* (http://rice.plantbiology.msu.edu/; http://www.ic4r.org/). Only some of these, as mentioned above, have been studied, and the functional significance of many others with variations in coding and non-coding regions is still not completely known. Rice genome contains seven SODs, four CuZn SODs (cytosolic, peroxisomal, and chloroplastic), two Fe SODs (chloroplastic), and a single mitochondrial Mn SOD, which generates a total of seven constitutive and seven alternative transcripts (http://rice.plantbiology.msu.edu/). The AS-transcripts are formed by events in the UTRs, coding regions, or both, indicating possible impacts on function at RNA or protein level (Saini *et al.*, 2021). The splicing pattern of the rice SODs are affected by different abiotic stress conditions (salinity, drought, metal, low temperature, and oxidative stress), suggesting that AS-mediated modulation of transcript levels can contribute toward to regulation of expression of all the three (Fe, Mn and CuZn type) SOD isoforms (Saini *et al.*, 2021).

In both *A. thaliana* and *O. sativa*, the Fe SODs undergo alternative splicing to generate alternative isoforms (Rice Genome Annotation Project, RGAP: http://rice.uga.edu/ and The Arabidopsis Information Resource, TAIR: https://www.arabidopsis.org). In *A. thaliana*, AS of *Atfsd3* (nucleoid-localized AtFSDs) produces two transcripts (*fsd3* and *fsd3s*) due to an intron retention (IR) event, leading to variation in the coding regions. Both the isoforms harbor SOD activity, however the smaller alternative isoform (AtFSD3S) anchors to a chloroplastic membrane (contains AS-introduced transmembrane region), and negatively impacts chloroplast development (Lee *et al.*, 2019). In *O. sativa*, the alternative splicing of OsFSD1 is modulated by different abiotic stress conditions, which can have structural and/or functional implications (Saini *et al.*, 2021). The AS-event in the coding region of *O. sativa Osfsd2* (homolog of *Atfsd3*) generates two transcripts (*Osfsd*-a and *Osfsd*-b) that show differential tissue- and stress-specific (light, cold) expression patterns at RNA levels, was also found to be enzymatically active (*in vitro*) despite substantial C-terminal truncation (Feng *et al.*, 2006).

In *A. thaliana* and *O. sativa*, the Mn SODs (*loci* AT3G10920 and LOC_Os05g25850, respectively) display different types of AS-events suggesting different fates and functional significance of the transcripts. In a study in *G. max*, the role of AS was also observed in the splicing difference in CCS and chloroplastic CuZn SOD (CSD2) in response to copper availability (Sagasti *et al.*, 2014). These limited studies highlight the importance of AS-generated SOD isoforms. The presence and dynamic regulation of multiple alternative transcripts suggest their importance in the regulation and/or functioning of SODs, however, many of these isoforms need to be investigated thoroughly.

6.13.4 Copper Chaperone for Superoxide Dismutase (CCS)–Mediated Regulation and Functioning of CuZn SODs

The levels of CuZn SOD (and other Cu-containing metalloenzymes) are also linked to the Cu status of the cell (Yamasaki *et al.*, 2009). Plants contain multiple mechanisms for uptake and translocation of metals to different locations (Printz *et al.*, 2016). Some elements (e.g., Zn^{2+}, Mn^{2+}, Fe^{2+}, Cu^{2+}) are important for stability, interactions, and catalysis of proteins/enzymes, particularly those involved in redox reactions (Holm *et al.*, 1996; Barber-Zucker *et al.*, 2017). Since certain metal ions can participate in redox cycling reactions leading to ROS-damage, control and targeted delivery of free metals to a particular site or target protein in the cell is facilitated by metalloproteins/metallochaperones (Rae *et al.*, 1999; Aguirre *et al.*, 2016). A specific metallochaperone, copper chaperone for SODs (CCS) delivers Cu to the active site of CuZn SODs (Rae *et al.*, 1999; Cohu *et al.*, 2009), and concomitantly, prevent redox cycling of free Cu between Cu(I) and Cu(II) states, and associated oxidative damage (Cohen and d'Arcy Doherty, 1987). Unlike, a wide distribution of CuZn SODs in different domains of life, CCS is not equally ubiquitous. The CCS is absent in many simple organisms, containing CuZn SODs, and is rather restricted to complex higher organisms including plants, which may also confer an advantage in unfavorable conditions (Dreyer and Shippers, 2019).

The CCS protein, identified first in *S. cerevisiae*, shows a conserved domain structure (Dreyer and Shippers, 2019) containing metallochaperone (I), SOD homologous (II), and short carboxyl-terminal peptide (III) domains (Schmidt *et al.*, 1999). Domain I and

III are important for the delivery of Cu cofactor via heteromeric interactions, while II (central domain) physically interacts with the CuZn SOD (Lamb et al., 2001). The CCS: CuZn SOD interaction also facilitates intra-molecular disulfide bond (-S-S-) formation converting the enzyme into an active form (Huang et al., 2012). The important features of CCS protein and mechanism of activation of CuZn SODs seem conserved among different eukaryotes; however, some CCS-independent alternative pathways also do exist in the way different CuZn SOD isoforms (cytosolic, chloroplastic, peroxisomal) are activated (Dreyer and Shippers, 2019).

The *A. thaliana* CCS gene (AtCCS, At1g12520) codes for 320 amino acid long constitutive CCS isoform (CCS-SV1), and two alternative isoforms (CCS-SV2 and CCS-SV3, *https://www.arabidopsis.org*). The AS-event results in loss of *N*-terminal chloroplast-targeting peptide, that is, transit peptide (TP) in both CCS-SV1 and CCS-SV2 (Fig. 6.9). The CCS-SV1 isoform is localized in chloroplast and involved in activation of chloroplastic CuZn SOD (CSD2) (Abdel-Ghany et al., 2005), while the other CCS isoforms lacking *N*-terminal signal may be involved in activation of cytosolic (CSD1) and peroxisomal (CSD3) CuZn SODs (Huang et al., 2012; Dreyer and Shippers, 2019). Interestingly, due to AS-event, the CCS-SV2 isoform lacks both chaperone domain (I) and *N*-terminal cTP region (Fig. 6.9), which may have important implications in the role of CCS in the interaction and activation of CuZn SODs. The *O. sativa* CCS gene (LOC_Os04g48410) codes for a constitutive CCS isoform similar to Arabidopsis CCS, in length (312 amino acids) and domain organization, however, AS-event generates only one alternative isoform. While the constitutive isoform (OsCCS-SV1, 312 amino acids) contains all domains, the alternative isoform (OsCCS-SV2, 249 amino acids) lacks domain II (SOD binding domain) and III C-terminal regions (Fig. 6.9). The AS-events affected the *O. sativa* OsCCS gene in a manner different than *A. thaliana*.

The AS can modulate the levels and function of CCS genes at two levels: (1) modulation of multiple CCS transcripts levels in response to different conditions, and (2) functional involvement/interference in CuZn SOD activation. Since the alternative splicing events impact the CCS differently in *A. thaliana* and *O. sativa*, its functional implications are likely to be different in these two, and other plant species. Furthermore, the cellular levels (and functions) of CCS are also regulated by miR398, which control the levels of all three CCS splice variants in *A. thaliana* (Beauclair et al., 2010). Under copper

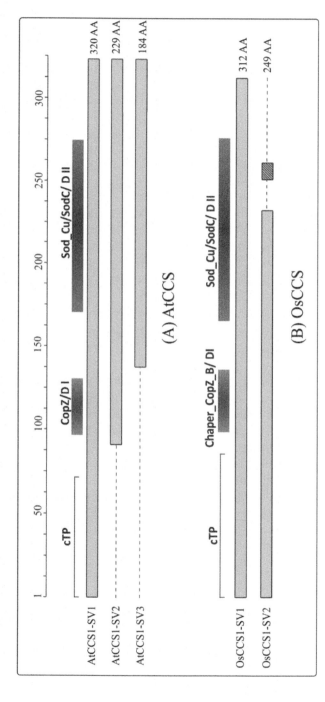

Figure 6.9 Comparison of outcome of alternative splicing on domain organization of CCS of *A. thaliana* (A) and *O. sativa* (B). Protein coding regions are indicated by gray boxes, dashed lines indicate regions removed by AS-events, gray boxes with different patterns indicate AS-incorporated alternative coding regions. Chloroplastic targeting peptide (cTP), Domain I (Copz/Chaper_CopZ_B, associated with metal delivery and chaperone function), and Domain II (DII, Sod_Cu/SodC, involved in interacting with CuZn SOD) are indicated in the figure as per analysis at Conserved Domain Database (CDD) database of NCBI.

limitation/deficiency the miR398 down-regulates the CCS (and CuZn SODs) to channelize the Cu to important cellular proteins (Abdel-Ghany and Pilon, 2008; Shahbaz and Pilon, 2019). Additionally, miR398-mediated down-regulation of CCS and CuZn SODs is also an important component of thermotolerance in Arabidopsis (Guan et al., 2013). In *A. thaliana*, the CuZn SODs are activated by either CCS-dependent (chloroplastic isoform, CSD2) or CCS-independent and (glutathione-dependent, peroxisomal isoform, CSD3) or both (cytosolic isoform, CSD1) the pathways (Huang et al., 2012). Direct CCS interaction-mediated SOD activation is quite intriguing; however, recently involvement of Ctr1 (a copper transporter) has also been shown, where initially formation of a stable CuZn SOD:CCS: Ctr1 heterotrimer is required for SOD activation, followed by dissociation of the complex, post-activation (Skopp et al., 2019). Such, interactions may also be involved in the activation CuZn SOD in other plants. Apart from CuZn SOD, Fe SOD also require a chaperone protein chaperonin 20 (CPN20), involved in the delivery of iron to the enzyme (Kuo et al., 2013).

6.13.5 Role of Posttranslational Modifications (PTMs) in SOD Functioning

The level and functional state of cellular proteins are continually altered in response to physiological needs and environmental perturbations. As seen in previous sections, SODs are regulated by multiple mechanisms that operate at different levels. The SODs are also affected by posttranslational modifications (PTMs), which affect the localization, assembly, function, signaling, and stability of cellular proteins (Yamakura and Kawasaki, 2010). The PTMs can occur at any region of the protein, display cellular compartment specificity, and affects diverse characteristics, for example, *N*-glycosylation (protein folding, sorting), *O*-glycosylation (structure, signaling), O-linked sugars (interaction, signaling, crosstalk), phosphorylation (function, signaling, localization), ubiquitination (degradation), etc. (Millar et al., 2019). The PTMs can introduce features/characteristics in proteins, other than solely based on their primary structure/sequence. Reports of PTMs on SOD isoforms from humans and yeast have shown enhancement of functional diversity and characteristics in different conditions (Yamakura and Kawasaki, 2010; Banks and Anderson, 2019). Some important PTM sites in human SOD1 are shown below in Fig. 6.10, where the conserved sites may indicate the possibility of similar PTMs and fates in plant CuZn SODs.

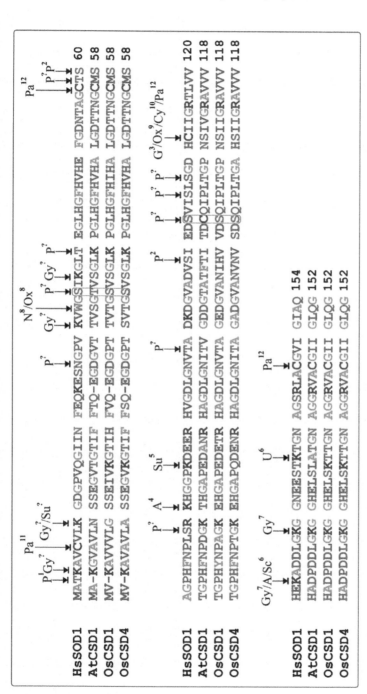

Figure 6.10 Multiple sequence alignment of cytosolic SODs of humans (HsSOD1), Arabidopsis (AtCSD1), and rice (OsCSD1 and OsCSD4), and important PTM sites in SOD1. P: phosphorylation, A: acetylation, Sc: succinylation, Su: Sumoylation, U: ubiquitination, Gy: glycation, Ox: oxidation, G: glutathionylation; Cy: cysteinylation, N: nitration; Pa: palmitoylation. The impact of some PTMs is indicated by superscript symbols:: 1: stabilizes dimer, 2: re-localization into the nucleus, 3: promotes subunit dissociation, 4: inactivates ROS scavenging activity, 5: enhanced stability, and propensity to aggregate, 6: ubiquitination occurs after aggregation, 7: enzyme deactivation, 8: enhanced aggregation, 9: misfolding, 10: protects from oxidation, 11: reduces enzyme activity, 12: maturation, membrane anchoring,?: unknown fate.

Posttranslational modifications involving phosphorylation of threonine/serine residues affect SOD function, dimerization, and its role as a transcription factor (Tsang et al., 2014; Banks and Anderson, 2019). Lysine residues can undergo different types of PTMs viz. succinylation, acetylation, sumoylation, ubiquitination, glycation with a wide range of effects (inactivation, enhanced stability, and aggregation) (Banks and Anderson, 2019). Residues such as cysteine and tryptophan are prone to redox modification like oxidation (cause misfolding, aggregation) and glutathionylation (destabilizes dimer and promotes aggregation), while cysteinylation protects the enzyme from oxidation and aggregation (Banks and Anderson, 2019). Some PTMs are also reversible viz. lysine acylation that affects SOD function and palmitoylation (S-acylation), which affects localization by targeting (and anchoring) it to the cell membrane (Antinone et al., 2013; Antinone et al., 2017).

Among the RNS, NO-mediated S-nitrosylation and tyrosine nitration modulate the properties and functions of proteins (Astier and Lindermayr, 2012), whereas $ONOO^-$-mediated nitration leads to partial/complete loss of activity of different SOD isoforms (Demicheli et al., 2007; Martinez et al., 2014). The $ONOO^-$-mediated nitration of tyrosine residues affected the AtFSD3 most, followed by AtFSD2 and AtFSD1 (Holzmeister et al., 2015). Furthermore, it is interesting to see that certain sites (Lys-10, Lys-122, Trp-33, City-112, Fig. 6.10) can undergo more than one type of PTM suggesting functional importance in diverse conditions. In plants, the studies on PTM-mediated effects on SODs are rather limited. Nitric oxide-mediated PTMs were found to affect different SOD isoforms in *A. thaliana*, differentially. While S-nitrosylation did not affect any isoform, NO-mediated tyrosine nitration inhibited the mitochondrial AtMSD (~90% loss in activity), AtCSD3 (peroxisomal), and AtFSD3 (chloroplastic) to a different extent (Holzmeister et al., 2015).

In Mn SOD, the tyrosine-nitration mediated impact on the accessibility to the substrate-binding site seems to be a conserved mechanism (Holzmeister et al., 2014). Interestingly, both NO-mediated nitration as well as S-nitrosylation inhibit CAT (a component of the antioxidant defense system, downstream to SODs) (Begara-Morales, 2016). Therefore, NO-mediated PTMs modulate antioxidant enzyme function/activity and serve as a control switch for ROS dynamics and H_2O_2-mediated cellular signaling (Begara-

Morales, 2016). Additionally, recent studies have shown the roles of additional proteins, which interact with SODs and modulate function. For example, AtMTM1 and AtMTM2 are involved in the Mn homeostasis function of *A. thaliana* Mn SOD (Hu et al., 2021), whereas EGY3 (a chloroplastic protein) stabilizes *A. thaliana* chloroplastic CuZn SOD and helps in chloroplastic ROS homeostasis (Zhuang et al., 2021). The PTMs modulate different characteristics of SODs, however, due to sequence differences among SOD homologs of different plants, the potential sites differ affecting modulation of structural/functional characteristics. Hence, certain PTM-mediated modifications (and associated fates) may not exist in plants, however, it is evident that plant SODs have many other potential sites that may be available for PTM-mediated modulation of function (Fig. 6.10). These potential PTM sites need to be investigated for their role in the regulation and functioning of plant SODs. A schematic representation of posttranslational regulation (mediated by ROS/RNS and metallochaperones) of SOD isoforms in different cellular compartments is shown in Fig. 6.11.

6.13.6 Genome Duplication–Mediated Copy Number Increase of Plant SOD Genes

Multiple isoforms of SODs have evolved due to the interplay of factors like the type of atmosphere (reducing/oxidizing), differential availability of metal cofactors, endosymbiosis, and certain genomic arrangements. An additional factor is more relevant to the plant genomes, as it is related to the generation of multiple gene copies (or paralogs) or gene families. Most plant genomes have undergone multiple genome duplication events (whole-genome duplications, segmental duplications, block duplications, etc.) during evolution (Barker et al., 2012). These events lead to increased copies of several genes, including stress-responsive genes, and also lead to the formation of gene families with functionally and/or structurally divergent members (Qiao et al., 2019). Genomic data of plants at PLAZA web server (https://bioinfromatics.psb.ugent.be/plaza/) has shown the presence of multiple copies of SOD genes in genomes of many monocots and dicots, due to inter-/intra-chromosomal block or tandem duplicated fragments in the genomes. These events affected all the three types of isoforms (Fe, Mn, and CuZn), to a different extent, however in general, the effect was more pronounced

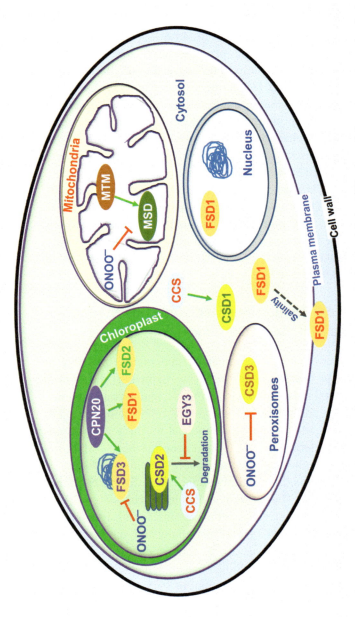

Figure 6.11 Schematic representation of posttranslational regulation of SODs localized to different cellular compartments in plants. The metallo-chaperones (CCS for Cu and CPN20 for Fe) activate respective SODs by delivering metal to the corresponding apo-SODs, while MTM transports Mn for Mn SOD activation. The EGY3 stabilizes the CSD2 by interacting with it, which prevents its degradation. Peroxynitrite inhibits the SOD activity localized in different compartments. Green colored arrow indicates activation, red lines indicate inactivation, and dashed arrows indicate specific response under certain conditions.

on CuZn SODs. Many plants genomes are also known to contain multiple Fe and Mn SOD genes (Tyagi et al., 2019). Prevalence of the block duplication events is generally more than the tandem or combined type events. It is evident that the species that have undergone multiple rounds of genome duplications (e.g., *S. spontaneum, T. aestivum, P. trichocarpa, G. max, P. bretscheneideri, C. clementina, M. domestica, V. vinifera*, etc.) harbor a higher number of CuZn SODs. Multiple copies might be important for the overall function and dynamics of the SODs in different compartments, for protection against oxidative stress, and ROS-mediated signaling. However, further experimental evidence is needed to find out, if gene copies are expressed, their divergence, and whether they harbor altered characteristics/functions, to enhance our understanding of the regulation and functioning of the SODs in plants.

In view of the information detailed above, it is clear that the regulation of superoxide dismutase is complex and operates at multiple levels, and it is not surprising considering the functional diversity of multiple isoforms of this important antioxidant enzyme. Information on mechanisms such as alternative splicing, posttranslational modifications, duplicated copies, etc. is still not complete and needs to be investigated thoroughly for better insights into the regulation and functioning of SODs in diverse functions, ranging from antioxidant defense to cellular signaling.

6.14 Stress Responsiveness of SODs

Most abiotic and biotic stress conditions disturb the cellular ROS homeostasis leading to oxidative stress as a result of the elevation of ROS and other reactive species (Miller et al., 2010; Hasanuzzaman et al., 2020). Elevated ROS levels affect almost all physiological processes occurring in different cellular compartments, causing localized oxidative damage, disruption of inter-organellar ROS-mediated communication, and leading to redox dysregulation in the cell (Janků et al., 2019). Under stress conditions, cellular antioxidant mechanisms are activated to minimize the ROS-mediated oxidative damage (Gill and Tuteja, 2010). SODs being the first line of defense against ROS-mediated damage are activated in most stress conditions (Tyagi et al., 2019). Abiotic stress conditions such as salinity, drought, heat, low temperature, salinity, radiation, heavy metals, etc. are known to alter cellular redox status due to enhanced ROS generation, leading to induction of SOD isoforms as a protective measure in plants (Mittler, 2006; Miller *et al.*, 2010; Mishra and Sharma, 2019; Tyagi *et al.*, 2019). Although the SOD genes contain *cis* elements responsive to stress conditions, these may also be regulated indirectly by other *trans* factors, and mechanisms including miR398, alternative splicing, or PTM-mediated regulation, that are also modulated by stresses (Sunkar *et al.*, 2012; You and Chan, 2015; Saini *et al.*, 2021). As multiple SODs are present in the cell, induction in their levels minimizes ROS-mediated damage in cellular compartments involved in oxidative metabolic reactions (Janků *et al.*, 2019). Additionally, SOD-mediated dismutation of $O_2^{\cdot-}$ also reduces the levels of other reactive species ROS/RNS, which helps in the restoration of an appropriate 'redox environment' for normal cellular functions (Miller, 2012; Cejudo *et al.*, 2021). Hence, different SOD isoforms have been utilized in genetic engineering approaches to enhance the tolerance of plants to different stress conditions (Mishra and Sharma, 2019; Tyagi *et al.*, 2019).

6.15 Biotechnological Applications of SODs for Stress Tolerance Enhancement

ROS are metabolic byproducts that are also essential for important cellular functions including signaling (Janků *et al.*, 2019). Most stress conditions elevate the cellular ROS levels resulting in detrimental oxidative damage, which can be alleviated by activation of antioxidant defense systems (Hasanuzzaman *et al.*, 2020; Rajput *et al.*, 2021). Transgenic experiments involving the overexpression of various antioxidant enzymes have been shown to minimize oxidative damage. Different transgenic plants overexpressing SODs (Fe, Mn, CuZn SODs) alone or in combination with other antioxidant enzymes have been extensively utilized for enhancement of tolerance against different stress conditions (Gill and Tuteja, 2010; Mishra and Sharma, 2019; Gill *et al.*, 2015; Chakradhar *et al.*, 2017; Rajput *et al.*, 2021; Tyagi *et al.*, 2019). An overview of some recent studies on transgenic applications of SOD isoforms for stress tolerance is provided in Table 6.2.

Table 6.2 List of recent transgenic studies involving overexpression of SODs for stress tolerance

S. No.	Source Plant Species	Target Species	SOD Isoform	Stress Condition	Reference
1.	Cucumis sativus	Arabidopsis thaliana	CuZn SOD	Salinity	(Zhou et al., 2018)
2.	Oryza sativa	Oryza sativa	CuZn SOD (chl)	Saline and sodic stress	(Guan et al., 2017)
3.	Solanum lycopersicum	Capsicum annum	CuZn SOD (chl)	MV and drought	(Chatzidimitriadou et al., 2009)
4.	Sedum alfredii	Arabidopsis thaliana	CuZn SOD	Oxidative stress (Cd)	(Li et al., 2017)
5.	Kandelia candel	Nicotiana tabacum	CuZn SOD (chl)	Salinity	(Jing et al., 2015)
6.	Pisum sativum	Nicotiana tabacum	CuZn SOD (Chl)	Low temperature, Light stress, Oxidative stress (MV)	(Gupta et al., 1993)
7.	Pisum sativum	Nicotiana tabacum	CuZn SOD (cyt)	Ozone stress	(Pitcher and Zilinskas, 1996)
8.	Arabidopsis thaliana	Nicotiana tabacum	Fe SOD (chl)	No major effect seen	(Van Camp et al., 1996)
9.	Triticum aestivum	Zea mays	Mn SOD	Oxidative stress (MV)	(Du et al., 2006)
10.	Triticum aestivum	Brassica napus	Mn SOD (mit)	Aluminum toxicity	(Basu et al., 2001)
11.	Nicotiana tabacum	Nicotiana tabacum	Mn SOD (chl)	Oxidative stress (MV)	(Slooten et al., 1995)

(*Continued*)

Table 6.2 (Continued)

S. No.	Source Plant Species	Target Species	SOD Isoform	Stress Condition	Reference
12.	Arachis hypogaea	Nicotiana tabacum	CuZn SOD (cyt)	Salinity drought	(Negi et al., 2015)
13.	Pisum sativum Spinacia oleracia	N. tabacum	CuZn SOD (cyt) APX (cyt)	Drought	(Faize et al., 2011)
14.	Saussurea involucrata	N. tabacum	CuZn SOD (per)	Drought, cold, and oxidative stress (MV)	(Zhang et al., 2017)
15.	Jatropa curcus	Arabidopisis thaliana	CuZn SOD (chl)	Salinity	(Liu et al., 2015)
16.	Solanum lycopersicum	Solanum tuberosum	CuZn SOD (cyt)	Oxidative stress (MV)	(Perl et al., 1993)
17.	Avicennia marina	Oryza sativa	CuZn SOD (cyt)	Salinity and oxidative stress	(Prashanth et al., 2008)
18.	Arabidopsis thaliana	Hordeum vulgare	Fe SOD (chl)	Oxidative stress	(Van Camp et al., 1996)
19.	Arabidopsis thaliana	Arabidopsis thaliana	Mn SOD	Salinity	(Wang et al., 2004)
20.	Oryza sativa	Oryza sativa	Mn SOD	Heat stress	(Shiraya et al., 2015)
21.	Pisum sativum	Oryza sativa	Mn SOD	Drought stress	(Wang et al., 2005)

S. No.	Source Plant Species	Target Species	SOD Isoform	Stress Condition	Reference
22.	Festuca arundinacea	Festuca arundinacea	CuZn SOD (chl) + APX (chl)	Oxidative stress (MV, H_2O_2, Cu, Cd, As)	(Lee et al., 2007)
23.	Prunus domestica	Prunus domestica	CuZn SOD (cyt)+ APX (cyt)	Salinity	(Diaz-Vivancos et al., 2013)
24.	Manihot esculenta	Manihot esculenta	CuZn SOD (cyt)+ Catalase (Per)	Shelf-life increase post-harvest produce (storage root)	(Xu et al., 2013a)
25.	Manihot esculenta	Manihot esculenta	CuZn SOD (cyt)+ APX (cyt)	Chilling and oxidative stress	(Xu et al., 2014)
26.	Manihot esculenta	Manihot esculenta	CuZn SOD (cyt)+ Catalase (Per)	Chilling and drought stress	(Xu et al., 2013b)
27.	Manihot esculenta	Manihot esculenta	CuZn SOD (cyt)+ Catalase (Per)	Mite resistance	(Lu et al., 2017)
28.	Potentilla atrosanguinea Rheum australe	Solanum tuberosum	CuZn SOD (cyt) + APX (cyt)	Salinity	(Shafi et al., 2017)

6.16 Industrial Applications of Plant SODs

SODs comprise an important group of antioxidant enzymes that confer oxidative stress protection in living systems. The SODs have immense importance in diverse applications with use as antioxidant supplements for the management of oxidative stress in certain conditions to a wide range of cosmetics products (Bafana et al., 2011; Tyagi et al., 2019; Stephenie et al., 2020). As the enzymes from the biological systems are optimized for the mild physiological environment, and not suitable for industrial treatment/conditions, they are often engineered to alter certain characteristics (stability, activity, specificity, etc.) required for desired applications (Jemli et al., 2014). For example, yeast SOD with stability at 45 °C was developed by such approaches (Lods et al., 2000). However, in recent years several plant SOD isoforms have been reported with characteristics like high thermostability, wide pH range, high specific activity (Carter and Thornburg, 2000; Lin et al., 2002; Khanna-Chopra and Sabarinath, 2004; Kumar et al., 2012; Kumar et al., 2014; Tuteja et al., 2015; Sanyal et al., 2018; Tyagi et al., 2019; Fesharaki-Esfahani et al., 2021). Some of the plant SODs may not need engineering interventions and can be utilized for appropriate industrial applications.

6.17 Conclusions

SODs have always been an important group of enzymes with crucial roles ranging from protection of aerobic life forms from oxidative damage to a diverse array of physiological functions including ROS homeostasis, and cellular signaling in diverse conditions. The SODs are highly conserved across eukaryotes, however, unlike animal isoforms, information on several aspects of plant SODs is relatively less known. SODs are crucial for important cellular mechanisms, and hence their regulation is complex and multi-layered. Complete understanding of posttranscriptional and posttranslational mechanisms in the regulation and functioning of plant SODs is still lacking. Furthermore, multiple SOD copies in many plants genomes due to genome duplication also add another dimension to regulation and functional diversification with the possibility of different or inter-linked fates. Future research in this area should address these important and relevant aspects for better insights into SOD regulation and functioning, in plants.

Abbreviations

$^1O_2$	Singlet oxygen
^3Chl	Chlorophyll triplet state
3D	Three dimensional
$^3O_2$	Triplet oxygen
ADH	Aldehyde dehydrogenase
AER	Alkenal/one oxidoreductase
AKR	Aldo-keto reductase
AO	Aldehyde oxidase
APX	Ascorbate peroxidase
AsA	Ascorbic acid
AS	Alternative splicing
ASH	Reduced ascorbate
ASS	Alternative splice site
At	*Arabidopsis thaliana*
CAT	Catalase
CCS	Copper chaperone for SOD
CS	Constitutive splicing
CSD	CuZn Superoxide dismutase
cTP	Chloroplastic targeting peptide
Ctr1	Copper transporter
CuAO	Copper amine oxidase
Cu	Copper
Cys	Cysteine
DHA	Dehydroascorbate
DHAR	Dehydroascorbate reductase
DNA	Deoxyribonucleic acid
ER	Endoplasmic reticulum
ES	Exon skipping
ETC	Electron transport chain
FAD	Flavin adenine dinucleotide
Fe-S	Iron-sulfur centers
Fe	Iron
FSD	Fe Superoxide dismutase
GAL	1-Galactono-γ lactone dehydrogenase

GOE	Great Oxygenation Event
GOPX	Guaiacol peroxidase
GOX	Glycolate oxidase
GPX	Glutathione peroxidase
GR	Glutathione reductase
GRx	Glutaredoxin
GSH	Glutathione (reduced)
GSNOR	S-Nitrosoglutathione reductase
GSSG	Glutathione (oxidized)
GST	Glutathione *S*-transferase
H_2O_2	Hydrogen peroxide
H_2S	Hydrogen sulfide
HNO_2	Nitrous acid
$HO_2^{\cdot}$	Peroxy radical
IR	Intron retention
KCN	Potassium cyanide
LOX	Lipoxygenase
MDHA	Monodehydroascorbate
MDHAR	Monodehydroascorbate reductase
MEE	Mutually exclusive exons
miR	MicroRNA
Mn	Manganese
MTM	Mn trafficking transporters for mitochondrial Mn SOD
Mya	Million years ago
N_2O_4	Dinitrogen tetroxide
NADH	Nicotinamide adenine dinucleotide (reduced)
NAD	Nicotinamide adenine dinucleotide
NADPH	Nicotinamide adenine dinucleotide phosphate (reduced)
NAPD	Nicotinamide adenine dinucleotide phosphate
NAT	Natural antisense transcript
Ni	Nickel
NR	Nitrate reductase
O_2	Molecular Oxygen
$O_2^{\cdot -}$	Superoxide
$ONOO^-$	Peroxynitrite
Os	*Oryza sativa*
OX	Oxalate oxidase
PAO	Polyamine oxidase
PAP	Plastid-encoded RNA polymerase associated proteins

PCD	programmed cell death
PCD	Programmed cell death
PEP	Plastic encoded RNA polymerase
POX	Peroxidase
PPO	Polyphenol oxidase
PRX	Peroxiredoxin
PS II	Photosystem II
PS I	Photosystem I
PTM	Posttranslational modification
PTS1	Peroxisomal targeting signal 1
PTS2	Peroxisomal targeting signal 2
RBOH	Respiratory burst oxidases homolog
RCS	Reactive Carbonyl Species
RNA	Ribonucleic acid
RNS	Reactive Nitrogen Species
ROS	Reactive Oxygen Species
RSOH	Sulfenic acid
RSS	Reactive Sulfur Species
RS·	Thiyl radical
SOD	Superoxide dismutases
SO	Sulfite oxidase
SPL	Squamosa promoter binding protein
SV	Splice variant
TRX	Thioredoxin
UV	Ultraviolet
XDH	Xanthine dehydrogenase
XOD	Xanthine oxidase
XOR	Xanthine oxidoreductase
Zn	Zinc
·OH	Hydroxyl radical
·NO$_2$	Nitrogen dioxide
·NO	Nitric oxide

References

Abdel-Ghany S. E., Burkhead J. L., Gogolin K. A., Andrés-Colás N., Bodecker J. R., Puig S., Peñarrubia L., Pilon M., *FEBS Lett.*, **579** (2005), 2307–2312.

Abdel-Ghany S. E., Pilon M., *J. Biol. Chem.*, **283** (2008), 15932–15945.

Aguirre G., Pilon M., *Front. Plant Sci.*, **12** (2016), 1250.

Alia P., Saradhi P., *J. Plant Physiol.*, **138** (1991), 554–558.

Alscher R. G., Erturk N., Heath L. S., *J. Exp. Bot.*, **53** (2002), 1331–1341.

Andreyev A. Y., Kushnareva Y. E., Starkov A. A., *Biochem. (Mosc.)*, **70** (2005), 200–214.

Antinone S. E., Ghadge G. D., Lam T. T., Wang L., Roos R. P., Green W. N., *J. Biol. Chem.*, **288** (2013), 21606–21617.

Antinone S. E., Ghadge G. D., Ostrow L. W., Roos R. P., Green W. N., *Sci. Rep.*, **7** (2017), 41141.

Apel K., Hirt H., *Annu. Rev. Plant Biol.*, **55** (2004), 373–399.

Araji S., Grammer T. A., Gertzen R., Anderson S. D., Mikulic-Petkovsek M., Veberic R., Phu M. L., Solar A., Leslie C. A., Dandekar A. M., Escobar M. A., *Plant Physiol.*, **164** (2014), 1191–1203.

Arnao M. B., Hernández-Ruiz J., *Melatonin Res.*, **2** (2019), 152–168.

Astier J., Gross I., Durner J., *J. Exp. Bot.*, **69** (2018), 3401–3411.

Astier J., Rasul S., Koen E., Manzoor H., Besson-Bard A., Lamotte O., Jeandroz S., Durner J., Lindermayr C., Wendehenne D., *Plant Sci.*, **181** (2011), 527–533.

Bafana A., Dutt S., Kumar A., Kumar S., Ahuja P. S., *J. Mol. Catal. B Enzym.*, **68** (2011), 129–138.

Banks C. J., Andersen J. L., *Redox Biol.*, **26** (2019), 101270.

Bannister J. V., Parker M. W., *Proc. Natl. Acad. Sci. U.S.A.*, **82** (1985), 149–152.

Bannister W. H., Bannister J. V., Barra D., Bond J., Bossa F., *Free Radic. Res. Commun.*, **12–13**(Pt 1), (1991), 349–361.

Barber-Zucker S., Shaanan B., Zarivach R., *Sci. Rep.*, **7** (2017), 16381.

Barondeau D. P., Kassmann C. J., Bruns C. K., Tainer J. A., Getzoff E. D., *Biochem.*, **43** (2004), 8038–8047.

Basu U., Good A. G., Taylor G. J., *Plant Cell Environ.*, **24** (2001), 1278–1269.

Beauclair L., Yu A., Bouché N., *Plant J.*, **62** (2010), 454–462.

Begara-Morales J. C., Sánchez-Calvo B., Chaki M., Valderrama R., Mata-Pérez C., Padilla M. N., Corpas F. J., Barroso J. B., *Front. Plant Sci.*, **7** (2016), 152.

Belén M., Uciel C., Siwaret A., Irina P. S., Claudia H., Rodolfo M. R., Blake C. M., Javier F. P., *Nucleic Acids Res.*, **46**(20), (2018), 10709–10723.

Bienert G. P., Møller A. L., Kristiansen K. A., Schulz A., Møller I. M., Schjoerring J. K., Jahn T. P., *J. Biol. Chem.*, **282** (2007), 1183–1192.

Biłas R., Szafran K., Hnatuszko-Konka K., Kononowicz A. K., *Plant Cell Tiss. Organ Cult.*, **127** (2016), 269–287.

Biswas M. S., Fukaki H., Mori I. C., Nakahara K., Mano J. I., *Plant J.*, **100** (2019), 536–548.

Bordo D., Djinovic K., Bolognesi M., *J. Mol. Biol.*, **238** (1994), 366–386.

Bouldin S. D., Darch M. A., Hart P. J., Outten C. E., *Biochem. J.*, **446** (2012), 59–67.

Bowler C., Van Camp W., Van Montagu M., Inzé D., *Crit. Rev. Plant Sci.*, **13** (1994), 199–218.

Boyer J. S., *Science* **218** (1982), 443–448.

Case A. J., *Antioxidants (Basel)*, **6** (2017), 82.

Caverzan A., Passaia G., Rosa S. B., Ribeiro C. W., Lazzarotto F., Margis-Pinheiro M., *Genet. Mol. Biol.*, **35** (2012), 1011–1019.

Cejudo F. J., Sandalio L. M., Van Breusegem F., *J. Exp. Bot.*, **72** (2021), 5785–5788.

Chakradhar T., Mahanty S., Reddy R. A., Divya K., Reddy P. S., Reddy M. K., Biotechnological perspective of reactive oxygen species (ROS)-mediated stress tolerance in plants, in *Reactive Oxygen Species and Antioxidant Systems in Plants: Role and Regulation under Abiotic Stress* (Khan M., Khan N., eds), Springer, Singapore, 2017.

Chatzidimitriadou K., Nianiou-Obeidat I., Madesis P., Perl-Treves R., Tsaftaris A., *Electron. J. Biotechnol.*, **12** (2009), doi: 10.2225/vol12-issue4-fulltext-10.

Chaudhary S., Khokhar W., Jabre I., Reddy A. S. N., Byrne L. J., Wilson C. M., Syed N. H., *Front. Plant Sci.*, **10** (2019), 708.

Chen C., Dickman M. B., *Proc. Natl. Acad. Sci. U.S.A.*, **102** (2005), 3459–3464.

Choudhury F. K., Rivero R. M., Blumwald E., Mittler R., *Plant J.*, **90** (2017), 856–867.

Cohen G. M., d'Arcy Doherty M., *Br. J. Cancer Suppl.*, **8** (1987), 46–52.

Cohu C. M., Abdel-Ghany S. E., Gogolin Reynolds K. A., Onofrio A. M., Bodecker J. R., Kimbrel J. A., Niyogi K. K., Pilon M., *Mol. Plant.*, **2** (2009), 1336–1350.

Corpas F. J., Barroso J. B., *Front. Plant Sci.*, **5** (2014), 97.

Corpas F. J., Barroso J. B., Carreras A., Quirós M., León A. M., Romero-Puertas M. C., Esteban F. J., Valderrama R., Palma J. M., Sandalio L. M., Gómez M., del Río L. A., *Plant Physiol.*, **136** (2004), 2722–2733.

Corpas F. J., Barroso J. B., del Río L. A., *Trends Plant Sci.*, **6** (2001), 145–150.

Corpas F. J., Río L. A. D., Palma J. M., *Plants (Basel)*, **8** (2019), 37.

Corpas F. J., González-Gordo S., Palma J. M., *Front. Plant Sci.*, **11** (2020), 853.

Das K., Roychoudhury A., *Front. Environ. Sci.*, **2** (2014), 53.

Dat J., Vandenabeele S., Vranová E., Van Montagu M., Inzé D., Van Breusegem F., *Cell. Mol. Life Sci.*, **57** (2000), 779–795.

Del Río L. A., Corpas F. J., Sandalio L. M., Palma J. M., Gómez M., Barroso J. B., *J. Exp. Bot.*, **53** (2002), 1255–1272.

Del Río L. A., *J. Exp. Bot.*, **66** (2015), 2827–2837.

Del Río L. A., Sandalio L. M., Corpas F. J., Palma J. M., Barroso J. B., *Plant Physiol.*, **141** (2006), 330–335.

Del Río L. A., Sandalio L. M., Palma J. M., Bueno P., Corpas F. J., *Free Radic. Biol. Med.* **13** (1992), 557–580.

Del Río L. A., Corpas F. J., López-Huertas E., Palma J. M., *Antioxidants and Antioxidant Enzymes in Higher Plants*, Springer, Cham. (2018).

Demicheli V., Quijano C., Alvarez B., Radi R., *Free Radic. Biol. Med.*, **42** (2007), 1359–1368.

Demidchik V., *Environ. Exp. Bot.*, **109** (2015), 212–228.

Diaz-Vivancos P., Faize M., Barba-Espin G., Faize L., Petri C., Hernández J. A., Burgos L., *Plant Biotechnol. J.*, **11** (2013), 976–985.

Dickinson B. C., Chang C. J., *Nat. Chem. Biol.*, **7** (2011) 504–511.

Dietz K.-J., Turkan I., Krieger-Liszkay A., *Plant Physiol.*, **171** (2016), 1541–1550.

Dixon D. P., Skipsey M., Edwards R., *Phytochemistry*, **71** (2010), 338–350.

Dreyer B. H., Schippers J., *Annu. Plant Rev.* **2** (2019), 1–36.

Du J., Zhu Z., Li W.-C., *J. Plant Physiol. Mol. Biol.*, **32** (2006), 57–63.

Dvořák P., Krasylenko Y., Ovečka M., Basheer J., Zapletalová V., Šamaj J., Takáč T., *Plant Cell Environ.*, **44** (2021), 68–87.

Eitinger T., *J. Bacteriol.*, **186** (2004), 7821–7825.

Elia L., Alain G., *Annu. Rev. Cell Dev. Biol.* **36** (2020), 291–313.

Eltayeb A. E., Kawano N., Badawi G. H., Kaminaka H., Sanekata T., Shibahara T., Inanaga S., Tanaka K., *Planta*, **225** (2007), 1255–1264.

Evans M. D., Dizdaroglu M., Cooke M. S., *Mutat. Res.*, **567** (2004), 1–61.

Faize M., Burgos L., Faize L., Piqueras A., Nicolas E., Barba-Espin G., Clemente-Moreno M. J., Alcobendas R., Artlip T., Hernandez J. A., *J. Exp. Bot.*, **62** (2011), 2599–2613.

Feng W., Hongbin W., Bing L., Jinfa W., *Plant Cell Rep.*, **24** (2006), 734–742.

Fink R. C., Scandalios J. G., *Biochem. Biophys.*, **399** (2002), 19–36.

Foyer C. H., Halliwell B., *Planta*, **133** (1976), 21–25.

Foyer C. H., Noctor G., *Plant Cell.*, **17** (2005), 1866–1875.

Fridovich I., *Arch. Biochem. Biophys.*, **247** (1986), 1–11.

Fridovich I., *Science*, **201** (1978), 875–880.

Gabbianelli R., Battistoni A., Polizio F., Carrì M. T., De Martino A., Meier B., Desideri A., Rotilio G., *Biochem. Biophys. Res. Commun.*, **216** (1995), 841–847.

Gallie D. R., Chen Z., *PLoS One*, **14** (2019), e0220078.

Ganie S. A., Reddy A. S. N., *Biology (Basel)*, **10** (2021), 309.

Garcia Y. M., Barwinska-Sendra A., Tarrant E., Skaar E. P., Waldron K. J., Kehl-Fie T. E., *PLoS Pathog.*, **13** (2017), e1006125.

Getzoff E. D., Tainer J. A., Weiner P. K., Kollman P. A., Richardson J. S., Richardson D. C., *Nature*, **306** (1983), 287–290.

Giles G. I., Nasim M. J., Ali W., Jacob C., *Antioxidants (Basel, Switzerland)*, **6** (2017), 38.

Gill S. S., Anjum N. A., Gill R., Yadav S., Hasanuzzaman M., Fujita M., Mishra P., Sabat S. C., Tuteja N., *Environ. Sci. Pollut. Res.*, **22** (2015), 10375–10394.

Gill S. S., Tuteja N., *Plant Physiol. Biochem.*, **48** (2010), 909–930.

Grace S. C., *Life Sciences,* **47** (1990), 1875–1886.

Gracz J., *BioTechnologia*, **1** (2016), 9–17.

Guan Q., Liao X., He M., Li X., Wang Z., Ma H., Yu S., Liu S., *PLoS ONE*, **12** (2017), e0186052.

Guan Q., Lu X., Zeng H., Zhang Y., Zhu J., *Plant J.,* **74** (2013), 840–851.

Gupta A. S., Heinen J. L., Holaday A. S., Burke J. J., Allen R. D., *Proc. Natl. Acad. Sci. U. S. A*, **90** (1993), 1629–1633.

Haak D. C., Fukao T., Grene R., Hua Z., Ivanov R., Perrella G., Li S., *Front. Plant Sci.*, **8** (2017), 1564.

Halliwell B., Gutteridge J. M. C., *Free Radicals in Biology and Medicine*, 3rd ed, Oxford University Press, Oxford, UK, 1999.

Halliwell B., Gutteridge J. M. C., *Free Radicals in Biology and Medicine,* 4th ed, Oxford University Press, New York, UK, 2007.

Halliwell B., *Plant Physiol.*, **141** (2006), 312–322.

Hasanuzzaman M., Bhuyan M., Zulfiqar F., Raza A., Mohsin S. M., Mahmud J. A., Fujita M., Fotopoulos V., *Antioxidants (Basel, Switzerland)*, **9** (2020), 681.

Hasanuzzaman M., Hossain M. A., Teixeira da Silva J. A., Fujita M., Plant responses and tolerance to abiotic oxidative stress: antioxidant defense is a key factor, in *Crop Stress and its Management: Perspectives and Strategies* (Bandi V., Shanker A. K., Shanker C., Mandapaka M., eds), Springer, Berlin, 2012.

He M., He C.-Q., Ding N.-Z., *Front. Plant Sci.*, **9** (2018), 1771.

Hollander-Czytko H., Grabowski J., Sandorf I., Weckermann K., Weiler E. W., *J. Plant Physiol.*, **162** (2005), 767–770.

Holm et al., *Chem. Rev.*, **96** (1996), 2239–2314.

Holzmeister C., Gaupels F., Geerlof A., Sarioglu H., Sattler M., Durner J., Lindermayr C., *J. Exp. Bot.*, **66** (2015), 989–999.

Hu S. H., Lin S. F., Huang Y. C., Huang C. H., Kuo W. Y., Jinn T. L. *Front. Plant Sci.*, **12** (2021), 690064.

Huang C.-H., Kuo W.-Y., Weiss C., Jinn T.-L., *Plant Physiol.*, **158** (2012), 737–746.

Jagadeeswaran G., Saini A., Sunkar R., *Planta*, **229** (2009), 1009–1014.

Jajic I., Sarna T., Strzalka K., *Plants (Basel)*, **4** (2015), 393–411.

Janků M., Luhová L., Petřivalský M., *Antioxidants (Basel, Switzerland)*, **8** (2019), 105.

Jemli S., Ayadi-Zouari D., Hlima H. B., Bejar S., *Crit. Rev. Biotechnol.*, **36** (2016), 246–258.

Jensen L. T., Culotta V. C., *J. Biol. Chem.*, **16** (2005), 41373–41379.

Jimenez A., Hernandez J. A., Pastori G., del Rio L. A., Sevilla F., *Plant Physiol.*, **118** (1998), 1327–1335.

Jing X., Hou P., Lu Y., Deng S., Li N., Zhao R., Sun J., Wang Y., Han Y., Lang T., Ding M., Shen X., Chen S., *Front. Plant Sci.*, **6** (2015), 1–13.

Kanematsu S., Asada K., *Arch. Biochem. Biophys.*, **195** (1979), 535–545.

Kar R. K., *Plant Signal. Behav.*, **6** (2011), 1741–1745.

Kaufmann K., Pajoro A., Angenent G., *Nat. Rev. Genet.*, **11** (2010), 830–842.

Kaur P., Handa N., Verma V., Bakshi P., Kalia R., Sareen S., Nagpal A., Vig A., Mir B. A., Bhardwaj R., Cross talk among reactive oxygen, nitrogen and sulfur during abiotic stress in plants, in *Reactive Oxygen, Nitrogen and Sulfur Species in Plants: Production, Metabolism, Signaling and Defense Mechanisms* (Hasanuzzaman M., Fotopoulos V., Nahar K., Fujita M., eds), John Wiley & Sons, Hoboken, 2019.

Kavi Kishor P. B., Sangam S., Amrutha R. N., Laxmi P. S., Naidu K. R., Rao K. R. S. S., Rao S., Reddy K. J., Theriappan P., Sreenivasulu N., *Curr. Sci.*, **88** (2005), 424–438.

Kliebenstein D. J., Monde R. A., Last R. L., *Plant Physiol.*, **118** (1998), 637–650.

Krieger-Liszkay A., Fufezan C. Trebst A., *Photosynthesis Res.*, **98** (2008), 551–564.

Kuo W. Y., Huang C. H., Jinn T. L., *Plant Signal. Behav.*, **8** (2013), e23074.

Laloum T., Martín G., Duque P., *Trends Plant Sci.*, **23** (2018), 140–150.

Lamb A. L., Torres A. S., O'Halloran T. V., Rosenzweig A. C., *Nat. Struct. Biol.*, **8** (2001), 751–755.

Larson R. A., *Phytochemistry*, **27** (1988), 969–978.

Lee S. H., Ahsan N., Lee K. W., Kim D. H., Lee D. G., Kwak S. S., Kwon S. Y., Kim T. H., Lee B. H., *J. Plant Physiol.*, **164**(12), (2007), 1626–1638.

Lee S., Joung Y. H., Kim J.-K., Do Choi Y., Jang G., *BMC Plant Biol.*, **19** (2019), 524.

Li H.-T., Jiao M., Chen J., Liang Y., *Acta Biochim. Biophys. Sin.*, **42** (2010), 183–194.

Li F., Vallabhaneni R., Yu J., Rocheford T., Wurtzel E. T., *Plant Physiol.*, **147** (2008), 1334–1346.

Li L., Yi H., Xue M., Yi M., *Ecotoxicology*, **26** (2017), 1181–1187.

Li Y.-F., Zheng Y., Addo-Quaye C., Zhang L., Saini A., Jagadeeswaran G., Axtell M. J., Zhang W., Sunkar R., *Plant J.*, **62** (2010), 742–759.

Li Y., Li X., Yang J., He Y., *Nat Commun.*, **11** (2020), 5351.

Li Z., Han X., Song X., Zhang Y., Jiang J., Han Q., Liu M., Qiao G., Zhuo R., *Front. Plant Sci.*, **8** (2017), 1010.

Ling Y., Serrano N., Gao G., Atia M., Mokhtar M., Woo Y. H., Bazin J., Veluchamy A., Benhamed M., Crespi M., Gehring C., Reddy A. S. N., Mahfouz M. M., *J. Exp. Bot.*, **69** (2018), 2659–2675.

Liu X., Hua X., Guo J., Qi D., Wang L., Liu Z., Jin Z., Chen S., Liu G., *Biotec. Lett.*, **30** (2008), 1275–1280.

Liu Z., Zhang W., Gong X., Zhang Q., Zhou L., *Genet. Mol. Res.*, **14** (2015), 2086–2098.

Lu F., Liang X., Lu H., Li Q., Chen Q., Zhang P., Li K., Liu G., Yan W., Song J., Duan C., Zhang L., *Sci. Rep.*, **7**(1), (2017), 1–13.

Lu Y., Feng Z., Bian L., Xie H., Liang J., *Funct. Plant Biol.*, **38** (2010), 44–53.

Mandelli F., Franco Cairo J. P., Citadini A. P., Büchli F., Alvarez T. M., Oliveira R. J., Leite V. B., Paes Leme A. F., Mercadante A. Z., Squina F. M., *Lett. Appl. Microbiol.* **57** (2013), 40–46.

Mano J., Biswas M. S., Sugimoto K., *Plants (Basel, Switzerland)*, **8** (2019), 391.

Marques A. T., Santos S. P., Rosa M. G., Rodrigues M. A., Abreu I. A., Frazão C., Romão C. V., *Acta Crystallogr. F. Struct. Biol. Commun.*, **70** (2014), 669–672.

Marquez Y., Brown J. W. S., Simpson C., Barta A., Kalyna M., *Genome Res.* **22** (2012), 1184–1195.

Martin M. V., Fiol D. F., Sundaresan V., Zabaleta E. J., Pagnussat G. C., *Plant Cell*, **25** (2013), 1573–1591.

Martin W., Russell M. J., *Philos. Trans. R. Soc. Lond., B, Biol. Sci.*, **358** (2003), 59–85.

Martinez A., Peluffo G., Petruk A. A., Hugo M., Piñeyro D., Demicheli V., Moreno D. M., Lima A., Batthyány C., Durán R., Robello C., Martí M. A., Larrieux N., Buschiazzo A., Trujillo M., Radi R., Piacenza L., *J. Biol. Chem.* **289** (2014), 12760–12778.

Martinez C., Baccou J. C., Bresson E., Baissac Y., Daniel J. F., Jalloul A., Montillet J. L., Geiger J. P., Assigbetsé K., Nicole M., *Plant Physiol.*, **122** (2000), 757–766.

Martinez C., Montillet J. L., Bresson E., Agnel J. P., Dai G. H., Daniel J. F., Geiger J. P., Nicole M., *Mol. Plant Microbe Interact.*, **11** (1998), 1038–1047.

McCord J. M., Fridovich I., *J. Biol. Chem.* **244** (1969), 6049–6055.

McCord J. M., Keele B. B., Fridovich I., *Proc. Natl. Acad. Sci. U. S. A.*, **68** (1971), 1024–1027.

McDowell J. M., Dangl J. L., *Trends Biochem. Sci.*, **25** (2000), 79–82.

Millar A. H., Heazlewood J. L., Giglione C., Holdsworth M. J., Bachmair A., Schulze W. X., *Annu. Rev. Plant Biol.*, **70** (2009), 119–151.

Miller A. F., *Febs Lett.*, **586** (2012), 585–595.

Miller G., Suzuki N., Ciftci-Yilmaz S., Mittler R., *Plant Cell Environ.*, **33** (2010), 453–467.

Mishra P., Sharma P., Superoxide dismutases (SODs) and their role in regulating abiotic stress induced oxidative stress in plants, in *Reactive Oxygen, Nitrogen and Sulfur Species in Plants: Production, Metabolism, Signaling and Defense Mechanisms* (Hasanuzzaman M., Fotopoulos V., Nahar K., Fujita M., eds), John Wiley & Sons Ltd, 2019.

Mittler R., *Trends Plant Sci.*, **11** (2006), 15–19.

Mittler R., Vanderauwera S., Suzuki N., Miller G., Tognetti V. B., Vandepoele K., Gollery M., Shulaev V., Van Breusegem F., *Trends Plant Sci.* **16** (2011), 300–309.

Mittler R., *Trends Plant Sci.* **22** (2017), 11–19.

Moller I. M., *Annu. Rev. Plant Physiol. Mol. Biol.*, **52** (2001), 561–591.

Morgan M. J., Lehmann M., Schwarzlander M., Baxter C. J., Sienkiewicz-Porzucek A., Williams T. C. R., Schauer N., Fernie A. R., Fricker M. D., Ratcliffe R. G., Sweetlove L. J., Finkemeier I., *Plant Physiol.*, **147** (2008), 101–114.

Mullineaux P. M., Rausch T., *Photosynthetic Res.* **86** (2005), 459–474.

Munné-Bosch S., *J. Plant Physiol.*, **162** (2005), 743–748.

Myouga F., Hosoda C., Umezawa T., Iizumi H., Kuromori T., Motohashi R., Shono Y., Nagata N., Ikeuchi M., Shinozaki K., *Plant Cell*, **20** (2008), 3148–3162.

Negi N. P., Shrivastava D. C., Sharma V., Sarin N. B., *Plant Cell Rep.*, **34** (2015), 1109–1126.

Neill S., Desikan R., Hancock J., *Curr. Opin. Plant Biol.*, **5** (2002), 388–395.

Ng D. W., Abeysinghe J. K., Kamali M., *Int. J. Mol. Sci.*, **19** (2018), 3737.

Niu L., Liao W., *Front. Plant Sci.*, **7** (2016), 230.

Op den Camp R. G., Przybyla D., Ochsenbein C., Laloi C., Kim C., Danon A., Wagner D., Hideg E., Gobel C., Feussner I., Nater M., Apel K., *Plant Cell*, **15** (2003), 2320–2332.

Palma J. M., Gupta D. K., Corpas F. J., Hydrogen peroxide and nitric oxide generation in plant cells: overview and queries, in *Nitric Oxide and Hydrogen Peroxide Signaling in Higher Plant*, Springer, Cham, 2019.

Panche A. N., Diwan A. D., Chandra S. R., *J. Nutr. Sci.*, **5** (2016), e47.

Patil V. S., Zhou R., Rana T. M., *Crit. Rev. Biochem. Mol. Biol.*, **49** (2014), 16–32.

Pelmenschikov V., Siegbahn P. E., *Inorg. Chem.*, **44** (2005), 3311–3320.

Perl A., Perl-Treves R., Galili S., Aviv D., Shalgi E., Malkin S., Galun, E., *Theor. Appl. Genet.*, **85** (1993), 568–576.

Perry J. J. P., Shin D. S., Getzoff E. D., Tainer J. A., *Biochim. Biophys. Acta.* **1804** (2010), 245–262.

Pilon M., Ravet K., Tapken W., *Biochim Biophys Acta.* **1807** (2011), 989–998.

Pinto E., Sigaud-kutner T., Leitao M. A., Okamoto O. K., Morse D., Colepicolo P., *J. Phycol.*, **39** (2003), 1008–1018.

Pitcher L. H., Zilinskas B. A., *Plant Physiol.*, **110** (1996), 583–588.

Podgórska A., Burian M., Szal B., *Front. Plant Sci.* **8** (2017), 1353.

Prashanth S. R., Sadhasivam V., Parida A., *Transgenic Res.*, **17** (2008), 281–291.

Printz B., Lutts S., Hausman J.-F., Sergeant K., *Front. Plant Sci.*, **7** (2016), 601.

Qiao X., Li Q., Yin H., Qi K., Li L., Wang R., Zhang S., Paterson A. H., *Genome Biol.* **20** (2019), 38.

Radi R., *Acc. Chem. Res.* **46** (2013), 550–555.

Rago A., Kouvaris K., Uller T., Watson R., *PLoS Comput. Biol.*, **15** (2019), e1006260.

Rajput V. D., Harish, Singh R. K., Verma K. K., Sharma L., Quiroz-Figueroa F. R., Meena M., Gour V. S., Minkina T., Sushkova S., Mandzheiva S., *Biology*, **10** (2021), 267.

Rasmusson A. G., Geisler D. A., Møller I. M., *Mitochondrion*, **8** (2008), 47–,60,

Reddy A. S., *Annu. Rev. Plant Biol.*, **58** (2007), 267–294.

Reddy A. S. N., Marquez Y., Kalyna M., Barta A., *Plant Cell*, **25** (2013), 3657–3683.

Reiter R. J., Tan D. X., Manchester L. C., Qi W., *Cell Biochem. Biophys.*, **34** (2001), 237–256.

Richter C., *Mutat. Res., DNAging: Genet. Instab. Aging.*, **275** (1992), 249–255.

Ryan K. C., Johnson O. E., Cabelli D. E., Brunold T. C., Maroney M. J., *J. Biol. Inorg. Chem.*, **15** (2010), 795–807.

Saddhe A. A., Malvankar M. R., Karle S. B., Kumar K., *Env. Exp. Bot.*, **161** (2019), 86–97.

Sagasti S., Bernal M., Sancho D., del Castillo M. B., Picorel R., *Funct. Plant Biol.*, **41** (2014), 144–155.

Saini A., Rohila J. S., Govindan G., Li Y.-F., Sunkar R., *Int. J. Mol. Sci.*, **22** (2021), 3997.

Saito M. A., Sigman D. M., Morel F. M. M., *Inorganica Chim. Acta.*, **356** (2003), 308–318.

Satomi M., Muller F., Beckman K. B., The basics of oxidative biochemistry, in *Oxidative Stress in Aging: From Model Systems to Human Diseases* (Miwa S., Beckman K. B., Muller F. L., eds), Humana Press, Totowa, 2008.

Scandalios G., Guan L., Polidoros A. N., Catalases in plants: gene structure, properties, regulation and expression, in *Oxidative Stress and the Molecular Biology of Antioxidants Defenses* (Scandalios J. G., ed), Cold Spring Harbor Laboratory Press, New York, 1997.

Schmidt A., Gube M., Kothe E., *J. Basic Microbiol.* **49** (2009), 109–118.

Schmidt M., Meier B., Parak F., *JBIC J. Biol. Inorg. Chem.* **1** (1996), 532–541.

Schmidt P. J., Rae T. D., Pufahl R. A., Hamma T., Strain J., O'Halloran T. V., Culotta V. C., *J. Biol. Chem.*, **274** (1999), 23719–23725.

Schulz G., Schirmer R. H., Sachsenheimer W., Pai E. F., *Nature*, **273** (1978), 120–124.

Shafi A., Pal A. K., Sharma V., Kalia S., Kumar S., Ahuja P. S., Singh A. K., *Plant Mol. Biol. Rep.*, **35** (2017), 504–518.

Shapiguzov A., Vainonen J. P., Wrzaczek M., Kangasjärvi J., *Front. Plant Sci.*, **3** (2012), 292.

Sharma P., Jha A. B., Dubey R. S., Oxidative stress and antioxidative defense system in plants growing under abiotic stresses, in *Handbook of Plant and Crop Stress* (Pessarakli M., ed), CRC Press, Taylor and Francis Publishing Company, Florida, 2010.

Sharma P., Jha A. B., Dubey R. S., Pessarakli M., *J. Bot.*, **2012** (2012), 217037.

Sheng Y., Abreu I. A., Cabelli D. E., Maroney M. J., Miller A. F., Teixeira M., Valentine J. S., *Chem. Rev.*, **114** (2014), 3854–3918.

Shiraya T., Mori T., Maruyama T., Sasaki M., Takamatsu T., Oikawa K., Itoh K., Kaneko K., Ichikawa H., Mitsui T., *Plant Biotechnol. J.*, **13** (2015), 1251–1263.

Singh K. B., *Plant Physiol.*, **118** (1998), 1111–1120.

Skopp A., Boyd S. D., Ullrich M. S., Liu L., Winkler D. D., *Biometals.*, **32** (2019), 695–705.

Shahbaz M., Pilon M., *Plants*, **8** (2019), 141.

Slooten L., Capiau K., Van Camp W., Van Montagu M., Sybesma C., Inze D., *Plant Physiol.* **107** (1995), 737–750.

Smirnoff N., Ascorbate, tocopherol and carotenoids: metabolism, pathway engineering and functions, in *Antioxidants and Reactive Oxygen Species in Plants* (Smirnoff N., ed), Blackwell Publishing Ltd., Oxford, 2005.

Srivastava V., Srivastava M. K., Chibani K., Nilsson R., Rouhier N., Melzer M., Wingsle G. *Plant Physiol.*, **149** (2009), 1848–1859.

Stephenie S., Chang Y. P., Gnanasekaran A., Esa N. M., Gnanaraj C., *J. Funct. Foods*, **68** (2020), 103917.

Sunkar R., Kapoor A., Zhu J.-K. *Plant Cell.*, **18** (2006), 2051–2065.

Sunkar R., Li Y.-F., Jagadeeswaran G. *Trends Plant Sci.*, **17** (2012), 196–203.

Szabados L., Savoure A., *Trends Plant Sci.*, **15** (2010), 89–97.

Szarka A., Horemans N., Kovacs Z., Grof P., Mayer M., Banhegyi G., *Physiol. Plant.*, **129** (2007), 225–232.

Takagi D., Takumi S., Hashiguchi M., Sejima T., Miyake C., *Plant Physiol.* **171** (2016), 1626–1634.

Takahashi M. A., Asada K., *Arch. Biochem. Biophys.* **226** (1983), 558–566.

Torres M. A., Dangl J. L., Jones J. D. G., *Proc. Natl. Acad. Sci. U.S.A.*, **99** (2002), 517–522.

Tounsi S., Feki K., Kamoun Y., Saïdi M. N., Jemli S., Ghorbel M., Alcon C., Brini F., *Plant Physiol. Biochem.* **142** (2019), 384–394.

Trovato M., Mattioli R., Costantino P., *Rendiconti Lincei*, **19** (2008), 325–346.

Tsang C. K., Liu Y., Thomas J., Zhang Y., Zheng X. F., *Nat. Commun.*, **5** (2014), 3446.

Tsuboi H., Kouda K., Takeuchi H., Takigawa M., Masamoto Y., Takeuchi M., Ochi H., *Br. J. Dermatol.*, **138** (1998), 1033–1035.

Tsukamoto S., Morita S., Hirano E., Yokoi H., Masumura T., Tanaka K., *Plant Physiol.*, **137** (2005), 317–327.

Turrens J. F., *J. Physiol.*, **552** (2003), 335–344.

Ushimaru T., Maki Y., Sano S., Koshiba K., Asada K., Tsuji H., *Plant Cell Physiol.*, **38** (1997), 541–549.

Waititu J. K., Zhang C., Liu J., Wang H., *Int. J. Mol. Sci.*, **21** (2020), 8401.

Wang F. Z., Wang Q. B., Kwon S. Y., Kwak S. S., Su W. A., *J. Plant Physiol.*, **162** (2005), 465–472.

Wang T., Song H., Zhang B.., Lu Q, Liu Z., Zhang S., Guo R., Wang C., Zhao Z., Liu J., Peng R., *3 Biotech*, **8** (2018), 486.

Wang Y., Ying Y., Chen J., Wang X., *Plant Sci.*, **167** (2004), 671–677.

Winkel-Shirley B., *Curr. Opin. Plant Biol.*, **5** (2002), 218–223.

Wolfe-Simon F., Grzebyk D., Schofield O., Falkowski P. G., *J. Phycol.*, **41** (2005), 453–465.

Wuerges J., Lee J.-W., Yim Y.-L., Kang S.-O., Carugo K. D., *Proc. Natl. Acad. Sci. U.S.A.*, **101** (2004), 8569–8574.

Xing Y., Cao Q., Zhang Q., Qin L., Jia W., Zhang J., *Plant Cell Physiol.*, **54** (2013), 1217–1227.

Xing Y., Chen W.-H., Jia W., Zhang J., *J. Exp. Bot.*, **66** (2015), 5971–5981.

Xu J., Duan X., Yang J., Beeching J. R., Zhang P., *Plant Physiol.*, **161** (2013a), 1517–1528.

Xu J., Duan X., Yang J., Beeching J. R., Zhang P., *Plant Signal. Behav.*, **8** (2013b), e24525.

Xu J., Yang J., Duan X., Jiang Y., Zhang P., *BMC Plant Biol.*, **14** (2014), 208.

Xu X. M., Lin H., Maple J., Björkblom B., Alves G., Larsen J. P., Møller S. G., *J. Cell Sci.*, **123** (2010), 1644–1651.

Yadav S., Gill S. S., Passricha N., Gill R., Badhwar P., Anjum N. A., Francisco J.-B. J., Tuteja N., *Plant Gene.*, **17** (2019), 100165.

Yamakura F., Kawasaki H., *Biochim. Biophys. Acta*, **1804** (2010), 318–325.

Yamano S., Maruyama T., *J. Biochem.*, **125** (1999), 186–193.

Yamasaki H., Abdel-Ghany S. E., Cohu C. M., Kobayashi Y., Shikanai T., Pilon M., *J. Biol. Chem.*, **282**(22), (2007), 16369–16378.

Yamasaki H., Hayashi M., Fukazawa M., Kobayashi Y., Shikanai T., *Plant Cell,* **21** (2009), 347–361.

Yogavel M., Mishra P. C., Gill J., Bhardwaj P. K., Dutt S., Kumar S., Ahuja P. S., Sharma A., *Acta Cryst.,* **D64** (2008), 892–901.

You J., Chan Z., *Front. Plant Sci.,* **6** (2015), 1092.

Youn H. D., Kim E. J., Roe J. H., Hah Y. C., Kang S. O., *Biochem. J.,* **318** (1996), 889–896.

Yu M., Lamattina L., Spoel S. H., Loake G. J., *New Phytol.,* **202** (2014), 1142–1156.

Zhu C., Ding Y., Liu H, *Physiol. Plant.,* **143** (2011), 1–9.

Zhuang Y., Wei M., Ling C., Liu Y., Amin A. K., Li P., Li P., Hu X., Bao H., Huo H., Smalle J., Wang S., *Cell Rep.,* **36** (2021), 109384.

Zigmantas D., Hiller R. G., Sundstrom V., Polivka T., *Proc. Natl. Acad. Sc.i U. S. A.,* **99**, (2002), 16760–16765.

Chapter 7

Peroxisomes from Higher Plants and Their Metabolic Diversity

Francisco J. Corpas and José M. Palma
Group of Antioxidants, Free Radicals, and Nitric Oxide in Biotechnology, Food and Agriculture. Department of Biochemistry, Cell and Molecular Biology of Plants, Zaidín Experimental Station (Spanish National Research Council, CSIC), C/Professor Albareda 1, 18008 Granada, Spain
javier.corpas@eez.csic.es

Peroxisomes are subcellular compartments that, in higher plants, are characterized to have versatile metabolic plasticity participating in a myriad of biochemical pathways including photorespiration, β-oxidation, glyoxylate cycle, biosynthesis of plant hormones (auxin and jasmonic acid), metabolism of purines, as well as the metabolism of reactive-oxygen and -nitrogen species (ROS and RNS) which includes signaling molecules (hydrogen peroxide and nitric oxide). Thus, plant peroxisomes are involved in all physiological processes from seed germination, plant development, leaf senescence, and flower and fruit ripening to the mechanisms of response to environmental adverse stressful conditions. Accordingly, this

---

Agricultural Biocatalysis: Enzymes in Agriculture and Industry
Edited by Peter Jeschke and Evgeni B. Starikov
Copyright © 2023 Jenny Stanford Publishing Pte. Ltd.
ISBN 978-981-4968-47-8 (Hardcover), 978-1-003-31310-6 (eBook)
www.jennystanford.com

chapter aims to provide a general overview of the great relevance of peroxisomes, organelles which in plants are less known than other organelles such as chloroplasts or mitochondria.

7.1 Introduction

The peroxisome is a cellular compartment that was first described metabolically in the 1960s in animal systems (de Duve *et al.*, 1960; de Duve and Baudhuin, 1966). At a morphological level, it is a very simple organelle made up of a simple membrane that surrounds a dense matrix that sometimes contains crystalline structures. In subsequent years, peroxisomes were found to exist in almost all types of eukaryotic cells including photosynthetic organisms (Beevers, 1979; Tolbert *et al.*, 1981; Islinger *et al.*, 2010; Corpas *et al.*, 2021). Figure 7.1 illustrates, at the level of electron microscopy, the appearance of a peroxisome in a pea leaf section that is in the vicinity of other organelles such as mitochondria and chloroplasts. However, the number of research manuscripts about plant peroxisomes is significantly lower in comparison with other subcellular compartments (Fig. 7.2).

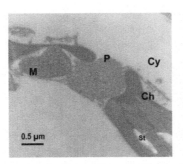

Figure 7.1 Representative electron micrograph of a thin section of pea leaf where it is possible to visualize the close position of peroxisome with a mitochondrion and a chloroplast. Ch, chloroplast; M, mitochondrion; P, peroxisome; Cy, cytosol; St, starch granule; V, vacuole. Bar = 0.5 μm.

The basic biochemical constituents of peroxisomes are the antioxidant enzyme catalase (Palma *et al.*, 2020) and hydrogen peroxide-generating flavin-oxidases. Additionally, plant peroxisomes have a versatile metabolism because their biochemical constituents may change depending on the organ/tissue, development stage, plant species, and environmental conditions (Hu *et al.*, 2012; Igamberdiev and Lea, 2002; Corpas *et al.*, 2017; 2018). Table 7.1 shows the main metabolic pathways which have been described in peroxisomes from higher plants. This diversity of pathways allows that plant peroxisomes to be involved in a wide range of physiological processes from seed germination to leaf senescence and fruit ripening, as well as in the mechanism of response to diverse adverse environmental conditions (Fig. 7.3).

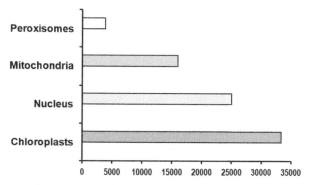

Figure 7.2 Number of publications about the main subcellular compartments in plants found in PubMed database (updated in September 2021).

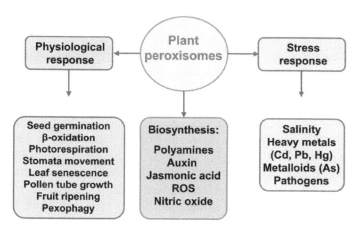

Figure 7.3 Summary of the main functions exerted by plant peroxisomes.

Table 7.1 Main metabolic pathways in which higher plant peroxisomes are involved

Peroxisomal pathways	Reference
Photorespiration	Mano and Nishimura, 2005; Florian et al., 2013; Sørhagen et al., 2013; Engqvist and Maurino, 2017
β-Oxidation of fatty acids	Tolbert and Essner, 1981; Kindl, 1993; Baker et al., 2006
Glyoxylate cycle	Eastmond and Graham, 2001; Pracharoenwattana, Cornah, and Smith, 2005
Biosynthesis of auxin (IAA)[a]	Spiess and Zolman, 2013; Jawahir and Zolman, 2021
Metabolism of ROS and RNS[b]	del Río et al., 1992; Corpas et al., 2017; 2019, 2021
Jasmonic acid (JA) and polyamine metabolism	Ono et al., 2012; Planas-Portell et al., 2013; Wang et al., 2019; Griffiths, 2020

[a]IAA, indole-3-acetic acid; [b]ROS, reactive oxygen species; RNS, reactive nitrogen species.

7.2 Photorespiration

Photorespiration is a metabolic pathway that takes place in the green tissue of plants. It involves the uptake of oxygen (O_2) with the concomitant release of carbon dioxide (CO_2) from diverse organic compounds which requires the participation of three organelles, chloroplasts, peroxisomes, and mitochondria (Peterhansel et al., 2010; Peterhansel and Maurino, 2011; Florian et al., 2013; Eisenhut et al., 2017). Initially, photorespiration might be considered a useless pathway because it reduces the photosynthetic carbon fixation by around 25%. However, this is an integrating pathway since, besides the association of three organelles, it allows the interaction of diverse metabolic including photosynthesis, nitrate assimilation, amino acid metabolism, and the tricarboxylic acid (TCA) cycle, and provides CO_2 when this gas lowers in the environment (Hodges et al., 2016; Busch, 2020). Furthermore, it could be a mechanism to dissipate the excess of energy to equilibrate the ATP and NADPH ratio (Busch, 2020; Zhang et al., 2020). Figure 7.4 outlines the main reaction of the photorespiration in the involved organelles.

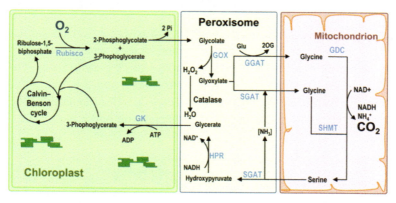

Figure 7.4 Photorespiratory pathway and its interconnection with photosynthetic Calvin–Benson cycle in higher plants implying the metabolic connection among chloroplasts, peroxisomes, and mitochondria in green tissues. Blue ink depicts the involved enzymes. Abbreviations: 2OG, 2-oxoglutarate; CAT, catalase; GDC, glycine decarboxylase complex; GGAT, glutamate:glyoxylate aminotransferase; GOX, glycolate oxidase; GK, glycerate kinase; HPR1, hydroxypyruvate reductase; OAA, oxaloacetate; Rubisco, ribulose 1,5-bisphosphate carboxylase/oxygenase; SGAT, serine-glyoxylate aminotransferase; SHMT, serine hydroxymethyltransferase.

A very fascinating aspect that facilitates the exchange of metabolites between the peroxisome and the other cell compartments is the dynamic movement of peroxisomes along actin filaments (Mano et al., 2002) and the physical interactions that occur between peroxisomes and chloroplasts depending on the light (light or dark phase of photosynthesis) that causes morphological changes of peroxisomes to optimize the exchange of metabolites (Oikawa et al., 2015; 2019; Corpas, 2015). Similar physical interactions have been also found between peroxisomes and lipid bodies during seed germination (Cui et al., 2016).

7.3 Fatty Acids β-Oxidation, Glyoxylate Cycle, and Auxin Metabolism

Fatty acid catabolism is made through the peroxisomal β-oxidation which is especially relevant in processes such as seed germination or leaf senescence (Baker et al., 2006). Thus, during seed germination, this pathway is indispensable to convert the stored lipids as triacylglycerides in carbohydrates necessary to seedling growth until they can start photosynthesis (Cui *et al.*, 2016). Once fatty acids have been activated through the action of acyl-CoA synthetase, the generated fatty acids acyl-CoA undertakes several rounds of β-oxidation in peroxisomes which implies three enzymes, acyl-CoA oxidase (ACX), multifunctional protein (MFP), and 3-ketoacyl-CoA thiolase (KAT) that finally renders acetyl-CoA (Poirier *et al.*, 2006; Arent *et al.*, 2010; Hielscher *et al.*, 2017; Jawahir and Zolman, 2021) (Fig. 7.5).

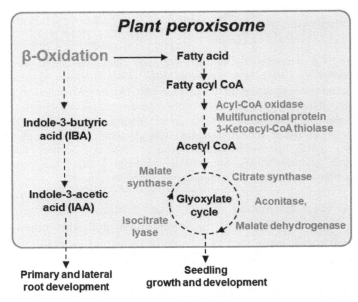

Figure 7.5 Peroxisomal β-oxidation in higher plants. Fatty acids are converted into fatty acids acyl-CoA which then undergoes several rounds of β-oxidation to obtain acetyl-CoA by the action of ACX, MFP, and KAT. This acetyl-CoA is then metabolized to sucrose which is required for seedling development by the action of the glyoxylate cycle which has five enzymes: citrate synthase, aconitase, malate dehydrogenase, isocitrate lyase, and malate synthase, being the last two exclusive located in peroxisomes. The β-oxidation of the indole-3-butyric acid (IBA) produces the auxin IAA which has signal properties to promote primary and lateral root development.

Another essential pathway involved in the process of seedling growth that functions coordinately with the β-oxidation is the glyoxylate cycle. This pathway, mostly similar to the TCA cycle present in the mitochondrion, allows combining the acetyl-CoA generated in the β-oxidation with glyoxylate to synthesize the carbohydrates required for seedling development. In this route, five enzymes are participating: three of them are similar to those of the TCA cycle (citrate synthase, aconitase, and malate dehydrogenase), but two are exclusive of peroxisomes, isocitrate lyase, and malate synthase (Cornah and Smith, 2002). The glyoxylate cycle allows generating carbon skeleton without the loss of carbon in the form of CO_2 (Dellero et al., 2016) (Fig. 7.5).

Peroxisomal β-oxidation is also involved in the generation of the IBA-derived IAA, an auxin involved in the regulation of primary and lateral root development (Strader et al., 2010; Schlicht et al., 2013; Spiess and Zolman, 2013; Sherp et al., 2018; Damodaran and Strader, 2019). Furthermore, the IAA signaling seems to also mediate stress tolerance (Kerchev et al., 2015).

7.4 Biosynthesis of Jasmonic Acid and Polyamine Metabolism

JA is a lipid-based signal molecule involved in an array of processes including seed germination, seedling growth, leaf senescence, fruit ripening, and in the response to various plant stresses including salinity, drought, and UV radiation, and providing a defense against pathogen infection and insect attacks (Dar et al., 2015; Kazan, 2015; Hu et al., 2017; Wasternack and Song, 2017; Griffiths, 2020). It is synthesized from α-linolenic acid by a route that involves the oxidation, cyclization, and shortening of the acyl chain that also implies the cooperation between the chloroplast and the peroxisome (Koo et al., 2006; León, 2013).

Polyamines (PAs) are aliphatic amines, being putrescine (Put), spermidine (Spd), and spermine (Spm) the most significant in plants. This group of molecules has a wide range of functions including cell division, organ development, leaf senescence, fruit development, and ripening, and in the response to abiotic stresses (Tiburcio et al., 2014; Chen et al., 2019; Gholizadeh and Mirzaghaderi, 2020; Gao et al., 2021). PAs are synthesized from arginine and ornithine by arginine decarboxylase and ornithine decarboxylase, respectively, but some peroxisomal enzymes such as copper-containing amine oxidases (CuAOs) and FAD-dependent polyamine oxidases (PAOs), have been shown to participate in PAs catabolism, and also in their back-conversion (Moschou et al., 2008; Fincato et al., 2011; Planas-Portell et al., 2013; Gholizadeh and Mirzaghaderi, 2020).

7.5 Metabolism of ROS and RNS

The name of peroxisomes was set because, since their biochemical characterization in the 1960s, it was found that this organelle had a high content of hydrogen peroxide (H_2O_2) generated by different oxidases such as GOX, ACX, urate oxidase, PA oxidase, CuAO, sulfite oxidase (SO), sarcosine oxidase, or superoxide dismutase (SOD) (Corpas et al., 2020a). Although H_2O_2 is the most abundant ROS in plant peroxisomes, there are other ROS, being together with the superoxide radicals ($O_2^{\bullet-}$) the most investigated (del Río et al., 1989; 1992; López-Huertas et al., 1999; Corpas FJ, Barroso, 2017). Figure 7.6 shows a model of the metabolism of ROS in peroxisomes where a relevant battery of antioxidant enzymes is involved including CAT, SOD, and components of the ascorbate-glutathione cycle such as APX, GR, or MDAR. Although for a long time ROS have been considered as disposable by-products of the oxidative metabolism of peroxisomes, today this concept has changed, and it is accepted that H_2O_2 exerts signaling functions, for example during stomatal movement (Yamauchi et al., 2019) and that superoxide can be used as a biochemical weapon against pathogens (Sørhagen et al., 2013).

Nitric oxide (NO) is a free radical which has a family of related molecules designated as RNS such as peroxynitrite ($ONOO^-$) or S-nitrosoglutathione (GSNO). The presence of NO in plant peroxisomes have been demonstrated by different experimental approaches including electron paramagnetic resonance (EPR) spectroscopy using the spin trap $Fe(MGD)_2$, ozone chemiluminescence, and fluorometric analysis with diaminofluorescein-2 diacetate (DAF-2 DA) as the fluorescence probe (Corpas et al., 2004; 2009; Corpas and Barroso, 2014, 2017). The relevance of these RNS is that they can mediate different PTMs of proteins including tyrosine nitration or S-nitrosation. Table 7.2 summarizes the plant peroxisomal protein targets identified so far which have undergone NO-derived PTMs. Tyrosine nitration involves the addition of a nitro group ($-NO_2$) to a tyrosine residue, it is a highly selective process and usually implies the loss of function of the target protein (Ferrer-Sueta et al., 2018). On the other hand, protein S-nitrosation comprises the covalent attachment of an NO group to the thiol (-SH) side chain of cysteine (Cys) from either protein or small peptides. These PTMs is considered cellular switch that allows regulating the function of the target proteins either positive or negatively (Corpas et al., 2020b).

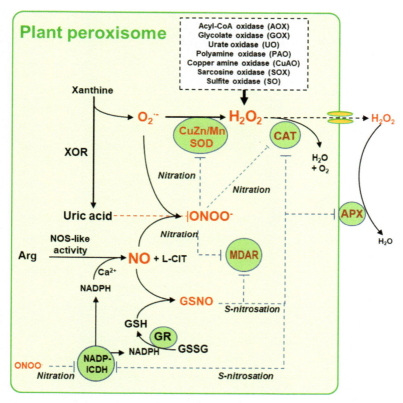

Figure 7.6 Model of the metabolism of ROS and RNS in plant peroxisomes. Peroxisomes have an important battery of H_2O_2-generating enzymes involved in diverse pathways. Xanthine oxidoreductase (XOR) activity produces uric acid which is the concomitant generation of superoxide radical ($O_2^{\bullet-}$) which is dismutated into H_2O_2 and O_2 by CuZn/Mn-superoxide dismutase (CuZn/Mn-SOD). The H_2O_2 pool is mainly decomposed by CAT, but also by the membrane-bound APX. An L-arginine (Arg)- and Ca^{2+}-dependent NOS-like activity generates L-citrulline (L-CIT) plus NO that can react chemically with $O_2^{\bullet-}$ to produce peroxynitrite ($ONOO^-$), a nitrating molecule that facilitates posttranslational modifications (PTMs) such as tyrosine nitration. NO can also interact with reduced glutathione (GSH) to form S-nitrosoglutathione (GSNO), a NO donor which mediates S-nitrosation. GSH is regenerated by GR which requires NADPH supplied by several NADPH-generating enzymes (NADPH-ICDH). Uric acid is an $ONOO^-$ scavenger, this being a mechanism of peroxisomal auto-regulation. With all these components, and according to reported data, the peroxisomal targets of NO-derived PTMs identified so far are CAT, CuZn-SOD, and monodehydroascorbate reductase (MDAR) which can undergo an inhibitory effect either by nitration or S-nitrosation. The red line denotes the inhibition effect. Reproduced from Corpas et al., 2021.

Table 7.2 Peroxisomal enzymes target of diverse PTMs whose activities are affected by either reactive oxygen, nitrogen, and sulfur species (ROS, RNS, and RSS)

Peroxisomal Enzyme	Pathway/ Reaction	PTM	Effect on Activity
Catalase (CAT)	H_2O_2 decomposition	Tyr-nitration S-nitrosation	Inhibition Inhibition
Monodehydroascorbate reductase (MDAR)	Ascorbate-glutathione cycle	Tyr-nitration S-nitrosation	Inhibition Inhibition
Hydroxypyruvate reductase (HPR)	Photorespiration	Tyr-nitration S-nitrosation	Inhibition Inhibition
Glycolate oxidase (GOX)	Photorespiration	S-nitrosation	Inhibition
CuZn-superoxide dismutase (CSD3)	$O_2^{\bullet-}$ dismutation	Tyr-nitration	Inhibition
Malate dehydrogenase (MDH)	Glyoxylate cycle	Tyr-nitration S-nitrosation	Inhibition Inhibition
Isocitrate lyase (ICL)	Glyoxylate cycle	S-nitrosation[a]	Not reported
Multifunctional protein AIM1 isoform	Fatty acid β-oxidation	S-nitrosation[a]	Not reported
Lon protease homolog 2	Peroxisomal protein import	S-nitrosation[a]	Not reported
NADP-isocitrate dehydrogenase	NADPH supply	Tyr-nitration S-nitrosation	Inhibition Inhibition

[a]Proteomic identification

It is remarkable the biochemical interactions between the metabolism of ROS and RNS in plant peroxisomes where there are mutual regulations to avoid an undesirable overproduction of these molecules under physiological situations (Fig. 7.6). However, it has been found that under stress conditions an overproduction of ROS and RNS may occur contributing to cellular nitro-oxidative stress which can trigger irreversible damages to the main macromolecules. The implication of peroxisomal nitro-oxidative metabolism has been found under physiological processes such as seed germination, leaf senescence (Pastori and del Río, 1997; Corpas et al., 2004; Ribeiro et al., 2017), pollen tube growth (Prado et al., 2004), or fruit ripening (Chaki et al., 2015; Palma et al., 2020), as well as under diverse stresses such as salinity (Corpas *et al.*, 1993; 2009; Guan *et al.*, 2015), cadmium (Romero-Puertas *et al.*, 1999; Corpas *et al.*, 2008; Corpas and Barroso, 2017), arsenic (Piacentini *et al.*, 2020), lead (Corpas and Barroso, 2017) and pathogen defense (Xu *et al.*, 2021), or in the presence of xenobiotic such as clofibrate (Palma *et al.*, 1991) and the herbicide 2,4-dichlorophenoxyacetic acid (2,4-D) (Hayashi *et al.*, 1998; Leterrier *et al.*, 2005; Rodríguez-Serrano *et al.*, 2014).

7.6 Pexophagy

This is a type of autophagy that allows the elimination of damaged peroxisomes (Young and Bartel, 2016). It is relevant under diverse circumstances, for example, when peroxisomes present in some organs undertake a metabolic transition. This eventuality takes place when cotyledons become green cotyledons and some enzymes of the glyoxylate cycle disappear whereas enzymes of photorespiration are activated (Kim *et al.*, 2013; Avin-Wittenberg and Fernie, 2014; Fahy *et al.*, 2017). Furthermore, ROS overproduction caused by CAT inhibition has been shown to induce pexophagy (Shibata *et al.*, 2013; Lee *et al.*, 2018), as well as during the interaction with some pathogenic fungi (Chen *et al.*, 2018).

7.7 Conclusions and Further Perspectives

Plant peroxisomes are characterized to have metabolic plasticity that is governed by the organ/tissue, the stage of development, and surrounding environmental conditions. Furthermore, another biochemical remarkable property of the plant peroxisomes is their implication in the biosynthesis of diverse molecules with signal properties, which indicates the dynamic interchange with other subcellular compartments being photorespiration as an excellent example, where chloroplasts, peroxisomes, and mitochondria interact. Thus, peroxisomes are implicated in almost all plant physiological processes as well as in the mechanism of response to adverse environmental conditions where the peroxisomal nitro-oxidative metabolism is exacerbated. Due to the diversity of biochemical pathways present in plant peroxisomes, they are attractive organelles because they could be used for biotechnological application in different areas such as those set to increase ROS metabolism to improve stress tolerance, or to favor the biosynthesis of designed polyunsaturated fatty acids or biodiesel (Kessel-Vigelius et al., 2013; Kechasov et al., 2020; Xu et al., 2021). Future research in peroxisomes will allow promising new and fascinating aspects of this versatile organelle.

Acknowledgments

FJC and JMP research is supported by a European Regional Development Fund cofinanced grant from the Spanish Ministry of Economy and Competitiveness (PID2019-103924GB-I00), the Plan Andaluz de Investigación, Desarrollo e Innovación (PAIDI 2020) (P18-FR-1359) and Junta de Andalucía (group BIO192), Spain.

Abbreviations

2OG	2-oxoglutarate
ACX	acyl-CoA oxidase
APX	ascorbate peroxidase
Arg	L-arginine
CAT	catalase
CuAO	copper amine oxidase
GDC	glycine decarboxylase complex
GGAT	glutamate: glyoxylate aminotransferase
GK	glycerate kinase
GOX	glycolate oxidase
GOX	glycolate oxidase
GR	glutathione reductase
GSNO	S-nitrosoglutathione
HPR	hydroxypyruvate reductase
IAA	indole-3-acetic acid
IBA	indole-3-butyric acid
JA	jasmonic acid
KAT	3-ketoacyl-CoA thiolase
MDAR	monodehydroascorbate peroxidase
MFP	a multifunctional protein
OAA	oxaloacetate
ONOO-	peroxynitrite

PAO	polyamine oxidase
PTMs	posttranslational modifications
Put	putrescine
RNS	reactive nitrogen species
ROS	reactive oxygen species
Rubisco	ribulose 1,5-bisphosphate carboxylase/oxygenase
SGAT	serine-glyoxylate aminotransferase
SHMT	serine hydroxymethyltransferase
SO	sulfite oxidase
SOD	superoxide dismutase
Spd	spermidine
Spm	spermine
TCA	tricarboxylic acid
UO	urate oxidase
XOR	xanthine oxidoreductase

References

Arent S., Christensen C. E., Pye V. E., Nørgaard A., Henriksen A., *J. Biol. Chem.* **285** (2010), 24066–24077.

Avin-Wittenberg T., Fernie A. R., *Mol. Plant* **7** (2014), 1257–1260.

Baker A., Graham I. A., Holdsworth M., Smith S. M., Theodoulou F. L., *Trends Plant Sci.* **11** (2006), 124–132.

Beevers, H.. *Ann. Rev. Plant Physiol.* **30** (1979), 159–193.

Busch F. A., *Plant J.* **101** (2020), 919–939.

Chaki M., Álvarez de Morales P., Ruiz C., Begara-Morales J. C., Barroso J. B., Corpas F. J., Palma J. M., *Ann. Bot.* **116** (2015), 637–647.

Chen D., Shao Q., Yin L., Younis A., Zheng B., *Front. Plant Sci.* **9** (2019), 1945.

Chen Y., Zheng S., Ju Z., Zhang C., Tang G., Wang J., Wen Z., Chen W., Ma Z., *Environ. Microbiol.* **20** (2018), 3224–3245.

Cornah J. E., Smith S. M., *Plant Peroxisomes* (Baker A., Graham I. A., eds), Springer, Dordrecht, 2002.

Corpas F. J., Barroso J. B., *Ann. Bot.* **113** (2014), 87–96.

Corpas F. J., Barroso J. B., Carreras A., Quirós M., León A. M., Romero-Puertas M. C., Esteban F. J., Valderrama R., Palma J. M., Sandalio L. M., Gómez M., del Río L. A., *Plant Physiol.* **136** (2004), 2722–2733.

Corpas F. J., Barroso J. B., del Río L. A., *Trends Plant Sci.* **6** (2001), 145–150.

Corpas F. J., Barroso J. B., *J. Cell Sci.* **131** (2018), jcs202978.

Corpas F. J., del Río L. A., Palma J. M., *J. Integr. Plant Biol.* **61** (2019), 803–816.

Corpas F. J., del Río L. A., Palma J. M., *Plants (Basel).* **8** (2019), 37.

Corpas F. J., del Río L. A., Palma J. M., *Subcell Biochem.* **89** (2018), 473–493.

Corpas F. J., Gómez M., Hernández J. A., del Río L. A., *J. Plant Physiol.* **141** (1993), 160–165.

Corpas F. J., González-Gordo S., Palma J. M., *Int. J. Mol. Sci.* **22** (2021), 2444.

Corpas F. J., Hayashi M., Mano S., Nishimura M., Barroso J. B., *Plant Physiol.* **151** (2009), 2083–2094.

Corpas F. J., *Nat. Plants.* **1** (2015), 15039.

Corpas F. J, González-Gordo S., Palma J. M., *Front. Plant Sci.* **11** (2020a), 853.

Corpas F. J., González-Gordo S., Palma J. M., *J. Biotechnol.* **324** (2020b), 211–219.

Corpas F. J., Palma J. M., Sandalio L. M., Valderrama R., Barroso J. B., del Río L. A., *J. Plant Physiol.* **165** (2008), 1319–1330.

Corpas, F. J., Barroso, J. B., *Nitric Oxide.* **68** (2017), 103–110.

Cui S., Hayashi Y., Otomo M., Mano S., Oikawa K., Hayashi M., Nishimura M., *J. Biol. Chem.* **291** (2016), 19734–19745.

Damodaran S., Strader L. C., *Front. Plant Sci.* **10** (2019), 851.

Dar T. A., Uddin M., Khan M. M. A., Hakeem K. R., Jaleel H., *Environ. Exp. Bot.* **115** (2015), 49–57.

De Bellis L., Picciarelli P., Pistelli L., Alpi A., *Planta* **180** (1990), 435–439.

de Duve C., Beaufay H., Jacques P., Rahman-Li Y., Sellinger O. Z., Wattiaux R., de Coninck S., *Biochim. Biophys. Acta* **40** (1960), 186–187.

de Duve C., Baudhuin P., *Physiol. Rev.* **46** (1966), 323–357.

del Río L. A., Fernández V. M., Rupérez F. L., Sandalio L. M., Palma J. M., *Plant Physiol.* **89** (1989), 728–731.

del Río L. A., Sandalio L. M., Palma J. M., Bueno P., Corpas F. J., *Free Radic. Biol. Med.* **13** (1992), 557–580.

Dellero Y., Jossier M., Schmitz J., Maurino V. G., Hodges M., *J. Exp. Bot.* **67** (2016), 3041–3052.

Eastmond P. J., Graham I. A., *Trends Plant Sci.* **6** (2001), 72–78.

Eisenhut M., Brautigam A., Timm S., Florian A., Tohge T., Fernie A. R., Bauwe H., Weber A. P., M., *Mol. Plant* **10** (2017), 47–61.

Engqvist M. K. M., Maurino V. G., *Methods Mol. Biol.* **1653** (2017), 137–155.

Fahy D., Sanad M. N., Duscha K., Lyons M., Liu F., Bozhkov P., Kunz H. H., Hu

J., Neuhaus H. E., Steel P. G., Smertenko A., *Sci. Rep.* **7** (2017), 39069.

Ferrer-Sueta G., Campolo N., Trujillo M., Bartesaghi S., Carballal S., Romero N., Alvarez B., Radi R., *Chem. Rev.* **118** (2018), 1338–1408.

Fincato P., Moschou P. N., Spedaletti V., Tavazza R., Angelini R., Federico R., Roubelakis-Angelakis K. A., Tavladoraki P., *J. Exp. Bot.* **62** (2011), 1155–1168.

Florian A., Araújo W. L., Fernie A. R., *Plant Biol.* (Stuttgart) **15** (2013), 656–666.

Gao F., Mei X., Li Y., Guo J., Shen Y., *Front. Plant Sci.* **12** (2021), 610313.

Gholizadeh F., Mirzaghaderi G., *PLoS One* **15** (2020), e0236226.

Griffiths G., *Essays Biochem.* **64** (2020), 501–512.

Guan Q., Wang Z., Wang X., Takano T., Liu S., *J. Plant Physiol.* **175** (2015), 183–191.

Hayashi M., Toriyama K., Kondo M., Nishimura M., *Plant Cell.* **10** (1998), 183–195.

Hielscher B., Charton L., Mettler-Altmann T., Linka N., *Methods Mol. Biol.* **1595** (2017), 291–304.

Hu J., Baker A., Bartel B., Linka N., Mullen R. T., Reumann S., Zolman B. K., *Plant Cell.* **24** (2012), 2279–2303.

Hu Y., Jiang Y., Han X., Wang H., Pan J., Yu D., *J. Exp. Bot.* **68** (2017), 1361–1369.

Igamberdiev A. U., Lea P. J., *Phytochemistry* **60** (2002), 651–674.

Islinger M., Cardoso M., Schrader M., *Biochim. Biophys. Acta (BBA) Bioenerg.* **1803**, (2010), 881–897.

Jawahir V., Zolman B. K., *Plant Physiol.* **185** (2021), 120–136.

Kazan K., *Trends Plant Sci.* **20** (2015), 219–229.

Kechasov D., de Grahl I., Endries P., Reumann S., *Front. Cell Dev. Biol.* **8** (2020), 593922.

Kerchev P., Mühlenbock P., Denecker J., Morreel K., Hoeberichts F. A., Van Der Kelen K., Vandorpe M., Nguyen L., Audenaert D., Van Breusegem F., *Plant Cell Environ.* **38** (2015), 253–265.

Kessel-Vigelius S. K., Wiese J., Schroers M. G., Wrobel T. J., Hahn F., Linka N., *Plant Sci.* **210** (2013), 232–240.

Kim J., Lee H., Lee H. N., Kim S. H., Shin K. D., Chung T., *Plant Cell* **25** (2013), 4956–4966.

Koo A. J., Chung H. S., Kobayashi Y., Howe G. A., *J. Biol. Chem.* **281** (2006), 33511–33520.

Lackus N. D., Schmidt A., Gershenzon J., Köllner T. G., *Plant Physiol.* (2021), kiab111.

León J., *Subcell Biochem.* **69** (2013) 299–313.

Leterrier M., Corpas F. J., Barroso J. B., Sandalio L. M., del Río L. A., *Plant Physiol.* **138** (2005), 2111–2123.

López-Huertas E., Corpas F. J., Sandalio L. M., del Río L. A., *Biochem. J.* **337** (1999), 531–536.

Mano S., Nakamori C., Hayashi M., Kato A., Kondo M., Nishimura M., *Plant Cell Physiol.* **43** (2002), 331–341.

Moschou P. N., Sanmartin M., Andriopoulou A. H., Rojo E., Sanchez-Serrano J. J., Roubelakis-Angelakis K. A., *Plant Physiol.* **147** (2008), 1845–1857.

Oikawa K., Hayashi M., Hayashi Y., Nishimura M., *J. Integr. Plant Biol.* **61**(2019), 836–852.

Oikawa K., Matsunaga S., Mano S., Kondo M., Yamada K., Hayashi M., Kagawa T., Kadota A., Sakamoto W., Higashi S., Watanabe M., Mitsui T., Shigemasa A., Iino T., Hosokawa Y., Nishimura M., *Nat. Plants* **1** (2015), 15035.

Ono Y., Kim D. W., Watanabe K., Sasaki A., Niitsu M., Berberich T., Kusano T., Takahashi Y., *Amino Acids* **42** (2012), 867–876.

Palma J. M., de Morales P. Á., del Río L. A., Corpas F. J., *Subcell. Biochem.* **89** (2018), 323–341.

Palma J. M., Garrido M., Rodríguez-García M. I., del Río L. A., *Arch. Biochem. Biophys.* **287** (1991), 68–74

Palma J. M., Mateos R. M., López-Jaramillo J., Rodríguez-Ruiz M., González-Gordo S., Lechuga-Sancho A. M., Corpas F. J., *Redox Biol.* **34 (**2020), 101525.

Pastori G. M., del Rio L. A., *Plant Physiol.* **113** (1997), 411–418.

Peterhansel C., Maurino V. G., *Plant Physiol.* **155** (2011), 49–55.

Peterhansel C., Horst I., Niessen M., Blume C., Kebeish R., Kürkcüoglu S., Kreuzaler F., *Arabidopsis Book* **8** (2010), e0130.

Piacentini D., Corpas F. J., D'Angeli S., Altamura M. M., Falasca G., *Plant Physiol. Biochem.* **148** (2020), 312–323.

Planas-Portell J., Gallart M., Tiburcio A. F., Altabella T., *BMC Plant Biol.* **13** (2013), 109.

Poirier Y., Antonenkov V. D., Glumoff T., Hiltunen J. K., *Biochim. Biophys. Acta* **1763** (2006), 1413–1426.

Pracharoenwattana I., Cornah J. E., Smith S. M., *Plant Cell* **17** (2005), 2037–2048.

Prado A. M., Porterfield D. M., Feijó J. A., *Development* **131** (2004), 2707–2714.

Ribeiro C. W., Korbes A. P., Garighan J. A., Jardim-Messeder D., Carvalho F. E. L., Sousa R. H. V., Caverzan A., Teixeira F. K., Silveira J. A. G., Margis-Pinheiro M., *Plant Sci.* **263** (2017), 55–65.

Rodríguez-Serrano M., Pazmiño D. M., Sparkes I., Rochetti A., Hawes C., Romero-Puertas M. C., Sandalio L. M., *J. Exp. Bot.* **65** (2014), 4783–4793.

Romero-Puertas M. C., McCarthy I., Sandalio L. M., Palma J. M., Corpas F. J., Gómez M., del Río L. A., *Free Radic. Res.* **31**(Suppl), (1999), S25–S31.

Schlicht M., Ludwig-Müller J., Burbach C., Volkmann D., Baluska F., *New Phytol.* **200** (2013), 473–482.

Sherp A. M., Westfall C. S., Alvarez S., Jez J. M., *J. Biol. Chem.* **293** (2018), 4277–4288.

Sørhagen K., Laxa M., Peterhänsel C., Reumann S., *Plant Biol.* (Stuttgart) **15** (2013), 723–736.

Spiess G. M., Zolman B. K., *Subcell. Biochem.* **69** (2013), 257–281.

Strader L. C., Culler A. H., Cohen J. D., Bartel B., *Plant Physiol.* **153** (2010), 1577–1586.

Tabak H. F., Braakman I., Distel B., *Trends Cell Biol.* **9** (1999), 447–453.

Tiburcio A. F., Altabella T., Bitrián M., Alcázar R., *Planta* **240** (2014), 1–18.

Tolbert N. E., *Annu. Rev. Biochem.* **50** (1981), 133–157.

Tolbert N. E., Essner E., *J. Cell Biol.* **91** (1981), 271s–283s.

Wang W., Paschalidis K., Feng J. C., Song J., Liu J. H., *Front. Plant Sci.* **10** (2019), 561.

Wasternack C., Song S., *J. Exp. Bot.* **68** (2017), 1303–1321.

Xu J., Padilla C. S., Li J., Wickramanayake J., Fischer H. D., Goggin F. L., *Mol. Plant Pathol.* **22** (2021), 727–736.

Yamauchi S., Mano S., Oikawa K., Hikino K., Teshima K. M., Kimori Y., Nishimura M., Shimazaki K. I., Takemiya A., *Proc. Natl. Acad. Sci. U.S.A.* **116** (2019), 19187–19192.

Young P. G., Bartel B., *Biochim. Biophys. Acta* **1863** (2016), 999–1005.

Zhang Z., Liang X., Lu L., Xu Z., Huang J., He H., Peng X., *BMC Plant Biol.* **20** (2020), 357.

Part III
Herbicide-Tolerant Traits

Chapter 8

Oxygenase Enzymes for Agricultural Biotechnology Applications

Clayton T. Larue
Bayer Crop Science, St. Louis, Missouri, USA
claton.larue@bayer.com

Agriculture biotechnologies have been an important part of our efforts to provide food, fiber, and fuel to a growing world population. One such application is the development of traits that can be integrated with crop plants to address a specific need. These traits can include an enzyme that performs a specific task in the crop plant. For example, herbicide tolerance traits can employ enzymes that act on selected herbicides to enable the use of a given herbicide during a cropping season. The oxygenase enzymes are an enzyme family that has been proven to be useful in developing several herbicide tolerance traits. In this chapter, monooxygenase and dioxygenase enzymes and their utility in agricultural biotechnology–based herbicide tolerance traits will be reviewed.

Agricultural Biocatalysis: Enzymes in Agriculture and Industry
Edited by Peter Jeschke and Evgeni B. Starikov
Copyright © 2023 Jenny Stanford Publishing Pte. Ltd.
ISBN 978-981-4968-47-8 (Hardcover), 978-1-003-31310-6 (eBook)
www.jennystanford.com

8.1 Introduction

Biotechnology applications for agriculture often depend on enzymes or proteins that can perform a variety of unique tasks. A widely employed biotechnology application is the generation and use of genetically modified organisms (GMOs) such as crop plants enhanced with the addition of a specific trait. For example, these traits can improve the quality of the crop, such as non-browning apples (Stowe and Dhingra, 2020) or improve agronomic characteristics of the crop such as improved pest and weed control (Mall et al., 2019). In this chapter, the focus will be on herbicide tolerance traits. Herbicide tolerance traits are biotechnology traits that enable the use of a specific herbicide or herbicide family in a cropping field during the growing season for a crop that would normally be sensitive to the herbicide application. The presence of the herbicide tolerance trait imparts a tolerance (in some scientific publications the term resistance is used) in the crop to the herbicide application, allowing the crop plant to continue to grow without injury while the targeted weeds are killed from the herbicide application. The use of herbicide tolerance traits, paired with the corresponding herbicide applications, has become a widely adopted tool for farmers to use as a part of an integrated weed control system in many world geographies.

Currently, herbicide tolerance traits that are commercially available or in advanced development typically follow one of two technical approaches (Fig. 8.1). In the first approach, the biotechnology trait utilizes an enzyme that deactivates the herbicide chemistry directly. This deactivation can be via the removal of a portion of the herbicide molecule or the addition of a functional group to the herbicide molecule that renders the compound inactive as an herbicide. One family of enzymes that have been used in multiple herbicide tolerance traits is the oxygenase enzymes. This family of enzymes will be the subject of this chapter and will be reviewed in more detail in the remainder of the chapter. However, it should be noted that other enzymes families can function to deactivate herbicides. For example, *pat* and *bar*, two genes that encode phosphinothricin acetyltransferase enzymes, acetylate the herbicide glufosinate resulting in herbicide deactivation (Wehrmann et al., 1996). Both of these genes have been used in the successful development of glufosinate tolerant crops.

The second approach utilizes an insensitive target, an alternate version of the molecular target of the herbicide that is not susceptible to the action of the herbicide chemistry (Fig. 8.1). While insensitive target herbicide tolerance traits will not be the focus of this chapter, it is important to note that this approach has also been successful. For example, tolerance to glyphosate in soybeans was engineered using CP4, an insensitive version of the enzyme 5-enolpyruvylshikimate-3-phosphate synthase (EPSPS) (Padgette *et al.*, 1995). Glyphosate inhibits the enzymatic function of the native EPSPS, however, the presence of the glyphosate-insensitive bacterial-derived CP4 EPSPS enables the enzymatic function to continue even in the presence of glyphosate and thus the plants are tolerant to the herbicide application. Recently, a similar approach was taken to engineer tolerance to a family of herbicides that inhibit the enzyme protoporphyrinogen IX oxidase (PPO), an enzyme in the chlorophyll and heme biosynthetic pathways. An herbicide insensitive PPO enzyme variant called H_N90 was identified from a microbial sourcing effort that is sequence diverse relative to native plant PPO enzymes but shows functional conservation and thus can perform the same enzymatic step in the chlorophyll and heme biosynthetic pathways as the native plant PPO enzyme. The expression of H_N90 in several crop plants was shown to provide tolerance to several PPO-inhibitor herbicides (Larue *et al.*, 2020).

The focus of this chapter will be on the oxygenase enzymes used in agriculture biotechnology for herbicide tolerance traits through an herbicide deactivation approach. Here, we will focus on two types of oxygenase enzymes, dioxygenases, and monooxygenases. Both dioxygenases and monooxygenases activate dioxygen and incorporate the oxygen atoms into the enzymatic products. Dioxygenases incorporate both of the oxygen atoms into the products and are often dependent on metal cofactors, such as ferrous metal ions, Fe(II) or Fe(III) (Bugg, 2003). One class of dioxygenases is the α-ketoglutarate-dependent dioxygenases. These enzymes are found across many life forms and are somewhat unusual in that generally only one of the oxygen atoms is transferred to the substrate that is being studied, while the other oxygen atom is transferred to the α-ketoglutarate co-substrate (which binds the ferrous metal ion to activate molecular oxygen) to generate succinate (Guengerich, 2015). These enzymes are now known to perform a wide variety of

248 | *Oxygenase Enzymes for Agricultural Biotechnology Applications*

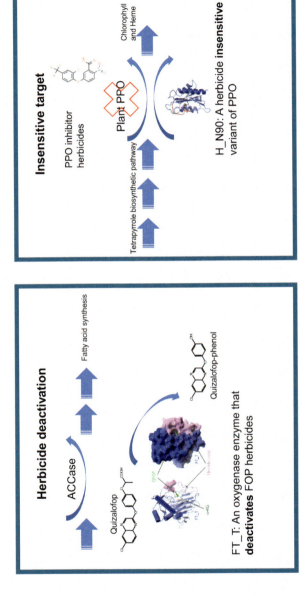

Figure 8.1 An overview of two alternative technical approaches for engineering biotechnological herbicide tolerance traits. In the herbicide deactivation technical approach, a biotechnological enzyme directly modifies the herbicide molecule, rendering the herbicide inactive. Here, the FT_T oxygenase enzyme deactivates the herbicide quizalofop. Deactivation of the herbicide allows the enzyme ACCase, which would normally be inhibited by the herbicide in sensitive plants, to continue to function in the fatty acid synthesis pathway. In the insensitive target approach, a biotechnological trait employs an insensitive alternate version of the molecular target for the herbicide. Here, the herbicide insensitive microbial PPO enzyme, H_N90, takes over for the native plant PPO enzyme that is inhibited by the herbicide application allowing the chlorophyll and heme biosynthetic pathways to continue uninterrupted.

reactions through C-H bond activation and thus play an important role in microbial natural product biosynthesis (Wu *et al.*, 2016). Monooxygenases catalyze the insertion of a single oxygen atom (from molecular oxygen) into the organic substrate performing a wide range of reactions, often with high substrate selectivity (Pazmiño *et al.*, 2010). Monooxygenases often depend on cofactors, which can be metal ions or compounds such as flavins and may also depend on partner co-enzymes. As will be explored in more detail in this chapter, both dioxygenases and monooxygenases have been successfully employed as the basis for herbicide tolerance traits.

8.2 Discovery and Early Development of Herbicide Tolerance Traits

The process of discovery, optimization, testing, and early development of a given oxygenase enzyme for use as an herbicide tolerance trait is often a complex, iterative process (Fig. 8.2). Here, an overview of the steps in a generalized representative process is outlined to enable the reader to better understand the process. However, this chapter is not designed to be a comprehensive review of the numerous techniques that could be employed in this process; the reader is encouraged to seek published reviews on the techniques that are of most interest for further information. Furthermore, the reader should understand that there are many variations with alternate steps, techniques, and pathways available to achieve the goal of the discovery of an herbicide tolerance trait. A successful discovery effort will modify what is presented here to best fit the biology and details of each trait that is being explored.

The first step to this process is sourcing relevant oxygenase enzymes. A variety of sources and techniques can be used to build a starting pool of test enzymes. A large diversity of oxygenase enzymes is found throughout life forms, with microbes and plants being successful sources in the examples discussed here. Sourcing strategies are generally designed to enrich genes of interest, to increase the chances for success. For example, sourcing strategies could employ microbial enrichments, information from literature sources, bioinformatic analysis, or characterization of plants showing varying degrees of resistance to herbicides. Additionally, enzyme engineering could be used to broaden the starting pool of genes of interest and variants.

250 | *Oxygenase Enzymes for Agricultural Biotechnology Applications*

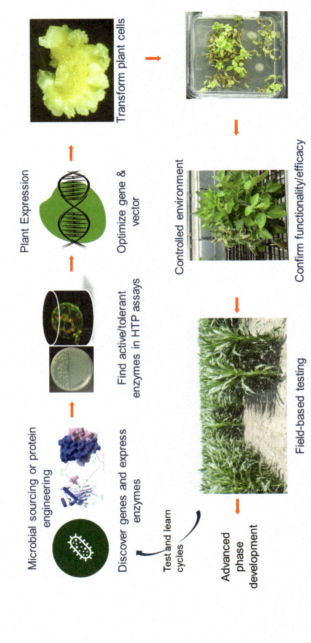

Figure 8.2 An overview of the discovery and early development processes for engineering herbicide tolerance traits.

After starting pools of enzymes have been identified, the next step is to screen these enzyme variants in a high-throughput manner. It is often the case that 1000s of variants will need to be screened to begin to narrow the pool to the best candidates (Larue *et al.*, 2019). One of the keys to success in the discovery process is the design of quality high-throughput (HT) assays. It is important to caution the reader that these HT assays often are still laborious as multiple parameters will need to be considered and that the outcome of the assays is unpredictable. Furthermore, while these assays will need to be designed to rapidly screen a large number of candidates, care should be taken to obtain the best information to inform results that may translate to what will ultimately be observed in whole plants. A successful HT assay screen will enable a significant narrowing of the pool of candidate enzymes to a smaller number of candidates suitable for screening in plants. However, it should be recognized that even with well-designed HT assays, success in these HT assays does not guarantee success when candidate enzymes are moved to testing in plant systems.

The next step is to screen these selected candidate enzymes in plants (generally as a transgene or as a gene-editing target). Screening in plants as a transgene requires designing expression vectors to ensure the enzyme is expressed in the proper tissues, developmental timing, and expression levels. Oftentimes these screens start using expression elements designed for medium to high expression levels across plant tissues throughout the growth of the plant. However, as the optimization process progress, discovery and fine-tuning of the expression elements is often as important as the optimization of the enzyme itself. With both transgene and gene editing–based approaches, plantlets expressing the gene of interest must be regenerated and then grown, often in a controlled environment setting such as greenhouses or growth chambers. A variety of molecular or biochemical assays should be considered to confirm the presence and expression of the gene/enzyme of interest.

Once plants expressing the candidate enzymes are generated, the plants can be screened with herbicide applications to assay for tolerance. Here there are a variety of methodologies that can be followed. One could first produce seed from the regenerated plants, and then screen a subset of the progeny (keeping segregation of the transgene/gene edit in mind). Alternatively, plants can be screened shortly after regeneration. If one follows this path, it is important to keep in mind that all the plants may die or be injured to the point that little or no seed is produced following the herbicide test, eliminating what could be controlled for in future experiments or plants that may have partial tolerance which could have been further characterized to provide a starting point for further optimization. Therefore, one could also consider herbicide treatments of only a subset of regenerated plants or screening of clonal cuttings or tissues such as leaf punches. Generally, herbicide screening can start at partial rates relative to the desired full rate and then increased through the optimization process.

Following successful identification of lead candidate enzymes in the whole plant, controlled environment screening, testing should advance to field-relevant conditions. As will be shown in one of the examples below, this step is essential to identify enzymes that are robust and can perform under a variety of field-relevant growing conditions for the crop of interest. Generally, for lead candidates that advance to this stage, a researcher will likely test the plants with multiple herbicide applications through the relevant timing window at rates above the expected rates in a variety of field settings, seasons, geographies, or cropping systems.

The final important point regarding this process is the test and learn iterative cycles. At every step during the process, the researcher should take time to gather the relevant data, review the data and look for ways in which this data could inform additional rounds of candidate selection or optimization. Designing and developing a robust herbicide tolerance trait requires repeating testing, optimization, and further selection to find the best combination of elements that represents the final field-ready trait. Shortcuts in these steps will almost certainly result in a trait needing improvements, with the shortcomings not always being immediately obvious. It is with this process that optimal herbicide tolerance traits can be discovered, developed, and advanced to a product that can be deployed in production agriculture.

8.3 Dioxygenases for FOP and 2,4-D Tolerance Traits

The aryloxyphenoxy-propionate (FOP) herbicides and 2,4-dichlorophenoxyacetic acid (2,4-D) herbicides have different modes of action (MoA) in a plant. The herbicide 2,4-D was first commercialized in the 1940s and acts as a synthetic auxin (Peterson *et al.*, 2016). This herbicide has been shown to directly interfere with the auxin sensing machinery within a plant cell resulting in an uncontrolled over-stimulation of the hormone signaling pathways and eventual plant death in sensitive plants (especially in the dicotyledonous/broadleaf weeds). The FOP herbicides are one chemical family within a broader Group 1 class of herbicides, which all act to inhibit the enzyme acetyl coenzyme A (CoA) carboxylase (ACCase) in the fatty acid synthesis pathway. The FOP herbicides, such as quizalofop, have been shown to inhibit the ACCase isoform that represents the majority of the enzymatic activity in the chloroplasts of the grasses (*Graminaceae*) resulting in strong herbicide activity in the grasses but not in the dicotyledonous plants, which mostly depend on an alternate insensitive ACCase isoform (Ruizzo and Gorski, 1988; Dehaye *et al.*, 1994; Herbert *et al.*, 1996). Despite the unique MoAs as herbicides, both herbicide families have shared portions of the chemical molecule, namely a phenoxy ring with an alkanoic acid attached via an ether linkage (Fig. 8.3). It is through these shared chemical moieties that a single enzyme was identified as an herbicide tolerance trait for both herbicides.

With the application or release of agriculture and industrial chemistries to soil and aquatic environments, microbes have acquired the ability to metabolize some of these compounds. One of the first enzymes characterized in metabolizing 2,4-D is a 2,4-D dioxygenase (2,4-dichlorophenoxyacetic acid/α-ketoglutarate dioxygenase; TfdA). TfdA was isolated from bacteria capable of utilizing 2,4-D as a carbon source and was characterized as an α-ketoglutarate-dependent dioxygenase that initiates the biodegradation pathway for 2,4-D (Amy *et al.*, 1985; Fukumori and Hausinger, 1993a; Fukumori and Hausinger, 1993b). However, further characterization of TfdA uncovered stereospecific enzymatic activity for this enzyme family (Saari *et al.*, 1999). TfdA was able to oxidize *(S)*-dichlorprop (a closely related compound to 2,4-D except for the presence of a chiral propionic acid side chain in place of the achiral side chain for 2,4-D), while activity from other isolates was found to be specific for the *(R)*-enantiomer. Additionally, work by Hogan *et al.* (2000) began to uncover a core set of residues characteristic of the α-ketoglutarate dependent dioxygenase enzyme family that help form the metallocenter and coordinate substrate binding.

Around the same time as the work was underway for TdfA, additional bacterial isolates were being uncovered that showed similar activity on 2,4-D or similar synthetic auxin herbicides (Horvath *et al.*, 1990; Wesendorf *et al.*, 2003). Two bacterial strains, *Sphingomonas herbicidovorans* MH and *Delftia acidovorans* MC1, were found to contain two dioxygenase enzymes: α-ketoglutarate dependent *(R)*-dichlorprop dioxygenase (RdpA) and α-ketoglutarate dependent *(S)*-dichlorprop dioxygenase (SdpA) that were able to enzymatically act on several synthetic auxin herbicide compounds of the corresponding enantiomers (Nickel *et al.*, 1997; Kohler, 1999; Schleinitz *et al.*, 2004; Müller *et al.*, 2006). The RdpA enzymes from both strains were found to be identical enzymes. While the overall sequence homology to TfdA was low, both RdpA and SdpA maintained the characteristic α-ketoglutarate dependent dioxygenase motif as proposed in Hogan *et al.* (2000). Detailed characterization of the enzymes demonstrated the α-ketoglutarate and ferrous cofactor-dependent nature of the enzymes and a strict enantiomer selectivity without any observed enzyme inhibition when supplied with the opposing enantiomer suggesting only the correct enantiomer is capable of binding in the active pocket (Müller *et al.*, 2006). Furthermore, substrate selectivity of RdpA was observed to be dependent mostly on the alkanoic acid side chain and relatively indifferent to the substituents on the aromatic ring (Müller *et al.*, 2006). Given that many of the agriculturally relevant herbicides containing this chemical signature (a phenoxy ring with an alkanoic acid attached via an ether linkage) are active as the *(R)*-enantiomer (the notable exception being 2,4-D, which has an achiral sidechain) and the forgiving nature of the enzyme to accept substrates with a variety of additional substituents on the aromatic ring, RdpA became a key target enzyme for agriculture biotechnology applications.

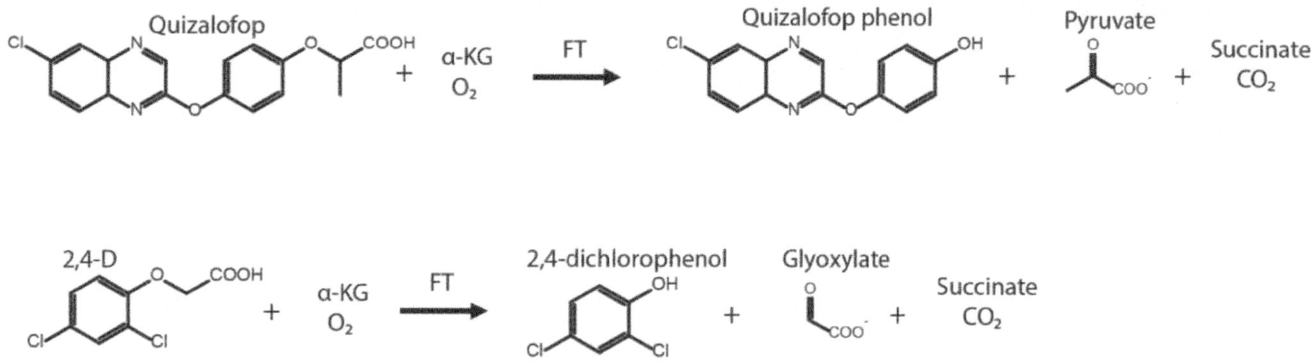

Figure 8.3 A schematic illustrating the oxygenase activity of the FT enzymes on selected herbicide molecules. Figure adapted from Larue et al., 2019.

The use of RdpA and SdpA in agriculture biotechnology was first demonstrated by Wright et al. (2010). In this work, RdpA from *S. herbicidivorans* (renamed by Wright et al. (2010) as aryloxyalkanoate dioxygenase-1 or AAD-1) and SdpA from *D. acidovorans* (renamed by Wright et al. (2010) as AAD-12) were further characterized and expressed in *Arabidopsis thaliana*, corn (maize) and soybean plants. Further characterization of the substrate specificity of these enzymes confirmed that these enzymes were selective based on the nature and chirality of alkanoic acid side chain, but forgiving regarding the substituents on the aromatic ring, including being able to accept members of the FOP herbicides which have additional ring structures as substituents on the aromatic ring (Wright et al., 2010). RdpA was transformed as a transgene into corn plants and plants expressing the transgene were screened with herbicide applications (Wright et al., 2010). These corn plants displayed tolerance to applications of both a FOP herbicide (quizalofop) and 2,4-D herbicide at rates that exceeded the typical field application rates. While 2,4-D injuries dicotyledonous (broadleaf) plants more than monocotyledonous (such as corn), corn will show malformation injury following 2,4-D applications at certain growth stages. SdpA demonstrated better enzymatic activity on 2,4-D relative to RdpA (Wright et al., 2010). Soybeans, being a dicotyledonous plant, are very sensitive to 2,4-D and this likely provided the rationale for using SdpA for the generation of transformed soybean plants. The soybean plants expressing SdpA showed tolerance to 2,4-D applications above normal field use rates (Wright et al., 2010). This work in both corn and soybeans nicely illustrates the potential value these dioxygenase enzymes could bring to agriculture biotechnology.

As mentioned earlier in this chapter, native enzymes, such as oxygenase enzymes, can be excellent starting points for structure-based and computational-assisted enzyme optimization efforts. This was the approach taken by Larue et al. (2019). In this work, the authors were interested in engineering optimized dioxygenase enzymes (called FT enzymes) based on the RdpA scaffold which would have robust activity on both members of the FOP herbicides and members of the synthetic auxins such as 2,4-D (Fig. 8.3). However, it was discovered during the optimization process that some engineered versions of the enzyme, and the RdpA starting scaffold, displayed poor enzyme stability at higher temperatures.

This was shown to be problematic when FT expressing plants were exposed to higher temperatures that were selected to mimic hot field environments often found in crop fields in many world geographies and challenged with herbicide applications (Larue et al., 2019). This new finding was used to inform additional enzyme optimization work in which heat stability was included as an optimization target. This large effort resulted in the engineering and identification of several optimized FT enzymes which showed significantly improved temperature stability as well as improved enzymatic parameters for selected herbicide chemistries (Larue et al., 2019). During optimization of the plant expression of the FT enzymes, it was discovered that the addition of a chloroplast targeting peptide to the expressed FT enzyme significantly improved the tolerance *in planta* to the FOP herbicides (such as quizalofop), and thus chloroplast targeting peptides were included for the FT variants tested in corn (Larue et al., 2019). However, the addition of chloroplast targeting peptides to the FT enzymes did not result in large changes in tolerance to 2,4-D herbicide applications in both corn and soybeans expressing these FT variants. The chloroplast targeting peptide is a short amino acid sequence located on the N-terminal end of the protein that acts as a cellular signal to import the protein to the chloroplast within the plant cell (Lee and Hwang, 2018). Both controlled environment and field-based testing of corn and soybean plants expressing FT enzyme variants displayed excellent tolerance to applications of quizalofop and 2,4-D herbicides above normal field rates (Larue et al., 2019). In addition, the tolerance remained remarkably robust even at elevated temperatures indicating that optimization efforts to heat stabilize the FT enzymes were successful. This work nicely illustrates that oxygenase enzymes may be amendable to enzyme engineering and optimization efforts to design new oxygenase variants with attractive properties for applied applications such as agriculture biotechnology.

8.4 Monooxygenase Enzyme for Dicamba Tolerance

Dicamba (3,6-dichloro-2-methoxy benzoic acid) is another synthetic auxin herbicide that began use as an herbicide in the 1960s. Similar to 2,4-D, dicamba disrupts normal hormone signaling pathways in plants resulting in plant death with dicotyledonous (broadleaf) weeds, in general, being more sensitive to the herbicide (Shaner, 2014). However, dicamba is chemically unique relative to some of the other synthetic auxins such as 2,4-D in that it does not contain an alkanoic acid side chain and instead contains a methoxy group.

The soil bacterium, *Pseudomonas maltophilia* DI-6, was characterized to survive on dicamba as a sole carbon source with the likely first step in the metabolism of dicamba to be the removal of the methyl group to produce 3,6-dichlorosalicylic acid (DCSA, Fig. 8.4) with an unidentified demethylase enzyme (Cork and Krueger, 1991; Yang *et al.*, 1994). Further characterization of this strain identified a megaplasmid carrying an *O*-demethylase as a part of a three-component enzyme system (Wang *et al.*, 1997; Herman *et al.*, 2005). This three-component enzyme system included a reductase, a ferredoxin, and an oxygenase enzyme which form a short electron transfer chain from reduced pyridine nucleotides (such as NADH, reduced nicotinamide adenine dinucleotide), through the ferredoxin to the non-heme iron-containing oxygenase. Sequence analysis and enzymatic characterization of the oxygenase revealed the oxygenase to be a Rieske (2Fe-2S) non-heme iron monooxygenase that converts dicamba into DCSA and formaldehyde in the presence of molecular oxygen and an active two enzyme electron handoff partner. This dicamba *O*-demethylase would become known as dicamba monooxygenase (DMO). A similar three-component system with activity on dicamba and vanillate was also uncovered in *Moorella thermoacetica* (Naidu and Ragsdale, 2001).

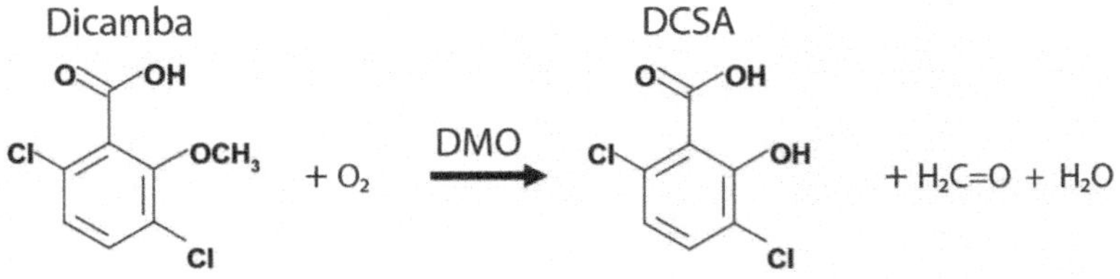

Figure 8.4 A schematic illustrating the oxygenase activity of the DMO enzyme on the dicamba herbicide molecule. Figure adapted from D'Ordine *et al.*, 2009.

Detailed structural enzymatic characterization of DMO was completed (D'Ordine *et al.*, 2009; Dumitru *et al.*, 2009). DMO was found to organize as a toroidal trimer with a head-to-tail arrangement; the non-heme iron center and the Rieske center are located on roughly opposite ends of the monomer (~48 Å apart) however, the non-heme iron center of one monomer is located in much closer proximity to the Rieske center of the adjacent monomer (~12 Å) likely enabling the electron transfer needed for catalysis. This would enable an electron transfer from the partner ferredoxin to the Rieske center to the non-heme iron center where molecular oxygen is activated to react with dicamba. DMO is unique relative to other Rieske oxygenases that act on aromatic substrates in that DMO oxygenates an exocyclic methyl group instead of directly on the aromatic ring. Additionally, while the domain housing the active site is smaller than other characterized Rieske oxygenases, the active site pocket was found to be larger than expected relative to similar oxygenases that act on larger hydrophobic substrates which may be in part due to the amphipathic nature of the dicamba substrate.

To determine if DMO can function as an herbicide tolerance trait in plants, Behrens *et al.* (2007) transformed Arabidopsis, tomato, tobacco, and soybean plants with a DMO transgene. One of the concerns would be if the DMO would be able to function in a plant cell without the native partner reductase and ferredoxin that would be found in the source bacterial strain. To address this concern, the authors fused a chloroplast targeting peptide to the *N*-terminal end of DMO to take advantage of the reduced ferredoxin naturally found in the plant chloroplasts. Although it was unknown if DMO would be able to accept electrons from a plant ferredoxin. However, plants expressing DMO in all four plant species showed tolerance to dicamba applications above normal field rates, suggesting that DMO could accept electrons from plant ferredoxins in the chloroplasts (Behrens *et al.*, 2007). Additionally, tobacco plants with DMO transformations directed to the chloroplast (DNA integration into the chloroplast genome instead of the nuclear genome) and selected to produce homoplastidic DMO-transformed chloroplasts also displayed robust dicamba tolerance, indicating that DMO can function if it is exclusively localized to the chloroplasts (as opposed to being transported into the chloroplasts posttranslation). Enzyme assays with recombinant DMO enzyme also demonstrated that DMO can function with isolated ferredoxin from spinach or a different bacterium, *Clostridium pasteurianum*, suggesting that DMO can accept electrons from a variety of ferredoxin partners (Behrens *et al.*, 2007). However, surprisingly, DMO transformations without a chloroplast targeting peptide into the nuclear genome also provided some tolerance to dicamba applications in tobacco (Behrens *et al.*, 2007). It is unclear what partner enzyme could provide electrons to DMO or if DMO was somehow translocated to the chloroplast via an unknown mechanism. While monocotyledonous plants such as corn are not as sensitive as dicotyledonous plants to dicamba applications, Cao *et al.* (2011) also demonstrated that corn expressing DMO showed less injury to dicamba applications illustrating that this enzyme can function, like the RdpA and FT enzymes, in both dicotyledonous and monocotyledonous plants as a robust herbicide tolerance trait.

8.5 Dioxygenase Enzyme for HPPD Inhibitor Tolerance

The 4-hydroxyphenyl-pyruvate dioxygenase (HPPD)-inhibitor herbicides inhibit the activity of the enzyme HPPD, an enzyme in the plastoquinone biosynthetic pathway (Shaner, 2014). Inhibition of plastoquinone biosynthesis disrupts the function of downstream enzymes in the carotenoid biosynthetic pathway, resulting in bleaching of new plant growth and eventual plant death in susceptible species. One family of HPPD-inhibitor herbicides includes the triketone HPPD-inhibitor herbicides which all maintain a conserved chemical scaffold. The HPPD-inhibitor class of herbicides represents a relatively new family of herbicides and research into new chemistries in this family of herbicides remains active (Ndikuryayo *et al.*, 2017). While this chapter focuses on oxygenase enzymes used as deactivation enzymes for herbicide tolerance traits, it is of interest to note that HPPD is a plant dioxygenase and overexpression of HPPD enzymes, which includes HPPD enzymes with reduced sensitivity to herbicide inhibition, has been successful in generating HPPD-inhibitor herbicide-tolerant plants.

HPPD-inhibitor herbicides are used in many cropping systems including rice. In rice, some elite lines have shown sensitivity to some triketone HPPD-inhibitor herbicides, such as benzobicyclon. Benzobicyclon is a pro-herbicide with its hydrolysate (BBC-OH) being the active molecule *in vivo*. To characterize the rice gene(s) responsible for the sensitivity to benzobicyclon, Maeda *et al.* (2019) undertook a map-based cloning effort with benzobicyclon tolerant and sensitive rice lines. In this effort, a single gene was identified and named HPPD-Inhibitor Sensitive 1 (HIS1). HIS1 contained conserved motifs suggesting it was an α-ketoglutarate-dependent dioxygenase. Additional mutant analysis, genotyping, and breeding cross-analysis confirmed that this gene was able to restore tolerance in sensitive, rice-breeding lines to benzobicyclon, and a short deletion in this gene in the modern *indica* variety parent cultivars is responsible for the herbicide sensitivity observed in some breeding lines (Maeda *et al.*, 2019). HIS1 is a member of a clade of plant α-ketoglutarate dependent dioxygenases with a currently uncharacterized function and members of this clade are found throughout the plant kingdom (Maeda *et al.*, 2019).

Transformation of benzobicyclon sensitive rice-breeding lines and *A. thaliana* (which is naturally sensitive to HPPD-inhibitor herbicides) confirmed that expression of HIS1 yielded plants with a tolerance to benzobicyclon and several other triketone HPPD-inhibitor herbicides such as mesotrione (Maeda *et al.*, 2019). Characterization of these HIS1 transformed rice lines showed an absence of BBC-OH which accumulated in sensitive lines. Further enzymatic characterization of HIS1 uncovered a ring hydroxylation on BBC-OH in an α-ketoglutarate and Fe^{2+} dependent manner (Fig. 8.5) (Maeda *et al.*, 2019). Further characterization by the authors demonstrated similar hydroxylation by HIS1 on several other triketone HPPD-inhibitor herbicides suggesting that HIS1 deactivates triketone HPPD-inhibitor herbicides as an α-ketoglutarate dependent dioxygenase via ring hydroxylation of the active herbicide molecule and thus can be a useful herbicide tolerance trait.

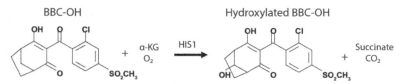

Figure 8.5 A schematic illustrating the oxygenase activity of the HIS1 enzyme on the benzobicyclon (BBC) herbicide molecule. Figure adapted from Maeda *et al.*, 2019.

8.6 Conclusion

In this chapter, three unique oxygenase families were discussed that had demonstrated utility as herbicide tolerance traits via a deactivation approach. These families represent both dioxygenases and monooxygenase and are enzymatically active on unique sets of herbicides. Some of the oxygenases discussed here were originally isolated from microbes but were found to function well in a plant cell. While this illustrates nicely that these enzymes can function in two very different cellular contexts, it is prudent to caution the reader that this should not be taken as a rule and should be carefully investigated with each new oxygenase enzyme. It is also prudent to caution the reader that it is also possible that a given oxygenase may enzymatically act on a given herbicide, but the product produced by this enzymatic activity may still retain activity (or retain partial activity) as an herbicide and thus full-plant tolerance to the herbicide may not be achieved despite good enzymatic activity within the plant cell. Again, this is something that must be carefully investigated during scientific endeavors. However, given the diversity of oxygenase enzymes that can be sourced from both prokaryotes and eukaryotes and given a broad range of substrates and reactions on these substrates that can be performed, it is likely that the oxygenases will remain a rich and fruitful source of enzymes for a variety of biotechnology applications within agriculture and beyond.

While this chapter is focused on the oxygenase enzymes used in herbicide tolerance traits, it is important for the reader to understand the utility and application in agriculture. While it is not possible to review or summarize the complex and continually evolving weed management practices here, a few key points will be made that directly relate to herbicide tolerance traits. The introduction of chemical herbicides for weed control in the mid-20th century brought a powerful new tool to weed control in agriculture. However, as with any new tool, weeds were able to adapt to the new selective pressure and weed resistance to many of these herbicides developed with time and continues to grow (Heap, 2021). The introduction of herbicide tolerance traits in the late 20th century added another tool to weed management programs for several crops in certain world regions and has been shown to bring value to agriculture (Carpenter, 2010). Often agriculture biotechnology traits are "stacked" in which one or more herbicide tolerance traits may be combined with one or more biotechnology traits for a different goal (such as insect control) within the same plant. This further adds value since it enables better control of multiple pests (such as weeds and insects) or within weed control may add value due to enabling different herbicides to be used on a single crop to address problematic weeds or enable better weed resistance management. However, as the rate of the commercial release of new herbicides with unique MoAs has slowed while the development of weed resistance continues, this has placed increasing emphasis on preserving the value of herbicide chemistries and integrated weed management programs. Weed management programs should include best management practices to reduce the risks of weed resistance to herbicides (Norsworthy *et al.*, 2012). These management practices directed for weed resistance should be a component of a holistic weed management practice that is tailored to a farmer's cropping systems, growing conditions, weed pressures, and sustainability goals.

References

Amy P. S., Schulke J. W., Frazier L. M., and Seidler R., *J. Appl. Environ. Microbiol.* **49**(5), (1985), 1237–1245.

Behrens M. R., Mutlu N., Chakraborty S., Dumitru R., Jiang W. Z., LaVallee B. J., Herman P. L., Clemente T. E., and Weeks D. P., *Science* **316** (2007), 1185–1188.

Bugg T. D. H., *Tetrahedron* **59** (2003), 7075–7101.

Cao M., Sato S. J., Behrens M., Jiang W. Z., Clemente T. E., and Weeks D. P., *J. Agric. Food Chem.* **59** (2011), 5830–5834.

Carpenter J. E., *Nat. Biotechnol.* **28**(4), (2010), 319–321.

Cork D. J., and Krueger J. P., *Adv. Appl. Microbiol.* **36** (1991), 1–66.

Dehaye L., Alban C., Job C., Douce R., and Job D., *Eur. J. Biochem.* **225** (1994), 1113–1123.

Dumitru R., Jiang W. Z., Weeks D. P., and Wilson M. A., *J. Mol. Biol.* **392** (2009), 498–510.

D'Ordine R. L., Rydel T. J., Storek M. J., Sturman E. J., Moshiri F., Bartlett R. K., Brown G. R., Eilers R. J., Dart C., Qi Y., Flasinski S., and Franklin S. J., *J. Mol. Biol.* **392** (2009), 481–497.

Fukumori F., and Hausinger R. P., *J. Bacteriol.* **175**(7), (1993a), 2083–2086.

Fukumori F., and Hausinger R. P., *J. Biolog. Chem.* **268**(32), (1993b), 24311–24317.

Guengerich F. P., *J. Biol. Chem.* **290**(34), (2015), 20700–20701.

Heap I. *The International Survey of Herbicide Resistant Weeds*. Available: www.weedscience.org. (Accessed 2021).

Herbert D. Price L. J., Alban C., Dehaye L., Job D., Cole D. J., Pallett K. E., and Harwood J. L., *Biochem. J.* **318** (1996), 997–1006.

Herman P. L., Behrens M., Chakraborty S., Chrastil B. M., Barycki J., and Weeks D. P., *J. Biol. Chem.* **280**(26), (2005), 24759–24767.

Hogan D. A., Smith S. R., Saari E. A., McCracken J., and Hausinger R. P., *J. Biolog. Chem.* **275**(17), (2000), 12400–12409.

Horvath M., Ditzelmüller G., Loidl M., and Streichsbier F., *Appl. Microbiol. Biotechnol.* **33** (1990), 213–216.

Kohler H. P. E., *J. Ind. Microbiol. Biotechnol.* **23** (1999), 336–340.

Larue C. T., Goley M., Shi L., Evdokimov A. G., Sparks O. C., Ellis C., Wollacott A. M., Rydel T. J., Halls C. E., Van Scoyoc B., Fu X., Nageotte J. R., Adio A. M., Zheng M., Sturman E. J., Garvey G. S., and Varagona M. J., *Pest Manag. Sci.* **75** (2019), 2086–2094.

Larue C. T., Ream J. E., Zhou X., Moshiri F., Howe A., Goley M., Sparks O. C., Voss S. T., Hall E., Ellis C., Weihe J., Qi Q., Ribeiro D., Wei X., Guo S., Evdokimov A. G., Varagona M. J., and Roberts J. K., *Pest Manag. Sci.* **76** (2020), 1031–1038.

Lee D. W., and Hwang I., Mol. Cell **41**(3), (2018), 161–167.

Maeda H., Murata K., Sakuma N., Takei S., Yamazaki A., Karim R., Kawata M., Hirose S., Kawagishi-Kobayashi M., Taniguchi Y., Suzuki S., Sekino K., Ohshima M., Kato H., Yoshida H., and Tozawa Y., *Science* **365**(6451), (2019), 393–396.

Mall T., Gupta M., Singh Dhadialla T., and Rodrigo S. Overview of biotechnology-derived herbicide tolerance and insect resistance traits in Plant Agriculture in Transgenic Plants: Methods and Protocols, *Methods in Molecular Biology*, Volume 1864 (Kumar S., *et al.* eds), Springer Nature, London, 2019.

Müller T. A., Fleischmann T., van der Meer J. R., and Kohler H.-P. E., *Appl. Environ. Microbiol.* **72**(7), (2006), 4853–4861.

Naidu D., and Ragsdale S. W., *J. Bacteriol.* **183**(11), (2001), 3276–3281.

Ndikuryayo F., Moosavi B., Yang W.-C., and Yang G.-F., *J. Agric. Food Chem.* **65** (2017), 8523–8537.

Nickel K., Suter M. J.-F., and Kohler H.-P. E., *J. Bacteriol.* **179**(21), (1997), 6674–6679.

Norsworthy J. K., Ward S. M., Shaw D. R., Llewellyn R. S., Nichols R. L., Webster T. M., Bradley K. W., Frisvold G., Powles S. B., Burgos N. R., Witt W. W., and Barrett M., *Weed Science* **12**(sp1), (2012), 31–62.

Padgette S. R., Kolacz K. H., Delannay X., Re D. B., LaVallee B. J., Tinius C. N., Rhodes W. K., Otero Y. I., Barry G. F., Eichholtz D. A., Peschke V. M., Nida D. L., Taylor N. B., and Kishore G. M., *Crop Science* **35** (1995), 1451–1461.

Pazmiño D. E. T., Winkler M., Glieder A., and Fraaije M. W., *J. Biotechnol.* **146** (2010), 9–24.

Peterson M. A., McMaster S. A., Riechers D. E., Skelton J., and Stahlman P. W., *Weed Technol.* **30**(2), (2016), 303–345.

Ruizzo M. A., and Gorski S. F., *Weed Science* **36** (1988), 713–718.

Schleinitz K. M., Kleinsteuber S., Vallaeys T., and Babel W., *Appl. Environ. Microbiol.* **70**(9), (2004), 5357–5365.

Shaner D. L. *Herbicide Handbook*, 10th edn, Weed Science Society of America, Lawrence, KS, 2014.

Stowe E., and Dhingra A. *Development of the Arctic® Apple in Plant Breeding Reviews*, Vol. 44 (Goldman I., ed), John Wiley and Sons, New York, 2020.

Wang X.-Z., Li B., Herman P. L., and Weeks D. P., *Appl. Environ. Microbiol.* **63**(4), (1997), 1623–1626.

Wehrmann A., Van Vliet A., Opsomer C., Botterman J., and Schulz A., *Nat. Biotechnol.* **14** (1996), 1274–1278.

Westendorf A., Müller R. H., and Babel W., *Acta Biotechnol.* **23**(1), (2003), 3–17.

Wright T. R., Shan G., Walsh T. A., Lira J. M., Cui C., Song P., Zhuang M., Arnold N. L., Lin G., Yau K., Russell S. M., Cicchillo R. M., Peterson M. A., Simpson D. M., Zhou N., Ponsamuel J., and Zhang Z., *Proc. Nat. Acad. Sci.* **107**(47), (2010), 20240–20245.

Wu L.-F., Meng S., and Tang G.-L., *Biochim. Biophys. Acta* **1864** (2016), 453–470.

Yang J., Wang X.-Z., Hage D. S., Herman P. L., and Weeks D. P., *Analyt. Biochem.* **219** (1994), 37–42.

Part IV
Plant Viruses

Chapter 9

P1 Leader Proteinases from the *Potyviridae* Family

Fabio Pasin[a,b] **and Hongying Shan**[c,d]

[a]*Institute of Molecular and Cellular Biology of Plants (IBMCP), Consejo Superior de Investigaciones Científicas – Universitat Politècnica de València (CSIC-UPV), Valencia, Spain*
[b]*School of Science, University of Padova, Padova, Italy*
[c]*College of Horticulture and Gardening, Tianjin Agricultural University, Tianjin, China*
[d]*State Key Laboratory for Biology of Plant Diseases and Insect Pests, Institute of Plant Protection, Chinese Academy of Agricultural Sciences, Beijing, China*
f.pasin@csic.es, 21-hy@163.com

P1 proteinases are located in the polyprotein leader region of most members of *Potyviridae*, the largest family of known RNA viruses. They show considerable sequence variability, but a chymotrypsin-like serine protease domain is conserved in their carboxy terminus, which is responsible for P1 self-cleavage from viral polyproteins. The proteinases are classified as Types A and B - functional groups with divergent biochemical properties and phylogeny. Besides their proteolytic activity, P1 proteinases act as host-range and symptom determinants and have roles in RNA silencing suppression and immune evasion. Characterization of P1 genetics and biochemical properties has been instrumental in the generation of early potyvirid-based biotechnologies. A follow-up systematic investigation of P1 diversity and evolution is predicted to spur the development of new antiviral strategies, as well as innovative biotechnology and synthetic biology devices.

9.1 Introduction

Proteolytic events regulate the virulence and fitness of many pathogenic agents of infectious diseases. Proteolysis of viral proteins is needed to activate diverse human viruses such as human immunodeficiency virus (HIV) and influenza virus (Hallenberger et al., 1992; Stieneke-Gröber et al., 1992); it has recently been implicated in host cell entry and tropism of severe acute respiratory syndrome coronavirus 2 (SARS-CoV-2), the agent of the pandemic disease syndrome COVID-19, and related pathogenic strains of human coronaviruses (Hoffmann et al., 2020; Hoffmann et al., 2018; Wrobel et al., 2020). Proteinases (also known as endopeptidases or endoproteases) are a class of proteases that catalyze peptide bond hydrolysis at internal positions of proteins or polyprotein substrates. They are common in viruses that, to increase their coding capacity, have evolved polyprotein synthesis as a genomic expression strategy (Dougherty and Semler, 1993; Mann and Sanfaçon, 2019; Rodamilans et al., 2018a). Viral proteinases are targets for therapeutic intervention, as well as the sources of tools for biotechnological and synthetic biology applications (Agbowuro et al., 2018; Chung and Lin, 2020).

Potyviridae is the largest family of known RNA viruses (realm *Riboviria*) (see the ViralZone and ICTV entries, Table 9.1), and comprises over 200 species assigned to the 12 genera *Arepavirus*, *Bevemovirus*, *Brambyvirus*, *Bymovirus*, *Celavirus*, *Ipomovirus*, *Macluravirus*, *Poacevirus*, *Potyvirus*, *Roymovirus*, *Rymovirus*, and *Tritimovirus*, of which *Potyvirus* is the most abundant (Wylie et al., 2017; Gibbs et al., 2020; International Committee on Taxonomy of Viruses, 2020). A revised phylogenomic reconstruction based on RNA-dependent RNA polymerase (RdRp) proteins includes *Potyviridae* in the picornavirus supergroup (phylum *Pisuriviricota*), along with single-stranded RNA viruses of plants (families *Secoviridae*, and *Solemoviridae*) as well as of humans and invertebrates (orders *Picornavirales* and *Nidovirales*), and multiple unclassified viruses identified in metagenomic surveys (Dolja et al., 2020).

Introduction | 271

Table 9.1 Biological databank resources for the study of *Potyviridae* P1 proteinases

Data	Databank[a]	Accession	Link[b]
Potyviridae molecular biology information	ViralZone	*Potyviridae*	https://viralzone.expasy.org/48
Potyviridae taxonomy	ICTV	Family: *Potyviridae*	https://talk.ictvonline.org/ictv-reports/ictv_9th_report/positive-sense-rna-viruses-2011/w/posrna_viruses/272/potyviridae-figures
Proteinase sequences	GenBank	P17767 | Plum pox virus P1	https://www.ncbi.nlm.nih.gov/protein/P17767.22?from=1&to=308
	GenBank	ASG92173.1 | Ugandan cassava brown streak virus P1	https://www.ncbi.nlm.nih.gov/protein/ASG92173.1?from=1&to=362
Protein functional information	UniProt	P17767 | Plum pox virus genome polyprotein	https://www.uniprot.org/uniprot/P17767
Peptidase class	MEROPS	S30.001 | *Potyvirus* P1 peptidase	https://www.ebi.ac.uk/merops/cgi-bin/pepsum?id=S30.001
Proteinase profiles	InterPro	IPR025910 | Plant viral polyprotein P1, serine peptidase domain	https://www.ebi.ac.uk/interpro/entry/InterPro/IPR025910/
		IPR002540 | Peptidase S30, polyprotein P1, *Potyvirus*	https://www.ebi.ac.uk/interpro/entry/InterPro/IPR002540/
	Pfam	PF01577 | Peptidase_S30	https://pfam.xfam.org/family/PF01577
		PF13611 | Peptidase_S76	https://pfam.xfam.org/family/PF13611
	Prosite	PS51871 | *Potyviridae* P1 protease domain profile	https://prosite.expasy.org/PS51871

[a]Databank references are as follows: GenBank (NCBI Resource Coordinators, 2018), InterPro (Blum *et al.*, 2021), ICTV (Lefkowitz *et al.*, 2018), MEROPS (Rawlings *et al.*, 2018), Pfam (Mistry *et al.*, 2021), Prosite (Sigrist *et al.*, 2013), UniProt (The UniProt Consortium *et al.*, 2021), ViralZone (Hulo *et al.*, 2011)
[b]Last accessed July 2021

Members of the family have a positive single-stranded RNA genome that is translated into polyproteins, which are in turn processed by virus-encoded proteinases to release mature subunits (Adams et al., 2005; Revers and García, 2015). The organization of the amino (N)-terminal region of the potyvirid polyproteins is highly variable (Cui and Wang, 2019), with the P1 proteinase and helper component proteinase (HC-pro) being the most common cistrons of this portion (Fig. 9.1A). A succession of eight mature proteins is present in the conserved central and carboxy (C)-terminal regions of potyvirid polyproteins - P3, 6 kDa protein 1 (6K1), cytoplasmic inclusion (CI) protein, 6 kDa protein 2 (6K2), viral genome-linked protein (VPg), nuclear inclusion protein A proteinase (NIa-pro), nuclear inclusion protein B (NIb), and coat protein (CP) (Revers and García, 2015). Frameshifting events on the P3 cistron generate the two additional proteins P3N-PIPO and P3N-ALT (Yang et al., 2021). Atypical domains are further encoded by potyvirids with unusual genomic patterns (Pasin et al., 2022). A HAM1 pyrophosphatase-like sequence is found between NIb and CP of a few potyvirid genomes (James et al., 2021). An alkylation B (AlkB) domain is present in P1 of blackberry virus Y (BlVY), the sole member of the genus *Brambyvirus* (Susaimuthu et al., 2008), and of the *Potyvirus* endive necrotic mosaic virus (ENMV; Table 9.2). The pretty interesting sweet potato potyviral ORF (PISPO) is present in the P1 cistron of sweet potato feathery mottle virus (SPFMV) and of related potyviruses (Clark et al., 2012). Bymoviruses lack P1 homologs and encode a tobacco mosaic virus-like CP, a domain not found in other potyvirids (Pasin et al., 2022).

Three classes of proteinases have been characterized in potyvirids - NIa-pro, HC-pro, and P1 (Adams et al., 2005). P1 proteinases are located in the polyprotein leader region of most *Potyviridae* members. They are generally present in one copy, but two copies are found in some ipomoviruses (Table 9.2). P1 is an accessory factor shown to be dispensable for infection of *Potyvirus* members (Verchot and Carrington, 1995a). No significant homology with its protease domain can be detected in viruses of *Arepavirus*, *Bevemovirus*, *Bymovirus*, *Celavirus*, and *Macluravirus*. Features of P1 proteinases from the *Potyviridae* family are described in this chapter.

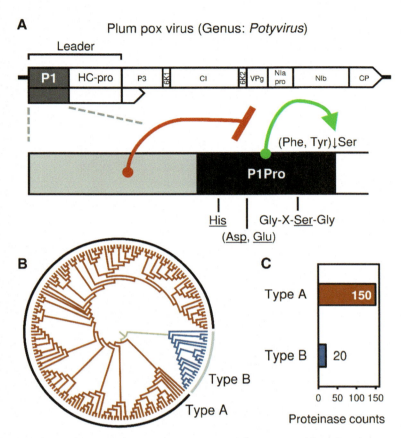

Figure 9.1 Genomic location, representative features, and functional groups of the P1 proteinases of *Potyviridae*. (A) Top, genomic diagram of plum pox virus, a reference potyvirid; the RNA genome and encoded polyproteins are represented as a line and arrowed boxes, respectively. Bottom, key features of the P1 proteinase; P1Pro, core serine protease domain; catalytic residues are underlined. The partially conserved cleavage site is shown; the green arrow indicates the self-cleavage activity and the T-shaped arrow indicates the autoinhibitory role of the *N* terminus. (B) Cladogram of the functional group's Types A and B. Reference isolates of recognized species were obtained from the International Committee on Taxonomy of Viruses (2020), and sequences with complete or near-complete genomic sequences were considered (n = 185). The P1 protease domains were identified by Prosite profile scan (Sigrist *et al.*, 2013); sequences (n = 170) were aligned and phylogeny inferred (Pasin *et al.*, 2022). (C) Abundance of Type-A and Type-B proteins within the *Potyviridae* family is shown (Pasin *et al.*, 2022).

Table 9.2 P1 diversity in genera of the *Potyviridae* family

Genus	Representative Species	Type	P1 Layout[a]	Atypical P1 Domains[b]
Potyvirus	Plum pox virus	A	P1/HC-pro/P3	n.r.
	Sweet potato feathery mottle virus	A	P1/HC-pro/P3	PISPO
	Endive necrotic mosaic virus	A	P1/HC-pro/P3	AlkB
Rymovirus	Ryegrass mosaic virus	A	P1/HC-pro/P3	n.r.
Unassigned	Common reed chlorotic stripe virus	A	P1/HC-pro/P3	n.r.
	Spartina mottle virus	A	P1/HC-pro/P3	n.r.
Ipomovirus	Sweet potato mild mottle virus	B	P1/HC-pro/P3	n.r.
	Cucumber vein yellowing virus	A, B	P1a/P1b/P3	n.r.
	Ugandan cassava brown streak virus	B	P1/P3	n.r.
Poacevirus	Triticum mosaic virus	B	P1/HC-pro/P3	n.r.
Tritimovirus	Wheat streak mosaic virus	B	P1/HC-pro/P3	n.r.
Roymovirus	Rose yellow mosaic virus	B	P1/HC-pro/P3	n.r.
Unassigned	Longan witches broom-associated virus	B	P1/HC-pro/P3	n.r.
Brambyvirus	Blackberry virus Y	B	P1/HC-pro/P3	AlkB
Arepavirus	Areca palm necrotic spindle-spot virus	–[c]	–	–

Genus	Representative Species	Type	P1 Layout[a]	Atypical P1 Domains[b]
Bevemovirus	Bellflower veinal mottle virus	–	–	–
Celavirus	Celery latent virus	–	–	–
Macluravirus	Maclura mosaic virus	–	–	–
Bymovirus	Barley yellow mosaic virus	–	–	–

[a]Cistrons flanking P1 proteins in potyvirid polyproteins; P3, first conserved cistron of the polyprotein central and C-terminal region
[b]PISPO, pretty interesting sweet potato potyviral ORF; AlkB, alkylation B; n.r., not reported
[c]No P1 homology can be detected in available sequences

9.2 P1 Diversity of the *Potyviridae* Genomes

The last of the *Potyviridae* proteinases to be identified (Verchot *et al.*, 1991; Mavankal and Rhoads, 1991), P1 has a chymotrypsin-like serine protease domain responsible for its autocatalytic release from viral polyproteins. P1 proteins of *Potyviridae* show large sequence variability and are classified as Type A and Type B (Fig. 9.1B) - functional groups with divergent biochemical properties and phylogeny (Rodamilans *et al.*, 2013; Pasin *et al.*, 2022).

Profiles based on hidden Markov models (HMM) are widely used resources for classifying sequences into protein families and domains. Identification of P1 and its catalytic domain in potyvirid sequences can be assisted by sensitive HMM profile searches (Table 9.1). The current Pfam database includes HMM profiles for detecting P1 proteins and their functional groups (Mistry *et al.*, 2021). Protease domains of Type-A proteinases are currently assigned to 'Peptidase_S30' (Pfam: PF01577), whereas 'Peptidase_S76' (Pfam: PF13611) includes most of those of Type B. Alternative protein classifiers such as those of the MEROPS, PROSITE, InterPro databases are available for detecting domain signatures of potyvirid P1 proteinases (Blum *et al.*, 2021; Rawlings *et al.*, 2018; Sigrist *et al.*, 2013).

The distribution of the P1 functional groups and their genomic layouts in potyvirids are heterogeneous (Table 9.2), but Type A dominates over Type B (Fig. 9.1C). A single copy of Type-A P1 is located at the extreme *N* terminus of polyproteins of all *Potyvirus* and *Rymovirus* members. A single Type-B P1 is located at the extreme *N* terminus of polyproteins of all *Poacevirus*, *Tritimovirus*, *Roymovirus*, and *Brambyvirus* members. In all six of these genera, polyproteins have a common *N*-terminal pattern of a single P1 of Type A or Type B followed by HC-pro and P3, the first cistron of the polyprotein conserved region. *Ipomovirus* members show a variety of genomic organizations and P1 patterns (Desbiez *et al.*, 2016; Dombrovsky *et al.*, 2014; Li *et al.*, 2008; Mbanzibwa *et al.*, 2009; Valli *et al.*, 2006). Polyprotein *N* termini of ipomoviruses include (*i*) a Type-B P1 followed by HC-pro and P3 in sweet potato mild mottle virus (SPMMV) and tomato mild mottle virus (TMMoV), (*ii*) a Type-A P1 followed by a Type-B P1 and P3 in cucumber vein yellowing virus (CVYV), squash vein yellowing virus (SqVYV), and *Coccinia* mottle virus (CocMoV), and (*iii*) a single Type-B P1 followed by P3 in Ugandan cassava brown streak virus (UCBSV) and cassava brown streak virus (CBSV).

9.3 Structural Properties and Proteolytic Activity of P1

The chymotrypsin-like serine protease domain conserved in the *C* terminus of Type-A and Type-B proteinases is responsible for the P1 self-cleavage (Fig. 9.1A). Viral clones that encode P1 mutants with proteolytic defects are not infectious; peptide bond hydrolysis between P1 and its downstream polyprotein cistron is thus essential for virus infectivity (Pasin *et al.*, 2014b; Verchot and Carrington, 1995b). Proteolysis takes place intramolecularly at the P1 *C*-terminal end by a *cis*-acting mechanism, and no *trans*-cleavage activity could be detected *in vitro* (Shan, 2018; Verchot *et al.*, 1992). Lack of *trans*-cleavage is hypothesized to be caused by trapping of the mature *C* terminus within the active cleft after the first proteolytic event (Verchot *et al.*, 1992). This phenomenon has been reported in several viral proteinases that undergo autoinhibition, such as the alphavirus serine protease togavirin and the potyvirid papain-like protease HC-pro (Choi et al., 1991; Guo et al., 2011).

Peptide bond hydrolysis occurs at the partially conserved motif (Phe, Tyr)-Ser, wherein Ser represents the first amino acid of the downstream cistron (Fig. 9.1A). The proteinase active site is formed by the catalytic triad typical of serine proteases, which comprises reactive serine, and histidine and aspartic- or glutamic-acid residues (Hedstrom, 2002). The triad is embedded within the conserved motif His-x_n-(Asp, Glu)- x_n-Gly-x-Ser-Gly, wherein the catalytic residues are underlined, and x represents any amino acid.

Proteins of Types A and B show different proteolytic properties. Characterization of tobacco etch virus (TEV) and tobacco vein mottling virus (TVMV) homologs revealed that Type-A proteinases are active *in planta* and wheat germ extracts, but lack detectable activity in animal systems (Carrington et al., 1990; Verchot et al., 1991; Mavankal and Rhoads, 1991; Thornbury et al., 1993). Verchot and coworkers (1992) used mixes of rabbit reticulocyte lysates and wheat germ extracts to show that the latter includes a heat-labile-positive factor associated with P1 activation. These results suggest that activation of Type-A P1 requires a plant co-factor, the identity of which is still unknown. In contrast to Type A, the Type B proteinases show robust self-cleavage *in planta*, but also in the rabbit reticulocyte lysate translation system and bacteria (Rodamilans et al., 2013; Shan et al., 2018); this evidence indicates their lack of plant co-factor requirements.

The *N*-terminal region of P1 is hypervariable both in length and sequence composition. Despite this diversity, bioinformatic analyses have identified conserved structural disorder that maps upstream of the protease domain (Pasin et al., 2014b). With CP and VPg, P1 displays the highest content of conserved disorder among potyviral proteins (Charon et al., 2016). The *N* terminus is not necessary for P1 self-cleavage (Rodamilans et al., 2013; Verchot et al., 1991). Fine analysis of the plum pox virus (PPV) P1 *N*-terminal deletions has allowed mapping of the minimal *C*-terminal protease domain (P1Pro) at single-amino acid resolution (Pasin et al., 2014b) (Fig. 9.1A).

Structural disorder-based mechanisms grant tight control of active and inactive states of several proteins and protein complexes (Trudeau et al., 2013), and disordered loops are known to autoinhibit serine proteases by shielding the catalytic triad from substrate access (Hedstrom, 2002). Co-factor binding, proteolytic events, or posttranslational modifications promote structural rearrangements that are reported to relieve autoinhibition and to be required for protein activation (Gohara and Di Cera, 2011; Trudeau et al., 2013). Assays used to map the proteolytic domain of PPV P1 further showed a gain-of-function phenotype of the core proteinase. The full-length PPV P1, a Type-A proteinase, lacks detectable activity in rabbit reticulocyte lysates; the core proteinase devoid of the *N*-terminal region was nonetheless proteolytically active both in wheat germ extracts and in rabbit reticulocyte lysates (Pasin et al., 2014b). The length of the PPV P1 *N* terminus directly affects the strength of the proteolytic autoinhibition (Shan et al., 2018). These data are consistent with a regulatory mechanism in which P1 proteolysis is autoinhibited by its *N* terminus (Fig. 9.1A), and autoinhibition relief by plant co-factor(s) activates the core proteinase for self-cleavage (Pasin et al., 2014b).

PPV P1 belongs to Type A, but the lack of plant co-factor requirements and the cleavage kinetics of its core proteinase resemble those of Type-B proteins. It is unknown whether the PPV protein represents a unique functional link between Types A and B, or if its regulatory mechanism is conserved in other Type-A proteinases (Shan et al., 2018).

9.4 P1 Proteins as Viral Suppressors of RNA Silencing

Viruses have evolved proteins to counter RNA silencing, a major antiviral immune defense of plants (Csorba et al., 2015). HC-pro of *Potyvirus* and *Rymovirus* members have multiple roles in immune evasion that include direct sequestration of small RNA molecules and inhibition of RNA silencing components (Valli et al., 2018; Yang et al., 2021). No functional motifs or functional homologs of *Potyvirus* HC-pro are found in members of *Ipomovirus*, *Poacevirus*, *Tritimovirus*, *Roymovirus*, and *Brambyvirus*, which specifically encode P1 proteins of Type B. Experimental evidence indicates that Type-B homologs act as suppressors that functionally replace the *Potyvirus* HC-pro in counteracting antiviral RNA silencing (Table 9.3). This activity was first identified in the *Ipomovirus* CVYV, which lacks HC-pro and encodes a tandem of proteolytic active P1 copies (Valli et al.,

2006). The *N*-terminal copy (P1a) is a Type-A homolog that shares common features to P1 of potyviruses (Shan *et al.*, 2015), whereas the *C*-terminal copy (P1b) belongs to Type B and displays strong silencing suppression activity (Valli *et al.*, 2006).

Follow-up investigation of other ipomoviruses and viruses of *Poacevirus* and *Tritimovirus* indicates that the silencing suppression activity of Type-B proteins is conserved. The ipomoviruses CBSV and UCBSV lack HC-pro and encode a single Type-B P1 proteinase that strongly suppresses RNA silencing (Mbanzibwa *et al.*, 2009). Both Type-B P1 and HC-pro cistrons are present in the *Ipomovirus* SPMMV, the poaceviruses sugarcane streak mosaic virus (SCSMV), and *Triticum* mosaic virus (TriMV), and the *Tritimovirus* wheat streak mosaic virus (WSMV). Their Type-B proteins have evolved to take over the RNA silencing suppressor functions originally identified in HC-pro of model potyviruses (Chen *et al.*, 2020; Giner *et al.*, 2010; Gupta and Tatineni, 2019a; Tatineni *et al.*, 2012; Young *et al.*, 2012). No experimental characterization has been reported for the Type-B homologs of *Roymovirus* and *Brambyvirus*.

No RNA silencing suppressor activity has been reported for Type-A proteins of the genera *Potyvirus* or *Rymovirus* (Revers and García, 2015; Young *et al.*, 2012). They nonetheless promote the HC-pro activity and viral fitness, possibly by enhancing viral polyprotein translation and HC-pro synthesis, or by evading hormone-based immune response activation (Martínez and Daròs, 2014; Pasin *et al.*, 2020; Tena Fernández *et al.*, 2013). Exceptionally, P1N-PISPO is an atypical product of Type-A cistrons that has been implicated in RNA silencing suppression of the *Potyvirus* SPFMV (Mingot *et al.*, 2016; Untiveros *et al.*, 2016).

Many biochemical mechanisms have evolved in plant viruses to avoid or counteract RNA silencing (Csorba *et al.*, 2015; Li and Wang, 2019), and some have been implicated in the silencing suppression of P1 and the frameshift product P1N-PISPO. Conserved Leu-*x*-(Lys, Arg)-Ala and putative zinc-finger motifs, and glycine-tryptophan (GW) dipeptides participate in this activity (Valli *et al.*, 2008; Valli *et al.*, 2011; Giner *et al.*, 2010; Mingot *et al.*, 2016; Untiveros *et al.*, 2016; Kenesi *et al.*, 2017; Gupta and Tatineni, 2019a; Gupta and Tatineni, 2019b). The *N*-terminal part of SPFMV P1 is essential for the silencing suppressor activity of P1N-PISPO (Clark *et al.*, 2012; Rodamilans *et al.*, 2021). The entire *C*-terminal protease domain or its proteolytic activity are not needed for silencing suppression of

Type-B homologs from the *Ipomovirus* SPMMV and the *Poacevirus* TriMV (Giner *et al.*, 2010; Gupta and Tatineni, 2019b).

Type-B homologs of CVYV and TriMV bind short RNA molecules; this activity correlated with their ability to antagonize RNA silencing and was linked to conserved zinc-finger motifs (Valli *et al.*, 2008; Gupta and Tatineni, 2019b). Other studies could not detect RNA binding, but in P1 sequences they identified GW motifs that resemble the Argonaute (AGO)-binding linear peptide motif conserved in metazoans and plants (Giner *et al.*, 2010). AGO proteins are core components of the RNA-induced silencing complex (RISC) and plant antiviral immunity (Carbonell and Carrington, 2015). GW dipeptides of SPMMV P1 guide AGO1 binding and RISC inhibition (Giner *et al.*, 2010; Kenesi *et al.*, 2017). The strict GW motif requirement for silencing suppression was confirmed for Type-B proteins of the genera *Ipomovirus*, *Poacevirus*, *Tritimovirus*, as well as for P1N-PISPO of the *Potyvirus* SPFMV (Giner *et al.*, 2010; Mingot *et al.*, 2016; Untiveros *et al.*, 2016; Kenesi *et al.*, 2017; Gupta and Tatineni, 2019a; Gupta and Tatineni, 2019b).

9.5 P1 Proteins as Host-Range and Symptom Determinants

Besides proteolytic and silencing suppressor activities, additional P1 roles have been reported in potyvirid infection (Table 9.3). P1 was identified as a host-range determinant. Genus-wide analysis of potyviral genome variation showed that the P1 cistron is a hypervariable area that accumulates non-synonymous nucleotide substitutions possibly linked to host adaptation (Nigam *et al.*, 2019). Recombination events within P1 have been detected and are suggested to have led to the emergence of novel isolates as well as potyvirid species with broad or altered host ranges (Desbiez *et al.*, 2017; Desbiez and Lecoq, 2004; Gibbs *et al.*, 2020; Glasa *et al.*, 2011; Jiang *et al.*, 2017). Experimental data using interspecific chimeric viruses of PPV and TVMV showed that P1 sequences determine host range (Salvador *et al.*, 2008b). A PPV portion including P1 was identified as a host-specific pathogenicity determinant through infection assays that used chimeric clones of isolates adapted to either woody or herbaceous hosts (Salvador *et al.*, 2008a).

Table 9.3 Major P1 features and roles in host–virus interactions

Genus	Virus[a]	Type	Features[b]	Reference
—	Several	A	Accumulation of non-synonymous nucleotide substitutions possibly linked to host adaptation	Nigam et al., 2019
—	Several	A	Conserved structural disorder	Charon et al., 2016; Pasin et al., 2014b
—	Several	A, B	Functional divergence of Types A and B	Rodamilans et al., 2013; Shan et al., 2018
—	Several	A	P1 recombination events	Desbiez et al., 2017; Desbiez and Lecoq, 2004; Gibbs et al., 2020; Glasa et al., 2011; Jiang et al., 2017
—	Several	A, B	Large sequence variability, evolutionary diversification and duplication	Pasin et al., 2022; Valli et al., 2007
—	Several	A, B	P1 cleavage site revision	Adams et al., 2005
Potyvirus	PPV	A	Avoidance of ABA- and SA-mediated defense activation	Pasin et al., 2020
			P1 self-cleavage autoinhibition defines host range	Shan et al., 2018
			Host-dependent autoinhibition of P1 self-cleavage	Pasin et al., 2014b

(Continued)

Table 9.3 (Continued)

Genus	Virus[a]	Type	Features[b]	Reference
			P1 proteolysis controls HC-pro activity	Pasin et al., 2014b
			P1 proteolysis controls virus infectivity	Pasin et al., 2014b
			Core P1 protease domain mapping	Pasin et al., 2014b
			Host-specific pathogenicity determinant	Maliogka et al., 2012; Nagyová et al., 2012; Salvador et al., 2008a
			Host-range determinant	Salvador et al., 2008b
	SPFMV	A	Identification and RNA silencing suppression of P1N-PISPO	Clark et al., 2012; Mingot et al., 2016; Untiveros et al., 2016; Rodamilans et al., 2018b; Rodamilans et al., 2021
			Host-range determinant	Salvador et al., 2008b
	TVMV	A	In vitro nucleic acid-binding activity	Brantley and Hunt, 1993
			P1 cleavage site mapping	Mavankal and Rhoads, 1991
	TuMV	A	G3BP-like protein colocalization and possible participation in stress granule formation	Reuper and Krenz, 2021
			Host-dependent proteolytic activation	Shan et al., 2018
			In vitro nucleic acid-binding activity	Soumounou and Laliberté, 1994

Genus	Virus[a]	Type	Features[b]	Reference
	TEV	A	Host ribosome binding and viral protein translation enhancement	Martínez and Darós, 2014
			Differential P1 accumulation during infection stages and rapid degradation	Martínez and Darós, 2014
			Lack of RNA silencing suppression	Young et al., 2012
			P1 proteolysis controls virus infectivity	Verchot and Carrington, 1995b
			Stimulation of viral genome amplification	Verchot and Carrington, 1995a
			P1 cleavage site mapping	Verchot et al., 1992
			Host-dependent proteolytic activation	Verchot et al., 1992
			P1 protease active site characterization	Verchot et al., 1992; Verchot et al., 1991
			P1 serine protease domain identification	Verchot et al., 1991
	PVA	A	Enhancement of HC-pro RNA silencing suppression activity	Rajamäki et al., 2005
			Interaction with viral replication complex proteins	Guo et al., 2001; Merits et al., 1999
			In vitro nucleic acid-binding activity	Merits et al., 1998
	PVY	A	HC-pro translation enhancement	Tena Fernández et al., 2013

(Continued)

Table 9.3 (Continued)

Genus	Virus[a]	Type	Features[b]	Reference
			Interaction with viral replication complex proteins	Arbatova et al., 1998
	CIYVV	A	P1 cleavage site mapping	Yang et al., 1998
			Overcoming eIF4E-mediated recessive resistance	Nakahara et al., 2010
	SMV	A	Rieske Fe/S protein interaction and possible symptom determinant	Shi et al., 2007
	ENMV	A	Identification of an AlkB domain	Pasin et al., 2022
Rymovirus	AgMV	A	Lack of RNA silencing suppression	Young et al., 2012
	HoMV	A	Lack of RNA silencing suppression	Young et al., 2012
Ipomovirus	UCBSV	B	Host-independent proteolytic activation	Shan et al., 2018
	SPMMV	B	RNA silencing suppression	Mbanzibwa et al., 2009
			RNA silencing suppression	Giner et al., 2010; Kenesi et al., 2017
	CVYV	A	Host-dependent proteolytic activation of P1a	Rodamilans et al., 2013; Shan et al., 2018; Shan et al., 2015
			P1a proteolysis controls the activity of downstream RNA silencing suppressors	Carbonell et al., 2012; Shan et al., 2015
			P1a proteolysis controls virus infectivity	Carbonell et al., 2012; Shan et al., 2015

Genus	Virus[a]	Type	Features[b]	Reference
		B	Sterol isomerase HYDRA1 interaction of P1b	Ochoa et al., 2019
			Host-independent proteolytic activation of P1b	Rodamilans et al., 2013
			RNA silencing suppression of P1b	Carbonell et al., 2012; Valli et al., 2008; Valli et al., 2006
Poacevirus	TriMV	B	RNA silencing suppression	Gupta and Tatineni, 2019b; Tatineni et al., 2012
	SCSMV	B	RNA silencing suppression	Bagyalakshmi and Viswanathan, 2020; Chen et al., 2020
Tritimovirus	WSMV	B	RNA silencing suppression	Gupta and Tatineni, 2019a; Young et al., 2012
			P1 cleavage site mapping	Choi et al., 2002
Brambyvirus	BlVY	B	RNA demethylation and possible genome integrity protection by the P1 AlkB domain	van den Born et al., 2008

[a]PPV, plum pox virus; SPFMV, sweet potato feathery mottle virus; TVMV, tobacco vein mottling virus; TuMV, turnip mosaic virus; TEV, tobacco etch virus; PVA, potato virus A; PVY, potato virus Y; ClYVV, clover yellow vein virus; SMV, soybean mosaic virus; ENMV, endive necrotic mosaic virus; AgMV, Agropyron mosaic virus; HoMV, Hordeum mosaic virus; UCBSV, Ugandan cassava brown streak virus; SPMMV, sweet potato mild mottle virus; CVYV, cucumber vein yellowing virus; SPMMV, sweet potato mild mottle virus; TriMV, Triticum mosaic virus; SCSMV, sugarcane streak mosaic virus; WSMV, wheat streak mosaic virus; BlVY, blackberry virus Y

[b]ABA, abscisic acid; SA, salicylic acid; G3BP, ras-GAP SH3 domain-binding protein; eIF4E, eukaryotic translation initiation factor 4E; AlkB, alkylation B

P1 is a determinant of symptom manifestation, and of activation of host defenses that involve salicylic acid (SA) and abscisic acid (ABA) signaling pathways (Maliogka et al., 2012; Nagyová et al., 2012; Pasin et al., 2020; Pasin et al., 2014b). A single P1 mutation identified in a clover yellow vein virus (ClYVV) isolate was sufficient to overcome *Potyvirus* recessive resistance in pea (Nakahara et al., 2010). Sequence variation and residue substitutions of PPV P1 were responsible for symptom development in woody and herbaceous hosts (Maliogka et al., 2012; Nagyová et al., 2012). Soybean mosaic virus (SMV) P1 was suggested to participate in symptom development through interaction with plant Rieske Fe/S proteins (Shi et al., 2007). Turnip mosaic virus (TuMV) P1 colocalizes with a G3BP-like protein and was suggested to participate in stress granule formation (Reuper and Krenz, 2021).

Type-A P1 proteinases are characterized by host-specific activation that is indispensable for virus infectivity (Pasin et al., 2014b; Verchot and Carrington, 1995b). P1-HC-pro fusion products lack RNA silencing suppressor activity, and viral clones that encode P1 proteolytic mutants were not infectious in wild-type plants but were rescued in hosts defective in antiviral RNA silencing components (Pasin et al., 2014b). The intrinsically disordered *N*-terminal region of PPV P1 has an antagonistic effect on protein proteolysis and release of downstream cistrons, whereas the P1 core protease domain (P1Pro) free of the *N*-terminal region lacks autoinhibition and plant co-factor dependency (Pasin et al., 2014b). Disruption of the autoinhibitory mechanism that controls PPV P1 proteinase activation by removal of the *N*-terminal region was shown to alter viral replication and disease severity, and to promote local infection in a non-permissive host (Pasin et al., 2014b; Shan et al., 2018; Pasin et al., 2020). P1Pro efficiently self-cleaves in cucumber, a non-permissive host for PPV in which the wild-type protein shows limited proteolysis. A PPV mutant clone that encodes P1Pro locally replicates at higher levels than the parental virus in cucumber, which indicates that incompatibility between P1 and host co-factor(s) is potentially involved in host restriction of potyviral infection (Shan et al., 2018). In alternative experimental designs, the PPV P1 cistron was replaced by P1a, the Type-A homolog from CVYV (Shan et al., 2015). P1a shows efficient self-cleavage in cucumber, a natural host for CVYV, and a PPV chimera that encodes P1a displays a high local replication level in this host. The use of *Nicotiana benthamiana* as an experimental host showed otherwise; P1a was characterized by limited self-cleavage and incomplete HC-pro release, and reduced replication levels of the chimeric PPV in this host. Accumulation of the chimeric virus was enhanced by co-expression of a heterologous silencing suppressor, or by insertion of an additional NIa-pro recognition site to rescue CVYV P1a processing defects and sustain the release of active HC-pro (Shan *et al.*, 2015). These results support a link between the host-dependent proteolytic activation of Type-A P1, the strength of viral silencing suppression, and the consequent proteinase contribution to host-range definition.

Plant viruses have evolved a variety of mechanisms to escape cellular antiviral responses and modulate disease severity (Mandadi and Scholthof, 2013; Paudel and Sanfaçon, 2018; Križnik *et al.*, 2020). Data obtained from the PPV-plant system have recently been summarized by a study model that connects several features of Type-A P1, namely (*i*) its autoinhibition and the host co-factor requirements for its proteolysis, (*ii*) the RNA silencing suppressor activity of the downstream cistron HC-pro and lack of infectivity of P1 catalytic mutants, and (*iii*) the roles described in host-range definition and symptom development (Pasin *et al.*, 2020). According to the proposed model and its supporting mathematical simulations, autoinhibited P1 self-cleavage regulates viral replication through controlled release of the functional silencing suppressor HC-pro, which depends on host co-factor availability. This regulatory mechanism would avoid excessive antiviral pathway inhibition and viral amplification, which could trigger host damage and phytohormone-mediated defense activation. Self-controlled proteolysis of Type-A P1 would thus allow to balance viral replication kinetics and the magnitude of host immune responses and to finally promote long-term viral fitness (Pasin *et al.*, 2020).

9.6 Additional P1 Functions

Type-A P1 has a large number of positively charged residues (Valli *et al.*, 2007). Recombinant proteins of TVMV, TuMV and potato virus A (PVA) are able to bind RNA, likely by electrostatic attraction (Brantley and Hunt, 1993; Merits *et al.*, 1998; Soumounou and Laliberté, 1994); the biological significance of this activity is unclear.

Type-A P1 is dispensable for potyviral infection and movement but is able to promote virus amplification (Verchot and Carrington, 1995a). The protein is suggested to participate in replication complex formation based on its interaction and colocalization with the viral helicase CI and P3 (Arbatova et al., 1998; Merits et al., 1999; Guo et al., 2001). TEV P1 stimulates the translation of viral proteins by physically interacting with the plant ribosomes, specifically by binding to the 60S ribosomal subunits during virus infection (Martínez and Daròs, 2014). The *Brambyvirus* BlVY encodes a large P1 with an atypical AlkB domain that catalyzes RNA demethylation, suggested to promote genome integrity through methylation damage repair (van den Born et al., 2008). AlkB was recently identified also in P1 of ENMV, a potyvirus (Pasin et al., 2022).

9.7 Biotechnologies of P1 Proteinases

Recombinant Type-A P1 proteins of TVMV, TuMV, and PVA were over-expressed in *Escherichia coli* and purified from insoluble fractions (Merits et al., 1998; Rodríguez-Cerezo and Shaw, 1991; Soumounou and Laliberté, 1994; Wisler et al., 1995); glutathione S-transferase fusions promoted solubility of TVMV P1 in *E. coli* (Brantley and Hunt, 1993). Expression of tagged versions of TEV P1 showed that the protein is rapidly degraded *in planta* (Martínez and Daròs, 2014). In contrast to Type A, CVYV P1b - a Type-B proteinase - shows good solubility in *E. coli* and high stability upon *in planta* over-expression (Valli et al., 2008).

Potyvirids have a great economic impact on agricultural production; their consequences range from crop yield reduction to total yield losses (Jiang et al., 2020; Jones and Naidu, 2019). Antiviral therapies with proteinase inhibitors are used to treat human virus infection to a clinically useful level (Agbowuro et al., 2018). Along with NIa-pro and HC-pro, P1 proteinases are potential objects of antiviral strategies for potyvirid control, since inhibition of their proteolytic activity impairs infectivity (Verchot and Carrington, 1995b; Pasin et al., 2014b; Shan et al., 2015).

Transgenic expression of P1 sequences or of self-complementary hairpin constructs that trigger RNA silencing of P1 were shown to confer plant resistance to potyviruses (Di Nicola-Negri et al., 2010; Di Nicola-Negri et al., 2005; García-Almodóvar et al., 2015; Mäki-

Valkama *et al.*, 2000; Moreno *et al.*, 1998; Wang *et al.*, 2015). A study of PPV P1 recently allowed the identification of ABA as an important component of plant immunity to potyvirids (Pasin *et al.*, 2020). Genetic manipulation of ABA signaling pathways or exogenous treatments of ABA synthetic analogs is a potential source of plant-engineered resistance to potyvirids (Alazem *et al.*, 2019; Cao *et al.*, 2017; González *et al.*, 2021; Manacorda *et al.*, 2021; Vaidya *et al.*, 2019; Zhang *et al.*, 2019).

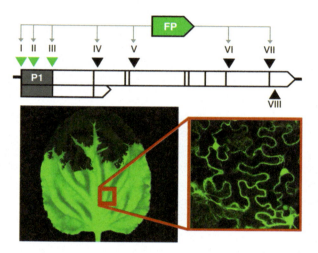

Figure 9.2 Potyvirid-based expression vectors for heterologous sequence delivery and expression in plants. Top, potyvirid genome diagram and insertion sites suitable for gene expression. Three sites are within or near the P1 cistron (Chen *et al.*, 2007; Majer *et al.*, 2015; Masuta *et al.*, 2000; Rajamäki *et al.*, 2005). Fluorescent protein (FP) gene shows a representative heterologous sequence; coat protein *N* terminus (VIII) has been used for heterologous peptide expression (Fernández-Fernández *et al.*, 1998; Sánchez *et al.*, 2013). Bottom left, FP was expressed in *Nicotiana benthamiana* using a potyviral vector and its fluorescence imaged; right, the subcellular distribution of FP expressed in leaf cells. Images adapted from Pasin *et al.* (2014a).

Plant viruses have been repurposed as expression vectors for biotechnology and synthetic biology applications (Abrahamian *et al.*, 2020; Khakhar and Voytas, 2021; Pasin *et al.*, 2019). The dissection of P1 biochemical properties has been instrumental in the development of plant expression vectors based on potyvirids (Fig. 9.2). In potyvirid vectors, heterologous sequences inserted within or upstream of P1, or between P1 and HC-pro have been successfully delivered and expressed in plants for recombinant protein and metabolite production, for gene silencing, and for reprogramming of crop traits (Choi *et al.*, 2002; Dolja *et al.*, 1992; Gammelgård *et al.*, 2007; Kelloniemi *et al.*, 2008; Majer *et al.*, 2015; Martí *et al.*, 2020; Masuta *et al.*, 2000; Rajamäki *et al.*, 2005; Tatineni *et al.*, 2011; Torti *et al.*, 2021; Xie *et al.*, 2021).

9.8 Conclusions

P1 is the most divergent among the potyvirid-encoded proteins, and its characterization has been instrumental in the generation of early potyvirid-based biotechnologies. Plant virus discovery has been revolutionized by advances in high-throughput sequencing technologies (Maclot *et al.*, 2020; Pasin *et al.*, 2019; Villamor *et al.*, 2019). Novel potyvirids are continuously being reported from the characterization of viral diseases of crop and wild species. For instance, divergent potyvirids have been isolated in umbelliferous vegetables from Italy (Rose *et al.*, 2019), in leguminous shrubs of Brazilian pastures (de Souza *et al.*, 2021), as well as in areca palm trees from China (Yang *et al.*, 2018). Recognized bymovirus species have been reported in a limited number of monocot hosts (Jiang *et al.*, 2020), but the recent identification of soybean leaf rugose mosaic virus indicates that the bymovirus host range is broader than previously thought (Ohki *et al.*, 2021). A combination of metaviromics and metatranscriptomics approaches and the facile access to underexplored geographical and ecological areas is predicted to favor the identification of new potyvirids with the unusual genomic organization. This will eventually refine our comprehension of P1 diversity and evolution, and spur the development of novel antiviral strategies as well as biotechnology and synthetic biology devices.

Further Reading

For those interested in obtaining in-depth knowledge of the content of this chapter, the authors recommend a review by Rohožková and Navrátil (2011), in which P1 was dubbed "mysterious protein." More recently, a family-wide inventory and evolutionary analysis of P1 and atypical protein domains encoded by *Potyviridae* members was reported by Pasin *et al.* (2022). Comprehensive reviews of potyvirus molecular biology were published by Revers and García (2015), and of the proteinases encoded by potyvirids and their cleavage specificities by Adams *et al.* (2005). The roles of virus-encoded proteinases in host-virus interactions were reviewed by Lei and Hilgenfeld (2017), Rodamilans *et al.* (2018a), and Mann and Sanfaçon (2019). The authors further recommend the works of Chung and Lin (2020) for a perspective on synthetic biology applications of (viral) proteinases, and of Pasin *et al.* (2019) for advances in reverse genetics and biotechnologies of plant viruses.

Acknowledgments

The authors are grateful to Catherine Mark for editorial assistance. F.P. is the recipient of a Juan de la Cierva-Incorporación contract (IJC2019-039970-I) from Ministerio de Ciencia e Innovación, Spain; H.S. is supported by the National Natural Science Foundation of China (grant 32001868), the Scientific Research Project of Tianjin Educational Commission, China (grant 2019KJ043), and State Key Laboratory for Biology of Plant Diseases and Insect Pests, China (open grant SKLOF202003).

References

Abrahamian P, Hammond RW, Hammond J, *Annu Rev Virol* **7** (2020), 513–535, doi:10.1146/annurev-virology-010720-054958.

Adams MJ, Antoniw JF, Beaudoin F, *Mol Plant Pathol* **6** (2005), 471–487, doi:10.1111/j.1364-3703.2005.00296.x.

Agbowuro AA, Huston WM, Gamble AB, Tyndall JDA, *Med Res Rev* **38** (2018), 1295–1331, doi:10.1002/med.21475.

Alazem M, Widyasari K, Kim K-H, *Viruses* **11** (2019), E879, doi:10.3390/v11090879.

Arbatova J, Lehto K, Pehu E, Pehu T, *J Gen Virol* **79** (1998), 2319–2323, doi:10.1099/0022-1317-79-10-2319.

Bagyalakshmi K, Viswanathan R, *VirusDisease* **31** (2020), 333–340, doi:10.1007/s13337-020-00618-7.

Blum M, Chang H-Y, Chuguransky S, Grego T, Kandasaamy S, Mitchell A, Nuka G, Paysan-Lafosse T, Qureshi M, Raj S, Richardson L, Salazar GA, Williams L, Bork P, Bridge A, Gough J, Haft DH, Letunic I, Marchler-

Bauer A, Mi H, Natale DA, Necci M, Orengo CA, Pandurangan AP, Rivoire C, Sigrist CJA, Sillitoe I, Thanki N, Thomas PD, Tosatto SCE, Wu CH, Bateman A, Finn RD, *Nucleic Acids Res* **49** (2021), D344–D354, doi:10.1093/nar/gkaa977.

Brantley JD, Hunt AG, *J Gen Virol* **74** (1993), 1157–1162, doi:10.1099/0022-1317-74-6-1157.

Cao M-J, Zhang Y-L, Liu X, Huang H, Zhou XE, Wang W-L, Zeng A, Zhao C-Z, Si T, Du J, Wu W-W, Wang F-X, Xu HE, Zhu J-K, *Nat Commun* **8** (2017), 1183, doi:10.1038/s41467-017-01239-3.

Carbonell A, Carrington JC, *Curr Opin Plant Biol* **27** (2015), 111–117, doi:10.1016/j.pbi.2015.06.013.

Carbonell A, Dujovny G, García JA, Valli A, *Mol Plant Microbe Interact* **25** (2012), 151–164, doi:10.1094/MPMI-08-11-0216.

Carrington JC, Freed DD, Oh C-S, *EMBO J* **9** (1990), 1347, doi:10.1002/j.1460-2075.1990.tb08249.x.

Charon J, Theil S, Nicaise V, Michon T, *Mol Biosyst* **12** (2016), 634–652, doi:10.1039/c5mb00677e.

Chen C-C, Chen T-C, Raja JAJ, Chang C-A, Chen L-W, Lin S-S, Yeh S-D, *Virus Res* **130** (2007), 210–227, doi:10.1016/j.virusres.2007.06.014.

Chen J-S, Liang S-S, Sun S-R, Damaj MB, Fu H-Y, Gao S-J, *Plant Pathol* **69** (2020), 1390–1400, doi:10.1111/ppa.13210.

Choi H-K, Tong L, Minor W, Dumas P, Boege U, Rossmann MG, Wengler G, *Nature* **354** (1991), 37–43, doi:10.1038/354037a0.

Choi I-R, Horken KM, Stenger DC, French R, *J Gen Virol* **83** (2002), 443–450, doi:10.1099/0022-1317-83-2-443.

Chung HK, Lin MZ, *Nat Methods* **17** (2020), 885–896, doi:10.1038/s41592-020-0891-z.

Clark CA, Davis JA, Abad JA, Cuellar WJ, Fuentes S, Kreuze JF, Gibson RW, Mukasa SB, Tugume AK, Tairo FD, *Plant Dis* **96** (2012), 168–185, doi:10.1094/pdis-07-11-0550.

Csorba T, Kontra L, Burgyán J, *Virology* **479–480** (2015), 85–103, doi:10.1016/j.virol.2015.02.028.

Cui H, Wang A, *Annu Rev Virol* **6** (2019), 255–274, doi:10.1146/annurev-virology-092818-015843.

Desbiez C, Lecoq H, *Arch Virol* **149** (2004), 1619–1632, doi:10.1007/s00705-004-0340-9.

Desbiez C, Verdin E, Tepfer M, Wipf-Scheibel C, Millot P, Dafalla G, Lecoq H, *Arch Virol* **161** (2016), 2913–2915, doi:10.1007/s00705-016-2981-x.

Desbiez C, Wipf-Scheibel C, Millot P, Verdin E, Dafalla G, Lecoq H, *Virus Res* **241** (2017), 88–94, doi:10.1016/j.virusres.2017.06.022.

Di Nicola-Negri E, Brunetti A, Tavazza M, Ilardi V, *Transgenic Res* **14** (2005), 989–994, doi:10.1007/s11248-005-1773-y.

Di Nicola-Negri E, Tavazza M, Salandri L, Ilardi V, *Plant Cell Rep* **29** (2010), 1435–1444, doi:10.1007/s00299-010-0933-6.

Dolja VV, Krupovic M, Koonin EV, *Annu Rev Phytopathol* **58** (2020), 23–53, doi:10.1146/annurev-phyto-030320-041346.

Dolja VV, McBride HJ, Carrington JC, *Proc Natl Acad Sci U S A* **89** (1992), 10208–10212, doi:10.1073/pnas.89.21.10208.

Dombrovsky A, Reingold V, Antignus Y, *Pest Manag Sci* **70** (2014), 1553–1567, doi:10.1002/ps.3735.

Dougherty WG, Semler BL, *Microbiol Rev* **57** (1993), 781–822, doi:10.1128/mr.57.4.781-822.1993.

Fernández-Fernández MR, Martínez-Torrecuadrada JL, Casal JI, García JA, *FEBS Lett* **427** (1998), 229–235, doi:10.1016/s0014-5793(98)00429-3.

Gammelgård E, Mohan M, Valkonen JPT, *J Gen Virol* **88** (2007), 2337–2346, doi:10.1099/vir.0.82928-0.

García-Almodóvar RC, Clemente-Moreno MJ, Díaz-Vivancos P, Petri C, Rubio M, Padilla IMG, Ilardi V, Burgos L, *Plant Cell Tissue Organ Cult* **120** (2015), 791–796, doi:10.1007/s11240-014-0629-7.

Gibbs AJ, Hajizadeh M, Ohshima K, Jones RAC, *Viruses* **12** (2020), 132, doi:10.3390/v12020132.

Giner A, Lakatos L, García-Chapa M, López-Moya JJ, Burgyán J, *PLoS Pathog* **6** (2010), e1000996, doi:10.1371/journal.ppat.1000996.

Glasa M, Malinowski T, Predajňa L, Pupola N, Dekena D, Michalczuk L, Candresse T, *Phytopathology* **101** (2011), 980–985, doi:10.1094/phyto-12-10-0334.

Gohara DW, Di Cera E, *Trends Biotechnol* **29** (2011), 577–585, doi:10.1016/j.tibtech.2011.06.001.

González R, Butković A, Escaray FJ, Martínez-Latorre J, Melero Í, Pérez-Parets E, Gómez-Cadenas A, Carrasco P, Elena SF, *Proc Natl Acad Sci U S A* **118** (2021), e2020990118, doi:10.1073/pnas.2020990118.

Guo B, Lin J, Ye K, *J Biol Chem* **286** (2011), 21937–21943, doi:10.1074/jbc.M111.230706.

Guo D, Rajamäki M-L, Saarma M, Valkonen JPT, *J Gen Virol* **82** (2001), 935–939, doi: 10.1099/0022-1317-82-4-935.

Gupta AK, Tatineni S, *Viruses* **11** (2019a), 472, doi:10.3390/v11050472.

Gupta AK, Tatineni S, *Virus Res* **269** (2019b), 197640, doi:10.1016/j.virusres.2019.197640.

Hallenberger S, Bosch V, Angliker H, Shaw E, Klenk H-D, Garten W, *Nature* **360** (1992), 358–361, doi:10.1038/360358a0.

Hedstrom L, *Chem Rev* **102** (2002), 4501–4524, doi:10.1021/cr000033x.

Hoffmann M, Hofmann-Winkler H, Pöhlmann S, *Activation of Viruses Host Proteases* (Böttcher-Friebertshäuser E., Garten W., and Klenk H. D.), Springer International Publishing, Cham, 2018, pp. 71–98.

Hoffmann M, Kleine-Weber H, Pöhlmann S, *Mol Cell* **78** (2020), 779–784.e5, doi:10.1016/j.molcel.2020.04.022.

Hulo C, de Castro E, Masson P, Bougueleret L, Bairoch A, Xenarios I, Le Mercier P, *Nucleic Acids Res* **39** (2011), D576–D582, doi:10.1093/nar/gkq901.

International Committee on Taxonomy of Viruses 2020, ICTV master species list 2019.v1 (MSL #35). Last accessed July 2021, https://talk.ictvonline.org/files/master-species-lists/m/msl/9601.

James AM, Seal SE, Bailey AM, Foster GD, *Mol Plant Pathol* **22** (2021), 382–389, doi:10.1111/mpp.13021.

Jiang C, Kan J, Ordon F, Perovic D, Yang P, *Theor Appl Genet* **133** (2020), 1623–1640, doi:10.1007/s00122-020-03555-7.

Jiang H, Li K, Dou D, Gai J, *Arch Virol* **162** (2017), 549–553, doi:10.1007/s00705-016-3123-1.

Jones RAC, Naidu RA, *Annu Rev Virol* **6** (2019), 387–409, doi:10.1146/annurev-virology-092818-015606.

Kelloniemi J, Mäkinen K, Valkonen JPT, *Virus Res* **135** (2008), 282–291, doi:10.1016/j.virusres.2008.04.006.

Kenesi E, Carbonell A, Lózsa R, Vértessy B, Lakatos L, *Nucleic Acids Res* **45** (2017), 7736–7750, doi:10.1093/nar/gkx379.

Khakhar A, Voytas DF, *Front Plant Sci* **12** (2021), 668580, doi:10.3389/fpls.2021.668580.

Križnik M, Baebler Š, Gruden K, *Curr Opin Virol* **42** (2020), 25–31, doi:10.1016/j.coviro.2020.04.006.

Lefkowitz EJ, Dempsey DM, Hendrickson RC, Orton RJ, Siddell SG, Smith DB, *Nucleic Acids Res* **46** (2018), D708–D717, doi:10.1093/nar/gkx932.

Lei J, Hilgenfeld R, *FEBS Lett* **591** (2017), 3190–3210, doi:10.1002/1873-3468.12827.

Li F, Wang A, *Trends Microbiol* **27** (2019), 792–805, doi:10.1016/j.tim.2019.05.007.

Li W, Hilf ME, Webb SE, Baker CA, Adkins S, *Virus Res* **135** (2008), 213–219, doi:10.1016/j.virusres.2008.03.015.

Maclot F, Candresse T, Filloux D, Malmstrom CM, Roumagnac P, van der Vlugt R, Massart S, *Front Microbiol* **11** (2020), 578064, doi:10.3389/fmicb.2020.578064.

Majer E, Navarro J-A, Daròs J-A, *Biotechnol J* **10** (2015), 1792–1802, doi:10.1002/biot.201500042.

Mäki-Valkama T, Pehu T, Santala A, Valkonen JPT, Koivu K, Lehto K, Pehu E, *Mol Breed* **6** (2000), 95–104, doi:10.1023/a:1009679609459.

Maliogka VI, Salvador B, Carbonell A, Sáenz P, San León D, Oliveros JC, Delgadillo MO, García JA, Simón-Mateo C, *Mol Plant Pathol* **13** (2012), 877–886, doi:10.1111/j.1364-3703.2012.00796.x.

Manacorda CA, Gudesblat G, Sutka M, Alemano S, Peluso F, Oricchio P, Baroli I, Asurmendi S, *Plant Cell Environ* **44** (2021), 1399–1416, doi:10.1111/pce.14024.

Mandadi KK, Scholthof K-BG, *Plant Cell* **25** (2013), 1489–1505, doi:10.1105/tpc.113.111658.

Mann K, Sanfaçon H, *Viruses* **11** (2019), 66, doi:10.3390/v11010066.

Martí M, Diretto G, Aragonés V, Frusciante S, Ahrazem O, Gómez-Gómez L, Daròs J-A, *Metab Eng* **61** (2020), 238–250, doi:10.1016/j.ymben.2020.06.009.

Martínez F, Daròs J-A, *J Virol* **88** (2014), 10725–10737, doi:10.1128/JVI.00928-14.

Masuta C, Yamana T, Tacahashi Y, Uyeda I, Sato M, Ueda S, Matsumura T, *Plant J* **23** (2000), 539–546, doi: 10.1046/j.1365-313x.2000.00795.x.

Mavankal G, Rhoads RE, *Virology* **185** (1991), 721–731, doi:10.1016/0042-6822(91)90543-K.

Mbanzibwa DR, Tian Y, Mukasa SB, Valkonen JPT, *J Virol* **83** (2009), 6934–6940, doi:10.1128/JVI.00537-09.

Merits A, Guo D, Järvekülg L, Saarma M, *Virology* **263** (1999), 15–22, doi:10.1006/viro.1999.9926.

Merits A, Guo D, Saarma M, *J Gen Virol* **79** (1998), 3123–3127, doi: 10.1099/0022-1317-79-12-3123.

Mingot A, Valli A, Rodamilans B, León DS, Baulcombe DC, García JA, López-Moya JJ, *J Virol* **90** (2016), 3543–3557, doi:10.1128/jvi.02360-15.

Mistry J, Chuguransky S, Williams L, Qureshi M, Salazar GA, Sonnhammer ELL, Tosatto SCE, Paladin L, Raj S, Richardson LJ, Finn RD, Bateman A, *Nucleic Acids Res* **49** (2021), D412–D419, doi:10.1093/nar/gkaa913.

Moreno M, Bernal JJ, Jiménez I, Rodríguez-Cerezo E, *J Gen Virol* **79**(Pt 11), (1998), 2819–2827, doi:10.1099/0022-1317-79-11-2819.

Nagyová A, Kamencayová M, Glasa M, Subr ZW, *Virus Genes* **44** (2012), 505–512, doi:10.1007/s11262-012-0726-9.

Nakahara KS, Shimada R, Choi S-H, Yamamoto H, Shao J, Uyeda I, *Mol Plant Microbe Interact* **23** (2010), 1460–1469, doi:10.1094/MPMI-11-09-0277.

NCBI Resource Coordinators, *Nucleic Acids Res* **46** (2018), D8–D13, doi:10.1093/nar/gkx1095.

Nigam D, LaTourrette K, Souza PFN, Garcia-Ruiz H, *Front Plant Sci* **10** (2019), 1439, doi:10.3389/fpls.2019.01439.

Ochoa J, Valli A, Martín-Trillo M, Simón-Mateo C, García JA, Rodamilans B, *Plant Cell Environ* **42** (2019), 3015–3026, doi:10.1111/pce.13610.

Ohki T, Kuroda T, Sayama M, Maoka T, *Arch Virol* **166** (2021), 1885–1892, doi:10.1007/s00705-021-05069-z.

Pasin F, Daròs J-A, Tzanetakis IE, *FEMS Microbiol Rev* (2022), fuac011, doi:10.1093/femsre/fuac011.

Pasin F, Kulasekaran S, Natale P, Simón-Mateo C, García JA, *Plant Methods* **10** (2014a), 22, doi:10.1186/1746-4811-10-22.

Pasin F, Menzel W, Daròs J-A, *Plant Biotechnol J* **17** (2019), 1010–1026, doi:10.1111/pbi.13084.

Pasin F, Shan H, García B, Müller M, San León D, Ludman M, Fresno DH, Fátyol K, Munné-Bosch S, Rodrigo G, García JA, *Plant Commun* **1** (2020), 100099, doi:10.1016/j.xplc.2020.100099.

Pasin F, Simón-Mateo C, García JA, *PLOS Pathog* **10** (2014b), e1003985, doi:10.1371/journal.ppat.1003985.

Paudel DB, Sanfaçon H, *Front Plant Sci* **9** (2018), 1575, doi:10.3389/fpls.2018.01575.

Rajamäki ML, Kelloniemi J, Alminaite A, Kekarainen T, Rabenstein F, Valkonen JPT, *Virology* **342** (2005), 88–101, doi:10.1016/j.virol.2005.07.019.

Rawlings ND, Barrett AJ, Thomas PD, Huang X, Bateman A, Finn RD, *Nucleic Acids Res* **46** (2018), D624–D632, doi:10.1093/nar/gkx1134.

Reuper H, Krenz B, *Virus Genes* **57** (2021), 233–237, doi:10.1007/s11262-021-01829-w.

Revers F, García JA, *Adv Virus Res* **92** (2015), 101–199, doi:10.1016/bs.aivir.2014.11.006.

Rodamilans B, Casillas A, García JA, *J Virol* **95** (2021), e0015021, doi:10.1128/jvi.00150-21.

Rodamilans B, Shan H, Pasin F, García JA, *Front Plant Sci* **9** (2018a), 666, doi:10.3389/fpls.2018.00666.

Rodamilans B, Valli A, García JA, *J Gen Virol* **94** (2013), 1407–1414, doi:10.1099/vir.0.050781-0.

Rodamilans B, Valli A, Mingot A, San León D, López-Moya JJ, García JA, *Sci Rep* **8** (2018b), 1–10, doi:10.1038/s41598-018-34358-y.

Rodríguez-Cerezo E, Shaw JG, *Virology* **185** (1991), 572–579, doi:10.1016/0042-6822(91)90527-I.

Rohožková J, Navrátil M, *J Biosci* **36** (2011), 189–200, doi:10.1007/s12038-011-9020-6.

Rose H, Döring I, Vetten H-J, Menzel W, Richert-Pöggeler KR, Maiss E, *J Gen Virol* **100** (2019), 308–320, doi:10.1099/jgv.0.001207.

Salvador B, Delgadillo MO, Sáenz P, García JA, Simón-Mateo C, *Mol Plant Microbe Interact* **21** (2008a), 20–29, doi:10.1094/MPMI-21-1-0020.

Salvador B, Saénz P, Yangüez E, Quiot JB, Quiot L, Delgadillo MO, García JA, Simón-Mateo C, *Mol Plant Pathol* **9** (2008b), 147–155, doi:10.1111/j.1364-3703.2007.00450.x.

Sánchez F, Sáez M, Lunello P, Ponz F, *J Biotechnol* **168** (2013), 409–415, doi:10.1016/j.jbiotec.2013.09.002.

Shan H, *Characterization of P1 Leader Proteases of the Potyviridae Family and Identification of the Host Factors Involved in Their Proteolytic Activity during Viral Infection*, Universidad Autónoma de Madrid, Spain, 2018.

Shan H, Pasin F, Tzanetakis IE, Simón-Mateo C, García JA, Rodamilans B, *Mol Plant Pathol* **19** (2018), 1504–1510, doi:10.1111/mpp.12640.

Shan H, Pasin F, Valli A, Castillo C, Rajulu C, Carbonell A, Simón-Mateo C, García JA, Rodamilans B, *Virology* **476** (2015), 264–270, doi:10.1016/j.virol.2014.

Shi Y, Chen J, Hong X, Chen J, Adams MJ, *Mol Plant Pathol* **8** (2007), 785–790, doi:10.1111/j.1364-3703.2007.00426.x.

Sigrist CJA, de Castro E, Cerutti L, Cuche BA, Hulo N, Bridge A, Bougueleret L, Xenarios I, *Nucleic Acids Res* **41** (2013), D344-D347, doi:10.1093/nar/gks1067.

Soumounou Y, Laliberté J-F, *J Gen Virol* **75** (1994), 2567–2573, doi:10.1099/0022-1317-75-10-2567.

de Souza JM, da Silva Fragoso KN, Orílio AF, Melo FL, Nagata T, Fernandes CD, Valério JR, Vilela Torres FZ, Amaral BB, Camargo Pereira TB, de Oliveira AS, Resende RO, *Virus Res* **293** (2021), 198257, doi:10.1016/j.virusres.2020.198257.

Stieneke-Gröber A, Vey M, Angliker H, Shaw E, Thomas G, Roberts C, Klenk HD, Garten W, *EMBO J* **11** (1992), 2407–2414, doi: 10.1002/j.1460-2075.1992.tb05305.x.

Susaimuthu J, Tzanetakis IE, Gergerich RC, Martin RR, *Virus Res* **131** (2008), 145–151, doi:10.1016/j.virusres.2007.09.001.

Tatineni S, McMechan AJ, Hein GL, French R, *Virology* **410** (2011), 268–281, doi:10.1016/j.virol.2010.10.043.

Tatineni S, Qu F, Li R, Morris TJ, French R, *Virology* **433** (2012), 104–115, doi:10.1016/j.virol.2012.07.016.

Tena Fernández F, González I, Doblas P, Rodríguez C, Sahana N, Kaur H, Tenllado F, Praveen S, Canto T, *Mol Plant Pathol* **14** (2013), 530–541, doi:10.1111/mpp.12025.

The UniProt Consortium, Bateman A, Martin M-J, Orchard S, Magrane M, Agivetova R, Ahmad S, Alpi E, Bowler-Barnett EH, Britto R, Bursteinas B, Bye-A-Jee H, Coetzee R, Cukura A, Da Silva A, Denny P, Dogan T, Ebenezer T, Fan J, Castro LG, Garmiri P, Georghiou G, Gonzales L, Hatton-Ellis E, Hussein A, Ignatchenko A, Insana G, Ishtiaq R, Jokinen P, Joshi V, Jyothi D, Lock A, Lopez R, Luciani A, Luo J, Lussi Y, MacDougall A, Madeira F, Mahmoudy M, Menchi M, Mishra A, Moulang K, Nightingale A, Oliveira CS, Pundir S, Qi G, Raj S, Rice D, Lopez MR, Saidi R, Sampson J, Sawford T, Speretta E, Turner E, Tyagi N, Vasudev P, Volynkin V, Warner K, Watkins X, Zaru R, Zellner H, Bridge A, Poux S, Redaschi N, Aimo L, Argoud-Puy G, Auchincloss A, Axelsen K, Bansal P, Baratin D, Blatter M-C, Bolleman J, Boutet E, Breuza L, Casals-Casas C, de Castro E, Echioukh KC, Coudert E, Cuche B, Doche M, Dornevil D, Estreicher A, Famiglietti ML, Feuermann M, Gasteiger E, Gehant S, Gerritsen V, Gos A, Gruaz-Gumowski N, Hinz U, Hulo C, Hyka-Nouspikel N, Jungo F, Keller G, Kerhornou A, Lara V, Le Mercier P, Lieberherr D, Lombardot T, Martin X, Masson P, Morgat A, Neto TB, Paesano S, Pedruzzi I, Pilbout S, Pourcel L, Pozzato M, Pruess M, Rivoire C, Sigrist C, Sonesson K, Stutz A, Sundaram S, Tognolli M, Verbregue L, Wu CH, Arighi CN, Arminski L, Chen C, Chen Y, Garavelli JS, Huang H, Laiho K, McGarvey P, Natale DA, Ross K, Vinayaka CR, Wang Q, Wang Y, Yeh L-S, Zhang J, Ruch P, Teodoro D, *Nucleic Acids Res* **49** (2021), D480–D489, doi:10.1093/nar/gkaa1100.

Thornbury DW, van den Heuvel JF, Lesnaw JA, Pirone TP, *J Gen Virol* **74** (1993), 2731–2735, doi:10.1099/0022-1317-74-12-2731.

Torti S, Schlesier R, Thümmler A, Bartels D, Römer P, Koch B, Werner S, Panwar V, Kanyuka K, von Wirén N, Jones JDG, Hause G, Giritch A, Gleba Y, *Nat Plants* **7** (2021), 159–171, doi:10.1038/s41477-021-00851-y.

Trudeau T, Nassar R, Cumberworth A, Wong ETC, Woollard G, Gsponer J, *Structure* **21** (2013), 332–341, doi:10.1016/j.str.2012.12.013.

Untiveros M, Olspert A, Artola K, Firth AE, Kreuze JF, Valkonen JPT, *Mol Plant Pathol* **17** (2016), 1111–1123, doi:10.1111/mpp.12366.

Vaidya AS, Helander JDM, Peterson FC, Elzinga D, Dejonghe W, Kaundal A, Park S-Y, Xing Z, Mega R, Takeuchi J, Khanderahoo B, Bishay S, Volkman BF, Todoroki Y, Okamoto M, Cutler SR, *Science* **366** (2019), eaaw8848, doi:10.1126/science.aaw8848.

Valli A, Dujovny G, García JA, *J Virol* **82** (2008), 974–986, doi:10.1128/jvi.01664-07.

Valli A, López-Moya JJ, García JA, *J Gen Virol* **88** (2007), 1016–1028, doi:10.1099/vir.0.82402-0.

Valli A, Martín-Hernández AM, López-Moya JJ, García JA, *J Virol* **80** (2006), 10055–10063, doi:10.1128/JVI.00985-06.

Valli A, Oliveros JC, Molnar A, Baulcombe D, García JA, *RNA* **17** (2011), 1148–1158, doi:10.1261/rna.2510611.

Valli AA, Gallo A, Rodamilans B, López-Moya JJ, García JA, *Mol Plant Pathol* **19** (2018), 744–763, doi:10.1111/mpp.12553.

van den Born E, Omelchenko MV, Bekkelund A, Leihne V, Koonin EV, Dolja VV, Falnes PØ, *Nucleic Acids Res* **36** (2008), 5451–5461, doi:10.1093/nar/gkn519.

Verchot J, Carrington JC, *J Virol* **69** (1995a), 3668–3674, doi:10.1128/jvi.69.6.3668-3674.1995.

Verchot J, Carrington JC, *J Virol* **69** (1995b), 1582–1590, doi:10.1128/jvi.69.3.1582-1590.1995.

Verchot J, Herndon KL, Carrington JC, *Virology* **190** (1992), 298–306, doi:10.1016/0042-6822(92)91216-H.

Verchot J, Koonin EV, Carrington JC, *Virology* **185** (1991), 527–535, doi:10.1016/0042-6822(91)90522-D.

Villamor DEV, Ho T, Al Rwahnih M, Martin RR, Tzanetakis IE, *Phytopathology* **109** (2019), 716–725, doi:10.1094/PHYTO-07-18-0257-RVW.

Wang A, Tian L, Brown DCW, Svircev AM, Stobbs LW, Sanfaçon H, *Acta Hortic* (2015), 77–84, doi:10.17660/actahortic.2015.1063.9.

Wisler GC, Purcifull DE, Hiebert E, *J Gen Virol* **76** (1995), 37–45, doi:10.1099/0022-1317-76-1-37.

Wrobel AG, Benton DJ, Xu P, Roustan C, Martin SR, Rosenthal PB, Skehel JJ, Gamblin SJ, *Nat Struct Mol Biol* **27** (2020), 763–767, doi:10.1038/s41594-020-0468-7.

Wylie SJ, Adams M, Chalam C, Kreuze J, López-Moya JJ, Ohshima K, Praveen S, Rabenstein F, Stenger D, Wang A, Zerbini FM, ICTV Report Consortium, *J Gen Virol* **98** (2017), 352–354, doi:10.1099/jgv.0.000740.

Xie W, Marty DM, Xu J, Khatri N, Willie K, Moraes WB, Stewart LR, *BMC Plant Biol* **21** (2021), 208, doi:10.1186/s12870-021-02971-1.

Yang K, Ran M, Li Z, Hu M, Zheng L, Liu W, Jin P, Miao W, Zhou P, Shen W, Cui H, *Arch Virol* **163** (2018), 3471–3475, doi:10.1007/s00705-018-3980-x.

Yang LJ, Hidaka M, Masaki H, Uozumi T, *Biosci Biotechnol Biochem* **62** (1998), 380–382, doi:10.1271/bbb.62.380.

Yang X, Li Y, Wang A, *Annu Rev Phytopathol* **59** (2021), doi:10.1146/annurev-phyto-020620-114550.

Young BA, Stenger DC, Qu F, Morris TJ, Tatineni S, French R, *Virus Res* **163** (2012), 672–677, doi:10.1016/j.virusres.2011.12.019.

Zhang T, Liu P, Zhong K, Zhang F, Xu M, He L, Jin P, Chen J, Yang J, *Biology* **8** (2019), E80, doi:10.3390/biology8040080.

Part V
Soil Enzymes

Chapter 10

Soil Enzymes: Distribution, Interactions, and Influencing Factors

Sesan Abiodun Aransiola,[a] Femi Afolabi,[a]
Femi Joseph,[b] and Naga Raju Maddela[c]

[a]*Bioresources Development Centre, National Biotechnology Development Agency (NABDA) Ogbomoso, Oyo State, Nigeria*
[b]*Federal University of Technology, Minna, Nigeria*
[c]*Department of Biological Sciences, Faculty of Health Sciences, Technical University of Manabí, Portoviejo 130105, Ecuador*
raju.maddela@utm.edu.ec

Soil is the topmost layer of the earth which consists of biologically active constituents including enzymes for diverse purposes. Enzymes are produced by different sources in the soil, these could be from microorganisms, plant roots and residues, and soil animals. Soil enzymes usually accumulate, stabilize or form complexes in the soil matrix. Biotic and abiotic factors determine the distributions of enzymes in the soil. Soil enzymes play decisive roles in carbon, phosphorous, and nitrogen cycling which provide important nutrients for plant growth promotion and incrementing the microbial metabolism. They are widely distributed in nature and are sensitive

---

Agricultural Biocatalysis: Enzymes in Agriculture and Industry
Edited by Peter Jeschke and Evgeni B. Starikov
Copyright © 2023 Jenny Stanford Publishing Pte. Ltd.
ISBN 978-981-4968-47-8 (Hardcover), 978-1-003-31310-6 (eBook)
www.jennystanford.com

to alteration in the soil ecosystem. A high concentration of chemical compounds that are end products of enzymatic reactions in soil may lead to inhibition of the activity of the enzyme connected with the chemical in question through a process called feedback inhibition. This chapter, therefore, takes into account the sources, distribution, and abundance of soil enzymes, the ecological stoichiometry of plant-soil-enzyme interactions, soil chemical properties versus soil enzyme activities, and the impact of anthropogenic factors on soil enzyme activities

10.1 Introduction

Soil can be described as a biologically active exhaustible resource for the sustainable production of crops. Or a natural environment consisting of a mixture of organic and inorganic components present in the gaseous, aqueous, and solid states (Sang-Hwan *et al.*, 2020). Food production, environmental efficiency, and worldwide ecological stability are influenced by the situation of the soil (Binkley and Fischer, 2012). The strategic role of soil enzymes in soil biogeochemical methods, soil fitness, and agricultural productiveness is well established (Kaur *et al.*, 2020). The quality of the soil determines the yield of crops and can be sustained by employing the right tools both to evaluate and predict changes in it (Almeida *et al.*, 2015). Ecological stoichiometry is the study of how the stability of energy and chemical elements influence living organisms and their interactions in their ecosystem based on the principle of energy conservation. It also includes how the organisms and their activities affect the balance of chemical elements in an environment (Liu and Sun, 2013). Since the mineral elements form the nutrients needed by living organisms (plants, microbes), most work done in this regard questions how nutrient availability in an ecosystem and nutrient demands of inhabitant living organisms affect nutrient circle, growth of organisms, and their interface with the abiotic and biotic environment. (Michał, 2020). Ecological stoichiometry of plant-soil-enzyme interactions aims to understand the effect of the interaction of plant and soil enzymes on soil mineral nutrients. Researchers are currently concentrating on carbon, nitrogen, phosphorus ratio (C:N:P) stoichiometry because these chemical elements constitute the most vital mineral nutrients in the soil (Sophie *et al.*, 2015). Their study is vital to understanding nutrient dynamics of soil organisms, sustainability, and nutrient cycling in the soil ecosystem. Hailiang *et al.* (2020). According to Dedmer *et al.* (2018), the efficiency of organic carbon usage by microorganisms in the soil increased with the reduced presence of nitrogen but decreased with increased nitrogen. This discovery suggests that the activity of decomposers in the soil depends on litter or debris and an adjustment from nitrogen to carbon limited the process of decomposition. Interaction between plant and soil enzymes primarily occurs at the rhizosphere. Rhizosphere stoichiometry is a key tool for assessing interactions between plant and soil. The change in soil enzymatic activity drives plant secondary succession (Lie *et al.*, 2021).

10.2 Source, Distribution, and Abundance of Soil Enzymes

Soil quality is determined by its physicochemical properties including its natural composition and modifications due to human use and management (Abbott and Murphy, 2003; Abioye *et al.*, 2017). Enzymes are a key part of these physicochemical factors. The quality of the soil especially concerning its health is the deciding factor for the availability of plant vitamins to enhance crop productivity and environmental quality. Microorganisms of various types and very importantly, enzymes determine the quality of the soil. The enzymes found in soil catalyze a lot of vital reactions that are key to various life processes of soil microorganisms which culminate in the conversion of organic matter to inorganic matter; thereby helping in the launch of nutrients for plant use and cycling. Soil enzymes are known to be sensitive and therefore respond quickly to changes in soil management practices and environmental conditions (Lemanowicz *et al.*, 2018). The activities of these enzymes are beneficial because they are indicators of the biological excellence of soils (Kompała-Bąba *et al.*, 2021). This is because they are operationally practical, very sensitive, clean to a degree, and more responsive to soil tillage and shape than different soil variables. Soil enzymes include but are not limited to β-glucosidase, cellulose, arylsulfatase, dehydrogenase, phosphatase, and urease, which play a vital role in the productivity of the agricultural ecosystem. Some of these enzymes help in the breakdown of organic matter like hydrolase, glucosidase while others are involved in nutrient mineralization like amidase, urease, phosphatase, sulfates (Kaur et al., 2020) These enzymes also perform an important part in agriculture through energy transfer by the decomposition of soil organic matter. This is why soil enzymatic activity is employed for accessing and managing the productivity of an ecosystem.

There are different sources of enzymes in the soil and they include; living or dead microbes, plant roots and residues, and soil animals (Kaur et al., 2020). Soil Enzymes usually accumulate, stabilize or form complexes in soil matrix (Rao et al., 2014) These complexes are formed with humus, clay, and humus-clay but without any association with viable cells. It is estimated that close to 40% to 60% of enzymatic activities in the soil may come from accumulated and stabilized enzymes (USDA, 2010). This means that enzymatic activities in the soil do not necessarily mean high microbial biomass or respiration. Consequently, enzyme activity in the soil is the cumulative effect of long-term stabilized enzymes and activities of viable cells at sampling. The only exception to this is dehydrogenase which can only be produced by viable cells. However, these enzymes occur in different forms in the soil as follows:

Form 1: Clay-related roles

(a) Many activities largely associated with clay
(b) Improved resistance to proteolysis and microbial attack
(c) The temperature of inactivation increases

Form 2: Role of organic matter

(a) Nitrogen compounds are more stable due to the presence of humus materials.
(b) Enzymes in this category exhibit pH and temperature changes.
(c) They are difficult to purify (bound to organic matter).

Form 3: Role of clay–organic matter complexes

(a) Lignin + bentonite (clay) protect enzymes against proteolytic attack, but not bentonite alone.
(b) Enzymes are bound to organic matter which is then bound to clay (Shonkor and Ajit, 2011).

Generally, enzymes are classified into two broad groups, depending on the quantity present in a cell. These are constitutive and inducible enzymes. Both are present in the soil. Constitutive enzymes are those enzymes that are constantly present in the soil in specific amounts irrespective of the metabolic state of the cell (Sang-Hwan *et al.*, 2020). Their availability and quantity are not affected by the addition of any specific substrate (pyro-phosphatase). There is a need for continuous synthesis because of their role in maintaining cell processes and structure such as glucose metabolism, amino acid metabolism, transcription, translations, and fatty acid metabolism. They are sometimes referred to as housekeeping enzymes (Kaur *et al.*, 2020). On the other hand, inducible enzymes are usually present in trace amounts and some cases, are not available at all. Their production is triggered by the availability of the substrate they act on amidase. They are produced only when needed by the cell hence the name adaptive enzymes.

Furthermore, enzymes are classified based on their site of action like endo-cellular or intracellular and exo-cellular or extracellular. Intracellular enzymes catalyze reactions both within and outside of the cell that produced them (urease and β-glucosidase). On the other hand, extracellular enzymes perform their functions outside of the cell producing them (proteinase and cellulase) (Bueis *et al.*, 2018; Kaur *et al.*, 2020).

Therefore, the distribution and abundance of any soil enzyme are determined by its type constitutive or adaptive on one hand and intracellular and extracellular on the other. For instance, urease, an extracellular enzyme that is responsible for the hydrolysis of urea to ammonia (NH_3) and carbon dioxide (CO_2), accounts for about 63% of total enzyme activity in soil (Bueis *et al.*, 2018).

There is however a strong need for further research into the hypothesis that extracellular enzymes from bacterial sources generally tend to have neutral/alkaline optima while fungal and plant extracellular enzymes have acidic optima, for example, phosphatase must be more extensively tested before pH optima can be reliably used to distinguish enzyme sources. It should be noted that this approach would be limited to certain enzymes (phosphatases, proteases) because many polysaccharide-hydrolyzing enzymes from bacteria and fungi have acidic pH optima (Cadwell, 2005).

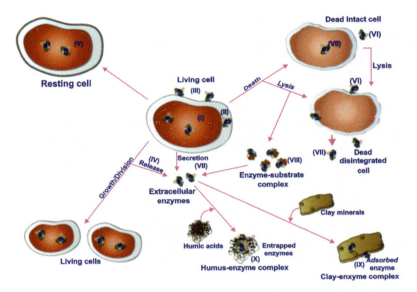

Figure 10.1 General view of soil enzyme. Locations of enzymes in soil adopted from Wallenstein and Burns, (2011) (i) functioning within the cytoplasm of microbial cells; (ii) restricted to the periplasmatic space of Gram-negative bacteria; (iii) located on the outer surface of cells with their active sites extending into the soil environment, contained within polysomes or retained by biofilms; (iv) situated within resting cells including fungal spores, protozoal cysts and bacterial endospores; (v) attached to entire dead cells and cell debris; (vi) leaking from intact cells or released from lysed cells; (vii) free in soil water; (viii) associated with enzyme substrate complexes; (ix) complexed with soil organic matter by absorption, entrapment or co-polymerization; (x) sorbed to the external and internal surfaces of clay minerals; and (xi) bound to condensed tannins (Burns et al., 2013).

The distribution and abundance of soil enzymes (Fig. 10.1) are usually dependent on some abiotic and biotic factors (Shonkor and Ajit, 2011). For example, soil enzymes function effectively at varying optimum pH and temperatures. It is well documented that the activity of phosphatase, arylsulfatase, and amidase involved in phosphorus, sulfur, and nitrogen cycling, respectively, is heavily related to variations in soil pH (USDA, 2010). The growth of microorganisms in the soil is also dependent on temperature and pH. It, therefore, means that the distribution or abundance of soil enzymes correlates to the presence of adequate viable cells in the soil per time (Abioye et al., 2015). The abundance or distribution of soil enzymes is also affected by the moisture content of the soil at any instant. The higher the moisture content, the higher the microbial activities and the higher the quantity of enzyme, drought, soil texture, and clay content have also been found to affect the abundance and distribution of soil enzymes (Cherukumali *et al.*, 2017). Clayey soils, as a result of their ability to store organic matter that promotes microbial communities, and forms clay-enzyme complexes, generally have a higher content of soil enzymes compared to any other type of soil. In contrast, sandy soils contain low quantity due to the low presence of organic matter and poor water holding capacity which do not support microbial growth. The presence or absence of plants in the soil also determines the abundance and distribution of enzymes this is because plant roots stimulate microbial activity due to the availability of exudates rich in substrates needed for their growth. This will consequently lead to the production of enzymes. The availability or otherwise of some chemical compounds that are end products of some enzymatic reactions can affect the distribution or abundance of such an enzyme. For example, phosphatase availability increases in phosphorus-deficient soil but decreases in soil with high phosphorus concentrations. In the same vein, urease presence may be suppressed by ammonia-based nitrogen fertilizer (Kaur *et al.*, 2020). Moreover, the activities of soil enzymes are dependent on the abundance and diversity of the microbial biomass. Also, the availability and activity of dehydrogenase are highly connected with the populations of soil microbes and the diversity of the microbial community structure, as it can only be produced by living cells (Kompała-Bąba *et al.*, 2021). Some researchers have also established that the composition of microorganisms in the soil can be changed depending on the diversity of the plant community (particularly the occurrence of dominant species) growing on it and the extent of the vegetation period (Bartelt-Ryser *et al.*, 2005; Kao-Kniffin *et al.*, 2007) Compaction may limit the availability of enzymes involved in nutrient mineralization because of decreased oxygen in the soil for those reactions or organisms requiring an aerobic environment. Conversely, anaerobic conditions from compaction or water saturation increase enzymatic reaction rates related to denitrification. The application of pesticides, herbicides, and insecticides containing heavy metals can reduce the availability of enzymes (e.g., amidase) due to their toxic effect on soil organisms and roots or direct inhibition of enzyme reactions. In terms of distribution, the availability of enzymes decreases with an increase in soil depth (Cherukumali *et al.*, 2017). Climatic factors such as elevated carbon dioxide, temperature, drought and soil management practices, and environmental conditions have been found to affect enzyme abundance and distribution (Cherukumali *et al.*, 2017). Farming practices such as mechanical tillage, cropping systems, and residues removal have been found to adversely affect enzymatic activities and availability (CeliKa *et al.*, 2011). While enzymatic availability and activity decrease with an increase in soil depth, management-induced differences are observed in reverse (Srinivasarao *et al.*, 2009). However, some enzymes such as acid and alkaline phosphatases, dehydrogenase, fluorescein diacetate (FDA) hydrolysis, β-glucosidase, and urease have demonstrated constancy irrespective of season and crop (Cabello *et al.*, 2011). The reduction in enzyme abundance and their potential activities may also be due to a decline in soil enzyme accumulation during prolonged drought (Pavani *et al.*, 2017). Also, the arylsulphatase enzymes, which are connected with the hydrolysis of organic sulfate ester with aromatic radical are produced by both plants and microorganisms, thereby influencing their abundance and distribution positively (Salazar, 2011).

The abundance and distribution of soil enzymes may also be determined by the type of enzyme and the predominance or otherwise of fungi in a given piece of land. This is because research has shown that 86% of cellulose in the soil is of fungal origin (Cadwell, 2005).

10.3 Ecological Stoichiometry of Plant-Soil-Enzyme Interactions

Organisms that can significantly modify the availability of environmental resources are termed ecosystem engineers (Andrew, 2019). Their activities cause changes in the soil biotic and abiotic materials, resulting in the maintenance, modification, or creation of habitat that would not have existed. The function and biodiversity of an ecosystem would be greatly reduced without the presence of an ecosystem engineer. (Houston, 2018). Ecosystem engineers are categorized as allogenic engineers and autogenic engineers (John, 2017).

Allogenic engineers mechanically transform materials which consequently leads to the modification of the environment (Houston, 2018). Autogenic engineer adjusts their environment by altering themselves. Plant, especially trees form this category of ecosystem engineers. As plants grow, their leaves, root, branches, and trunks provide new habitats for other organisms (John, 2017).

Thus, changes in the physical and chemical properties of the soil at the rhizosphere are influenced by plants (living or dead). This could in turn influence the performance of plants in that soil environment (Archana and Rao, 2021). In all, organisms living in an ecosystem control their function. Ecosystem processes are determined by the functional characteristics of the constituent organisms and not really by the number of species or individuals present. The richness of species and functional group individually influence biomass buildup (Changting *et al.*, 2011).

10.3.1 Role of Plant in Soil Health

Change in plant species composition modifies resources availability for soil microbial community, which consequently modifies their function and composition. Such changes in the composition and function of microbial communities influence soil carbon and nitrogen circle (Minghui *et al.*, 2019). Diverse microbial communities present in the soil facilitate important processes that control soil ecosystem carbon, nitrogen, phosphorus, and sulfur cycling. The presence of growth-limiting resources profiles the composition of the plant community. While the availability of resources needed by soil microbial communities is limited by the organic compounds in detritus (dead roots and leaves) (Changting *et al.*, 2011).

Plant species diversity and biomass have a great impact on enzyme activity. Dominant species of plants in a habitat influence the kind of soil enzymes that are predominant in that habitat (Xiao *et al.*,

2017). According to Agnieszka et al. (2021), alkaline phosphatase and dehydrogenase activity doubles in soil dominated by grass species compared with forbs-dominated soil. Grasses, via their root systems, are more efficient in increasing enzyme activity compared to other herbaceous plant species (David, 2013). About one-third of the earth's surface is covered by woodland and forest. Both of which play important role in world carbon repossession and nutrient cycling. The forest environment is extremely heterogeneous. The forest dominant trees affect the soil physicochemical properties of the soil via root exudates and litter. This, in turn, alters the structure of the soil microbial community with a consequential impact on soil enzyme activity (Haifeng, 2018).

10.3.2 Plant-Soil-Enzyme Relationship and Soil Health

Soil enzymes perform crucial roles in the biochemical functioning and conservation of the soil ecosystem (Swati et al., 2018). They catalyze the biochemical reactions that are vital to key soil processes of microbes, stabilization of soil structure, decomposition, and organic matter production (Burak, 2020). Soil enzymes are also vital in the cycling of nutrients such as carbon by enzyme invertase, nitrogen by urease and protease, as well as phosphorus by phosphatase (Haifeng et al., 2018). The activities of enzymes in the soil are primarily of microbial origin. Enzymes could exist intracellularly, associated with the producing cell, or as free enzymes (extracellularly). Extracellular enzymes are active outside the parent cell. Plants and microorganisms produce and secrete enzymes into their environment mainly for survival (Małgorzata, 2014). Extracellular enzymes facilitate the degradation of plant materials and other soil organic matter into simple compounds that can be assimilated by plants (Irene et al., 2019). Soil enzymes are the best pointer for soil health because their change is easily noticeable than other soil health parameters, therefore, it provides an early indication of the shift in soil health (Shonkor and Ajit, 2010). Factors that disturb plant-soil-microorganism interaction (Fig. 10.2), will consequently limit or promote soil enzyme activity and productivity (Swati et al., 2018). Soil enzymes analysis aids to establish a relationship between microbial activity and soil fertilization and measures the stage of ecosystem succession (Sanjoy et al., 2011).

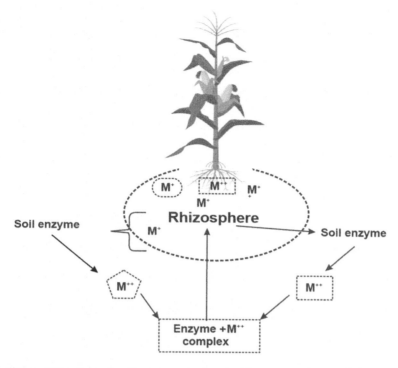

Figure 10.2 Role of soil enzymes in sustainable crop production (adapted from Dotiya *et al.* (2019).

10.3.2.1 Soil urease

Soil enzymes are associated with varied soil components (Małgorzata, 2014). The enzyme urease is involved in the degradation of urea (mainly nitrogenous) into CO_2 and NH_3 (Burak, 2020). Urease is a nitrogen-related extracellular enzyme, it, therefore, has an affinity for soil habitat with deposits of nitrogen-related biomass (Irene *et al.*, 2019). The accessibility of nitrogen in urea as fertilizer for plant growth is largely facilitated by urease. However, long-term use of nitrogen-based fertilizers on soil decreased urease activities in the soil, compared to soil that is left unfertilized (Burak, 2020). Studies have shown that the activity of urease with soil organic carbon had negative correlations. Thus, plants that release a very high amount of carbon with little or no nitrogen into the soil will negatively affect urease activities in the soil (Changting *et al.*, 2011).

10.3.2.2 Soil invertase

Invertase is responsible for the conversion of sucrose to fructose and glucose. It is also partly responsible for the degradation of soil-plant debris (Maddela *et al.*, 2016). The activity of invertase is dependent on its substrate, sucrose. Sucrose, a byproduct of photosynthesis, is one of the most abundant sugar found in plants. Sucrose plays a fundamental role in the biological functions of plants as well as their response to stress in the environment (Luis *et al.*, 2019).

10.3.2.3 Soil phosphatase

Phosphatases are involved in the hydrolysis of organic phosphorus to inorganic polyphosphate which exists in the soil and is needed for phosphorus recycling in soil that is deficient in phosphorus (Sanjoy *et al.*, 2011). According to Sanjoy *et al.* (2011), soil vegetation cover influences the phosphatase activity in the soil. The remnants of the dead organism such as dead plants or animals are the primary substrate on which phosphatase acts to produce phosphorus (Joanna, 2018). Phosphorus is deficient in the forest ecosystem and its presence in the soil is dependent on the abundance of phosphorus in plant litter (Joanna, 2018). Phosphatase speed up the hydrolysis of the phosphate ester bond, thereby releasing phosphate which is assimilated by the plant (Nannipieri *et al.*, 2011). In the soil rhizosphere, acid phosphatase is dominantly higher compared to neutral phosphatase and decreases with increased distance from tree stem (Sanjoy *et al.*, 2011).

10.4 Soil Chemical Properties Versus Soil Enzyme Activities

Microbes present in soil are involved in the cycling of carbon, phosphorous, nitrogen, sulfur, and other nutrients (Kaur and Gosal, 2017). These activities of microbes are affected by environmental factors also (Kaur and Gosal, 2015). Similarly, Soil enzymes play crucial roles in carbon (C), phosphorous (P), and nitrogen (N) cycling which provides important nutrients for plant growth promotion and incrementing the microbial metabolism. They are widely distributed in nature and are sensitive to alteration in the soil ecosystem. Different fertilization did not significantly influence the activity of soil enzymes at depths of 0–30 cm and 30–60 cm. However, when evaluating results, regardless of the depths of sampling, it was found that application of NPK (sodium, phosphorus, and potassium) + FYM (farmyard manure) stimulated the activity of glucosidases, and application of NPK inhibited the activity of arylsulphatases (Ladislav *et al.*, 2019). Soil enzymes can be employed in revealing ecosystem disruptions, and have been used as tools to determine biogeochemical cycles, organic matter (OM), degradation, and soil remediation. Thus, they can represent soil quality, especially in combination with other physical or chemical properties. Soil enzymes are also used as ecological indicators of soils affected by contamination, such as toxic trace elements (TTEs), stress conditions, and management practices (Polyak *et al.*, 2018; Khalid *et al.*, 2017). Of recent, it has also been demonstrated that they can as well indicate the correctness or otherwise of biochemical reactions in any given soil (Liang *et al.*, 2014; Yang *et al.*, 2016).

In general, the concentration of TTEs negatively correlates with soil enzyme activity. Consequently, discriminating pollution levels, have been investigated through soil enzyme assays designed to detect TTE pollution in soils (Sang-Hwan *et al.*, 2020). However, it has been impossible so far to determine the mode of this inhibition whether direct, reduction of enzyme synthesis or release or combination of both. Further studies also showed that some soil enzyme activities which were seriously inhibited by TTEs gradually became more active with time. This phenomenon may be attributed to microbial resistance, as sudden exposure of microorganisms to TTEs has been established to cause a significant decrease in enzyme activity. Some of the microorganisms later adapt to the polluted environment and recover their enzyme synthesis and activity (Sang-Hwan *et al.*, 2020).

When there is a high concentration of chemical compounds that are end products of enzymatic reactions in soil, it can lead to inhibition of the activity of the enzyme connected with the chemical in question through a process called feedback inhibition. For instance, soil that is deficient in phosphorus will trigger phosphatase activity and vice versa. In the same vein, urease activity may be suppressed by ammonia-based nitrogen fertilizer because ammonium is the product of urease activity (USDA, 2010). Bueis *et al.* (2018) reported that soil enzymatic activities, especially for dehydrogenase, urease, catalase, and microbial biomass C and N were higher in the calcareous soils under *Pinus halepensis* than in the acidic soils under *Pinus sylvestris*. It has also been demonstrated that enzyme activity is influenced by the OM content of the soil. This explains why a higher enzymatic activity is usually recorded in forest soil when compared to tillage soil (Bloriska *et al.*, 2017). The activities of soil enzymes are affected by the pH of the soil. Enzymes are more stable at optimum pH. Irreversible denaturation occurs at extremely high or low pH where the soil enzymes get destroyed (Kaur *et al.*, 2020). This is because enzymes are proteins and the functional groups of amino acids are sensitive to pH and can lead to conformational and chemical changes of amino acids essential for binding and catalysis. Enzyme activities can also be affected by pH when it causes the concentration of inhibitors or activators in the soil solution (Dicka *et al.*, 2000). Pavani *et al.* (2017) reported that the apparent pH optimum for clay observed enzymes is generally 1 or 2 pH units into the alkaline side of the pH scale. This shift in the optimum pH to higher values is believed to be due to the Bronsted acidity at clay surface which is usually significantly greater than in bulk solution (Pavani *et al.*, 2017). Shahariar *et al.* (2021) reported a non-significant impact of groundwater salinity on the activities of extracellular enzymes activities (EEAs). It has also been revealed that urease, alkaline phosphatase, and catalase activities, are significantly affected by nitrogen, organic carbon (OC), soil salinity, and pH (Guangminga *et al.*, 2017). Soil OM is another component of the soil that affects the activities of soil enzymes. The microbial biomass of soil is directly proportional to the OM in the soil. It, therefore, means the more the organic matter of soil, the higher the enzymatic activities and vice versa (Kaur *et al.*, 2020). Liu *et al.*, 2017 reported that catalase, urease, and alkaline phosphatase activities are negatively correlated to soil salinity, pH, N, P, potassium (K) while they are positively correlated to TN (total nitrogen) and soil organic matter (SOM). It was also observed by Pavani *et al.* (2017) that soil moisture has a profound influence on the production of soil enzymes and nutrient availability. The use of contaminated wastewater that is high in salinity, pH, electrical conductivity, and toxic elements has been reported to cause a reduction in the population of microorganisms and activities of soil enzymes, especially dehydrogenase and phosphatase (Tripathi *et al.*, 2008).

Bueis *et al.* (2018) reported that the activities of enzymes like dehydrogenase, alkaline phosphatase, urease, catalase, and fluorescein diacetate hydrolysis reaction were significantly correlated with OM and nutrient-related parameters such as easily oxidizable carbon (C), total organic C to total N ratio, available P, total N, cation exchange capacity, and calcium (Ca). It is established that soils with high base saturation percentage also have high pH; it, therefore, means that the activities of soil enzymes are affected in the same pattern as with pH. Also, significant positive correlations were found between the activity of dehydrogenase and alkaline phosphatase with pH, available P, soil moisture, and water holding capacity, and negative correlations between the activity of urease and soil OC (Kompała-Bąba *et al.*, 2021). An increase in soil sodicity increases the activities of antioxidant enzymes like catalase and superoxide dismutase while peroxidase and nitrate reductase decline (Singh *et al.*, 2014). However, Lemanowicz *et al.* (2019) reported inconsistent salt-affected soil effects on soil enzyme activity.

10.5 Impact of Anthropogenic Factors on Soil Enzyme Activities

Large quantities of pollutants enter into the soil which is attributed to two major sources, one is anthropogenic activities, and another is urbanization. Different varieties of soil contaminants are regularly being reported, such as heavy metals (Qin *et al.*, 2021), microplastics (Mbachu *et al.*, 2021), engineered nanomaterials (Zhu *et al.*, 2019), petroleum hydrocarbons (Maddela *et al.*, 2015), pesticides (Raju and Venkateswarlu, 2014; Maddela and Venkateswarlu, 2018g), polycyclic aromatic hydrocarbons (Yu *et al.*, 2019), military metals (Skalny *et al.*, 2021), contaminants of emerging concern (García Valverde *et al.*, 2021), fluorides (Rizzu *et al.*, 2021), antibiotics (Lyu *et al.*, 2020), trace metals (Luo *et al.*, 2012), synthetic microfibers (Singh *et al.*, 2020), etc. According to recent statistics (https://www.rubbishplease.co.uk/blog/land-pollution-facts-statistics/), there is nearly 200,000 tons of food waste/day is generated in the USA, where an average American produces 4.5 lbs of waste a day. Similarly, 0.1 million km^2 of cultivated land has been highly polluted in China. Thus, the annual environmental burden of hazardous waste across the globe is 400 million tons (RP, 2016). Interestingly, veterinary medicine is weakly absorbed by the animals, thus 30–90% of these substances are excreted easily from the animals and accumulated in the animal manure (Zhou *et al.*, 2019). It is noteworthy that the use of animal manure as a fertilizer in agricultural lands is a common practice in low- and middle-income countries. It should be remembered that the pollutants entering into the soil system have potential ecotoxicity. For instance, certain types of pollutants have long time persistence in the environment up to several years, therefore, their (e.g., insecticides (DDT) and aldrin) harmful potential is increased by 70,000 times (RP, 2016), which has a significant impact on soil microecology. Soil pollution by antibiotics has been extended up to the development of antibiotic resistance in the soil ecosystem, which has a significant impact on the human health perspective (Wang *et al.*, 2021). Soil arsenic was found to affect badly *Enchytraeus crypticus* in different characters such as morphology, body tissue, survival, reproduction, growth, antioxidant enzymes (catalase (CAT), peroxidase (POD), superoxide dismutase (SOD), and peroxidation malondialdehyde MDA) (Li *et al.*, 2021). Certain types of emerging contaminants (ECs) (phthalates, bisphenol A, polybrominated diphenyl ethers) are widely used in plastics in making the final products more effective, however, these ECs are easily released into the environment upon the degradation of plastics in the environment and have extremely harmful to flora and fauna (Rai *et al.*, 2021). In some cases, soil pollutants may not show adverse effects on the organisms but may have bioaccumulation propensities. For example, manganese released from the ancient metallurgical waste has a strong propensity to accumulate in the soil-dwelling invertebrates (snails) (Petitjean *et al.*, 2021), which implies that this type of pollutants has significant ecotoxicity effects even one millennium after their deposition. Microtox test has confirmed the severe effects of lead, zinc, and TPH (total petroleum hydrocarbons) on microbial community structure (Khudur *et al.*, 2018). Furthermore, co-contamination may have even more toxicity than the individual contaminants. For example, TPHs and heavy metal co-contamination was found to show elevated associated toxicity on the soil microorganisms (Khudur *et al.*, 2018). The above insights imply that the soil system is subjected to a great level of pollution by a wide variety of pollutants, which exert significant adverse effects on soil flora and fauna, which leads to severe effects on soil microecology (Abioye *et al.*, 2019).

Soil enzymes are highly sensitive to many factors including but not limited to tanning effluents, fuel oil, urban waste storage depot effluents (Trasar-Cepeda *et al.*, 1998), SOM (Kandeler *et al.*, 1999a), moisture (Bergstorm *et al.*, 1998), temperature (Tscherko *et al.*, 2001), cultivation practices (Bandick and Dick, 1999), fertilization (Ross *et al.*, 1995 and Ajwa *et al.*, 1999), and burning (Ajwa *et al.*, 1999). On the other side, soil enzyme activities may not be affected by certain substances (e.g., wastewater treatment plant effluents on freshwater sediment) (Montuelle and Volat, 1998), and some may stimulate the enzyme activities (e.g., food waste compost, Kim *et al.*, 2002). Soil protease activity was found to be stimulated by metal-contaminated sewage sludge (Achberger and Ohlinger, 1988), cotton ginning mills effluents (Narasimha *et al.*, 1997), pig slurry (Plaza *et al.*, 2002) which might be due to the presence of nutritional values of these substances for soil microflora. However, herbicides (Pahwa and Bajaj, 1999), insecticides (Omar and Abd-Alla, 2000), OM (Ladd and Butler, 1969), crude oils (Walker *et al.*, 1975) the fungicide chlorothalonil (Singh *et al.*, 2002), etc. have strong inhibitory effects on soil protease activity. Different pollutants that have stimulatory and inhibitory effects on different soil enzyme activities have been depicted in Tables 10.1 and 10.2, respectively.

Table 10.1 Stimulatory effects of different anthropogenic factors on soil enzyme activities

Enzyme	Stimulatory Effect
Soil cellulase	Textile and sugar industry effluents (Khanan and Oblisami, 1990)
	Cotton ginning mill effluents (Narasimha *et al.*, 1997)
	Solid urban waste (Ramakrishna parama *et al.*, 2002)
	Sodium-based black liquor from fiber pulping for paper making (Xiao *et al.*, 2005)
	Paper mill effluent and amendment addition (Chinnaiah *et al.*, 2002)
	Monocrotophos, quinalphos, and cypermethrin (insecticides) (Gundi *et al.*, 2007)
	Tridemorph and captan (fungicides) (Srinivasulu and Rangaswamy, 2006)

(*Continued*)

Table 10.1 (Continued)

Enzyme	Stimulatory Effect
Soil amylase	Cypermethrin (insecticide) (Tu, 1982)
	Effluents released from pulp and paper mill (Kannan and Oblisami, 1990)
	Cotton ginning mill effluents (Narasimha et al., 1997)
	Pressmud plus paper mill effluents (Chinnaiah et al., 2002)
	Baythroid (insecticide) (Lodhi et al., 2000)
	Monocrotophos, quinalphos and cypermethrin (Ghandhi et al., 2007)
Soil invertase	Pulp and paper mills effluents (Chinnaiah et al., 2002)
	Cotton ginning mill effluents (Narasimha et al., 1997)
	Hexachlorocyclohexane (insecticide) and its isomers (Srimathi and Karanth, 1989)
	Baythroid (insecticide) (Lodhi et al., 2003)
	Glyphosate and paraquat (herbicides) (Gianfreda and Sannino, 1993; Sannino and Gianfreda, 2001)
Soil urease	Baythroid (insecticide) (Lodhi et al., 2000)
	Glyphosate and paraquat herbicides) (Sannino and Gianfreda, 2001)
	Chlorimuron-ethyl (herbicide) and furadan (insecticide/nematicide) (Yang et al., 2006)
Soil acid phosphatase	Brominal (herbicide), Selecron (insecticide) (Omar and Abdel-Sater, 2001)
Soil alkaline phosphatase	Brominal (herbicide) and selecron (insecticide) (Omar and Abdel-Sater, 2001)

Table 10.2 Inhibitory effects of different anthropogenic factors on soil enzyme activities

Enzyme	Inhibitory Effect
Soil cellulase	Cement dust from cement industries (Shanthi, 1993)
	Crude oils (Walker et al., 1975)
	Fenamiphos (nematicide), 930 mg kg^{-1} (Ross and Speir, 1985)
	Baythroid (insecticide) (Lodhi et al., 2000)

Soil amylase	Imidacloprid (insecticide) (Tu, 1995)
	Dimethoate (insecticide) (Mandic et al., 1997)
	Chlorothalonil (fungicide) (Singh et al., 2002)
	Metsulfuron-methyl (herbicide) at 5 µg g^{-1} (Ismail et al., 1998)
Soil invertase	Toluene (Kiss and Peteri, 1959)
	Insecticides (El Hamady and Sheloa, 1999)
	Cement dust from cement industries (Shanthi, 1993)
	Soil organic matter (Malcolm and Vaughan, 1979)
	Monosulfuron (herbicide) (Yong-hong and Yu-bao, 2005)
	Carbaryl (insecticide) and atrazine (herbicide) (Gianfreda and Sannino, 1993)
Soil urease	Malathion, accothion and thimet (insecticides) (Lethbridge and Burns, 1976)
	Metsulfuron-methyl (herbicide) at 5 µg g^{-1} (Ismail et al., 1988)
	Diazinon(insecticide) (Ingram et al., 2005)
	Acetamiprid (insecticide) (Singh and Kumar, 2008)
	Omethoate (insecticide/acaricide) (Xiang et al., 2009)
	Chlorothalonil fungicide) (Yu et al., 2006)
	Amitraz, tebupirimphos and aztec (insecticides) (Tu, 1995)
	Dimethomorph (fungicide) (Wu et al., 2010)
Soil acid phosphatase	Glyphosate (herbicide) (Sannino and Gianfreda, 2001)
	Propiconazole (fungicide), profenofos (insecticide), and pretilachlor (insecticide) (Kalam et al., 2004)
	Acetamiprid (insecticide) (Yao et al., 2006)
	Chlorothalonil (fungicide) (Yu et al., 2006)
	Cyfluthrin, imidacloprid, tebupirimphos, aztec, and amitraz (insecticides) (Tu, 1995)
Soil alkaline phosphatase	Chlorothalonil (fungicide) (Yu et al., 2006)
	Glyphosate (herbicide) (Sannino and Gianfreda, 2001)
	Propiconazole (fungicide) (Kalam et al., 2004)
	Acetamiprid (insecticide) (Yao et al., 2006)
Soil arylamidase and myrosinase activities	5.0–10.0 kg ha^{-1} of acetamiprid and carbofuran (insecticides) (Mohiddin et al., 2015)

Regarding soil enzyme responses to the sugar industry effluents, enzymes of C-, N- cycling enzymes have responded differently to incubation time and effluent concentration (Maddela et al., 2017). When soils were treated with sugar industry effluents, soil protease activity has been increased with increasing the incubation periods from 0 to 30 days, later activity was dropped (Nagaraju, 2009; Naga Raju et al., 2017d). Furthermore, the highest soil protease activity (0.38–2.50 mg tyrosine g^{-1} soil) was observed at 100% concentration of the effluent that of lower concentration (10 and 50%) effluent (Naga Raju et al., 2017d). Cellulase activity in the sugar industry effluent treated soil was increased until 30 days incubation, later activity was declined with an increase in the incubation period (Nagaraju et al., 2009; Naga Raju et al., 2017b). However, from a quantitative point of view, higher (100%) and lower concentrations (10%) of effluent showed lesser cellulase activity than at 50% effluent concentration in the soil. Regarding soil incubation study, the response of soil amylase response to sugar industry effluents was very similar to that of soil cellulase activity (Naga Raju et al., 2017a), however, higher concentrations of the effluents (i.e., 50 and 100%) have shown less activity than at lower concentration of the effluent (i.e., 10%). Similarly, soil invertase has shown the highest activity at 30 days incubation in the soil treated with the sugar industry effluents (Naga Raju et al., 2017c), and the enzyme was found to be inhibited at higher concentrations of effluents (50% and 100%).

Response of soil enzyme activities to acephate and buprofezin alone and in combination (graded concentrations) and single and repeated applications have been investigated and reported recently (Maddela and Venkateswarlu, 2018g). Soil cellulase activity was stimulated after single (240–350% ↑ at 5.0 µg g^{-1}) and repeated applications of acephate (Raju and Venkateswarlu, 2014; Maddela and Venkateswarlu, 2018b), but the single application of buprofezin has resulted in a slight increase (40–140%) in the enzyme activity. Furthermore, the addition of NPK (nitrogen, phosphorous, potassium) has not affected the effects of acephate and buprofezin on soil cellulase activities. Regarding graded concentrations of acephate and buprofezin, combinations of acephate and buprofezin at lower concentrations showed synergistic reactions, and higher concentrations showed antagonistic insecticide interactions (Maddela and Venkateswarlu, 2018b). Therefore, such type of consistent results of soil cellulase to insecticides are very useful in toxicity studies. There was a significant increment (5–67%) in soil amylase acidity in the soils treated with lower concentrations (2.5–7.5 µg g^{-1}) of either acephate or buprofezin, but the activity was badly affected at 10.0 µg g^{-1} of either of the two insecticides (Raju and Venkateswarlu, 2014; Maddela and Venkateswarlu, 2018a). But the addition of NPK has stimulated the soil amylase activity by 60–240% at lower concentrations of the above insecticides. Similar to soil cellulase, a combination of two insecticides at higher concentrations have caused antagonistic effects (Raju and Venkateswarlu, 2014). Regarding soil invertase response to a single application of acephate or buprofezin, though the activity was tremendously increased (>209%) at concentrations up to 7.5 µg g^{-1} soil, activities have been decreased by 45% at 10 µg g^{-1} soil (Raju and Venkateswarlu, 2014; Maddela and Venkateswarlu, 2018c). Parallel results have been reported for NPK-amended soils. On the other side, a combination of acephate + buprofezin at 7.5 or 10 µg g^{-1} soil has exhibited antagonistic responses on soil invertase activity both in NPK-amended and unamended soils (Raju and Venkateswarlu, 2014; Maddela and Venkateswarlu, 2018c). The responses of soil proteases (Maddela and Venkateswarlu, 2018e), urease (Maddela and Venkateswarlu, 2018f) and phosphatases (Maddela and Venkateswarlu, 2018d) to single and repeated concentrations and graded concentrations of two insecticides in NPK-amended and unamended soils have been depicted in the Tables 10.3 and 10.4. These results imply that repeated applications of the insecticides have exhibited adverse effects on measured enzymatic activities in NPK-amended and unamended soils. Hence, repeated applications of insecticides should be minimized to protect soil fertility. Soil application of acephate or buprofezin at higher rates has greatly affected the activities of several enzymes in unamended or NPK-amended soils. This warrants the judicious use of insecticides at recommended doses only. Insecticide combinations, at higher concentrations, resulted in an interaction leading to a significant antagonistic effect on activities of all the soil enzymes tested.

Table 10.3 Activities of soil enzymes as influenced by single and repeated applications of buprofezin and acephate

Enzyme	NPK amendments	No. of applications					
		Buprofezin			Acephate		
		Single	Two	Three	Single	Two	Three
Cellulases	Without	↑	↑	↓	↑	↑	↓
	With	↑	↑	↑	↑	↑	↓
Amylase	Without	↑	↓	↓	↑	↓	↓
	With	↑	↓	↓	↑	↓	↓
Invertase	Without	↑	↓	↓	↑	↓	↓
	With	↑	↓	↓	↑	↓	↓
Proteases	Without	↑	↑	↓	↑	↑	↓
	With	↑	↑	↓	↑	↑	↓
Urease	Without	↑	↑	↓	↑	↑	↓
	With	↑	↓	↓	↑	↓	↓
Acid phosphatase	Without	↑	↑	↓	↑	↑	↓
	With	↑	↑	↓	↑	↑	↓

Note: Green and red arrows indicate enzyme stimulation and inhibition, respectively.

Table 10.4 Interaction effects of buprofezin and acephate on different soil enzyme activities

Enzyme	NPK amendments	Buprofezin			Acephate		
		A	B	C	A	B	C
Cellulases	Without	2.5 – 7.5*	5	10	2.5 – 7.5	5	10
	With	2.5 – 7.5	5	10	2.5 – 7.5	5	10
Amylase	Without	2.5 – 7.5	7.5	10	2.5 – 7.5	5	10
	With	2.5 – 7.5	7.5	10	2.5 – 7.5	7.5	10
Invertase	Without	2.5 – 7.5	5	10	2.5 – 7.5	5	10
	With	2.5 – 7.5	5	10	2.5 – 7.5	5	10
Proteases	Without	2.5 – 7.5	5	7.5, 10	2.5 – 7.5	5	10
	With	2.5 – 7.5	5	10	2.5 – 7.5	5	10
Urease	Without	2.5 – 7.5	5	10	2.5 – 7.5	5	7.5, 10
	With	2.5 – 7.5	5	10	2.5 – 7.5	5	10
Acid phosphatase	Without	2.5 – 7.5	5	10	2.5 – 7.5	5	10
	With	2.5 – 7.5	5	10	2.5 – 7.5	5	10

Note: A - Stimulation, B - Optimal activity, C - Inhibition.
*$\mu g\ g^{-1}$ soil (Raju and Venkateswarlu, 2014; Maddela and Venkateswarlu, 2018g).

10.6 Conclusions

Soil enzymes can originate from different sources such as microorganisms (both live and dead), soil animals, and plant roots. Activities of these enzymes are highly sensitive to the fluctuating factors in the soil, thus soil enzymes can serve as sensitive indicators of microclimatic change in the soil. As the soil enzymes are the key actors of biogeochemical cycles (e.g., C, N, P, S, and Fe) and subsequent maintenance of soil fertility. However, a global anthropogenic burden on soil greatly affects the activities of soil enzymes, this not only affects soil fertility but also threatens the terrestrial food chain and human health. In this direction, we paid special to four areas in this chapter: (*i*) source, distribution, and abundance of soil enzymes, (*ii*) ecological stoichiometry of plant-soil-enzyme interactions, (*iii*) soil chemical properties versus soil enzyme activities, and (*iv*) impact of anthropogenic factors on soil enzyme activities. The major findings are as follows - enzymatic activities in the soil do not necessarily mean high microbial biomass or respiration; enzyme activity in the soil is the cumulative effect of long-term stabilized enzymes and activities of viable cells at sampling; plant species diversity and biomass have a great impact on enzyme activity; physicochemical characteristics of soil and anthropogenic burden of soil have the greatest impact on the soil enzyme activities, and industrial effluents (e.g., sugar industry) and insecticides (e.g., acephate and buprofezin) have exhibited detrimental effects on the selected enzyme activities in a dose-dependent manner. These insights are certainly useful to researchers and industrialists in understanding the enzyme responses to changes in soil microecology. Also, we think that these insights are useful to the policymakers to redesign the pollution guidelines to protect the soil ecosystem, food insecurity, and human health.

Acknowledgments

We are grateful to Late Prof. Dr. Peter Grunwald for considering and inviting us to be part of this prestigious project. We are deeply saddened by Prof. Dr. Peter Grunwald's passing in December 2020. This chapter has been dedicated to him.

References

Abioye O. P., Aina P. F., Ijah U. J. J., Arasnsiola S.A., *Journal of Taibah University for Science*, **13**(1), (2019), 628-638.

Abioye O. P., Iroegbu V. T., Aransiola S. A., *Journal of Environmental Science and Technology*, **1994**, (2015).

Abioye O. P., Ijah U. J. J., Aransiola S. A., Phytoremediation of soil contaminants by biodiesel plant *Jatropha curcas*, in *Phytoremediation Potential of Bioenergy Plants* (Bauddh K., *et al.*, eds), Springer Nature Singapore Pte Ltd, 2017.

Achberger K., Ohlinger R., *Poster presentation at EC. EWPCA.* Symposium, Amesterdam, (1988).

Agnieszka K. B., Wojciech B., Edyta S., Agnieszka B., Aon M. A., Cabello M. N., Sarena D. E., Colaneri A. C., Franco M. G., Burgos J. L., Cortassa S. I., *Applied Soil Ecology*, **18** (2001), 239-254.

Ajwa H. A., Dell C. J., Rice C. W., *Soil Biology & Biochemistry*, **31** (1999), 769-777.

Andrew H. A., *Ecosystem Engineers*, Oxford Bibliographies, (2019).

Archana M., Rao K. S., India, SpringerOpen, 2021.

Bartelt-Ryser J., Joshi J., Schmid B., Brandl H., Balser T., *Plant Ecology*, **7** (2005), 27-49.

Bergstrom D. W., Montreal C. M., Millette J. A., King D. J., *Soil Science Society of America Journal*, **62** (1998), 1302-1308.

Bueis T., María B. T., Felipe B., Valentín P., Adele M., *Annals of Forest Science*, **75** (2018), 34.

Burak K., *Cukurova University*, 2020.

Burns R. G., DeForest J. L., Marxsen J., Sinsabaugh R. L., Stromberger M. E., Wallenstein M. D., Weintraub M. N., Zoppini A., *Soil Biology & Biochemistry*, **58** (2013), 216-234.

Cadwell A. B., *Pedobiologia*, **49** (2005), 637—644.

Celika I., Barut Z. B., Ortasa I., Goka M., Demirbasa A., Tuluna Y., Akpinara C., *International Journal of Plant Production*, **5** (2011), 237-254.

Changting W., Genxu W., Wei L., Pengfei W., *Hindawi*, (2011).

Cherukumalli S. R., Minakshi G., Sumanta K., Susheelendra D., *India. Encyclopedia of Soil Science*, 3rd edn, **6** (2017).

Chinnaiah U., Palaniappan M., Augustine S., *Rehabilitation of Paper Mill Effluent Polluted Soil Habitat and Indian Experience.* Poster presentation, Paper No. 770, Symposium No. 24, (2002).

David H. M., *The Rhizosphere: Roots, Soil and Everything in Between*, Knowledge Project, (2013).

Dedmer B. V., James J. E., Adam C. M., Robert W. S., James B. C., *Frontiers in Microbiology*, (2018).

Dicka W. A., Chenga L., Wangb P., *Soil Biology & Biochemistry*, **32** (2000), 915–1919.

Dotaniya M. L., Aparna K., Dotaniya C. K., Singh M., Regar K. L., Enzymes in food biotechnology; production, applications, and future prospects, in *Role of Soil Enzymes in Sustainable Crop Production*, (2019), pp. 569–589.

El Hamady S. E. E., Sheloa M. K. A. A., *Arab Univ. J. Agric. Sci.* **7**(2), (199), 561–574.

García Valverde M., Martínez Bueno M. J., Gómez-Ramos M. M., Aguilera A., Gil García M. D., Fernández-Alba A. R., *Science of The Total Environment*, **782** (2021), 146759.

Gianfreda L., Sannino F., *Pesticide Science*, **39** (1993), 237–244.

Gundi V. A. K. B., Viswanath B., Chandra M. S., Kumar V. N., Reddy B. R., *Ecotoxicology and Environmental Safety*, **68** (2007), 278–285.

Haifeng Z., Yang L., Zhang J., Chen Y., *ResearchGate*, 2018.

Houston C., *The Orianne Society*, 2018.

Ingram C. W., Coyne M. S., Williams D. W., *Journal of Environmental Quality*, **34** (2005), 1573–1580.

Irene C., Helen S., Richard D. B., *Soil Biology & Biochemistry*, NCBI, **134** (2019), 72–77.

Ismail B. S., Yapp K. F., Omar O., *Australian Journal of Soil Research*, **36** (1998), 449–456.

Joanna L., *Environmental Science and Pollution Research*, SpringerLink, **25** (2018), 33773–33782.

John M., *WorldAtlas*, (2017).

Kalam A., Tah J., Mukherjee A. K., *Journal of Environmental Biology*, **25** (2004), 201–208.

Kandeler E., Luxhoi J., Tscherko D., Magid J., Soil Biol. Biochem. **31** (1999a), 1171–1179.

Kannan K., Oblisami G., *Soil Biology & Biochemistry* **22** (1990b), 923–927.

Kao-Kniffin J. T., Balser T. C., *Soil Biology & Biochemistry* **39** (2007), 517–525.

Kaur J., Satwant K. G., Samiksha K., *Soil Enzymes: An Agricultural Perspective*, Lambert Academic Publishing, vol. 61, (2020).

Khalid S., Shahid M., Khan Niazi N., Murtaza B., Bibi I., Dumat C., *Journal of Geochemical Exploration*, **182** (2017), 247–268.

Khudur L. S., Gleeson D. B., Ryan M. H., Shahsavari E., Haleyur N., Nugegoda D., Ball A. S., *Environmental Pollution*, **243** (2018), 94–102.

Kim Y. W., Kim K. Y., Lee J. J., Shim J. H., Park R. D., Kim K. S., Sohn B. K., Chung S. J., *Poster presentation, Paper No. 921, Symposium No. 24. 17th WCSS*, (2002).

Kiss S., Peterfi Jr. *Biologia*. **2** (1959), 179 (cited in C.M. Tu, Chemosphere. 11:909–914).

Ladd J. N., Butler J. H. A., *Australian Journal of Soil Research*, **7** (1969), 241–251.

Ladislav H., Lukáš H., Roman H., Josef T., Hana B., Jan P., *Sustainability*, **11** (2019), 3251.

Lemanowicz J., Siwik-Ziomek A., Koper J., *International Journal of Environmental Science and Technology*, **16** (2019), 3309–3316.

Lethbridge G., Burns R. G., *Soil Biology and Biochemistry*, **8** (1976), 99–102.

Li S., Jia M., Li Z., Ke X., Wu L., Christie P., *Ecotoxicology and Environmental Safety*, **207** (2021), 111218.

Liang Q., Gao R., Xi B., Zhang Y., Zhang H., *Water Management*, **135** (2014), 100–108.

Lie X., Guobin L., Peng L., Sha X., *ScienceDirect*, (2021).

Liu C., Sun X., *ScienceDirect*, (2013).

Liu G., Zhang X., Wang X., Shao H., Yang J., Wang X., *Agriculture, Ecosystems and Environment*, **237** (2017) 274–279.

Lodhi A., Malik N. N., Mahmood T., Azam F., *Pakistan Journal of Biological Sciences*, **3** (2000), 868–871.

Luo X.-S., Yu S., Zhu Y.-G., Li X.-D., *Science of The Total Environment*, **421–422** (2012), 17–30.

Lynn B., Gabriela W., *Scientific Reports* **11** (2021), 5155.

Lyu J., Yang L., Zhang L., Ye B., Wang L., *Environmental Pollution*, **266** (2020), 115147.

Maddela N. R., Narasimha G., Rangaswamy V., *Soil Invertase*, SpringerLink, (2016), pp. 41–46.

Maddela N., Golla N., Vengatampalli R., Springer International Publishing Switzerland (2017).

Maddela N., Masabanda M., Leiva-Mora M., *Water Science and Technology*, **71** (2015), 1554–1561.

Maddela N. R., Venkateswarlu K., Impact of acephate and buprofezin on soil amylases, in *Insecticides–Soil Microbiota Interactions* (Maddela N. R., Venkateswarlu K., eds), Springer International Publishing, Cham, (2018a), pp. 41–48.

Maddela N. R., Venkateswarlu K., impact of acephate and buprofezin on soil cellulases, in *Insecticides–Soil Microbiota Interactions* (Maddela N. R., Venkateswarlu K., eds), Springer International Publishing, Cham, (2018b), pp. 33–40.

Maddela N. R., Venkateswarlu K., Impact of acephate and buprofezin on soil invertase, in *Insecticides–Soil Microbiota Interactions* (Maddela N. R., Venkateswarlu K., eds), Springer International Publishing, Cham, (2018c), pp. 49–56.

Maddela N. R., Venkateswarlu K., Impact of acephate and buprofezin on soil phosphatases, in *Insecticides–Soil Microbiota Interactions* (Maddela N. R., Venkateswarlu K., eds), Springer International Publishing, Cham, (2018d), pp. 75–86.

Maddela N. R., Venkateswarlu K., Impact of acephate and buprofezin on soil proteases, in *Insecticides–Soil Microbiota Interactions* (Maddela N. R., Venkateswarlu K., eds), Springer International Publishing, Cham, (2018e), pp. 57–64.

Maddela N. R., Venkateswarlu K., Impact of acephate and buprofezin on soil urease, in *Insecticides–Soil Microbiota Interactions* (Maddela N. R., Venkateswarlu K., eds), Springer International Publishing, Cham, (2018f), pp. 65–73.

Maddela N. R., Venkateswarlu K., *Insecticides–Soil Microbiota Interactions*, Springer International Publishing, (2018g).

Malcolm R. E., Vaughan D., *Soil Biology & Biochemistry* **11** (1979), 65–72.

Małgorzata B., *Encyclopedia of Agrophysics*, 2014.

Mandic L., Dukic D., Govedarica M., Kovic S. S., *Czeckoslevensko Vocarstvo* **31** (1997), 177–184.

Mbachu O., Jenkins G., Kaparaju P., Pratt C., *Science of The Total Environment*, **780** (2021), 146569.

Minghui L., Xin S., Yanbo H., Fujuan F., *BMC Microbiology,* 19(1), (2019).

Mohiddin G. J., Srinivasulu M., Maddela N. R., Manjunatha B., Rangaswamy V., Kaiser A. R. K., Rueda O. D., *Environmental Monitoring and Assessment*, **187** (2015), 1–9.

Montuelle B., Volat B., *Ecotoxicology and Environmental Safety*, **40** (1998), 154–159.

Naga Raju M., Golla N., Vengatampalli R., *Soil Amylase* (Maddela N. R., Golla N., Vengatampalli R., eds), Springer International Publishing, Cham, (2017a), pp. 31–39.

Naga Raju M., Golla N., Vengatampalli R., Soil Cellulase, in *Soil Enzymes: Influence of Sugar Industry Effluents on Soil Enzyme Activities* (Maddela N. R., Golla N., Vengatampalli R., eds), Springer International Publishing, Cham, (2017b), pp. 25–30.

Naga Raju M., Golla N., Vengatampalli R., Soil Invertase, in *Soil Enzymes: Influence of Sugar Industry Effluents on Soil Enzyme Activities* (Maddela N. R., Golla N., Vengatampalli R., eds), Springer International Publishing, Cham, (2017c), pp. 41–46.

Naga Raju M., Golla N., Vengatampalli R., Soil Protease, in *Soil Enzymes: Influence of Sugar Industry Effluents on Soil Enzyme Activities* (Maddela N. R., Golla N., Vengatampalli R., eds), Springer International Publishing, Cham, (2017d), pp. 19–24.

Nagaraju M., Narasimha G., Rangaswamy V., *Ecology, Environment and Conservation,* **15** (2009), 217–222.

Nagaraju M., Narasimha G., Rangaswamy V., *International Biodeterioration & Biodegradation,* **63** (2009), 1088–1092.

Nannipieri P., Giagnoni L., Landi L., Renella G., *Soil Biology,* 26, Springer-Verlag, Berlin Heidelberg (2011).

Narasimha G., M. Phil. Dissertation submitted to Sri Krishnadevaraya University, Anantapur, (1997).

Omar S. A., Abdel-Sater M. A., *Water, Air and Soil Pollution,* **127** (2001), 49–63.

Pahwa S. H., Bajaj K., *Indian Journal of Weed Science* **31** (1999), 148–150.

Pavani G., Chandrasekhar P. R., Padmaja G., Naveen K., *International Journal of Current Microbiology and Applied Science,* 16 (2017), 3081–3087.

Petitjean Q., Choulet F., Walter-Simonnet A. V., Mariet A. L., Laurent H., Rosenthal P., de Vaufleury A., Gimbert F., *Chemosphere,* **277** (2021), 130337.

Plaza C., Garcia-Gil J. C., Soler-Revira P., Polo A., *Poster presentation. Centro de Ciencias Medioambientales (CSIC), Madrid, Espana* (2002).

Polyak Y. M., Bakina L. G., Chugunova M. V., Mayakina N. V., Gerasimov A. O., Bure V. M., *International Biodeterioration & Biodegradation,* **126** (2018), 57–68.

Qin G., Niu Z., Yu J., Li Z., Ma J., Xiang P., *Chemosphere,* **267** (2021), 129205.

Rai P. K., Lee J., Brown R. J. C., Kim K. H., *Journal of Hazardous Materials,* **403** (2021), 123910.

Raju M. N., Venkateswarlu K., *Environmental Monitoring and Assessment*, **186** (2014), 6319–6325.

Ramakrishna Parama V. R., Venkatesha M., Bhargavi M. V., *Poster presentation, Paper No. 904, Symposium No. 24. 17th WCSS* (2002).

Rao M. A., Scelza R., Acevedo F., Diez M. C., Gianfreda L., *Chemosphere*, **107** (2014), 145–162.

Rizzu M., Tanda A., Cappai C., Roggero P. P., Seddaiu G., *Science of the Total Environment*, **787** (2021), 147650.

Ross D. J., Speir T. W., *Soil Biology and Biochemistry*, **17** (1985), 123–136.

Ross D. J., Speir T. W., Kettles H. A., Mackay A. D., *Soil Biology And Biochemistry*, **27** (1995), 1431–1443.

Rubbish Please, *Land Pollution Facts and Statistics*, January 28, 2016, https://www.rubbishplease.co.uk/blog/land-pollution-facts-statistics/ accessed 28 June 2021.

Salazara S., Sánchezb L. E., Alvareza J., Valverdea A., Galindoc P., Igualc J. M., Peixa A., Santa-Reginaa I., *Ecological Engineering*, **37** (2011), 1123–1131.

Sang-Hwan L., Min-Suk K., Jeong-Gyu K., Soon-Oh K., *Sustainability*, **12** (2020), 8209.

Sanjoy K., Chaudhuri S., Subodh K. M., *ResearchGate*, (2011).

Sannino F., Gianfreda L., *Chemosphere*, **45** (2001), 417–425.

Shahariar S., Helgason B., Soolanayakanahally R., *Wetlands*, **41** (2021), 31.

Shanthi M., M. Phil dissertation, Sri Krishnadevaraya University, Anantapur (1993).

Shonkor K. D., Ajit V., *Springer Linger*, (2010), 25–42.

Shonkor K. D., Ajit V., *Soil Biology*, **22** (2005).

Shonkor K. D., Ajit V., *Soil Biology* **22**(2011),

Singh B. K., Allan W., Denis J. W., *Environmental Toxicology and Chemistry*, **21** (2002), 2600–2605.

Singh D. K., Kumar S., *Chemosphere*, **71** (2008), 412–418.

Singh R. P., Mishra S., Das A. P., *Chemosphere*, **257** (2020), 127199.

Skalny A. V., Aschner M., Bobrovnitsky I. P., Chen P., Tsatsakis A., Paoliello M. M. B., Djordevic A. B., Tinkov A. A., *Environmental Research*, (2021), 111568.

Sophie Z. B., Katharina M. K., Maria M., Josep P., *Ecological Monographs*, **85** (2015), 133–155.

Srimathi M. S., Karanth M. G. K., *Journal of Soil Biology and Ecology*, **9** (1989), 65–71.

Srinivasarao C., Chary G. R., Venkateswarlu B., Vittal K. P. R., Prasad J. V. N. S., Kundu S., Singh S. R., Gajanan G. N., Sharma R. A., Deshpande A. N., Patel J. J., Balaguravaiah G., *Central Research Institute for Dryland Agriculture (ICAR): Hyderabad* (2009), 102.

Srinivasulu M., Rangaswamy V., *African Journal of Biotechnology*, **5** (2006), 175–180.

Swati J., Balaram M., Mishra P. N., *SpringerLink*, (2018), 179–192.

Trasar-Cepeda C., Leiros M. C., Seoane S., Gil-Sortres F., *Soil Pollution*, **26** (1998), 100–106.

Tu C. M., *Chemosphere*, **2** (1982), 909–914.

Tu C. M., *Journal of Environmental Science and Health, Part B. Pesticides, Food Contaminants, and Agricultural Wastes*, **30** (1995), 289–306.

USDA Natural Resources Conservation Service, *Soil Quality Indicators*, **10** (2010).

Wallenstein M. D., Burns R. G., Ecology of extracellular enzyme activities and organic matter degradation in soil: a complex community-driven process, in *Methods of Soil Enzymology* (Dick R. P., ed), Soil Science Society of America, Madison, Wisconsin, USA (2011), pp. 35–55.

Walker J., Austin H., Colwell R., *The Journal of General and Applied Microbiology*, **21** (1975), 27.

Wang F., Fu Y. H., Sheng H. J., Topp E., Jiang X., Zhu Y. G., Tiedje J. M., *Current Opinion in Environmental Science & Health*, **20** (2021), 100230.

Wu Y., Kong, F., Wu D., Yan Z., Chen Z., Deng T., *Bioinformatics and Biomedical Engineering (iCBBE)*, 14th International Conference on 18–20 June, Chengdu (2010), pp. 1–3.

Xiang H. W., Li Z. F., Xia T. H., *Journal Scientia Agricultura Sinica*, **42** (2009), 4282–4287.

Xiao Y. W., Yuan G., Jiang W., *Journal of Plant Interactions*, **12** (2017), 533–541.

Xiao C., Fauci M., Bezdicek D. F., McKean W. T., Pan W. L., *Soil Science Society of America Journal*, **70** (2005), 72–77.

Yang J. S., Yang F. L., Yang Y., Xing G. L., Deng C. P., Shen Y. T., Luo L. Q., Li B. Z., Yuan H. L., *Environmental Pollution*, **213** (2016), 760–769.

Yang C., Sun T., He W., Chen S., *Ying Yong Sheng Tai Xue Bao*, **17** (2006), 1354–1356.

Yao X., Min H., Lu Z., Yuan, H., *European Journal of Soil Biology,* **42** (2006), 120–126.

Yong-hong L. I., Yu-bao G. A. O., *Nongye Huanjing Kexue Xuebao,* **24** (2005), 1176–1181.

Yu H., Li T., Liu Y., Ma L., *Chemosphere,* **230** (2019), 498–509.

Yu Y. L., Shan M., Fang H., Wang X., Chu X. Q., *Journal of Agricultural and Food Chemistry,* **54** (2006), 10070–10075.

Zhou Z., Ma J., Liu X., Lin C., Sun K., Zhang H., Li X., Fan G., *Chemosphere,* **223** (2019), 196–203.

Zhu Y., Xu F., Liu Q., Chen M., Liu X., Wang Y., Sun Y., Zhang L., *Science of The Total Environment,* **662** (2019), 414–421.

Chapter 11

Carbon-, Nitrogen-, Phosphorus-, and Sulfur-Cycling Enzymes and Functional Diversity in Agricultural Systems

Avijit Ghosh,[a] Ranjan Paul,[b] Abhijit Sarkar,[c] M. C. Manna,[d] Sudeshna Bhattacharjya,[c] Khurshid Alam,[e] Sourav Choudhury,[e] and Prithusayak Mondal[f]

[a]*ICAR-Indian Grassland and Fodder Research Institute, Jhansi 284 003, Uttar Pradesh, India*
[b]*ICAR-National Bureau of Soil Survey and Land Use Planning, Nagpur 440 033, Maharashtra, India*
[c]*ICAR-Indian Institute of Soil Science, Bhopal 462 038, Madhya Pradesh, India*
[d]*Rajendra Prasad Central Agricultural University, Pusa 848 125, Bihar, India*
[e]*ICAR-Indian Agricultural Research Institute, New Delhi 110 012, India*
[f]*Regional Research Station (Terai Zone), Uttar Banga Krishi Viswavidyalaya, Cooch Behar 736165, West Bengal, India*
avijitghosh19892@gmail.com, avijit.ghosh@icar.gov.in

Soil enzymes are a category of enzymes whose habitats are the soil and play an important role in the maintenance of soil biodiversity, physical and chemical properties, fertility, and soil quality on an

---

Agricultural Biocatalysis: Enzymes in Agriculture and Industry
Edited by Peter Jeschke and Evgeni B. Starikov
Copyright © 2023 Jenny Stanford Publishing Pte. Ltd.
ISBN 978-981-4968-47-8 (Hardcover), 978-1-003-31310-6 (eBook)
www.jennystanford.com

ongoing basis. All soils comprise a community of enzymes that decide the metabolic processes of soils, which in turn depend on their physical, chemical, microbiological, and biochemical properties. In soil carbon (C), nitrogen (N), phosphorus (P), and sulfur (S) are the major nutrients that are cycled biologically with the help of soil enzymes. As, the levels of enzymes in soil systems vary in concentrations, largely because each type of soil has varying amounts of organic matter, the structure, and behavior of its living organisms, and the strength of biological processes, the concentrations of these nutrients also vary. Identifying sustainable soil management practices through analyzing soil biological, chemical, and physical indicators of management practices being followed in an agroecosystem will help in optimizing a favorable system needed for sustaining the crop and soil productivity of a particular ecosystem.

11.1 Introduction

Soil enzymes are a category of enzymes whose habitats are the soil and play an important role in the maintenance of soil biodiversity, physical and chemical properties, fertility, and soil quality on an ongoing basis. In the ultimate process of organic matter decomposition in the soil environment, these enzymes perform important biochemical roles (Ghosh *et al.*, 2019). They are effective in catalyzing many essential reactions required for soil microorganism life processes and soil structure stabilization, organic waste decomposition, organic matter formation, and nutrient cycling, thereby playing an important role in agriculture. All soils comprise a community of enzymes that decide the metabolic processes of soils, which in turn depend on their physical, chemical, microbiological, and biochemical properties. In soil carbon (C), nitrogen (N), phosphorus (P), and sulfur (S) are the major nutrients that are cycled biologically with the help of soil enzymes. As, the levels of enzymes in soil systems vary in concentrations, largely because each type of soil has varying amounts of organic matter, the structure, and behavior of its living organisms, and the strength of biological processes, the concentrations of these nutrients also vary. In practice, biochemical reactions are primarily caused by the catalytic contribution of microorganisms to enzymes and variable substrates that function as energy sources. These enzymes may include amylase, arylsulfatases, β-D- glucosidase, cellulose, chitinase, dehydrogenase, phosphatase, protease, and urease released from plants, animals, organic compounds, and microorganisms and soils. The enzymes (a) control release of nutrients into the soil through organic matter degradation, (b) control microbial activities in soils, and (c) act as sensitive indicators of ecological change.

11.2 Carbon-Cycling Enzymes and Their Mechanisms

11.2.1 Amylase

An amylase is a group of enzymes responsible for starch hydrolyzes (Ross, 1976). Amylase is commonly found in both soils and plants with various properties and activities (Ladd and Butler, 1969; Ladd and Butler, 1972). Soil amylase breaks down polysaccharides like starch to glucose (Singaram and Kamalakumari, 2000) (Fig. 11.1). Amylases are usually adaptive and extracellular. The ability of microorganisms to form amylases depends upon the type of starch. Amylases consist of two types: α-amylase and β-amylase (Pazur, 1965; Thoma et al., 1971). The α-amylase is synthesized by soil macro- and microorganisms and also by plants. It breaks the starch molecules by hydrolyzing the α-(1–4) glycosidic bonds (Pazur, 1965). The β-amylase is mostly secreted by plants, and it removes glucose disaccharide from "the non-reducing end of the starch" (Thoma et al., 1971). Depolymerization of amylose leads to the formation of maltose which is converted to glucose by the mediation of the enzyme α-glucosidase so that starch is transformed ultimately to glucose (Fig. 11.1).

Soil amylases activity in soil is affected by substrates quality, type of vegetation, management practices, fungal and bacterial populations, temperature, moisture soil types, and soil pH (Ross and Roberts, 1970; Pancholy and Rice, 1973; Ross, 1975; Sinsabaugh and Linkins, 1987; Joshi et al., 1993). Amylases contribute little toward soil carbon cycling, as soil organic inputs contain a small amount of starch.

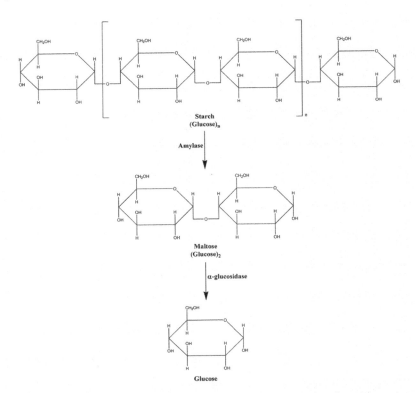

Figure 11.1 Breakdown of starch molecules by amylase and α-glucosidase.

11.2.2 β-Glucosidase

β-Glucosidase breaks glycosidic bonds in the glucosides produced by the decomposition of plant residues by cellulases and amylases (Martinez and Tabatabai, 1997). The glucose produced by β-glucosidase action on glucosides is an essential energy source for soil microbes (Esen, 1993). In soil environments, it is a ubiquitous and major enzyme (Tabatabai, 1994). β-Glucosidase is very sensitive to change in soil pH, soil management practices, and soil heavy metals content (Deng and Tabatabai, 1995; Bergstrom et al., 1998; Leirós et al., 1999; Acosta-Marténez and Tabatabai, 2000; Ndiaye et al., 2000; Madejón et al., 2001). Therefore, many researchers had suggested using this enzyme as an indicator of change in soil biological activity caused by soil acidification, past biological activity and to measure the soil organic matter stabilization capacity (Ndiaye et al., 2000; Madejón et al., 2001).

11.2.3 Cellulase and Hemicellulase

Cellulases catalyze the decomposition of insoluble cellulose into simple, water-soluble monosaccharides like β-glucose or shorter polysaccharides or oligosaccharides (Deng and Tabatabai, 1994) (Fig. 11.2). Complete degradation of cellulose requires cellulases, which consist of three types of enzymes viz. endoglucosidase or endo-1,4-β-glucanase, exo-glucosidase or exo-1,4-β-glucanase and β-glucosidase. Endoglucosidase breaks the cellulose chains arbitrarily and exo-1,4-β-glucanase breaks the cellulose by removing oligosaccharides from the non-reducing end of the carbohydrate chain. In contrast, the breakdown of cellulose to glucose is done by β-D-glucosidase by hydrolyzing water-soluble cellodextrins and cellobiose (Alef and Nannipieri, 1995). There are two possible mechanisms for substrate cleavage. Cellulase may cause random splitting of long cellulose molecules or cellobiose units may be removed from the terminal end of the chain. The microbial cell is impermeable to the cellulose molecule (Alexander, 1977). Therefore, the organism secretes extracellular cellulase for converting insoluble material into soluble sugar which penetrates the cell membrane.

Plant debris is the major contributor of cellulases while soil fungi and bacteria contribute a little amount toward the total cellulases in soil (Richmond, 1991). As cellulase decomposes the abundantly found organic compound in the soil, that is, cellulose, it plays an important role in soil carbon (C) cycling (Eriksson et al., 1990). Production of cellulase as extracellular enzymes in the soil is affected by various soil properties like soil moisture content, soil temperature and soil pH (Rubidge, 1977; Srinivasulu and Rangaswamy, 2006), oxygen content, and the trace elements from some pesticides (Petker and Rai, 1992; Arinze and Yubedee, 2000). The quality, quantity, composition, and location of the substrate in the soil profile also affect the cellulose production by microbes in soil (Gomah, 1980; Linkins et al., 1984; Hope and Burns, 1987), water, and. Soil fungal and bacterial populations can have a positive effect on soil cellulase activity (Joshi et al., 1993).

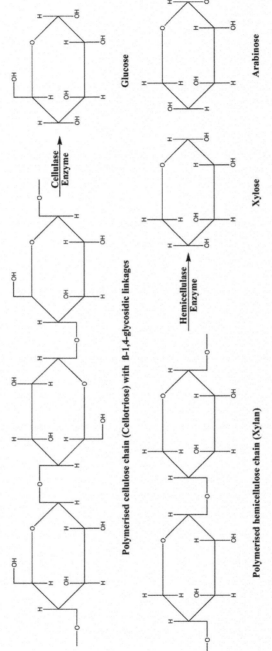

Figure 11.2 Hydrolysis of polymerized cellulose and polymerized hemicellulose chains.

The enzymes that catalyze the hemicellulose breakdown are broadly termed hemicellulases (Alexander, 1977). A variety of hemicellulases are found inside different organisms present in the soil. Hemicellases mainly act on the complex polysaccharide like xylan and yield simpler polysaccharides like xylose and arabinose (Fig. 11.2).

11.2.4 Ligninase

Lignins are the third most abundant polysaccharides (10–30% of dry weight) of plant tissues after cellulose (15–60%) and hemicellulose (10–40%) (Coyne, 1999). Lignin is composed of complex polymeric structures which depolymerized to simple aromatic substances such as vanillin and vanillic acid by the action of ligninase (Fig. 11.3). Ligninases are extracellular and mostly produced from fungi (Paul and Clark, 1996). The white-rot fungi are the most active lignin decomposing microorganisms resulting in the decomposition of all lignin-containing wood components (Paul and Clark, 1996).

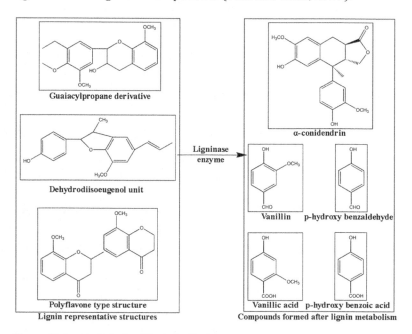

Figure 11.3 Hydrolysis of lignin by ligninase.

11.2.5 Invertase

Invertase belongs to the hydrolase enzyme group and converts sucrose to glucose and fructose. Invertase is predominantly present in plants, soil microorganisms, and animals (Alef and Nannipieri, 1995). It decomposes carbohydrate polymers to releases simpler sugars and facilitate carbon transformations. It also increases soluble nutrients content in the soil by mediating complex soil organic matter decomposition. Therefore, soil invertase enzyme activity can also be used as a soil carbon-cycling index (Sardans *et al.*, 2008).

11.2.6 Laccase

Laccases are multicopper phenoloxidases. These enzymes are found in fungi, bacteria, insects, and some higher plants. Laccases have low substrate specificity. They can oxidize various organo-pollutants such as polychlorinated biphenyls, polycyclic aromatic hydrocarbons, agrochemicals, and synthetic dyes, inorganic compounds like iron–cyanide complexes and iodine (Sinsabaugh, 2010; Eichlerová *et al.*, 2012). Laccases, along with other soil extracellular enzymes decompose lignin and other polyphenols added to soils. Therefore, laccases also play an essential role in soil carbon cycling (Eichlerová *et al.*, 2012).

11.2.7 Pectinase

Pectic substances are minor polysaccharides that contain <1% of the dry matter of plant tissues. Pectic substances are found in the middle lamella of plant tissues (Alexander, 1977). Pectic substances consist of three types: (a) protopectin (water-insoluble), (b) pectin (water-insoluble) and (c) pectic acids (water-soluble). After incorporating within the soil, these pectic substances undergo depolymerization by the action of three classes of enzymes, that is, protopectinases, (b) pectin methyl esterases (PMEs), and (c) polygalacturonases (PGs). Protopectinase decomposes protopectin with the formation of soluble pectin (Fig. 11.4). PME hydrolysases decompose the methyl ester linkage of pectin to yield pectic acid and methanol. The PG destroys the galacturonic acid linkages of pectin and pectic acid with the release of smaller chains and free galacturonic acid.

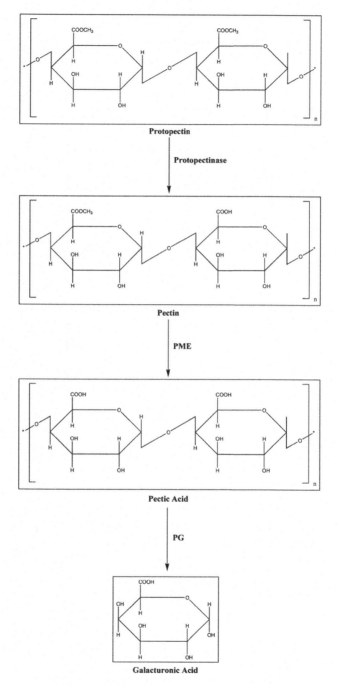

Figure 11.4 Hydrolysis of protopectin by protopectinase, pectin by PME, and pectic acid by PG.

11.3 Nitrogen-Cycling Enzymes and Their Mechanisms

11.3.1 Soil Protease

Proteases are extensively present in soils with a multitude of actions (Hayano, 1986). Proteases consist of a group of enzymes that hydrolyze peptide bonds in proteins to release short peptide-like polypeptides and oligopeptides, which further degrade amino acids (Handa et al., 2000). These enzymes are secreted by plants, soil microorganisms, and soil animals and found to be associated with the soil colloidal fractions (organic and inorganic colloids) (Nannipieri et al., 1996). So generally, protease is extracellular in nature and functions (Burns, 1982). Humocarbohydrate complex in soil partially contributes toward protease activities in soil (Batistic et al., 1980). Soil microbes use amino acids (released by protein hydrolysis) as nitrogen sources and mineralized these to ammonia. The released ammonia adds to plant-available nitrogen (N). Therefore, nitrogen mineralization and plant-available N in soils are dependent on soil protease activity (Moreno et al., 2003; Stevenson, 1986).

11.3.2 Urease

Urease enzymes "hydrolyze urea into ammonia and carbon dioxide" (Fazekasova, 2012) and during the urea hydrolyzes process, the soil pH increases (Fig. 11.5). The urease enzyme is ubiquitous and is secreted by most of the soil microbes and plant roots (Burns, 1986). It acts both as an extra- and intracellular enzyme (Mobley and Hausinger, 1989). It increases the ammoniacal nitrogen concentration after urea fertilization, and the soil nitrogen dynamics are prominently affected by the urease enzyme (Byrnes and Amberger, 1988). Thus, urease activity in soil is used as an index of N mineralization (Nannipieri et al., 2012). Cropping history, soil organic matter content, soil depth, soil temperature, presence of heavy metals, and agricultural management practices like application soil amendments influence urease activity in the soils (Tabatabai, 1977; Bremner and Mulvaney, 1978; Yang et al., 2006). Various reports suggested that extracellular urease stabilized on soil colloids contributes more toward total urease activity in the soil. Extracellular urease associated with soil organo-mineral complexes showed better stability as compared to urease present in the soil solution (Burns, 1986). Nannipieri *et al.* (1978) extracted humus-urease complexes from soil and found them resistant against the proteolytic attack and extreme temperature, while intracellular urease (extracted from microorganisms or plants) showed rapid degradation by soil proteolytic enzymes (Zantua and Bremner, 1977).

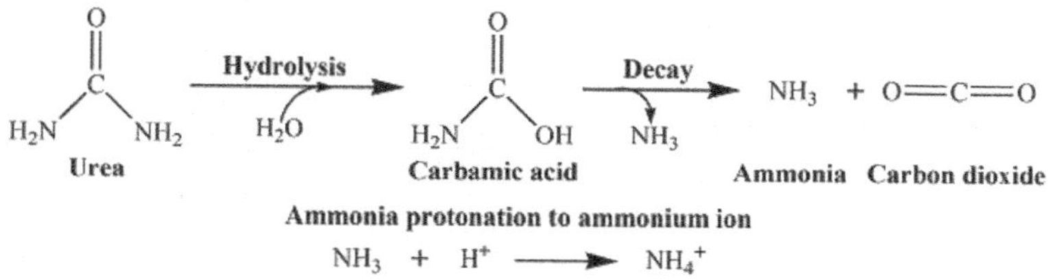

$$\underset{\text{Urea}}{H_2N-\overset{\overset{O}{\|}}{C}-NH_2} \xrightarrow[H_2O]{\text{Hydrolysis}} \underset{\text{Carbamic acid}}{H_2N-\overset{\overset{O}{\|}}{C}-OH} \xrightarrow[NH_3]{\text{Decay}} \underset{\text{Ammonia}}{NH_3} + \underset{\text{Carbon dioxide}}{O=C=O}$$

Ammonia protonation to ammonium ion
$$NH_3 + H^+ \longrightarrow NH_4^+$$

Figure 11.5 Hydrolysis of urea by urease.

11.3.3 Chitinase

Chitinase enzymes catalyze the hydrolysis of chitin (Fig. 11.6). For complete degradation of chitin, a compound consisting of N-acetyl-β-glucosaminidase, chitobiase, and chitinase is required. N-acetyl-β-glucosaminidase is essential in the mineralization of nitrogen from chitin; therefore, it is used as an indicator of soil chitinase activity (Olander and Vitousek, 2000). The major fraction of soil chitinases are mostly produced by fungi, and a little fraction is contributed by bacteria (Gooday, 1994).

11.4 Phosphorus-Cycling Enzymes and Their Mechanisms

11.4.1 Phosphatase Enzymes

Phosphatase enzymes play a significant role in the soil organic phosphorus (P) transformation (Dalal, 1977; Acosta-Martínez and Tabatabai, 2011). Phosphatases convert structurally unavailable

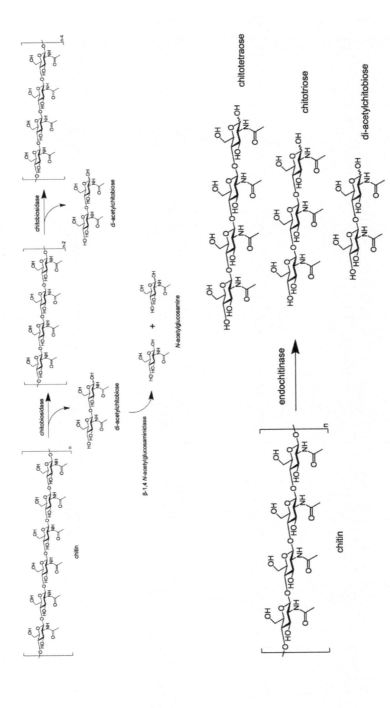

Figure 11.6 Hydrolysis of chitin by endochitinase.

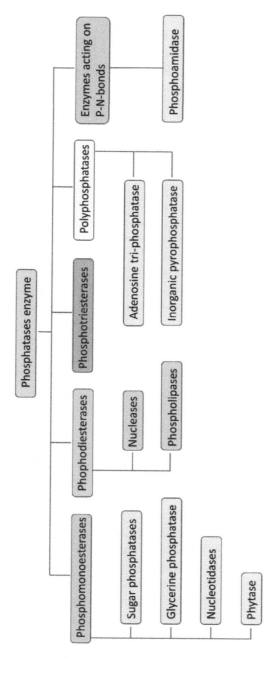

Figure 11.7 Different phosphatase enzymes in soils (Florkin and Stotz, 1964; Tabatabai, 1994; Acosta-Martínez and Tabatabai, 2011).

organic P into bioavailable phosphate ions ($H_2PO_4^-$ and HPO_4^{2-}), which can be taken up by plants and soil microbes. These phosphatase enzymes are excreted by plant roots and soil microbes. However, soil microbes excreted phosphatases dominated in soil and the activity is higher in rhizospheric soils than in bulk soil. Based on the number of ester bonds present in the substrate, the phosphatase enzymes are further classified as phosphomonoesterases, phosphodiesterases, and phosphotriesterases. Different types of reported phosphatases are classified and presented in Fig. 11.7.

11.4.2 Phosphomonoesterases

Phosphomonoesterase enzymes are often denoted by the term phosphatases and this is the most studied phosphatase group of enzymes. The phosphomonoesterase enzymes catalyze the hydrolysis of phosphomonoesters like phenyl phosphate, β-naphthyl phosphate, β-glycerophosphate, and *para*-nitrophenyl phosphate. Among these phosphomonoesters, *para*-nitrophenyl phosphate is the most used substrate for the determination of phosphomonoesterases activities. Based on the substrate specificity and optimum working pH, phosphatases are denoted as acid phosphatases and alkaline phosphatases. The pH dependency determines the availability of acid phosphatases and alkaline phosphatases. The range of alkaline soil pH triggers alkaline phosphatase activities; even pH 11.0 has been chosen as the optimum pH for the determination of alkaline phosphatase activities in the laboratory. On contrary, acid phosphatase activities predominated in acid soils. The optimum pH for laboratory determination is pH 6.5. Therefore, the activity depends greatly on soil management practices. Dick (1997) suggested that phosphatase activities are one of the most sensitive indicators to assess the performance of the P-cycle, which is directly related to land management and ecological restorations. Changes in phosphatase activities demarcate changes in crop cultivation and management practices (Acosta-Martínez *et al.*, 2004). Application of crop residues or manure increase the organic phosphorus (P) fractions in soil, which subsequently promotes phosphatase activities (Acosta-Martínez *et al.*, 2004; Acosta-Martínez and Tabatabai, 2011; Sarkar *et al.*, 2020). However, phosphatase enzymes are intended to adsorb on the reactive surfaces of soil colloids and entrapped in humus substances (Nannipieri et al., 2010). According to Dick and Tabatabai (1993), the soil pH at which proper acid phosphatase/alkaline phosphatase activity ratio is constant could be considered as the optimum pH level for crop production.

It has been reported that acid phosphatase is excreted by plant roots and soil microbes; however, the alkaline phosphatase is only excreted by the soil microbes (Beever and Burns, 1980; Sarkar et al., 2017). Among soil microbes, fungi have the major contributor to phosphatase activities. Arbuscular mycorrhizal fungi (AMF) are similarly efficient to produce phosphatase enzymes (Acosta-Martínez et al., 2008). The kinetics of acid and alkaline phosphatases are greatly varied compared to other soil extracellular enzymes. The apparent Michaelis-Menten constant (K_m) of alkaline phosphatases ranges between 0.4 to 4.9 mM; while the K_m for acid phosphatases ranges between 1.3 and 4.5 mM (Acosta-Martínez and Tabatabai, 2011). From the analysis of protein concentrations, it was confirmed that alkaline phosphatase is more efficient in catalyzing the hydrolysis of phosphomonoesters than acid phosphatase (Klose and Tabatabai, 2002). However, increased orthophosphate significantly reduced the phosphatase enzyme activity and rate kinetics (Ekenler and Tabatabai, 2003).

11.4.3 Phosphodiesterases

Phosphodiesterases are the second-most studied phosphatase group of enzymes. Phosphodiesterases are most important for the decomposition of fresh organic phosphorus (P) sources like plant residues and animal residue because phosphodiesterases are catalyzing the hydrolysis of phospholipids (Cosgrove, 1967) and nucleic acids (Razzell and Khorana, 1959; Acosta-Martínez and Tabatabai, 2000). The phosphodiester bond is the backbone of the strands of nucleic acids. Typically, the phosphodiester bond is the linkage between the 3rd carbon atom of a sugar moiety and the 5th carbon atom of another sugar moiety (deoxyribose in DNA and ribose in RNA). In the phosphodiester linkage, the phosphate group is negatively charged at pH 7.0 and the pK_a value is near zero. Enzymes that catalyze the hydrolysis of phosphodiester bonds are called phosphodiesterases. Phosphodiesterases are also known as cyclic nucleotide phosphodiesterases and the phosphodiesterase group of enzymes comprising of nucleases (deoxyribonuclease, ribonuclease), phospholipases, autotaxin, sphingomyelin phosphodiesterase, etc.

In the soil system, the apparent K_m of phosphodiesterases ranges between 1.3 and 2.0; whereas the activation energy of phosphodiesterases is ~37 kJ mol^{-1}. In soil medium the Vant-Hoff Q_{10} factor of phosphodiesterases is 1.7, that is, phosphodiesterase enzymes increased the hydrolysis rate by 1.7 times with each 10 ^{0}C temperature rise (Browman and Tabatabai, 1978; Acosta-Martínez and Tabatabai, 2011). It has been also described that phosphodiesterase activity increased two times with the increase in soil pH from 4.5 to 7.0 (Acosta-Martínez and Tabatabai, 2000; Ekenler and Tabatabai, 2003). Some common phosphodiesterase inhibitors are theophylline and papaverine (Boswell-Smith *et al.*, 2006). In general, manure treatment increase phosphodiesterase activities; however, application of tillage reduced the enzyme activities (Parham *et al.*, 2002; Deng and Tabatabai, 2003). Contradictorily, it has been reported that tillage does not have a significant impact on phosphodiesterase activities (Ekenler and Tabatabai, 2003).

11.4.4 Phosphotriesterases

Organophosphates (OPs) are organophosphorus compounds used as pesticides in agricultural systems. The group of pesticides accounts for more than 38% of global pesticide consumption and these OPs have triester bonds. It was found, that strains of amino acids isolated from *Pseudomonas diminuta* and *Flavobacterium spp.* are capable to hydrolyze the triester linkages of organophosphate molecules. These amino acid strains are known as phosphotriesterase enzymes. Other than these, phosphotriesterases have been successfully isolated from *Sphingobium sp.*, *Brevundimonas diminuta*, and *Agrobacterium radiobacter* (Gotthard *et al.*, 2013; Bigley *et al.*, 2016). Phosphotriesterases are metalloenzymes, which are also known as aryl dialkylphosphatases. Based on their substrate specificity phosphotriesterases are classified into parathion hydrolase and parathion arylesterase (insecticide parathion as substrate), paraoxonase (insecticide paraoxon as substrate). These enzymes activate the water molecule for a nucleophilic attack, which increases the electrophilic properties of phosphates and leads to their disintegration (Raushel and Holden, 2000). Dumas and Raushel (1990) reported that the catalytic activity of phosphotriesterases pretends a plateau in pH 7.0 and above; however, in acidic pH, its activity significantly decreased.

In the sequence of phosphoric acid esterification, monoester, diester, and triester bonds formed and hydrolysis of these ester bonds released phosphates and alcohols (or phenols). The activity of phosphomonoesterases, phosphodiesterases, and phosphotriesterases are well established and the reaction steps (Fig. 11.8) are well known (Acosta-Martínez and Tabatabai, 2011).

11.4.5 Polyphosphates

Phosphate ions are tetrahedral in structure, where phosphorus (P) is in the center and oxygen and hydroxy groups are adjacent groups. Polyphosphates are esters or salts of phosphoric acid, where multiple phosphate ions are linked together through sharing terminal or apical oxygens. Based on this, polyphosphate structures can be classified into linear chain polyphosphates and cyclic polyphosphates. Through sharing of the terminal oxygen atom with adjacent phosphate groups linear chain polyphosphates are formed. Whereas, sharing of the apical oxygen atom resulted in the formation of cyclic polyphosphates. Polyphosphate esters like adenosine triphosphate (ATP) and adenosine diphosphate (ADP) are involved in energy storage during photosynthesis (Dick and Tabatabai, 1983; Acosta-Martínez and Tabatabai, 2011). Polyphosphatases are enzymes that catalyze the hydrolysis of polyphosphates and are very much abundant in nature like the phosphatase group of enzymes. Polyphosphatases that catalyze the hydrolysis of pyrophosphates to orthophosphates are referred to as inorganic pyrophosphatases (Acosta-Martínez and Tabatabai, 2011). An enzyme-kinetic study in a furrow surface soil revealed that activation energy varies from 32 to 43 kJ mol^{-1} and the apparent K_m value ranges between 20 to 51 mM. Manure treatment, as well as neutral soil pH, is optimum for the functionality of polyphosphatases enzymes (Dick and Tabatabai, 1983). Different polyphosphatases and probable reactions are depicted in Fig. 11.9.

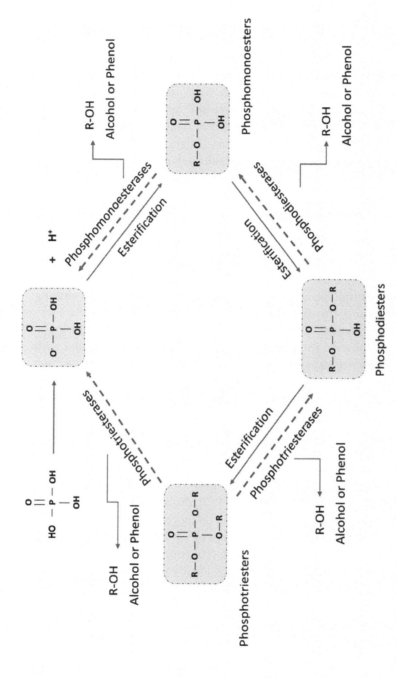

Figure 11.8 Cyclic functional relationships among phosphomonoesterases, phosphodiesterases, and phosphotriesterases (Tabatabai, 1994; Raushel and Holden, 2000; Acosta-Martínez and Tabatabai, 2011).

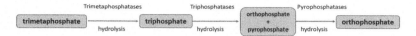

Figure 11.9 Different polyphosphatases and their hydrolysis (Tabatabai and Dick, 1979; Busman and Tabatabai, 1984; Acosta-Martínez and Tabatabai, 2011).

11.4.6 Phosphoamidase

Phosphoamidases belong to the hydrolase family that catalyzes the hydrolytic cleavage of *N*-phosphocreatine and produces phosphoric acid and creatine. Because of this phosphoamidase enzymes are also known as creatine phosphatases or phosphamide hydrolases (Müller *et al.*, 2009).

11.5 Sulfur-Cycling Enzymes and Their Mechanisms

11.5.1 Aryl Sulfatases

Ester sulfate is the most labile form of organic sulfur (S) in the soil system and comprises more than 50% of the organic S fraction. Sulfatases catalyze the hydrolysis of ester sulfates. Thus, sulfatases are often named sulfohydrolases. Though there are several types of sulfohydrolases (alkyl sulfatases, steroid sulfatases, glucosulfatases, chondro sulfatases, mycosulfatases) that occur in nature, arylsulfatases are the most dominant and mostly studied sulfohydrolases in this area (Klose *et al.*, 2011; Hettle *et al.*, 2018). Arylsulfatases cause cleavage in the S-O linkage of ester sulfate in the presence of water molecules. This reaction is irreversible. Although arylsulfatase is found in plants, fungi, bacteria, and animals, microorganisms are believed to be the main source for this enzyme in soil (Fitzgerald, 1978; Germida *et al.*, 1992).

Optimum soil pH for better arylsulfatase activities is ranging between 5.5 and 6.2 (Tabatabai and Bremner, 1970; Germida *et al.*, 1992; Tabatabai, 1994). Trasar-Cepeda *et al.* (2007) reported that arylsulfatase activity increased with increasing temperature up to 57°C and arylsulfatases activities become inactivate from 60 to 70°C (Tabatabai and Bremner, 1971). The apparent K_m of arylsulfatases ranges from 0.2 to 5.7 mM (Tabatabai and Bremner, 1971; Thornton and McLaren, 1975).

A brief of the reactions involved in the S-cycle and responsible enzymes are listed in Table 11.1.

Table 11.1 Summary of enzymes involved in the S-cycle in soil

Sulfur Compounds	Reactions	Enzyme Involved
Inorganic sulfur (S)	Sulfate to hydrogen sulfide	Sulfate reductase
	Sulfite to hydrogen sulfide	Sulfite reductase
	Elemental S to hydrogen sulfide	Sulfur reductase
	Thiosulfate to hydrogen sulfide Thiosulfate to sulfite	Thiosulfate reductase
	Thionate to hydrogen sulfide Polysulfide to hydrogen sulfide	Polysulfide reductase
	Thiosulfate to thiocyanate Thiosulfate to sulfite	Rhodanese
	Elemental S to sulfite	Sulfur oxygenase
	Thiosulfate to tetrathionate	Thiosulfate oxidase
	Tetrathionate to sulfate Tetrathionate to elemental sulfur	Tetrathionate hydrolase
	Trithionate to sulfite Trithionate to sulfate	Trithionate hydrolase
Organic sulfur (S)	Thiocyanate to carbonylsulfide	Thiocyanate hydrolase
	Djenkolic acid to carbon disulfide	S-alkyl cysteine lyase
	Cystine to thiocysteine Thiocysteine to hydrogen sulfide	Cystathionine lyases
	Carbonylsulfide to hydrogen sulfide	Carbonic anhydrase
	Ester sulfates to sulfates	Arylsulfatase
	Cysteine to cysteine sulfinic acid Cysteine to cysteic acid	Cysteine dioxygenase

Source: Compiled and modified from Scherer, 2001; Tabatabai, 2005; Klose *et al.*, 2011; Hettle *et al.*, 2018.

11.6 Microbial Functional Diversity in Agrosystems

Microbial biodiversity has been indicative of the richness of species which include plants, animals, and microorganisms, whereas microbial diversity is the part that includes protozoa, fungi, fauna, and bacteria. Different types of microorganisms present in soil are assigned different roles by the nature, such as some are active in nutrient cycling while others are in the suppression of diseases and used as biocontrol agents. In an agroecosystem nutrient, cycling is very diverse from an unmanaged ecosystem because of agricultural practices such as crop rotation, nutrient management, and application of fertilizers and agrochemicals. Different management practices and biocontrol treatments affect the soil microbial community. In the case of unmanaged ecosystems, wide losses and gain of nutrients occur. Many studies have shown that agricultural and management practices such as agroforestry, organic farming, etc. pose the least soil perturbation. Reduced tillage and crop rotation exert positive implications on the community structure, composition, abundance, and richness of specific groups of the organism (e.g., AMF, earthworms) and soil microbial diversity. Fatty acid methyl ester analysis/phospholipid-derived fatty acid (FAME/PLFA) profiling, molecular genetic profiling, functional profiling techniques, catabolic profiling based on substrate utilization, community-level physiological profiling, Simpson Diversity Index, Hannon Diversity Index, etc. are widely used for the quantification of soil functional diversity.

11.7 Conclusions and Future Prospects

Microbial diversity is the key element required for maintaining soil health. The crop and soil management practices of an agroecosystem need to be customized to harbor favorable microbial communities essentially needed to perform soil processes and sustain crop and soil productivity. Microbial diversity maintains soil health by suppressing the population of disease-causing organisms, improves nutrient cycling, etc. and can be enhanced by soil amendments and management practices such as conservation tillage, composting/

organic amendments, manuring, and fertilizers, crop rotation/crop sequences, etc. Identifying sustainable soil management practices through analyzing soil biological, chemical, and physical indicators of management practices being followed in an agroecosystem will help in optimizing a favorable system needed for sustaining the crop and soil productivity of a particular ecosystem.

References

Acosta-Martínez V., Tabatabai M. A. Enzyme activities in a limed agricultural soil. *Biol. Fertil. Soils*, **31** (2000), 85–91.

Acosta-Martínez V., Acosta–Mercado D., Sotomayor-Ramírez D., Cruz-Rodríguez L. Microbial communities and enzymatic activities under different management in semiarid soils. *Appl. Soil Ecol.*, **38** (2008), 249–260. doi:10.1016/j.apsoil.2007.10.012.

Acosta-Martínez V., Tabatabai M. A. Phosphorus cycle enzymes, in *Methods of Soil Enzymology* (Dick R. P., ed), Soil Science Society of America, Madison, WI, USA, (2011).

Acosta-Martínez V., Zobeck T. M., Allen V. Soil microbial, chemical and physical properties in continuous cotton and integrated crop-livestock systems. *Soil Sci. Soc. Am. J.*, **68** (2004), 1875–1884. doi:10.2136/sssaj2004.1875.

Alef K., Nannipieri P. Cellulase activity, in *Methods in Applied Soil Microbiology and Biochemistry* (Alef K., Nannipieri P., eds), Academic, San Diego, CA, 1995, pp. 345–349.

Alexander M. *Introduction to Soil Microbiology*, Wiley, New York, 1977, pp. 50–150.

Alori T. A., Glick B. R., Babalola O. O. Microbial phosphorus solubilization and its potential for use in sustainable agriculture. *Frontiers Microbiol.*, **8** (2017), 971.

Arinze A. E., Yubedee A. G. Effect of fungicides on Fusarium grain rot and enzyme production in maize (*Zea mays* L.). *Glob. J. Appl. Sci.*, **6** (2000), 629–634.

Batistic L., Sarkar J. M., Mayaudon J. Extraction, purification and properties of soil hydrolases. *Soil Biol. Biochem.*, **12** (1980), 59–63.

Beever R. E., Burns D. J. W. Phosphorus uptake, storage and utilization by fungi. *Adv. Bot. Res.*, **8** (1980), 128–129.

Bergstrom D. W., Monreal C. M., King D. J. Sensitivity of soil enzyme activities to conservation practices. *Soil Sci. Soc. Am. J.*, **62** (1998), 1286–1295.

Bigley A. N., Xiang D. F., Ren Z., Xue H., Hull K. G., Romo D., Raushel F. M. Chemical mechanism of the phosphotriesterase from *Sphingobium* sp. starin TCM1, an enzyme capable of hydrolyzing organophosphate flame retardants. *J. Am. Chem. Soc.*, **137** (2015), 8388–8391. doi: 10.1021/jacs.5b12739.

Bohn H. L., Barrow N. J., Rajan S. S. S., Parfitt R. L. Reactions of inorganic sulfur in soils, in *Sulfur in Agriculture* (Tabatabai M. A., ed), Agronomy Monograph 27, ASA, CSSA, and SSSA, Madison, WI, (1986), pp. 233–249.

Boswell-Smith V., Spina D., Page C. P. Phosphodiesterase inhibitors. *Br. J. Pharmacol.*, **147** (2006), S252–S257.

Bremner J. M., Mulvaney R. L. Urease activity in soils, in *Soil Enzymes* (Bums R. G., ed), Academic, London, 1978, pp. 149–196.

Browman M. G., Tabatabai M. A. Phosphodiesterase activity of soils. *Soil Sci. Soc. Am. J.*, **42** (1978), 284–290. doi: 10.2136/sssaj1978.03615995004200020016x.

Burns R. G. Enzyme activity in soil: location and a possible role in microbial ecology. *Soil Biol. Biochem.*, **14** (1982), 423–427.

Burns R. G. Interaction of enzymes with soil mineral and organic colloids, in *Interactions of Soil Minerals with Natural Organics and Microbes* (Huang P. M., Schnitzer M., eds), *Soil Sci. Soc. Am.*, Madison, 1986, pp. 429–452.

Busman L. M., Tabatabai M. A. Determination of trimetaphosphate added to soils. *Commun. Soil Sci. Plant Anal.*, **15** (1984), 1257–1268. doi:10.1080/00103628409367555.

Byrnes B. H., Amberger A. Fate of broadcast urea in a flooded soil when treated with N-(n-butyl) thiophosphoric triamide, a urease inhibitor. *Fertilizer Res.*, **18** (1988), 221–231.

Cosgrove D. J. Metabolism of organic phosphate in soil, in *Soil Biochemistry* (McLaren A. D., Peterson G. H., eds), vol. 1, Marcel Dekker, New York, 1967, pp. 216–288.

Coyne M. S. *Soil Microbiology: An Exploratory Approach*, Delmar Pub., 1999.

Dalal R. C. Soil organic phosphorus. *Adv. Agron.*, **29** (1977), 83–117. doi:10.1016/S0065-2113(08)60216-3.

Dao T. H. Extracellular enzymes in sensing environmental nutrients and ecosystem changes: ligand mediation in organic phosphorus cycling, in *Soil Enzymology, Soil Biology* (Shukla G., Varma A., eds), Springer-Verlag, Berlin, Heidelberg, 2004. doi: 10.1007/978-3-642-14225-3_5.

Deng S. P., Tabatabai M. A. Effect of tillage and residue management on enzyme activities in soils: phosphatases and arylsulfatase. *Biol. Fertil. Soils*, **24** (1997), 141–146. doi:10.1007/s003740050222.

Deng S. P., Tabatabai M. A. Cellulase activity of soils. *Soil Biol. Biochem.*, **26** (1994), 1347–1354.

Deng S. P., Tabatabai M. A. Cellulase activity of soils: effect of trace elements. *Soil Biol. Biochem.*, **27** (1995), 977–979.

Dick R. P. Soil enzyme activities as integrative indicators of soil health, in *Biological Indicators of Soil Health* (Pankhurst C. E., Doube B. M., Gupta V. V. S. R., eds), CABI, Wallingford, New York, pp. 121–153.

Dick W. A., Tabatabai M. A. Activation of soil pyrophosphate by metal ions. *Soil Biol. Biochem.*, **15** (1983), 359–363. doi:10.1016/0038-0717(83)90084-6.

Dick W. A., Tabatabai M. A. Significance and potential uses of soil enzymes, in *Soil Microbial Ecology: Applications in Agricultural and Environmental Management* (Metting F. B., ed), Marcel Dekker, New York, 1993, pp. 95–127.

Dumas D. P., Durst H. D., Landis W. G., Raushel F. M., Wild J. R. Inactivation of organophosphorus nerve agents by the phosphotriesterase from *Pseudomonas diminuta. Arch. Biochem. Biophys.*, **277** (1990), 155–159.

Eichlerová I., Šnajdr J., Baldrian, P. Laccase activity in soils: considerations for the measurement of enzyme activity. *Chemosphere*, **88** (2012), 1154–1160.

Ekenler M., Tabatabai M. A. Responses of phosphatases and arylsulfatase in soils to liming and tillage systems. *J. Plant Nutr. Soil Sci.*, **166** (2003), 281–290. doi:10.1002/jpln.200390045.

Eriksson K. E. L., Blancbette R. A., Ander P. Biodegration of cellulose, in *Microbial and Enzymatic Degradation of Wood and Wood Components* (Eriksson K. E. L., Blancbette R. A., Ander P., eds), Springer, New York, 1990, pp. 89–180.

Esen A. *β-Glucosidases-biochemistry and Molecular Biology*, ACS symposium series 533, American Chemical Society, Washington, DC, 1993, pp. 9–17.

Fazekasova D. *Evaluation of Soil Quality Parameters Development in Terms of Sustainable Land Use: Sustainable Development Authoritative and Leading Edge Content for Environmental Management*, In Tech, Rijeka, 2012.

Fitzgerald J. W. Naturally occurring organosulfur compounds in soil, in *Sulfur in the Environment* (Nriagu J. O., ed), John Wiley & Sons, New York, 1978, pp. 391–443.

Florkin M., Stotz E. H., (eds.). *Comprehensive Biochemistry*, Elsevier North-Holland, New York, 1967, pp. 126–134.

Germida J. J., Wainwright M., Gupta V. V. S. R. Biochemistry of sulfur cycling in soil, in Soil Biochemistry (Stotzky G., Bollag J. M., eds), vol. 7, Marcel Dekker, New York, pp. 1–38.

Ghosh A., Singh A. B., Kumar R. V., Manna M. C., Bhattacharyya R., Rahman M. M., Sharma P., Rajput P. S., and Misra S. Soil enzymes and microbial elemental stoichiometry as bio-indicators of soil quality in diverse cropping systems and nutrient management practices of Indian vertisols, *Appl. Soil Ecol.*, **145** (2020), 103304.

Gomah A. M. CM-cellulase activity in soil as affected by addition of organic material, temperature, storage and drying and wetting cycles. *Zeitschrift fuer Pflanzenernaehrung und Bodenkunde*, **143** (1980), 349–356.

Gooday G. W. Physiology and microbial degradation of chitin and chitosan, in *Biochemistry of Microbial Degradation* (Ratledge C., ed), Springer, Dordrecht, 1994, pp. 279–312.

Gotthard G., Hiblot J., Gonzalez D., Elias M., Chabriere E. Structural and enzymatic characterization of the Phosphotriesterases OPHC2 from *Pseudomonas pseudoalcaligenes*. *PloS One*, **8** (2013), e77995.

Handa S. K., Agnihothri M. P., Kulshresta G. Effect of pesticides on soil fertility, in *Pesticide Residue Analysis and Significance*, Research Periodicals and Publishing House, New Delhi, 2000, pp. 184–198.

Hayano K. Cellulase complex in tomato field soil: introduction localization and some properties. *Soil Biol. Biochem.*, **18** (1986), 215–219.

Hettle A. G., Vickers C., Robb C. S., Liu F., Withers S. G., Hehemann J. H., Boraston A. B. The molecular basis of polysaccharide sulfatase activity and a nomenclature for catalytic subsites in this class of enzyme. *Structure*, **26** (2018), 747–758.

Hope C. F. A., Burns R. G. Activity, origins and location of cellulases in a silt loam soil. *Biol. Fert. Soils*, **5** (1987), 164–170.

Joshi S. R., Sharma G. D., Mishra R. R. Microbial enzyme activities related to litter decomposition near a highway in a sub-tropical forest of North east India. *Soil Biol. Biochem.*, **25** (1993), 1763–1770.

Klose S., Bilen S., Tabatabai M. A., Dick W. A. Sulfur cycle enzymes, in *Methods of Soil Enzymology* (Dick R. P., ed), Soil Science Society of America, Madison, WI, USA, 2011, pp. 125–159.

Klose S., Tabatabai M. A. Response of phosphomonoesterases in soils to chloroform fumigation. *J. Plant Nutr. Soil Sci.*, **165** (2002), 429–434.

Ladd J. N., Butler J. H. A. Inhibition and stimulation of proteolytic enzyme activities by soil humic acids. *Austr. J. Soil Res.*, **7** (1969), 253–261.

Ladd J. N., Butler J. H. A. Short-term assays of soil proteolytic enzyme activities using proteins and peptide derivatives as substrates. *Soil Biol. Biochem.*, **4** (1972), 19–30.

Leiros M. C., Trasar-Cepeda C., Garcia-Fernandez F., Gil-Sotres F. Defining the validity of a biochemical index of soil quality. *Biol. Fertil. Soils*, **30** (1999), 140–146.

Lemanowicz J. Activity of selected enzymes as markers of ecotoxicity in technogenic salinization soils. *Environ. Sci. Pollut. Res.*, **26** (2019), 13014–13024. https://doi.org/10.1007/s11356-019-04830-x.

Linkins A. E., Melillo J. M., Sinsabaugh R. L. Factors affecting cellulase activity in terrestrial and aquatic ecosystems, in *Current Perspectives in Microbial Ecology* (Klug M. J., Reddy C. A., eds), American Society of Microbiology, Washington, 1984, pp. 572–579.

Madejon E., Burgos P., Lopez R., Cabrera F. Soil enzymatic response to addition of heavy metals with organic residues. *Biol. Fertil. Soils*, **34** (2001), 144–150.

Martinez C. E., Tabatabai M. A. Decomposition of biotechnology by-products in soils. *J. Environ. Qual.*, **26** (1997), 625–632.

Mobley H. L. T., Hausinger R. P. Microbial urease: significance, regulation and molecular characterization. *Microbiol. Rev.*, **53** (1989), 85–108.

Moreno J. L., Garcia C., Hernandez T. Toxic effect of cadmium and nickel on soil enzymes and the influence of adding sewage sludge. *Eur. J. Soil Sci.*, **54** (2003), 377–386.

Müller I. B., Knöckel J., Eschbach M. L., Bergmann B., Walter R. D., Wrenger C. Secretion of an acid phosphatase provides a possible mechanism to acquire host nutrients by *Plasmodium falciparum*. *Cell. Microbiol.*, **13** (2011), pp. 259–273. https://doi.org/10.1111/j.1462-5822.2010.01426.x.

Nannipieri P., Giagnoni L., Landi L., Renella G. Role of phosphatase enzymes in soil, in *Phosphorus in Action* (Bunemann E. K., et al., eds), Springer, Berlin, Heidelberg, 2011, pp. 215–243. doi:10.1007/978-3-642-15271-9_9.

Nannipieri P., Ceccanti B., Cervelli S., Sequi P. Stability and kinetic properties of humus-urease complexes *Soil Biol. Biochem.*, **10** (1978), 143–147.

Nannipieri P., Sequi P., Fusi P. Humus and enzyme activity, in *Humic Substances in Terrestrial Ecosystems* (Piccolo A., ed), Elsevier, New York, 1996, pp. 293–328.

Nannipieri P., Landi L., Giagnoni L., Renella, G. Past, present and future in soil enzymology, in *Soil Enzymology in the Recycling of Organic Wastes and Environmental Restoration, Environmental Science and Engineering* (Trasar-Cepeda C., Hernandez T., Garcia C., Rad C., Gonzalez-Carcedo S., eds), Springer-Verlag, Berlin, 2012, pp. 1–17.

Ndiaye E. L., Sandeno J. M., McGrath D., Dick R. P. Integrative biological indicators for detecting change in soil quality. *Am. J. Altern. Agric.*, **15** (2000), 26–36.

Olander L. P., Vitousek P. M. Regulation of soil phosphatase and chitinase activity by N and P availability. *Biogeochem.*, **49** (2000), 175–191.

Pancholy S. K., Rice E. L. Soil enzymes in relation to old field succession: amylase, cellulose, invertase, dehydrogenase and urease. *Soil Sci. Soc. Am. J.*, **37** (1973), 47–50.

Parham J. A., Deng S. P., Raun W. R., Johnson G. V. Long-term cattle manure application in soil. I. Effect on soil phosphorus levels, microbial biomass C, and dehydrogenase and phosphatases activities. *Biol. Fertil. Soils*, **35** (2002), 328–337.

Paul E. A., Clark F. E., (eds.). *Soil Microbiology and Biochemistry*, 2nd edn, Academic Press, San Diego, 1996.

Pazur J. H. Enzymes in the synthesis and hydrolysis of starch, in *Starch: Chemistry and Technology, Vol. 1 Fundamental Aspects* (Whistler R., Paschall E. F., eds), Academic Press, New York, 1965, pp. 133–175.

Petker A. S., Rai P. K. Effect of fungicides on activity, secretion of some extra cellular enzymes and growth of *Alternaria alternate*. *Indian J. Appl. Pure Biol.*, **7** (1992), 57–59.

Raushel F. M., Holden H. M. Phosphotriesterase: an enzyme in search of its natural substrate. *Adv. Enzymol. Relat. Areas Mol. Biol.*, **74** (2000), 51–93.

Razzell W. E., Khorana H. G. Studies on polynucleotides: III. Enzymatic degradation. Substrate specificity and properties of snake venom phosphodiesterase. *J. Biol. Chem.*, **234** (1959), 2105–2113.

Richmond P. A. Occurrence and functions of native cellulose, in *Biosynthesis and Biodegradation of Cellulose* (Haigler C. H., Weimer P. J., eds), Dekker, New York, 1991, pp. 5–23.

Ross D. J. Invertase and amylase activities in ryegrass and white clover plants and their relationships with activities in soils under pasture. *Soil Biol. Biochem.*, **8** (1976), 351–356.

Ross D. J. Studies on a climosequence of soils in tussock grasslands-5. Invertase and amylase activities of topsoils and their relationships with other properties. *NZ. J. Sci.*, **18** (1975), 511–518.

Ross D. J., Roberts H. S. Enzyme activities and oxygen uptakes of soils under pasture in temperature and rainfall sequences. *J. Soil Sci.*, **21** (1970), 368–381.

Roy T., Biswas D. R., Datta S. C., Sarkar A. Phosphorus release from rock phosphate as influenced by organic acid loaded nanoclay polymer composites in an alfisol. *Proceed. National Acad. Sci. India Sec. B: Biol. Sci.*, **88** (2018), 121–132.

Rubidge T. The effect of moisture content and incubation temperature upon the potential cellulase activity of John Innes no. 1 soil (ISSN. 0020-6164). *Int. Biodeterior. Bul.*, **13** (1977), 39–44.

Sardans J., Peñuelas J., Estiarte M. Changes in soil enzymes related to C and N cycle and in soil C and N content under prolonged warming and drought in a Mediterranean shrubland. *Appl. Soil Ecol.*, **39** (2008), 223–235.

Sarkar A., Saha M., Meena V. S. Plant beneficial rhizospheric microbes (PBRMs): prospects for increasing productivity and sustaining the resilience of soil fertility, in *Agriculturally Important Microbes for Sustainable Agriculture* (Meena V., Mishra P., Bisht J., Pattanayak A., eds), Springer, Singapore, 2017, https://doi.org/10.1007/978-981-10-5589-8_1.

Sarkar A., Saha M., Roy T., Biswas S. S., Mandal A. Phytobiomes: role in nutrient stewardship and soil health, in *Phytobiomes: Current Insights and Future Vistas* (Solanki M., Kashyap P., Kumari B., eds), Springer, Singapore, 2019, https://doi.org/10.1007/978-981-15-3151-4_1.

Scherer H. W. Sulphur in crop production-invited paper. *Eur. J. Agron.*, **14** (2001), 81–111. doi:10.1016/S1161-0301(00)00082-4.

Sharma S. B., Sayyed R. Z., Trivedi M. H., Gobi T. A. Phosphate solubilizing microbes: sustainable approach for managing phosphorus deficiency in agricultural soils. *Springer Plus*, **2** (2013), 1–14.

Singaram P., Kamala K. Effect of continuous application of different levels of fertilizers with farm yard manure on enzyme dynamics of soil. *Madras Agricul. J.*, **87** (2000), 364–365.

Sinsabaugh R. L. Phenol oxidase, peroxidase and organic matter dynamics of soil. *Soil Biol. Biochem.*, **2** (2010), 391–404.

Sinsabaugh R. L., Linkins A. E. Inhibition of the *Trichoderma viride* cellulase complex by leaf litter extracts *Soil Biol. Biochem.*, **19** (1987), 719–725.

Srinivasulu M., Rangaswamy V. Activities of invertase and cellulase as influenced by the application of tridemorph and captan to groundnut (*Arachis hypogaea*) soil. *Afr. J. Biotechnol.*, **5** (2006), 175–180.

Stevenson F. J. The phosphorus cycle, in *Cycles of Soils: Carbon, Nitrogen, Phosphorus, Sulfur, Micronutrients*, Stevenson F. J., eds), John Wiley & Sons, Inc., 1999, pp. 231–280.

Stevenson F. J., Cole M. A., (eds). *Cycles of Soil-Carbon, Nitrogen, Phosphorus, Sulfur, Micronutrients*, Wiley Inter. Science Publ., John Wiley & Sons, New York, 1986.

Tabatabai M. A., Dick W. A. Distribution and stability of pyrophosphatase in soils. *Soil Biol. Biochem.*, **11** (1979), 655–659. doi:10.1016/0038-0717(79)90035-X.

Tabatabai M. A. Chemistry of sulfur in soils, in *Chemical Processes in Soils* (Tabatabai M. A., Sparks D. L., eds), SSSA Book Ser. 8. ASA and SSSA, Madison, WI, 2005, pp. 193–226.

Tabatabai M. A., Bremner J. M. Arylsulfatase activity of soils. *Soil Sci. Soc. Am. Proc.*, **34** (1970), 225–229. doi:10.2136/sssaj1970.03615995003400020016x.

Tabatabai M. A., Bremner J. M. Michaelis constant of soil enzymes. *Soil Biol. Biochem.*, **3** (1971), 317–323. doi:10.1016/0038-0717(71)90041-1.

Tabatabai M. A. Effect of trace elements on urease activity in soils. *Soil Biol. Biochem.*, **9** (1977), 9–13.

Tabatabai M. A. Soil enzymes, in *Methods of Soil Analysis, Part 2. Microbiological and Biochemical Properties* (Weaver R. W., Angle J. S., Bottomley P. S., eds), SSSA Book Series no. 5, Soil Science Society America, Madison, WI, 1994, pp. 775–833.

Thoma J. A., Spradlin J. E., Dygert S. Plant and animal amylases, in *The Enzymes* (Boyer P. D., ed), International Society of Soil-Science, Netherlands, 1971, pp. 115–189.

Thornton J. I., McLaren A. D. Enzymatic characterization of soil evidence. *J. Forensic Sci.*, **20** (1975), 674–692.

Trasar-Cepeda C., Gil-Sotres F., Leirós M. C. Thermodynamic parameters of enzymes in grassland soils from Galicia, NW Spain. *Soil Biol. Biochem.*, **39** (2007), 311–319. doi:10.1016/j.soilbio.2006.08.002.

Yang Z., Liu S., Zheng D., Feng S. Effects of cadmium, zinc and lead on soil enzyme activities *J. Environ. Sci.*, **18** (2006), 1135–1141.

Zantua M. I., Bremner J. M. Stability of urease in soils. *Soil Biol. Biochem.*, **9** (1977), 135–140.

Part VI
Bioremediation

Chapter 12

Bioremediation: Removal of Polycyclic Aromatic Hydrocarbons from Soil

Zdeněk Košnář, Johanka Wernerová, Petr Frühbauer, and Pavel Tlustoš

Department of Agro-Environmental Chemistry and Plant Nutrition, Czech University of Life Sciences Prague, Kamýcká 129, 165 00, Prague 6, Suchdol, Czech Republic
kosnarz@af.czu.cz

Polycyclic aromatic hydrocarbons (PAHs) are ubiquitous organic contaminants that consist of two or more benzene rings. PAHs may pose serious threats to the environment and biota due to their toxic, mutagenic, teratogenic, and carcinogenic properties. Biological treatments are considered an environmental option to clean up polluted soil with PAHs. The natural attenuation approach usually leads to a negligible PAH removal. Phytoremediation of PAH-contaminated soil increases the removal of PAHs with low and medium molecular weight from the soil. Using ligninolytic fungi cultivated on organic waste materials in bioremediation (mycoremediation) could be a very promising approach how

Agricultural Biocatalysis: Enzymes in Agriculture and Industry
Edited by Peter Jeschke and Evgeni B. Starikov
Copyright © 2023 Jenny Stanford Publishing Pte. Ltd.
ISBN 978-981-4968-47-8 (Hardcover), 978-1-003-31310-6 (eBook)
www.jennystanford.com

to remove PAHs from the soil. Plant-assisted mycoremediation treatment significantly enhances the removal of PAHs with high molecular weight by higher ligninolytic enzymes activity in the soil. Cultivation of maize plants in association with *Pleurotus ostreatus* grown on the wood substrate could be a very promising *in situ* bioremediation strategy for PAH-contaminated agricultural soils. Bioaccumulation factors of PAHs are low suggesting a negligible PAH uptake from soil by maize roots therefore its aboveground biomass does not represent any environmental risk.

12.1 Introduction

12.1.1 General Description of Polycyclic Aromatic Hydrocarbons (PAHs)

More than a hundred organic compounds belong to the group of polycyclic aromatic hydrocarbons (PAHs). These compounds represent persistent organic pollutants (POPs), which are widely distributed in the environment as a consequence of human industrialization (Bignal *et al.*, 2008). They have been extensively studied for the last decades because PAHs may cause serious health risks and can negatively impact the environment even at very low exposure doses (Bamforth and Singleton, 2005).

PAHs are lipophilic compounds that consist of 2–7 fused benzene rings in linear, angular, or cluster arrangements with toxic, mutagenic, teratogenic, and carcinogenic properties (IARC, 2010). This arrangement predicts their resistance in the environment, also called persistence, as they are very recalcitrant to most degradation processes. The recalcitrance of PAHs is caused by the high resonance energy that stabilizes their aromatic ring systems, which makes them mostly resistant to nucleophilic attack. Therefore, they tend to accumulate mainly in soils, sediments, and organic wastes such as sewage sludge (Johnsen *et al.*, 2005).

Their boiling and melting points are usually high, which is also the reason why they mainly occur in solid forms, and they have a very low aqueous solubility, which is reflected in their hydrophobic property. With an increasing number of aromatic benzene rings in the PAH compound, the water solubility decreases, and that is the reason why PAHs are more resistant to oxidation and reduction processes. On the other hand, PAHs are highly lipophilic, which allows them high solubility in lipids and organic solvents (Wilson and Jones, 1992). PAHs are known for their coexistence with other inorganic and organic pollutants, like heavy metals (Cd, Cr, Pb, Ni, Zn, etc.) or other hydrocarbons, such as C_{10}–C_{40} alkanes (Gan *et al.*, 2009).

The most frequent formation mechanism of PAHs is pyrolysis and subsequent pyro-synthesis during the incomplete combustion of organic matter under low-oxygen conditions (McGrath *et al.*, 2001). Usually, high temperatures during the combustion can form free radicals of organic matter by breaking hydrocarbon bonds, which then react between each other or condensate to form PAH compounds (Ravindra *et al.*, 2008). According to Palma (2013), PAH compounds are formed by a direct combination of fused aromatic rings. Kaisalo *et al.* (2015) suggested the role of radical addition reactions of ethylene and acetylene with aromatic rings in the formation and sequential growth of PAHs (Fig. 12.1).

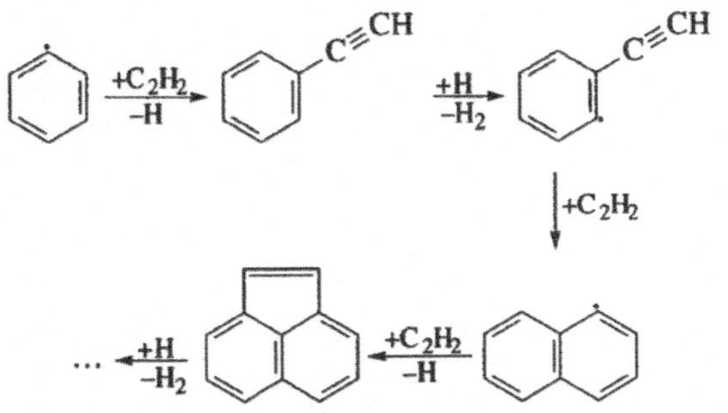

Figure 12.1 Formation of PAHs from benzene ring, as suggested by Frenklach *et al.* (1985).

Different PAH structures are strongly dependent on the physicochemical properties of combusted biomass, such as moisture, and operating conditions of combustion, like oxygen content and combustion speed (Ross *et al.*, 2002).

There are hundredths of PAH compounds and methyl, hydroxy, nitro, and other PAH derivates, therefore lists of most common and significant compounds of PAHs were done, to make research more complex and comparable. In 1970, the US EPA (United States Environmental Protection Agency) listed 16 individual PAH compounds (Fig. 12.2) as the most common and highest priority pollutants in the environment (Liu et al., 2001). The list of 16 basic PAHs is abbreviated in many studies as 16 US EPA PAHs (Vernoux et al., 2011). Some other studies show only a list of 12 PAHs according to the European Union guidance, which is known as 12 EU PAHs (Miguel et al., 2005).

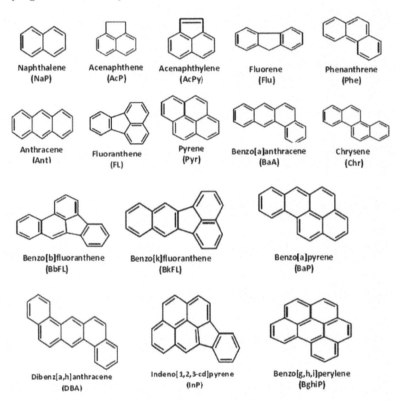

Figure 12.2 Chemical structures of 16 individual US EPA PAHs (Wang et al., 2019).

For better evaluation of environmental toxicity, other lists were introduced, for instance, 40 ENV PAHs, which include 40 individual PAH compounds present in the environment (Wise et al., 2014). Individual 16 US EPA PAHs (denoted as 16 PAHs) for screening in environmental matrixes are commonly available in one solution mix, which can be purchased for laboratory testing and screening (Andersson and Achten, 2015).

12.1.2 Basic Description of 16 Individual US EPA PAHs

The physical and chemical properties, distribution, and behavior of individual 16 PAHs in the environment vary considerably with the PAH molecular weight and number of rings. The basic properties of individual 16 PAHs are shown in Table 12.1. The lower molecular weight PAHs containing 2–3 rings are relatively mobile in the environment, whereas the medium molecular weight PAHs containing 4 rings and the higher molecular weight PAHs containing 5–7 rings are relatively non–mobile. With increasing molecular weight, the melting point, boiling point, and lipophilicity of PAHs grow with respect to log K_{OW} (octanol-water partition coefficient), and the water solubility decreases, suggesting an increased solubility in lipid compounds (Eisler, 2000).

Naphthalene is the simplest PAH compound with two benzene rings. It usually appears in a solid form. This PAH compound, with the lowest molecular weight of all 16 PAHs, is the most acutely toxic. When ingested, naphthalene causes acute hemolytic anemia, inflicts neurological damage, and damages the liver. Naphthalene has also been classified as a probable carcinogen by the International Agency for Research on Cancer (IARC) (Agoun-Bahar *et al.*, 2019). Naphthalene makes approximately 10% of coal on a weight basis, and it is the most abundant PAH compound in coal tar. It can also be found in biomass ashes at a relatively high amount (Košnář *et al.*, 2016). Naphthalene can be derived from petroleum hydrocarbons (Kairbekov *et al.*, 2019).

Acenaphtylene consists of three fused hydrocarbon rings. It is commonly present as solid particles of yellow color with no fluorescence (Griesbaum *et al.*, 2000). The toxicity of acenaphthylene has been defined by the no-observed-effect-level (NOEL) in rats, which was estimated as 4 mg kg^{-1} day^{-1} (Tanabe *et al.*, 2017). Acenaphtylene is mostly present in coal tar (about 2% by weight) and can be industrially produced from acenaphthene by gas-phase dehydrogenation (Griesbaum *et al.*, 2000).

Table 12.1 Basic physical and chemical properties of 16 US EPA PAHs (Shen, 2016)

	NB	MW	BP	MP	WS	VT	HC	logK$_{OW}$
Naphthalene	2	128.18	209	80	31.5	$1.1 \cdot 10^1$	43.0	3.37
Acenaphtylene	2	152.20	290	124	3.93	$8.9 \cdot 10^{-1}$	11.6	4.00
Acenaphthene	2	154.20	252	108	3.93	$2.9 \cdot 10^{-1}$	24.0	3.92
Fluorene	2	166.23	276	119	1.98	$8.0 \cdot 10^{-2}$	8.50	4.18
Phenanthrene	3	178.24	326	136	1.15	$2.5 \cdot 10^{-2}$	4.00	4.57
Anthracene	3	178.24	326	136	0.075	$1.1 \cdot 10^{-3}$	6.00	4.54
Fluoranthene	3	202.26	369	166	0.206	$1.1 \cdot 10^{-3}$	0.66	5.22
Pyrene	4	202.26	369	166	0.132	$5.5 \cdot 10^{-4}$	1.10	5.18
Benz[a]anthracene	4	228.30	400	177	0.009	$1.5 \cdot 10^{-5}$	0.102	5.91
Chrysene	4	228.30	400	177	0.002	$6.1 \cdot 10^{-7}$	0.106	5.86
Benzo[b]fluoranthene	4	252.32	461	209	0.002	$2.1 \cdot 10^{-5}$	0.054	5.80
Benzo[k]fluoranthene	4	252.32	430	194	0.0008	$1.3 \cdot 10^{-7}$	0.111	6.00
Benzo[a]pyrene	5	252.32	461	209	0.004	$7.5 \cdot 10^{-7}$	0.009	6.04
Dibenz[a,h]anthracene	5	278.36	487	218	0.0006	$4.3 \cdot 10^{-10}$	0.007	6.75
Indeno[1,2,3-cd]pyrene	5	276.34	498	233	0.0005	$1.0 \cdot 10^{-10}$	0.003	6.50
Benzo[g,h,i]perylene	6	276.34	467	218	0.0003	$1.4 \cdot 10^{-10}$	0.001	6.50

NB = number of benzene, MW = molecular weight, BP = boiling point (°C), MP = melting point (°C), WS = water solubility at 25 °C (mg L^{-1}), VT = vapor tension at 25 °C (Pa), HC = Henry's law constant (Pa·m^3/mol), logK$_{OW}$ = octanol–water partition coefficient.

Acenaphthene also has three rings, and its structure is similar to acenaphthylene, as they can be produced from each other by dehydrogenization or hydrogenization. Acenaphthene has similar properties as acenaphthylene, but acenaphthene is a more saturated compound (Stibala et al., 2019). Acenaphthene is commonly used for the production of pesticides (fungicides, insecticides), dyes, or plastics. Therefore, it could be a possible source of PAH contamination in anthropogenic soil, and many studies have been conducted to investigate the degradation of acenaphthene in soil (Mallick, 2019).

Fluorene is also a three-ring PAH compound and is sometimes named 9*H*-fluorene. Fluorene forms a white solid structure that exhibits a characteristic, aromatic odor similar to that of naphthalene. It can be synthesized from diphenylmethane by dehydrogenation, or it can be derived from coal tar (Griesbaum *et al.*, 2000). Also, its derived compounds could be used in the pharmaceutical industry or the preparation of dyes. Polymerization of fluorene produces polyfluorene polymers, which are electroluminescent (Shin *et al.*, 2006).

Phenanthrene is formed with three benzene rings, and it appears as a transparent solid or solid form of pale yellow. Phenanthrene is used in the pharmaceutical industry as well as in pesticide or dye production. Phenanthrene is usually used as a model PAH compound for bioremediation studies, as it biodegrades relatively well (Fanesi *et al.*, 2018).

Anthracene is also formed of three benzene rings and is colorless, but under the exposure of UV light, it can emit a blue fluorescence. It occurs in coal tar in an amount of 1.5% by weight. When the skin is directly exposed to anthracene or when it is ingested, it causes inflammation. Long-term exposure to anthracene causes a higher cancer risk and mutations, but it has been proven only in the case of rats so far. Nevertheless, anthracene is added to the compound list of extreme concerns of environmental threats (Griesbaum *et al.*, 2000).

Fluoranthene consists of four rings, and it is a colorless or yellow solid named after its fluorescence under UV light. It is usually present in coal tar pitch of a few percent. Fluoranthene has been confirmed as a carcinogenic compound to mice by the IARC. It is also a compound of high concern due to its toxicity and environmental persistence (Boström *et al.*, 2002).

Pyrene is a PAH compound of four benzene rings. It is very commonly used as a model PAH compound for degradation by many researchers even if it is hydrophobic, bioaccumulative, and resistant in the environment (Klankeo et al., 2009). Pyrene has not been proven as a carcinogenic compound but can stimulate the carcinogenic properties of other PAHs, such as benzo(a)pyrene. Quinones are compounds formed when pyrene is metabolized, and their metabolites are a greater threat to the biota than pyrene itself (Wei et al., 2017).

Benz(a)anthracene belongs to the group of four benzene ringed PAH compounds and is considered by IARC as a probable carcinogenic compound. It is highly acutely toxic, bioaccumulative, and a chemically stable compound. Therefore, it is recalcitrant to degradation in soil (Rachna et al., 2019).

Chrysene is formed of four benzene rings, and it is a yellow gold-colored solid compound. Its name comes from "chrȳsós," which means gold in Greek. It can usually be found bonded to tetracene in the environment. Their mixture has an orange/yellow color, but pure chrysene is colorless. Chrysene is probably carcinogenic. It could be derived from tobacco smoke, and it is also present in coal tar or creosote (Ojha et al., 2019).

Benzo(b)fluoranthene is a PAH compound consisting of 5 rings, and it is a yellow solid powder. This compound is usually present in coal tar, petrol exhausts, tobacco and cigarette smoke, and many other pyrolytic products. Benzo(b)fluoranthene is suspected to be a human carcinogen (Eisler, 2000).

Benzo(k)fluoranthene is a 5-ring yellow solid compound similar to benzo(b)fluoranthene. Like other PAHs, it is mainly formed by the incomplete combustion of organic matter and could be found in coal tar, petrol exhausts, and industrial waste products. It is industrially produced only for research purposes. As well as benzo(b)fluoranthene, it does not have a practical use, and it is also suspected to be carcinogenic to humans (Eisler, 2000).

Benzo(a)pyrene has five benzene rings, and it is classified as a human carcinogen by the IARC. Its diol epoxide metabolites bind to DNA, resulting in mutations. Therefore, this PAH compound is the most studied in the last decades. It can be found in coal tar, tobacco smoke, and many foods, especially grilled meats, as it is mainly formed from the incomplete combustion of organic matter at temperatures ranging from 300 °C to 600 °C (Guerreiro *et al.*, 2016).

Dibenz(*a*,*h*)anthracene consists of five fused benzene rings of crystalline structure, and it is present in coal tar, exhaust, and smoke. Dibenzo(*a*,*h*)anthracene is considered a mutagen, a suspected carcinogen to humans. This PAH compound is mainly used only for the investigation of tumorigenesis. (Eisler, 2000).

Indeno(1,2,3-*cd*)pyrene is a six-ring PAH compound with toxic, mutagenic, and carcinogenic properties. Due to its high molecular weight, it is highly hydrophobic and recalcitrant to degradation processes in the environment (Ojha *et al.*, 2019).

Benzo(*g*,*h*,*i*)perylene, also consisting of six rings, appears as a white or colorless solid. It has the highest molecular weight of all 16 US EPA PAHs, which causes a high persistence in the environment due to its accumulative properties. This PAH compound has no practical use, and it is often used only for analytical purposes. It has also been classified as carcinogenic and teratogenic (Griesbaum *et al.*, 2000).

12.1.3   Sources of PAHs in the Environment

The main sources of PAH are natural and anthropogenic, where anthropogenic ones (Fig. 12.3) can be seen as the most significant source of PAH forming in the last decades (Wilcke, 2000). Several ways can lead to the formation of PAHs. In general, the way in which PAHs form can affect their amount and kind. The pyrogenic way occurs when organic matter is burned at high temperatures with low or no oxygen such that pyrolysis takes place. The pyrolysis temperature usually starts from 200 °C and reaches over 1000 °C. Some examples of pyrolysis are the distillation of coal into coke or breaking petroleum into hydrocarbons with lower molecular weight. The most general source of pyrolysis is the incomplete combustion of fossil fuels in power plants or traffic. On the other hand, PAHs can also be formed during the incomplete combustion of biomass for the production of heat and electricity as well as during forest fires, which is happening at a much bigger scale in comparison to other PAH sources and is unintentional (Adams *et al.*, 2015).

Mohseni-Bandpei et al. (2019) investigated PAH formation after the combustion of medical wastes, which is commonly destroyed by pyrolysis. They concluded that fewer PAHs were formed when the particles for pyrolysis were smaller. PAHs can even be formed under lower temperatures than in pyrolysis, 100–150 °C, in processes named petrogenic. An example of a petrogenic substance is crude oil. Because crude oil is used extensively, it can get into the environment by oil spills, tank leaks, or by many machines that run on fossil fuels. The least known PAH production is the biological source. It is known that PAHs can also be formed biologically by bacteria and plants, but this is negligible in comparison to fossil fuel combustion (Ravindra et al., 2008).

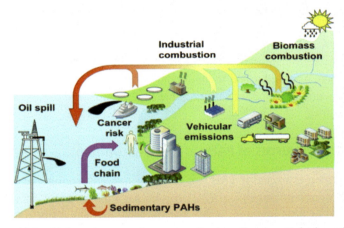

Figure 12.3 Main anthropogenic sources of polycyclic aromatic hydrocarbons in the environment (Balgobin and Singh, 2019).

All PAH origins mentioned above can be considered natural or anthropogenic. Crude oil formation, forest fires, and other natural cases of incomplete combustion, or bacterial/algal processes are natural sources, while crude oil spills, fossil fuel combustion, and other industrial combustion processes are considered anthropogenic sources (Abdel-Shafy and Mansour, 2015). The release of PAHs from these sources is mainly seasonally dependent. In winter, there is more biomass combusted, producing emissions of particulate matter containing pollutants. In summer, the major sources are forest fires and industrial processes, which are not as seasonally dependent (Han et al., 2020). Adverse conditions of burning processes, mainly known as incomplete combustion, can lead to the accumulation of PAHs in biomass ashes (Chagger *et al.*, 1998). The yields of PAHs vary considerably between the bottom and fly ashes (Košnář *et al.*, 2016). Masto *et al.* (2015) observed that the total PAH content in biomass ashes can be around 193 mg kg^{-1} at a temperature of 850 °C.

Another source of PAH formation by humans, which should not be forgotten, is food and its heat-treatment, such as grilling and baking. The amounts of PAHs formed depend on temperature, time, certain ingredients, and the food preparation method (Darwish *et al.*, 2019). PAHs are also a common part of various edible oils and flavorings (Gong *et al.*, 2019). A study published by Adesina *et al.* (2020) also takes smoking into account, as smoke contains carcinogenic PAHs. Singh *et al.* (2018) analyzed lung cancer risk among coal/coke industry workers, many of whom smoke. This leads to the suggestion that they were not able to evaluate the data satisfactorily, as smoking could be affecting them.

Ship traffic, oil spills, or urban runoffs are the main sources of water contamination by PAHs. The end sinks of water PAH contamination are river or lake sediments. PAHs found in sediments are persistent because they can be tightly sorbed on sediment organic matter, which causes immobilization of PAHs due to their physicochemical properties, like low water solubility and many others. River bottoms and swamps located downstream near urban areas or locations with frequent ship transport are examples of sediments that are highly contaminated by PAHs (Brown and Peake, 2005). Fine sediments like clay or silt usually contain lower amounts of PAHs than large-size fraction sediments because PAHs can't go through easily and have lower organic matter content (Wang *et al.*, 2001).

PAHs were also found in the snow, which can be much more easily investigated in comparison to air. PAHs present in the air do not undergo as many bioremediation processes as in soil (Birk *et al.*, 2017).

12.1.4 Emissions of PAHs in the Environment

In 2010, the estimated global anthropogenic emission of 16 PAHs was about 620 t. Carcinogenic benzo(*a*)pyrene was 3.2 t of this amount and was formed by the following sources: urban burning

76%, industrial burning 6.7%, traffic 4.3%, metal industry 3.4%, waste combustion 1.0%, and other sources 8.4% (Kim *et al.*, 2013). Newly produced PAHs by pyrolytic or petrogenic sources are emitted directly as a vapor or bonded on solid particles, also called particulate matter, to the atmosphere, from which they can be easily ingested (Ghanavati *et al.*, 2019). PAHs are hydrophobic compounds, and they have a relatively low vapor pressure; therefore, PAHs bond to particulate matter in the atmosphere. There are several differences between the vapor pressures of individual particular PAHs, meaning they present in different concentrations in vapor and sorbed to solid particles. This is also dependent on the moisture and temperature conditions of the atmosphere (Lawal, 2017). It is assumed that over 40 million people in Europe are exposed to pollutants at levels over the maximum recommended amounts (Baklanov *et al.*, 2007).

12.1.5 Soil Contamination by PAHs

The deposition of PAHs from the atmosphere occurs through their precipitation from air to the soil or water, where they can become more bioavailable, further metabolize, and accumulate in microorganisms, plants, and animals, including humans. Due to the PAH properties, PAHs tend to be accumulated only in the top layer (0–30 cm) of soil. Some PAHs can also be discharged into soil and water as leftover waste from industrial processes that have not been safely removed (Aydin *et al.*, 2017). Therefore, soils collected near urban and industrial areas were most contaminated by PAHs in the range from 1 to 10 mg kg^{-1} dry weight (dw), while natural background PAHs in the soil are 10 times lower (Wilcke, 2000).

Holoubek *et al.* (2009) focused on the presence of PAHs in forest soils, particularly at higher elevations above sea level. The PAH concentration strongly correlated with a high content of organic carbon in these soils. A high hydrophobic character and/or stable poly-condensed aromatic structures determine their sequestration to the soil particle by their sorption onto organic matter. This results in the low bioavailability of PAHs and less biodegradation in soil. Therefore, the PAH presence in soil is prolonged, which promotes the phenomenon known as "soil aging of PAHs" (Yap *et al.*, 2010). Environmental aging of PAHs leads to their accumulation in environmental media, such as agricultural soils (García-Sánchez *et al.*, 2018), river sediments (Dvořák *et al.*, 2017), and organic wastes, such as sewage sludges from wastewater treatment plants (Vácha *et al.*, 2005). Serious contamination of soil by fly ash around dumpsites has been reported by Nam *et al.* (2008). They found that the PAH content in soils of Western European countries ranged significantly from 0.009–11.2 mg kg^{-1} dw.

The content of PAHs in Central European arable soils range from 0.03 to 4.1 mg kg^{-1} dw (Maliszewska-Kordybach *et al.*, 2009). Thus, agricultural areas should receive satisfactory attention concerning PAHs contamination because the preventive limit of total PAHs is 1 mg kg^{-1} dw for arable soils in the Czech Republic (Public Notice No. 153, 2016). Nevertheless, the limit of PAH content in soils is different for many European countries. The Swedish EPA has developed generic guidelines for PAHs in soils. For sensitive land use, the limits are set to 0.3 mg kg^{-1} dw for carcinogenic PAHs (the sum of benzo(a)anthracene, chrysene, benzo(b)fluoranthene, benzo(k)fluoranthene, dibenz(a,h)anthracene, indeno(1,2,3-*cd*)pyrene) and 20 mg kg^{-1} dw for non-carcinogenic PAHs (Johansson and van Bavel, 2003). The legal limit of PAHs in organic amendments/fertilizers used in agriculture is 1–4 mg kg^{-1} dw. Furthermore, organic residues as soil amendments can be used in the United States and Canada only if the soil background PAH value is lower than 0.1 mg kg^{-1} dw (CCME, 2008; Roy *et al.*, 2018).

12.1.6 Impact of PAHs on Animal and Human Health

Research interest in environmental monitoring of PAH has increased recently because PAHs can be absorbed and assimilated by plants from the soil, water, and air and subsequently enter the food chain of animals and humans (Park *et al.*, 2012). When sorbed to particulate matter in the atmosphere, PAHs are able to travel for long distances in the atmosphere from their origin. Some studies have shown that PAHs have been observed in places very far from the place of their formation, such as polar regions or tropical forest areas. Unfortunately, the global PAH content has greatly increased in the last three decades (Kuppusamy *et al.*, 2016).

Depending on the PAH concentration and exposure length, effects can be acute or chronic. Acute symptoms are nausea, vomiting and diarrhea, eye irritation, skin irritation, and inflammation. Chronic results of long-term exposure to PAHs include mutation and damage of DNA, cancer, defects of the immune system, damage of organs, such as liver, kidney, and lungs, and asthma (Kim et al., 2013).

Concerning the harmful effects of PAHs on the environment and biota (microorganisms, plants, animals, and humans), they are proven to be toxic compounds. The toxicity of PAHs depends on many factors, like chemical structure, physicochemical properties, and environmental conditions.

Some PAHs are known to have carcinogenic, teratogenic, and mutagenic properties. According to seven US EPA PAHs, such as benz(*a*)anthracene, benzo(*a*)pyrene, benzo(*b*)fluoranthene, benzo(*k*)fluoranthene, chrysene, dibenz(*a,h*)anthracene, and indeno(1,2,3-*cd*)pyrene, they are probable human carcinogens (Gao et al., 2018). Due to their lipophilicity, they can be accumulated in lipid tissues and organs as well. PAHs can get into animals by inhalation, ingestion, or through the skin. From there, they are released into the whole animal system (Juhasz and Naidu, 2000). Due to their chemical structure, which is given by the angular arrangement of the compounds, they bind to nucleotides and also produce DNA-damaging byproducts, like quinones, diol epoxides, or radical cations of PAHs (Gao et al., 2018). Darwish et al. (2019) observed that a higher content of PAHs found in grilled meat induces mutagenesis and causes a higher production of ROS (reactive oxygen species) in cells, which could cause cell damage.

The carcinogenicity of some PAHs is the most discussed risk for animals and humans (Haritash and Kaushik, 2009). Especially, PAHs are toxic to birds and aquatic organisms as they are very sensitive to low amounts of toxic PAH, which cause tumors as well as immunity and reproductive diseases. Invertebrate organisms living in soil are not usually affected by soil PAH contamination unless the soil is contaminated by really high PAH loads (Abdel-Shafy and Mansour, 2015). A study published by Tong et al. (2018) showed that a relatively high amount of PAHs can be ingested through hand-to-mouth activities by 6- to 12-year-old children. Children are known for their bad hygienic habits and can ingest indoor solid particles or outdoor soil by their hand-to-mouth and object-to-mouth activities, where there can be high soil PAH pollution, especially in cities and urban areas. Workers that are exposed to high PAH concentrations at their workplace, like foundries, mines, and many other places, are in danger of developing skin or lung cancer (Singh *et al.*, 2018). People living in urban areas with massive traffic and air pollution are in danger of respiratory, cardiovascular, or neurological diseases (Guilbert *et al.*, 2018).

Food consumption is considered a major possibility for the entry of PAHs into the animal and human body (Domingo and Nadal, 2015). Since PAHs can be accumulated in plants, vegetables, and other crops from PAH polluted soil, one can be contaminated by their ingestion (Ray *et al.*, 2012). The PAH content in food ranges from 0.01 to 1 µg kg^{-1} dw, while in smoked food, the PAH concentration can reach up to 200 µg kg^{-1} dw (Abdel-Shafy and Mansour, 2015).

Soils are considered sinks of PAHs, and it is important to be aware when using soil for agriculture. Biota can be contaminated by PAH from all environmental media; therefore, it is crucial to keep finding ways to remove PAHs from the environment, especially from PAH-contaminated soil used in agriculture (Srogi, 2007).

12.2 Conventional Remediation of Soils Contaminated by PAHs

PAHs are considered persistent organic pollutants, and therefore, their removal from the environment, especially from the soil, is not so simple. When not intentionally using any remediation technique, they can be naturally degraded with the help of autochthonous soil microorganisms and plants, but at a very slow rate. A recent study showed that during the first year of soil contamination by PAHs, the natural PAH degradation progress is the most effective, but later, the degradation potential gradually slows down (Harmsen and Rietra, 2018).

There are several known ways of removing PAHs from contaminated areas, depending on the type of environmental media and PAH compound that needs to be removed (Sakshi, 2019). Contaminated soils can be excavated from the contaminated site, taken away, and then treated (*ex situ* remediation), for instance, by washing with mixtures of co-solvents. The soil can also undergo many other non-biological treatments, which can take place *in situ* (on a contaminated site) or *ex situ* (off a contaminated site). Overall, these remediation strategies, categorized as physical and chemical degradation, are expensive and often non-ecological (Cunningham et al., 1995).

Processes involving the effect of light radiation or heat are considered physical processes of degradation. They can occur naturally by sunlight on the surface of contaminated soils as well as artificially under laboratory conditions (Kuppusamy et al., 2016).

Chemical degradation occurs when PAHs are oxidized by various chemical reagents. Most using chemicals are ozone and Fenton's reagent the solution of hydrogen peroxide (H_2O_2) with ferrous iron (FeII) as a catalyst that is used to oxidize organic contaminants (Gan et al., 2009). The fact that chemicals used for chemical degradation are toxic for microorganisms causes that subsequent natural remediation is much slower because soil microorganisms must be re-established (Flotron et al., 2004).

Using proper chemical oxidants in a well-estimated concentration can help to catalyze the degradation of highly persistent PAHs with a high molecular weight, like benzo(a)pyrene, which can further be degraded by bacteria with high effectiveness. This remediation technique of contaminated soil by pre-oxidation, however, needs a good description of the site properties to estimate the dose of oxidants correctly (Xu et al., 2018).

Since the soil is usually still unsuitable for further agricultural use, it is advisable to recover these soils by planting low-maintenance plants and fast-growing trees, like poplars or willows (Vervaeke et al., 2001).

Following ways of PAH degradation, described below, show that the most efficient and inexpensive way could be the biological removal of PAHs (bioremediation), which provides, in general, excellent results of PAH removal from contaminated soil (Sakshi et al., 2019).

12.3 Bioremediation of Soil Contaminated by PAHs

When using plants as well as microorganisms (bacteria, fungi) for the remediation of soil or other PAH-contaminated environmental media, these techniques are collectively called bioremediation. In comparison with other remediation methods, bioremediation has several advantages. It can be seen as an environment friendly, sustainable, and relatively affordable method that produces great results (Sakshi *et al.*, 2019). In general, microorganisms in the bioremediation process alter the soil chemistry, and symbiosis can be established where fungi usually support bacteria, which can further support plants or crops growing thereby increasing nutrient bioavailability with their metabolism (Aydin *et al.*, 2017). The crucial precondition for bacteria, fungi, or plants to be able to metabolize persistent organic contaminants such as PAHs in their catabolic activity in using these xenobiotics for the mineralization as an energy source (Acevedo-Sandoval *et al.*, 2018).

Microorganisms and plants can be added artificially to the PAH-contaminated soil, which is called bioaugmentation. Another bioremediation method, biostimulation, means supporting microorganisms and plants with nutrients to achieve better growth conditions in the bioremediation process (Treu and Falandysz, 2017). Other important factors that can affect the rate at which the PAHs are removed from polluted soil involve the concentration of organic pollutants, its bioavailability, and physical and chemical properties of the site at which the bioremediation takes place, like moisture and temperature. Also, other chemicals and nutrients that are present in the soil play an important role in the bioremediation process. They establish suitable conditions for oxidation/reduction (electron acceptors like oxides of manganese and iron, nitrate, sulfate) and support microbial growth in the soil. All these basic characteristics always have to be considered since they have a strong impact on the results of any decontamination method (Adams *et al.*, 2015).

The most crucial requirement for the sufficient removal of PAHs from contaminated soil is its bioavailability to the autochthonous microorganisms and plants involved in their biodegradation. The bioavailability of PAHs in the soil is, to some extent, driven by other chemicals that are present. Ukalska-Jaruga *et al.* (2019) observed a correlation between soil organic matter (SOM) fractions and PAH concentration. SOM fractions that most influenced the bioavailability were humins and black carbon. These fractions effectively increased the sorption onto SOM, and therefore, the persistence of PAHs also increased, as they were prone to be less biodegradable. Microorganisms, plants, and higher biota can increase the bioavailability of PAHs in soil. Gomez-Eyles *et al.* (2010) found that earthworms are able to increase soil PAH mobility by over 40%, which is another factor that directly influences the bioremediation of soil on the field.

Individual PAHs mostly have different removal rates. PAH compounds containing more benzene rings are, in general, more difficult to degrade than those with less benzene rings. Recently, research has significantly progressed such that the removal of 2–4 ring PAHs has been successful, studies of 5 ring benzo(a)pyrene and other high molecular, has gradually expanded (Samanta *et al.*, 2002).

12.3.1 Phytoremediation of Soil Contaminated by PAHs

Phytoremediation can be considered the degradation of PAHs by photosynthesizing organisms, mostly higher plants. Green plants can either help to decontaminate or immobilize organic pollutants, such as PAHs, in the soil so they no longer hold an environmental risk, or plants can remove PAHs in various ways, as suggested in Fig. 12.4.

However, the contamination level must be manageable for a plant, or else it will not thrive and effectively bioremediate the soil (Cunningham *et al.*, 1995). To some extent, plants can cope with polluted soil by releasing root exudates such as amino acids, organic acids, carbohydrates, or even plant enzymes. Since contaminated soils can often also lack one or more necessary nutrients, plants tend to shift their conditions by these plant exudates and are able, for example, to attract supportive bacteria or other microorganisms or increase nutrient solubility and their bioavailability (Carvalhais *et al.*, 2010).

Individual PAH compounds have very low water solubility due to their lipophilic character. Therefore, PAHs tend to accumulate in lipid tissues very easily or can be adsorbed to the plant surface from where they get into the food chain. PAHs in the vapor state can also get in plants through stomata present on leaves. Generally, plants with larger surface areas can contain more surface-bounded PAHs. Very few surface-bound PAHs can be removed by only washing the plant; conversely, PAHs that are incorporated into lipid tissues are almost impossible to be removed. This phenomenon is called the immobilization of PAHs by plants (Srogi, 2007).

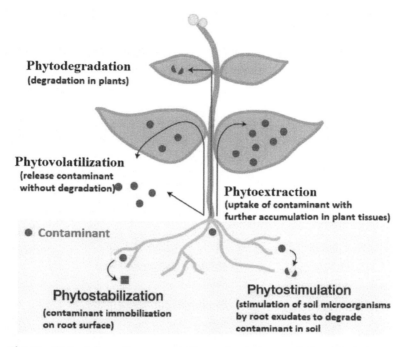

Figure 12.4 Schematic presentation of phytoremediation techniques (modified from Abdel-Shafy and Mansour, 2018).

Some organisms such as lichens can be used as information about environmental contamination and bioaccumulation of PAHs. Herzig et al. (2019) investigated selected PAHs in several lichen samples in Switzerland between 1995 and 2014. They found that the concentration of selected persistent organic pollutants, including PAHs, went down over time by 40–80% on average in all sites tested. This suggests that restrictions/regulations of these pollutants have a positive impact on the environment. Unfortunately, near roads and industrial sites, the concentration of these contaminants can even increase.

Not all PAHs are easily extractable from soil and taken up and accumulated by plants. Several plants were tested for bioremediation of PAHs in soil (Table 12.2). Only PAHs with low and medium molecular weight (2–4 ring PAHs) can be translocated from the root to the shoots through the plant transpiration stream, or they can be bounded in lipid tissues. Higher molecular weight PAHs (5–6 ring

PAHs) are usually adsorbed onto the outer layer of plant roots. A study focused on the uptake of PAHs by using plants such as maize, sunflower, and fast-growing trees of poplars and willows support the facts mentioned above. The plants were grown on fertilized PAH polluted soil for two years, after which they were harvested and further analyzed for the PAH content. The study concluded that PAHs were most efficiently absorbed by willow roots. Phenanthrene was accumulated even in above-ground biomass, while pyrene was only found in the roots (Kacálková and Tlustoš, 2010).

Table 12.2 The most common plants used in the phytoremediation of PAHs in soil (Gan et al., 2009; Kacálková and Tlustoš, 2010; Košnář et al., 2020)

Anethum graveolens L.	Melilotus officinalis Lam.
Avena barbata Pott.	Myriophyllum aquaticum Verdc.
Avena sativa L.	Oryza sativa L.
Bidens frondosa L.	Panicum bisulcatum Thunb.
Brassica napus L.	Panicum virgatum L.
Cucurbita pepo L. ssp. pepo	Phragmitis australis Adans.
Cynodon dactylon L.	Pinus banskiana Lamb.
Dactylis glomerate L.	Populus nigra x P. maximowiczii Henry.
Digitaria ciliaris Koeler.	Mimosa monancistra Benth.
Festuca arundinacea Schreb.	Pueraria lobata Willd.
Festuca rubra L.	Raphanus sativus L.
Helianthus annuus L.	Salix × smithiana Willd.
Lolium multiflorum Lam.	Schizachyrium scoparium Nash.
Lolium perenne L.	Spinacia oleracea L.
Lotus corniculatus L.	Trifolium pretense L.
Lupinus polyphyllus Lindl.	Trifolium repens L.
Medicago sativa L.	Zea mays L.

Another study showed that spinach as the experimental plant in the bioremediation of PAHs in soil was successful in the uptake of PAH from contaminated soil. Therefore, there is a high risk of PAH biomagnification through the ingestion of spinach biomass cultivated on PAH polluted soil (Chen et al., 2019).

The influence of PAHs on plants varies. In most cases, they inhibit their growth, due to their negative impact on seed germination and ability to affect the growth of plant tissues and therefore, the whole plant biomass. In a recent study, when *Lolium perenne* was exposed to soil contaminated by a PAH mixture, it showed a decrease in biomass yield in comparison to the control and *Medicago sativa* (Afegbuy and Batty, 2018).

Aranda *et al.* (2013) established an experiment to investigate whether soil PAHs can inhibit the root growth of plants in association with fungi. They studied four different individual PAH compounds in the soil in which carrots were planted (*Daucus carota* L.), which they colonized with *Rhizophagus custos*. After 7 weeks, root colonization, soil PAH content, and root dry weight were analyzed, and it was found that mycorrhizal fungi stimulated root growth by 30–40%. Surprisingly, anthracene had no effect at all, but phenanthrene inhibited root growth by 60% with a concentration of 60 µmol L^{-1}. When doubling the concentration, root growth was reduced to 80–92%.

Many species of grasses and legumes and even fast-growing trees such as poplars and willows are capable of not only accumulation but also biodegradation of PAHs (Mueller and Shann, 2006). Plants can be used directly in large fields (*in situ*) with surface contamination where other remediation approaches would not be as suitable, economical, or ecological. Besides that, plants always co-exist and cooperate with other organisms like bacteria and fungi, and are also able to remove organic pollutants, such as PAHs. Enzymes released by plant roots were identified as dehalogenases, nitro-reductases, and ligninolytic extracellular peroxidases and laccases. These enzymes usually catalyze several reactions in soil, which lead to the degradation of PAHs. Since these enzymes get secreted off the roots into the contaminated soil and function outside of the plant in the rhizosphere, enzymes can operate even after the plant dies or has been harvested (Haritash and Kaushik, 2009).

Overall, it has been concluded that planted soils usually show a higher removal rate of PAHs than contaminated soils with no plants by 30–40% (Reilley *et al.*, 1996). This can be supported by the study by Han *et al.* (2016). In that study, they used ryegrass for the phytoremediation of soil contaminated by petroleum hydrocarbons. The amount of organic pollutants in the soil was reduced by nearly 30%. The study also showed that adding biochar as a soil amendment did not significantly enhance the removal of the pollutant. Nevertheless, using ryegrass significantly helped to bioremediate contaminated soils by petroleum hydrocarbons.

In another study, four Korean plant species were used in an 80-day experiment for the bioremediation of selected soil PAHs. At the end of the experiment, the phenanthrene content was reduced in the soil by 99%, and the pyrene content decreased by up to 94%, which was significantly higher than in unplanted soil (Lee *et al.*, 2007).

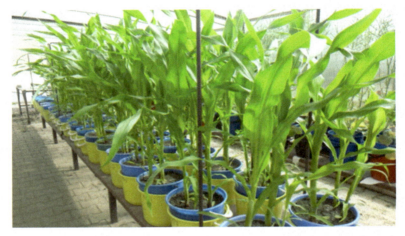

Figure 12.5 Phytoremediation of soil amended with biomass fly ash contaminated by PAHs using maize (photo by Košnář, 2018).

Košnář *et al.* (2018) conducted a 120-day pot experiment to compare the ability of natural attenuation and phytoremediation using maize (*Zea mays* L.) to remove PAHs from soil amended with PAHs-contaminated biomass fly ash (Fig. 12.5). The PAH removal from ash-treated soil was also compared with artificially PAH-contaminated soil. The removal of individual PAHs from the soil ranged from 4.8–87.8% within the experiment. The natural attenuation of soil led to a negligible total PAH removal. Phytoremediation was the most efficient approach for PAH removal, while the highest removal was observed in the case of ash-treated soil. The content of low molecular weight PAHs and the total PAHs in this treatment significantly decreased over the entire experiment by 47.6% and 29.4%, respectively. The tested level of 1600 µg PAH kg^{-1}

soil dw had no adverse effects on maize growth or the biomass yield. In addition, the PAHs were detected only in maize roots, and their bioaccumulation factors were significantly lower than 1, suggesting very negligible PAH uptake from soil by maize roots. The results showed that PAHs originating from ash were similarly susceptible to the removal of PAHs from artificially contaminated soil. The presence of maize significantly boosted the PAH removal from the soil, and its aboveground biomass did not represent any environmental risk.

In another study by Košnář and Tlustoš (2018), phytoremediation using maize assisted by compost or vermicompost amendments was the most appropriate treatment for the bioremediation of soil contaminated by PAHs derived from biomass fly ash. A higher removal of low molecular weight PAHs than medium and high molecular weight PAHs within the same treatment were observed. The total PAH content in the planted soil with compost or vermicompost decreased in a range between 62.9–64.9%. There were no significant differences between the compost and vermicompost amendments on the total removal of ash-borne PAHs. The PAH content derived by ash did not have an adverse effect on maize cultivation and the yield of maize biomass. The contribution of PAH removal by maize roots on total PAH removal from soil was negligible. This led to the suggestion that maize significantly boosted PAH removal only in bulk soil. The harvested maize shoots did not represent any environmental risk, as the PAH content was below 10 µg kg^{-1} dw.

Using fast-growing trees of willows (*Salix viminalis* L. 'Orm') has also proven to be effective in the bioremediation of PAHs in soil. In a 1.5 year experiment, willows helped remove PAHs from the soil as well as oils and heavy metals. In this study, PAHs in soil decreased significantly in comparison to the bare soil, while removal of oils and heavy metals was not significant (Vervaeke et al., 2003).

In a study by Košnář et al. (2020), a three-year experiment was conducted to investigate the use of willows of *Salix × smithiana* Willd. in the phytoremediation of soil contaminated by PAHs of ash origin (Fig. 12.6). The total removal of ash PAHs in the phytoremediation was 50.9%, while the ash PAHs were removed in natural attenuated soil by 9.9%. Low and medium molecular weight ash and spiked PAHs were susceptible to be removed at higher rates than PAHs with a high molecular weight. Lower bioaccumulation factors of 16 PAHs were observed in shoots than in roots of willow plants.

Relative removal of PAHs by *Salix × smithiana* in phytoremediation was significantly less than 1%, suggesting that the contribution of *Salix × smithiana* to extract PAHs from soil was negligible, and the PAH degradation occurred mainly in soil. Phytoremediation using *Salix × smithiana* could be seen as feasible and environmentally friendly bioremediation of arable soils impacted by PAH contaminated biomass fly ash.

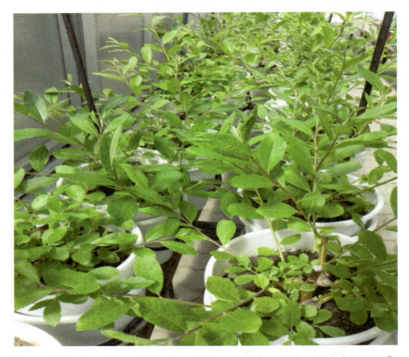

Figure 12.6 Long-term phytoremediation of soil amended with biomass fly ash contaminated by PAHs using willows (photo by Košnář, 2020).

A study by Bandowe *et al.* (2019) showed that using plant combinations involved in PAH biodegradation is very effective. A more diverse combination of plants supports the soil microbiome more effectively, especially bacteria; therefore, the PAH content in soil decreases faster. Another way to deal with high toxicity for plants when soil contamination loads are high is to alter the plant composition by using favorable plant species that grow well together and support the growth of the microbiome in the soil. In the work by

Xie *et al.* (2018), bristle grass and alfalfa were used separately and together as well. When plants were grown separately, the growth of both plants was significantly inhibited by the soil contaminant, but when grown together, the bacterial activity and contaminant removal were significantly boosted.

Using plants to help stabilize and remove PAHs has shown a great potential for bioremediation of contaminated soil. Besides PAH biodegradation, plants enhance nutrients in the soil and provide surface coverage, further improving the soil quality and environment. However, this strategy could have many disadvantages as well, one of these is the fact, that there are different results in greenhouse experiments (*ex situ* phytoremediation) and on the field (*in situ* phytoremediation). The reasons for these differences are not always discovered (Gerhardt *et al.*, 2008).

Another disadvantage is the relatively low speed of soil decontamination as well as sensitivity to the concentration of pollutants in the soil because, at some concentrations, the plants stop growing when the soil is heavily contaminated. Phytoremediation of soil also showed the greatest potential when combined with other bioremediation approaches. Therefore, soil phytoremediation is often combined with bioaugmentation of bacteria, fungi, and organic waste materials containing microorganisms involved in PAH biodegradation and many others (Gerhardt *et al.*, 2008).

12.3.2 Bacterial Remediation of Soil Contaminated by PAHs

Bacteria are known to accept PAHs as their source of energy. By rule, PAH compounds with a lower number of aromatic rings are degraded more easily than high molecular weight PAHs containing more than 4 benzene rings. Highly PAH-contaminated soils also possess higher numbers of bacteria and show a higher removal activity than soils with lower concentrations of organic pollutants such as PAHs. Since different PAHs have different solubility in water, some PAHs become bioavailable more easily in soil solution than others, which mainly depends on their molecular weight. In Table 12.3, a list of the main bacteria to use for bioremediation of PAHs is shown (Cerniglia, 1993).

Table 12.3 List of selected polycyclic aromatic hydrocarbons utilizing bacteria (Cerniglia, 1993)

Acinetobacter calcoaceticus	Vibrio sp.
Acinetobacter sp.	Agmenellum quadruplicatum
Aeromonas sp.	Anabaena sp.
Alcaligenes denitrificans	Amphora sp.
Alcahgenes faecalis	Aphanocapsa sp.
Arthrobacter pomogenes	Chlorella autotrophica
Bacillus cereus	Chlorella sorokiniana
Beijerinckia sp.	Chlamydomonas angulosa
Corynebacterium renale	Coccochloris elabens
Flavobacterium sp.	Cylindrotheca sp.
Micrococcus sp.	Dunahella tertiolecta
Moraxella sp.	Nlicrocoleus chthonoplastes
Mycobacterium sp.	Navicula sp.
Nocardia sp.	Nitzschia sp.
Pseudomonas cepacia	Nostoc sp.
Pseudomonas fluorescens	Oscdlatoria sp. (strain JCM)
Pseudomonas paucimobilis	Oscillatona sp. (strain MEV)
Pseudomonas putlda	Porphyridium cruentum
Pseudomonas testeroni	Selenastrum capricomutum
Pseudomonas vesicularis	Synedra sp.
Rhodococcus sp.	Ulva fasciata
Staphylococcus auriculans	Streptomyces sp.
Streptomyces griseus	Vibrio sp.

The mechanism that bacteria are using for the degradation of PAHs differs for aerobic and anaerobic bacteria. Aerobic processes of PAH degradation, which are more common for the soil environment, are shown in Fig. 12.7. In general, aerobic degradation of PAHs starts with the oxidation of aromatic ring(s) using dioxygenases or cytochrome P_{450} monooxygenases through PAH intermediates such as arene oxides, phenols, and dihydrodiols, to carbon dioxide and water or several PAH conjugates (glucosides, glucuronides, sulfates, etc.) (Bamforth and Singleton, 2005).

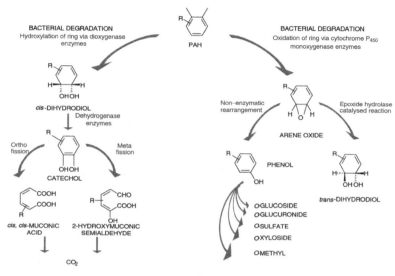

Figure 12.7 The main pathways for polycyclic aromatic hydrocarbon degradation by bacteria (modified from Bamforth and Singleton, 2005).

Bacterial degradation of PAHs has been extensively studied in the last decades. The time that the PAHs remain in the soil also affects their desorption speed. When PAHs are bioavailable for bacteria, their effectiveness in degradation can be very large, thus up to the total amount of PAHs can be removed. In a recent study, the bacterium *Bacillus kochii* was used in the bioremediation of soil contaminated by phenanthrene in relation to the influence of soil salinity on bacteria. The phenanthrene concentration of 50 mg kg^{-1} dw with 1.5% salinity was removed by 98%. When soil salinity was increased, the PAH degradation efficiency decreased (Feizi et al., 2019).

Many studies have been focused on finding bacterial genes responsible for soil PAH degradation to control catabolic pathways during its degradation more precisely and to be able to effectively assume PAH metabolites formed during the degradation (Habe and Omori, 2014).

An interesting and very promising way to effectively use bacteria for bioremediation of PAH-contaminated soil is to use genetically modified bacterial strains to enhance their ability to degrade PAH. In some cases, bacteria allow complete degradation of organic compounds; for example, modified *Pseudomonas putida* can metabolize benzene, toluene, and *p*-xylene with no metabolic intermediates. The disadvantages of this bioremediation approach are ethical aversions towards genetically modified organisms (GMO) as well as insufficient data to distinguish between the degradation impact of GMO bacteria on their own and the whole microbiome of contaminated soil because these results often remain unclear (Adams *et al.*, 2015). For instance, the biodegradation of benzo(*a*) pyrene, as suggested by Nzila *et al.* (2021), is shown in Fig. 12.8.

The combination of more bacterial strains capable of PAH biodegradation into one consortium has also been proven to be beneficial. In a recent study, three different bacterial strains were used for biodegradation of chrysene, which is a very recalcitrance PAH compound to its complete mineralization. The combined bacterial consortium removed and mineralized chrysene very effectively even in the presence of other PAHs and heavy metals (Vaidya *et al.*, 2018).

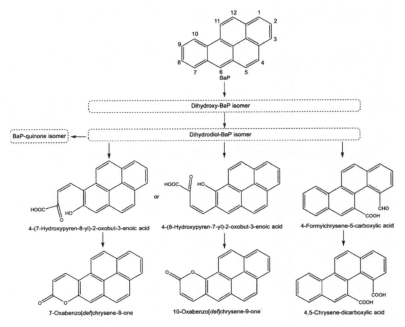

Figure 12.8 Suggested pathways for the biodegradation of carcinogenic benzo(*a*)pyrene by bacteria *Staphylococcus haemoliticus* strain 10SBZ1A (Nzila, 2021).

The rhizosphere is a soil environment near plant roots where bacteria and roots cooperate. It provides perfect conditions for PAH biodegradation. In fact, most of the PAH biodegradation in planted soil takes place there. Many extracellular enzymes can be released by plants roots, which make PAHs in the soil more bioavailable to the soil microbiome. On the other hand, bacteria present in the soil make soil nutrients more available for plant intake, making all soil organisms more prosperous (Kotoky et al., 2017).

12.3.3 Mycoremediation of Soil Contaminated by PAHs

Mycoremediation means using fungi (Table 12.4) cultivated on organic substrates (Fig. 12.9) in the bioremediation of soil. Mycoremediation of PAH-contaminated soil can be seen as a cost-effective and environment-friendly approach, as well as in cooperation with other bioremediation techniques like phytoremediation or bioaugmentation (Li et al., 2012).

Table 12.4 List of selected ligninolytic and non-ligninolytic fungi used in the mycoremediation of soil contaminated by PAHs (Acevedo et al., 2011; Cerniglia, 1993; Novotný et al., 2004; Ting et al., 2011)

Ligninolytic Fungi	Non-ligninolytic Fungi
Phanerochaete chrysosporium Burds.	*Aspergillus niger* Tiegh.
Trametes versicolor (L.) Lloyd	*Candida tropicalis* (Castell.) Berkhout
Pleurotus ostreatus (Jacq. ex Fr.) P. Kumm.	*Chrysosporium pannorum* (Link) S. Hughes
Irpex lacteus (Fr.) Fr.	*Cunninghamella elegans* Lendn.
Coriolopsis polyzona (Pers.) Ryv.	*Gliocladium* Corda
Bjerkandera adusta (Willd.) P. Karst.	*Mortierella verrucosa* Linnem.
Anthracophyllum discolor (Mont.) Singer	*Neurospora crassa* Shear & B.O. Dodge
Pycnoporus cinnabarinus (Jacq.) P. Karst.	*Penicillium* Link
Ganoderma lucidum (Curtis) P. Karst.	*Trichoderma viride* Pers.
Naematoloma frowardii (Speg.) E. Horak	*Rhizoctonia solani* J.G. Kühn

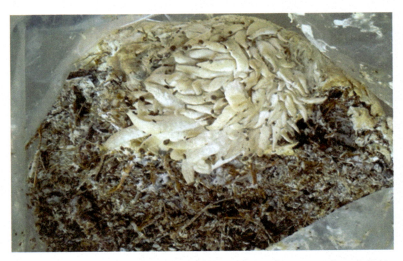

Figure 12.9 Ligninolytic fungi of *Pleurotus ostreatus* grown on a wood chip substrate (photo by Košnář, 2019).

Compared to bacteria, fungi do not use PAHs as their carbon and energy source. Instead, fungi break PAH compounds into simple and less toxic compounds by their enzymes as a side effect of fungi metabolism. Fungi species can be sorted into two main groups, ligninolytic and non-ligninolytic, and both fungi groups can oxidize PAHs, though the ligninolytic fungi are much more effective in PAH degradation. Therefore, most studies have focused on them (Cerniglia, 1993). Nevertheless, there have been some works where fungi were grown in contaminated soil under very low oxygen conditions using PAHs as a sole carbon source (Silva *et al.*, 2008). However, the number of fungi strains that can grow under these extreme conditions is very low (Aydin *et al.*, 2017). The activity of fungal enzymes varies slightly among different species of fungi and is mostly affected by the physical and chemical properties of the soil. High humidity, low pH, and temperature are the main factors affecting how fast and whether fungal enzymes will be active (Tuor *et al.*, 1995).

One of the strongest advantages of fungi, which makes them often more appropriate for PAH biodegradation than bacteria or plants, is the ability to access soil pores with their mycelium. Fungi mycelium can relocate sources and solve more complex issues like mechanical obstacles in the soil or local lack of nutrients (Treu and Falandysz, 2017).

Some non-ligninolytic fungi (Table 12.4), such as *Ascomycetes* and *Zygomycetes*, can remove highly persistent benzo(*a*)pyrene more effectively than bacteria. These fungi species grow well at neutral pH, and therefore, they could be a good option in a field condition. However, their metabolic pathways are not well known. Not much research has been focused on their metabolites and their possible effects on the soil environment; thus, further research needs to be conducted (Marco-Urrea *et al.*, 2015).

Ligninolytic fungi can be sorted into two main groups, brown rot and white rot fungi, which are the only ones able to decompose organic polymers like lignin (Rabinovich *et al.*, 2003). White rot fungi produce highly nonspecific ligninolytic enzymes, such as lignin peroxidases, laccases, or manganese peroxidases; therefore, they are also capable of PAH degradation (Aydin *et al.*, 2017; Haritash and Kaushik, 2009). Laccases work as catalysts for the initial reaction, which leads to the formation of quinones - PAH derivatives, which can be further oxidized by peroxidases and then completely mineralized (Pozdnyakova *et al.*, 2018). These ligninolytic enzymes are extracellular, which means that they can easily access pollutants with low bioavailability. The contaminated soil is usually enhanced by the media containing lignin, like milled wood used as feed by fungi, to support its growth during bioremediation using fungi (Pickard *et al.*, 1999). The metabolic pathways of PAH degradation by ligninolytic and non-ligninolytic fungi are suggested in Fig. 12.10.

However, about half of the fungal strains can produce a high concentration of persistent metabolite anthraquinone within the biodegradation of anthracene. A lower concentration of PAH metabolites or none at all were produced in the degradation of benzo(*a*)pyrene (Fig. 12.11). Several PAH metabolites during the bioremediation of PAH-contaminated soil were not estimated. For instance, oxygenated derivatives of PAHs can be formed during the incomplete combustion of organic matter, but they can occur as metabolites of PAHs (Lundstedt *et al.*, 2007).

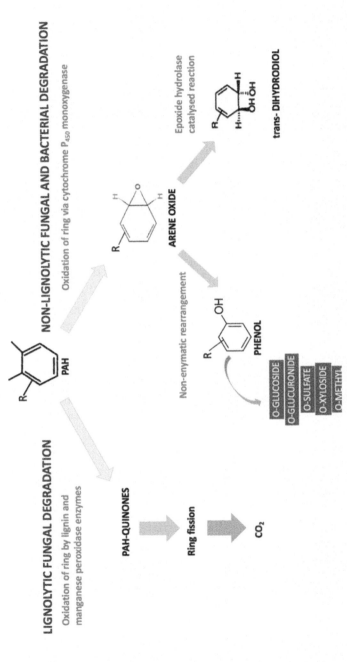

Figure 12.10 Main pathways for polycyclic aromatic hydrocarbon degradation by fungi (Aydin et al., 2017).

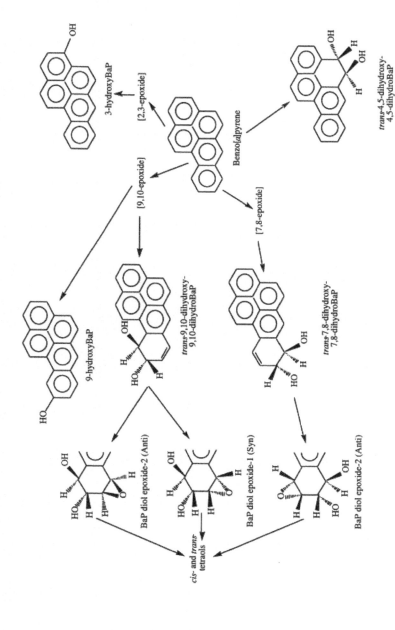

Figure 12.11 Fungal biodegradation products of benzo(*a*)pyrene as suggested by Juhasz and Naidu (2000).

Pozdnyakova *et al.* (2018) analyzed ligninolytic enzymes secreted by *Pleurotus ostreatus* and *Agaricus bisporus* in soil with the presence of 3-ring PAHs, where *P. ostreatus* produced both laccase and peroxidase enzymes, which are considered to be more efficient in PAH degradation, concerning the metabolites of PAHs. They found that when only laccase was present in the soil, the PAH metabolites were accumulated rather than further enzymatically biodegraded. Further degradation occurred if both laccase and peroxidase enzymes were present in the soil together, making *P. ostreatus* more suitable for fungal remediation. In another study, Pozdnyakova *et al.* (2016) focused on the biodegradation and metabolites of fluorene and fluoranthene during mycoremediation using *P. ostreatus*. The results showed a similar trend, where laccase and peroxidase subsequently helped to oxidize initial PAHs as well as their metabolites.

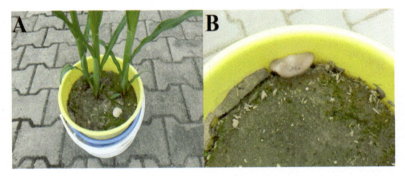

Figure 12.12 Mycoremediation assisted phytoremediation (A) and only mycoremediation of PAH contaminated soil by *P. ostreatus* (photo by Košnář, 2019).

Košnář *et al.* (2019) established a 120-days experiment to compare the removal of PAHs from agricultural soil by natural attenuation, phytoremediation, mycoremediation, and plant-assisted mycoremediation approaches (Fig. 12.12) in relation to the extracellular enzyme activities in soil. The PAH removal by natural attenuation was negligible. Phytoremediation using maize enhanced only the removal of low and medium molecular PAHs. The *P. ostreatus* cultivated on a 30–50 mm wood chip substrate used in mycoremediation was the most successful in removing the majority of the PAHs. Therefore, a total removal of PAHs of 36% was observed. When using the same fungal substrate together with maize in plant-assisted mycoremediation of soil, the removal of total PAHs was not statistically different from the previous soil mycoremediation. However, the combination of phytoremediation with mycoremediation boosted fungal biomass, microbial, and manganese peroxidase activity in soil significantly, which strongly correlated with the removal of total PAHs in soil.

Acevedo-Sandoval *et al.* (2018) studied the degradation of 10 different PAHs in a bioremediation experiment using *P. ostreatus* and *Ochrobactrum intermedium*. When the PAH-contaminated soil was amended by these fungi, fluoranthene, indene(1,2,3-*cd*)pyrene, and benzo(*g,h,i*)perylene were completely removed after 50, 80, and 50 days, respectively. Other PAHs in the mixture also decreased significantly after 110 days of the experiment, with the following removal efficiency: anthracene by 96%, pyrene by 86%, chrysene by 98%, and benzo(*a*)anthracene by 98%. The experiment also included treatments with both organisms tested separately, but the results showed that they are more efficient in PAH removal when they are used in a mixture.

In another study, the ability of fungi of *P. ostreatus* to remove PAHs in mycoremediation of soil was tested and compared to the natural attenuation of soil by naturally present bacterial colonies. *P. ostreatus* was able to significantly remove PAHs and also to support the bacterial growth, further helping with bioremediation. The removal rates of PAHs obtained in this experiment showed that low molecular weight PAHs were removed from the soil more easily. PAHs were dissipated in the soil as follows: 86–96% of 2-ring PAHs, 63–72% of 3-ring PAHs, 32–49% of 4-ring PAHs, and 31–38% of 5 and 6-ring PAHs (Byss *et al.*, 2008).

An aged creosote-contaminated soil is often recalcitrant to bioremediation by plants or bacteria due to unfavorable living conditions for these organisms. However, a work presented by Eggen and Majcherczyk (1997) showed that, in this case, using ligninolytic fungi can be a successful bioremediation approach. In their experiment, aged benzo(*a*)pyrene was removed by 28% in the first month of the mycoremediation of soil using *P. ostreatus* and spiked benzo(*a*)pyrene was reduced by 40% after the same time. At the end of the experiment, only 1% of benzo(*a*)pyrene was completely mineralized to CO_2, which was nearly 10 times more than in the unamended soil with no *P. ostreatus*.

Several different approaches of bioremediation of creosote-contaminated soil, such as natural bacterial bioremediation, biostimulation, or mycoremediation using *P. ostreatus*, were compared by García-Delgado *et al.* (2014). The mycoremediation of soil was the most efficient bioremediation strategy of PAHs in soil. The mycoremediation of soil showed the highest microbial growth. Only the mycoremediation of soil using *P. ostreatus* achieved a lower PAH content in the soil, which was below the level required by the Spanish legislation for contaminated soils.

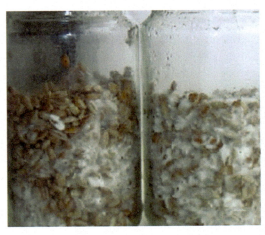

Figure 12.13 Cultivation of ligninolytic fungi *C. leave* on barley seeds (photo by Košnář, 2018).

A pot experiment was conducted by García-Sánchez *et al.* (2018) to comparatively evaluate four different strategies, including natural attenuation, mycoremediation by using *Crucibulum leave*, phytoremediation using maize plants, and phytoremediation assisted mycoremediation using *C. leave*, for the bioremediation of an aged PAH contaminated soil after 180 days. *C. leaves* were cultivated on barley seeds, further serving as a soil amendment (Fig. 12.13). The phytoremediation approach removed 2–3 and 4 ring PAHs significantly higher than natural attenuation and mycoremediation strategies. However, the largest decrease in the 4, 5–6 rings PAHs occurred after the phytoremediation was combined with mycoremediation. Sixteen PAHs, except fluorene and dibenzo[*a,h*]anthracene, were found in maize roots, whereas naphthalene, phenanthrene, anthracene, fluoranthene, and pyrene were accumulated in the shoots in both phytoremediation and phytoremediation assisted mycoremediation treatments. A higher PAH content in maize biomass was accumulated during the combination of phytoremediation and mycoremediation treatment than in the phytoremediation treatment without *C. leaves*. The bioaccumulation and translocation factors were significantly less than 1, indicating that phytostabilization of PAHs on maize roots or phytodegradation in plant cells occurred rather than phytoextraction of PAHs from the soil. The microbial biomass, activity, and ergosterol content were significantly boosted in the microbial-assisted phytoremediation treatment in comparison to the other treatments after 180 days.

The results described above suggest that ligninolytic white-rot fungi are successful in the removal of PAHs. However, some studies have suggested that when the initial PAH content was about 500 mg kg^{-1} dw, the fungi remain in an inactive state, while bacteria involved in biodegradation can keep growing. Also, the soil containing fungi solely with no or low bacteria colonies does not create a favorable environment for fungi to remove PAHs effectively (Canet *et al.*, 2000).

Winquist *et al.* (2013) compared PAH bioremediation by fungi and bacteria in laboratory and field conditions. In laboratory conditions, most of the PAH removal was caused by fungi, but in field experiments by bacteria. More work in field conditions still needs to be conducted because the differences between laboratory and *in situ* field bioremediation experiments are often non-negligible.

12.4 Conclusions

We have elucidated that the biodegradation of PAHs in soils is achievable with plant and microbial metabolism. The examples mentioned above show that relying on autochthonous microorganisms in PAH degradation was not as reliable, as the bioremediation treatments were generally more efficient than the control. Some authors reported that phytoremediation could promote microbial growth and degradation of PAHs in soil rather than the accumulation of PAHs by plants. Some authors reported that the presence of organic waste materials in soil enhanced the phytoremediation of soil PAHs. Many authors showed that amended soils by bacteria and fungi can serve as biocatalysts, which lead to the degradation of PAHs in soil. In addition, some authors investigated a combination of bioremediation approaches to further enhance the potential of more robust technology. Therefore, these studies provide novel evidence that microbe-assisted phytoremediation could be an environmentally sound management approach for the treatment of soils contaminated by PAHs. However, further research is required to develop potential *in situ* bioremediation technologies that will be effective and successful, especially in the removal of high molecular weight PAHs in field conditions.

Acknowledgment

This work was supported by the Czech Ministry of Agriculture (QK1710379) and by the European Regional Development Fund (project NUTRISK no. CZ.02.1.01/0.0/0.0/16_019/0000845). The contribution of authors to this chapter is as follows: Zdeněk Košnář (85%), Johanka Wernerová (5%), Petr Frühbauer (5%), and Pavel Tlustoš (5%).

References

Acevedo F., Pizzul L., del Pilar Castillo M., Cuevas R., Diez M. C. *J. Hazard. Mater.*, **185** (2011), 212–219.

Acevedo-Sandoval O., Gutiérrez-Alcantara E. J., Perez-Balan R., Rodriguez-Vázquez G., Zamorategui-Molina A., Tirado-Torres D. *Appl. Ecol. Environ. Res.*, **16** (2018), 3815–3829.

Adams G. O., Fufeyin P. T., Okoro S. E., Ehinomen I. *Int. J. Environ. Bioremediat. Biodegrad.*, **3** (2015), 28–39.

Adesina O. A., Nwogu A. S., Sonibare J. A. *Ecotox. Environ. Safe.*, **208** (2020), 111604.

Abdel-Shafy H. I., Mansour M. S. M. Phytoremediation for the elimination of metals, pesticides, PAHs, and other pollutants from wastewater and soil, in *Phytobiont and Ecosystem Restitution*, Springer, Singapore, 2018.

Abdel-Shafy H. I., Mansour M. S. M. *Egypt. J. Pet.*, **25** (2015), 107–123.

Afegbuya S. L., Batty L. C. *Environ. Sci. Pollut. Res.*, **25** (2018), 18596–18603.

Agoun-Bahar S., Djebbar R., Achour T. N., Abrous-Belbachir O. *Environ. Technol.*, **40** (2019), 3713–3723.

Andersson J. T., Achten, C. *Polycycl. Aromat. Compd.*, **35** (2015), 330–354.

Aranda E., Scervino J. M., Godoy P., Reina R., Ocampo J. A., Wittich R. M., García-Romera I. *Environ. Pollut.*, **181** (2013), 182–189.

Aydin S., Karaçay H. A., Shahi A., Gökçe S., Ince B., Ince O. *Fungal Biol. Rev.*, **31** (2017), 61–72.

Baklanov A., Hänninen O., Slørdal L. H., Kukkonen J., Bjergene N., Fay B., Finardi S., Hoe S. C., Jantunen M., Karppinen A., Rasmussen A., Shouloudis A., Sokhi R. S., Sørensen J. H., Ødegaard V. *Atmos. Chem. Phys.*, **7** (2007), 855–874.

Balgobin A., Singh N. R. *Sci. Total Environ.*, **664** (2019), 474–486.

Bamforth S. M., Singleton I. *J. Chem. Technol. Biotechnol.*, **80** (2005), 723–736.

Bandowe B. A. M., Leimer S., Meusel H., Velescu A., Dassen S., Eusenhauer N., Hoffmann T., Oelmann Y., Wilcke W. *Soil Biol. Biochem.*, **129** (2019), 60–70.

Bignal K. L., Langridge S., Zhou J. L. *Atmos. Environ.*, **42** (2008), 8863–8871.

Birk S. J., Cho S., Taylor E., Yi Y., Gibson Y. Y. *Sci. Total Environ.*, **603–604**, 570–583.

Boström C. E., Gerde P., Hanberg A., Jernstrom B., Johansson C., Kyrklund T., Rannug A., Tornqvist M., Victorin K., Westerholm R. *Environ. Health Perspect.*, **110** (2002), 451–488.

Brown J. N., Peake B. M. *Sci. Total Environ.*, **359** (2005), 145–155.

Byss M., Elhottová D., Tříska J., Baldrian P. *Chemosphere*, **73** (2008), 1518–1523.

CCME *Canadian Soil Quality Guidelines*, **229** (2008), 9781896997797.

Canet R., Birnstingl J. G., Malcolm D. G., Lopez-Real J. M., Beck A. J. *Bioresour. Technol.* **76** (2000), 113–117.

Carvalhais L. C., Dennis P. G., Fedoseyenko D., Hajirezaei M. R., Borriss R., von Wirén N. *J. Plant Nutr. Soil Sci.*, **174** (2011), 3–11.

Cerniglia C. E. *Curr. Opin. Biotechnol.*, **4** (1993), 331–338.

Cunningham S. D., Berti W. R., Huang J. W. *Trends Biotechnol.*, **13** (1995), 393–397.

Chagger H. K., Kendall A., McDonald A., Pourkashanian M., Williams A. *Appl. Energy*, **60** (1998), 101–114.

Chen J., Xia X., Wang H., Zhai Y., Xi N., Lin H., Wen W. *J. Hazard. Mater.*, **379** (2019), 120831.

Darwish W. S., Chiba H., El-Ghareeb W. R., Elhelaly A. E., Hui S. *Food Chem.*, **290** (2019), 114–124.

Domingo J. L., Nadal M. *Food Chem. Toxicol.*, **86** (2018), 144–153.

Dvořák T., Száková J., Vondráčková S., Košnář Z., Holečková Z., Najmanová J., Tlustoš P. *Soil Sediment Contam.*, **26** (2017), 584–604.

Eisler R. Polycyclic aromatic hydrocarbons, in *Handbook of Chemical Risk Assessment: Health Hazards to Humans, Plants, and Animals, Organics vol. 2*, Lewis Publishers, Boca Raton, Florida, 2000.

Eggen T., Majcherczyk A. *Int. Biodeterior. Biodegrad.*, **41** (1997), 111–117.

Fanesi A., Zegeye A., Mustin C., Cébron A. *Front. Microbiol.*, **9** (2018), 2999.

Field J. A., de Jong E., Costa G. F., de Bont J. A. M. *Appl. Environ. Microbiol.* **58** (1992), 2219–2226.

Feizi R., Jorfi S., Takdastan A. *Environ. Eng. Manag. J.*, **7** (2019), 23–30.

Flotron V., Delteil C., Padellec Y., Camel V. *Chemosphere*, **59** (2004), 1427–1437.

Frenklach M., Clary D. W., Gardiner Jr., W. C., Stein S. E. *Symp. (Int.) on Combust.*, **20** (1985), 885–901.

Gan S., Lau E. V., Ng H. K. *J. Hazard. Mater.*, **172** (2009), 532–549.

Gao P., de Silva E., Hou L., Denslow N. D., Xiang P., Ma L. Q. *Environ. Int.*, **119** (2018), 466–477.

García-Delgado C., Alfaro-Barta I., Eymar E. *J. Hazard. Mater.*, **285** (2014), 259–266.

García-Sánchez M., Košnář Z., Mercl F., Aranda E., Tlustoš P. *Ecotoxicol. Environ. Saf.*, **147** (2018), 165–174.

Gerhardt K. E., Huang X. D., Glick B. R., Greenberg B. M. *Plant Sci.*, **176** (2008), 20–30.

Ghanavati N., Nazarpour A., Watts M. J. *Catena*, **177** (2019), 246–259.

Gomez-Eyles J. L., Sizmur T., Collins C. D., Hodson M. E. *Environ. Pollut.*, **159** (2010), 616–622.

Gong G., Wu S., Wu X. *LWT – Food. Sci. Technol.*, **116** (2019), 108510.

Griesbaum K., Behr A., Biedenkapp D., Voges H. W., Garbe D., Paetz C., Collin G., Mayer D., Höke H. *Hydrocarbons. Ullman's Encyclopadia of Industrial Chemistry*, Wiley-VCH, Weinheim, 2000.

Guerreiro C. B. B., Horálek J., de Leeuw F., Couvidat F. *Environ. Pollut.*, **214** (2016), 657–667.

Guilbert A., De Cremer K., Heene B., Demoury C., Aerts R., Declerck P., Brasseur O., Van Nieuwenhuyse A. *Sci. Total Environ.*, **649** (2018), 620–628.

Habe H., Omori T. *Biosci. Biotechnol. Biochem.*, **67** (2014), 225–243.

Han T., Zhao Z., Bartlam M., Wang Y. *Environ. Sci. Pollut. Res.*, **23** (2016), 21219–21228.

Haritash A. K., Kaushik C. P. *J. Hazard. Mater.*, **169** (2009), 1–15.

Herzig R., Lohmann N., Meier R. *Environ. Sci. Pollut. Res.*, **26** (2019), 10562–10575.

Harmsen J., Rietra R. P. J. J. *Chemosphere*, **207** (2018), 229–238.

Holoubek I., Dusek L., Sanka M., Hofman J., Cupr P., Jarkovsky J., Zbiral J., Klanova J. *Environ. Pollut.*, **157** (2009), 3207–3217.

IARC (International Agency for Research on Cancer). *IARC Monographs on the Evaluation of Carcinogenic Risks to Humans 92 International Agency for Research on Cancer*, Lyons, France, 2010.

Johansson I., van Bavel B. *Sci. Total Environ.*, **311** (2003), 221–231.

Johnsen A. R., Wick L. Y., Harms H. *Environ. Pollut.*, **133** (2005), 71–84.

Juhasz A. L., Naidu R. *Int. Biodeterior. Biodegrad.*, **45** (2000), 57–88.

Kacálková L., Tlustoš P. *Cent. Eur. J. Biol.*, **6** (2010), 223–235.

Kairbekov Z. K., Smagulova N. T., Malonetnev A. S. *Coke and Chem.*, **62** (2019), 593–597.

Kaisalo N. K., Koskinen-Soivi M. L., Simell P. A., Lehtonen J. *Fuel*, **153** (2015), 118–127.

Kim K. H., Jahan S. A., Kabir E., Brown R. J. C. *Environ. Int.*, **60** (2013), 71–80.

Klankeo P., Nopcharoenkul W., Pinyakong O. *J. Biosci. Bioeng.*, **108** (2009), 488–495.

Košnář Z., Částková T., Wiesnerová L., Praus L., Jablonský I., Koudela M., Tlustoš P., *J. Environ. Sci.*, **76** (2019) 249–258.

Košnář Z., Mercl F., Perná I., Tlustoš P. *Sci. Total Environ.*, **563–564** (2016), 53–61.

Košnář Z., Mercl F., Tlustoš P., *Ecotoxicol. Environ. Saf.*, **153**, (2018), 16–22.

Košnář Z., Mercl F., Tlustoš P. *Environ. Pollut.*, **264** (2020), 114787.

Košnář Z., Tlustoš P., *Plant Soil Environ.*, **64** (2018), 88–94.

Kotoky R., Rajkumari J., Pandey P. *J. Environ. Manage.*, **217** (2018), 858–870.

Kuppusamy S., Thavamani P., Venkateswarlu K., Lee Y. B., Naidu R., Mergharaj M. *Chemosphere*, **168** (2016), 944–968.

Lawal A. T. *Cogent Environ. Sci.*, **3** (2017).

Lee S. H., Lee W. S., Lee C. H., Kim J. G. *J. Hazard. Mater.*, **153** (2007), 892–898.

Li X., Wu Y., Lin X., Zhang J., Zeng J. *Soil Biol. Biochem.*, **47** (2012), 191–197.

Liu K., Han W., Pan W. P., Riley J. T. *J. Hazard. Mater.*, **84** (2001), 175–188.

Lundstedt S., White P. A., Lemieux C. L., Lynes K. D., Lanbert I. B., Oberg L., Haglund P., Tysklind M. *Ambio*, **36** (2007), 475–485.

Mallick S. *Chemosphere*, **219** (2019), 748–755.

Maliszewska-Kordybach B., Smreczak B., Klimkowicz-Pawlas A. *Sci. Total Environ.*, **407** (2009), 3746–3753.

Marco-Urrea E., García-Romera I., Aranda E. *New Biotech.*, **32** (2015), 620–628.

Masto R. E., Sarkar E., George J., Jyoti K., Dutta P., Ram L. C. *Fuel Process. Technol.*, **132** (2015), 139–152.

McGrath T., Sharma R., Hajaligol M. *Fuel*, **80** (2001), 1787–1797.

Mohseni-Bandpei A., Majlesi M., Rafiee M., Nojavan S., Nowrouz P., Zolfagharpour H. *Chemosphere*, **227** (2019), 277–288.

Miguel A. H., Eiguren-Fernandez A., Sioutas C., Fine P. M., Geller M., Mayo P. R. *Aerosol Sci. Technol.*, **39** (2005), 415–418.

Mueller K. E., Shann J. R. *Chemosphere*, **64** (2006), 1006–1014.

Nam J. J., Thomas G. O., Jaward F. M., Steinnes E., Gustafsson O., Jones K. C. *Chemosphere*, **70** (2008), 1596–1602.

Novotný Č., Svobodová K., Erbanová P., Cajthaml T., Kasinath A., Lang E., Šašek V., *Soil Biol. Biochem.*, **36** (2004), 1545–1551.

Nzila A., Musa M. M., Sankara S., Al-Momani M., Xiang L., Li Q. X. *PLoS One*, **16** (2021), e0247723.

Ojha N., Mandal S. K., Das N. *3Biotech*, **9** (2019), 86.

Palma C. F. *Appl. Energy*, **111** (2013), 129–141.

Park N. D., Rutherford P. M., Thring R. W., Helle S. S. *Chemosphere*, **86** (2012), 427–432.

Pickard M. A., Roman R., Tinoco R., Vazquez-Duhalt R. *Appl. Environ. Microbiol.*, **65** (1999), 3805–3809.

Pozdnyakova N., Dubrovskaya E., Chernyshova M., Makarov O., Golubev S., Balandina S., Turkovskaya O. *Fungal Biol.*, **122** (2018), 363–372.

Pozdnyakova N. N., Chernyshova M. P., Grinev V. S., Landesman E. U., Koroleva O. V., Turkovskaya O. V. *Appl. Biochem. Microbiol.*, **52** (2016), 621–628.

Public Notice No. 153, *Legal Code of The Czech Republic*, 2016, 2692–2699.

Rabinovich M. L., Bolobova A. V., Vasil'chenko L. G. *Appl. Biochem. Microbiol.*, **40** (2003), 1–17.

Rachna Rani M., Shanker U. *J. Photochem. Photobiol. A Chem.*, **381** (2019), 111861.

Ravindra K., Sokhi R., Van Grieken R. *Atmos. Environ.*, **42** (2008), 2895–2921.

Ray S., Khillare P. S., Kim K. H., Brown J. C. *Environ. Eng. Sci.*, **29** (2012), 1008–1019.

Reilley K. A., Banks M. K.., Schwab A. P., *J. Environ. Qual.*, **25** (1996), 212–219.

Ross A. B., Jones J. M., Chaiklangmuang S., Pourkashanian M., Williams A., Kubica A., Andersson J. T., Kerst M., Danihelka P., Bartle K. D. *Fuel*, **81** (2002), 571–582.

Roy M., Roychowdhuryp R., Mukherjee P. *Pedosphere*, **28** (2018), 561–580.

Sakshi, Singh S. K., Haritash A. K. *Int. J. Environ. Sci. Technol.*, **16** (2019), 6489–6512.

Samanta S. K., Singh O. V., Jain R. K. *Trends Biotechnol.*, **20** (2002), 243–248.

Silva I. S., Grossman M., Durrant L. R. *Int. Biodeterior. Biodegrad.*, **63** (2008), 224–229.

Singh A., Kamal R., Ahamed I., Wagh M., Bihari V., Sathian B., Kesavachandran C. N., *Occup. Med.*, **68** (2018), 255–261.

Shen, H., *Polycyclic Aromatic Hydrocarbons. Their Global Atmospheric Emissions, Transport, ang Lung Cancer Risk*, Springer-Verlag, Berlin, 2016.

Shin J., Choi D., Shin D. M. *Mol. Cryst. Liq. Cryst. Sci. Technol. Sect.*, **370** (2001), 17–22.

Srogi K. *Environ. Chem. Lett.*, **5** (2007), 169–195.

Stibala R., Indhumathi S., Krishnakumar R. V., Srinivasan N. *Acta Cryst. E.*, **75** (2019), 1456–1462.

Tanabe S., Kobayashi K., Matsumoto M., Serizawa H., Igarashi T., Yamada T., Hirose A. *Fundam. Toxicol. Sci.*, **4** (2017), 247–259.

Ting W. T. E., Yuan S. Y., Wu S. D., Chang B. V. *Int. Biodeterior. Biodegrad*, **65** (2011), 238–242.

Tong R., Yang X., Zhang H., Cheng M., Wu C. *Hum. Ecol. Risk Assess.*, **24** (2018), 1673–1693.

Tuor U., Winterhalter K., Fiechter A. *J. Biotechnol.*, **41** (1995), 1–17.

Treu R., Falandysz J. *J. Environ. Sci. Health Part B-Pestic.*, **52** (2017), 148–155.

Ukalska-Jaruga A., Smreczak B., Klimkowicz-Pawlas A. *J. Soils Sediments*, **19** (2018), 1890–1900.

Vaidya S., Devpura N., Jain K., Madamwar D. *Front. Microbiol.*, **9** (2018), 1333.

Vervaeke P., Luyssaert S., Mertens J., De Vos B., Speelers L., Lust N. *Biomass Bioenerg.*, **21**, (2001), 81–90.

Vervaeke P., Luyssaert S., Mertens J., Meers E., Tack F. M. G., Lust N. *Environ. Pollut.*, **126** (2003), 275–282.

Vernoux A., Malleret L., Asia L., Doumenq P., Theraulaz F. *Environ. Res.*, **111** (2011), 193–198.

Vácha R., Horváthová V., Vysloužilová M. *Plant Soil Environ.*, **51** (2005), 12–18.

Wang X., Zhang Y. X., Chen R. F. *Mar. Pollut. Bull.*, **42** (2001), 1139–1149.

Wang S. W., Hsu K. H., Huang S. C., Tseng S. H., Wang D. Y., Cheng H. F. *J. Food Drug Anal.*, **27** (2019), 815–824.

Wei K., Yin H., Peng H., Liu Z., Lu G., Dang Z. *Chemosphere*, **178** (2017), 80–87.

Wilcke W. *J. Plant Nutr. Soil Sci.*, **163** (2000), 229–248.

Wilson S. C., Jones K. C. *Environ. Pollut.*, **8** (1992), 229–249.

Winquist E., Björklöf K., Schultz E., Räsänen M., Salonen K., Anasonye F., Cajthaml T., Steffen K. T., Jørgensen K. S., Tuomela M. *Int. Biodeterior. Biodegrad.*, **86** (2013), 238–247.

Wise S., Sander L., Schantz M. *Polycycl. Aromat. Compd.*, **35** (2014), 187–247.

Xie W., Li R., Li X., Liu P., Yang H., Wu T., Zhang Y. *Ecotox. Environ. Safe.*, **161** (2018), 763–768.

Xu S., Wang W., Zhu L. *Sci. Total Environ.*, **653** (2018), 1293–1300.

Yap C. L., Gan S. N., Ng H. K. *J. Hazard. Mater.*, **177** (2010), 28–41.

Part VII
Biochemical Conversion

Chapter 13

Enzymatic Saccharification of Lignocellulosic Biomass

Madhavi Latha Gandla, Chaojun Tang, Carlos Martín, and Leif J. Jönsson
Department of Chemistry, Umeå University, SE-901 87, Umeå, Sweden
leif.jonsson@umu.se

The abundance of lignocellulosic biomass and efforts to reduce the dependency on fossil resources to produce fuels and chemicals has led to an increased interest in enzymes partaking in the saccharification of lignocellulosic polysaccharides, primarily cellulose. Enzymatic saccharification of lignocellulosic polysaccharides has developed into a dynamic area covering both research on fundamental aspects of newly discovered enzyme activities and the development of innovative full-scale industrial processes based on biochemical conversion.

Agricultural Biocatalysis: Enzymes in Agriculture and Industry
Edited by Peter Jeschke and Evgeni B. Starikov
Copyright © 2023 Jenny Stanford Publishing Pte. Ltd.
ISBN 978-981-4968-47-8 (Hardcover), 978-1-003-31310-6 (eBook)
www.jennystanford.com

13.1 Introduction

Recent centuries have been characterized by the large-scale exploitation of finite fossil resources, such as coal and oil, for the production of energy and chemicals. Recent estimates indicate that fossil fuels account for annual emissions of roughly 30 Gt carbon dioxide and indicate end-dates for oil and natural gas in the 2060s (Abas *et al.*, 2015). Concerns regarding the negative effects of the utilization of fossil resources on the environment and concerns regarding energy security have invigorated research and development regarding the use of renewable resources, such as biomass, to produce energy, biofuels, and other biobased products.

A recent estimate of the total biomass resources on earth (Bar-On *et al.*, 2018) found that plants accounted for around 450 Gt C, or ~80%, out of a total of around 550 Gt C biomass. Furthermore, terrestrial biomass was estimated to account for 470 Gt C, that is, roughly 85% of the total biomass (Bar-On *et al.*, 2018). The vast majority of plant biomass is found in terrestrial environments, and the main part of that is vascular plants, while other types of plants, such as mosses, lichens, green algae, and seaweed, account for minor portions.

Secondary cell walls of vascular plants consist of lignocellulose (Kumar *et al.*, 2016; Meents *et al.*, 2018). The main constituents of lignocellulose (on a dry-matter basis) are cellulose, hemicelluloses, and lignin. Whereas both cellulose and hemicelluloses are polysaccharides, lignin is an aromatic polymer consisting of phenylpropane units (Ralph *et al.*, 2019). Lignified tissues of vascular plants form vessels that are essential for the transport of water and solutes between roots and leaves and other tissues. This permits vascular plants to reach considerable heights and compete successfully in stratified terrestrial ecosystems. In contrast, plants such as mosses rely on surface absorption and diffusion and do not require lignin (Roberts *et al.*, 2012).

Microorganisms and enzymes involved in the degradation of lignocellulosic materials are highly relevant in nature as well as in society. Research on enzymes involved in saccharification of lignocellulose polysaccharides was accelerated after the characterization of fungi and bacteria involved in the deterioration of cotton textiles in programs initiated in the USA during World War II

(Reese *et al.*, 1950). Microbial species were collected from tropical and subtropical areas where warm and humid conditions contributed to the rapid deterioration of cotton-based textiles. Fungal isolate QM6a, later known as strain *Trichoderma reesei* QM6a, was collected from Bougainville Island in the Solomon Islands and later became a very important organism for research on enzymes partaking in the degradation of cellulose and hemicelluloses (Druzhinina and Kubicek, 2016).

Although enzymes involved in the saccharification of cellulose and hemicelluloses are of interest in many different application areas, this chapter is devoted to the use of such enzymes for saccharification of lignocellulosic biomass to produce biobased commodities through biochemical conversion. The following sections cover lignocellulosic biomass as a substrate, biodegradation of lignocellulose, microbial enzymes with a focus on saccharification of cellulose, and application of such enzymes in an industrial context.

13.2 Lignocellulosic Biomass

Lignocellulosic biomass is the cell wall material resulting from photosynthetic processes in vascular plants. Although lignocellulosic materials are commonly associated exclusively with forest and agricultural residues, they go far beyond that simple classification. Lignocellulosic biomass also covers (*i*) non-edible parts of cereals and other food crops, (*ii*) wastes of non-food agricultural products, (*iii*) forest and wood processing residues, (*iv*) dedicated herbaceous energy crops and short rotation woody species, and (*v*) the cellulosic fraction of municipal solid waste.

Lignocellulosic polysaccharides, primarily cellulose and hemicelluloses, typically account for around 60–70% of the dry weight of biomass, while lignin roughly accounts for 20–40%, but those values can range widely depending on the biomass type. In Table 13.1, the composition of several lignocellulosic materials is shown. It includes the softwood species Norway spruce (*Picea abies*) and Scots pine (*Pinus sylvestris*), the hardwoods silver birch (*Betula pendula*) and hybrid aspen (*Populus tremula* × *tremuloides*), as well as sugarcane bagasse, a major by-product of industrial processing of sugar cane (*Saccharum officinarum*), and the residual straw from wheat (*Triticum aestivum*) harvesting. As shown in Table 13.1, cellulose is the main component of most types of lignocellulosic biomass, and its content is quantitatively comparable in most of the materials. Furthermore, cellulose is qualitatively uniform in different biomass types (Fengel and Wegener, 1989). On the other hand, hemicelluloses and lignin of different materials show important differences regarding both the fractions of the biomass and the monomer composition.

Plant cellulose is a homopolysaccharide composed of glucose units arranged linearly and linked by β-1,4-glycosidic bonds (Fengel and Wegener, 1989). Cellulose chains can reach a degree of polymerization (DP) as high as 15 000, and they are organized in a compact supramolecular structure, consisting of rigid microfibrils stabilized by hydrogen bonds (Fig. 13.1A) as well as by hydrophobic interactions (Lindman et al., 2021). Such an arrangement provides a high degree of crystallinity, which contributes to giving cellulose a low reactivity toward chemicals and enzymes and to making it insoluble in many solvents. There are also amorphous regions (Fig. 13.1B). Although amorphous regions represent a minor part of the cellulose macromolecule, they are important for chemical and enzymatic processing (Ciolacu et al., 2011).

In contrast to cellulose, hemicelluloses are branched heteropolysaccharides, and their DP is relatively low (up to around 200). Hemicelluloses have low crystallinity, and, consequently, they are reactive toward hydrolysis under mild conditions. Hemicelluloses are composed of units of both hexose and pentose sugars, and they also contain acetyl groups and uronic acid moieties. Hemicelluloses from different types of plants have different compositions. Softwood hemicelluloses are rich in hexose units, such as units of mannose, glucose, and galactose. Hexosans, such as *O*-acetyl-galactoglucomannan (Fig. 13.1C), are the main hemicelluloses in softwood. In contrast, hardwood hemicelluloses are mostly pentosans, and *O*-acetyl-4-*O*-methylglucurono-D-xylan (Fig. 13.1D) are the main constituents. As in hardwood, pentosans, such as arabino-(*O*-acetyl-4-*O*-methylglucurono)-D-xylan (Fig. 13.1E), are major hemicelluloses in *Gramineae* (*Poaceae*) (Xiao et al., 2001), that is, grasses.

Table 13.1 Main components of different types of lignocellulosic biomass

Biomass	Cellulose	Hemicelluloses	Lignin	Extractives	Minerals	Reference
Norway spruce	42.7	18.6[a]	29.5[b]	1.2	0.1	Normark et al., 2016
Scots pine	42.7	23.5[a]	29.5	4.5	0.2	Normark et al., 2014
Silver birch	38.8	27.7[c]	28.5	1.7	N.D.	Wang et al., 2018
Hybrid aspen	44.0	22.8[c]	24.8	0.8	N.D.	Wang et al., 2018
Sugarcane bagasse	42.2	27.67[c]	21.6	5.6	2.8	Rocha et al., 2015
Wheat straw	39.8	24.37[c]	22.8	5.1	4.7	Ilanidis et al., 2021b

[a]Mannan as the main constituent
[b]Klason lignin
[c]Xylan as the main constituent

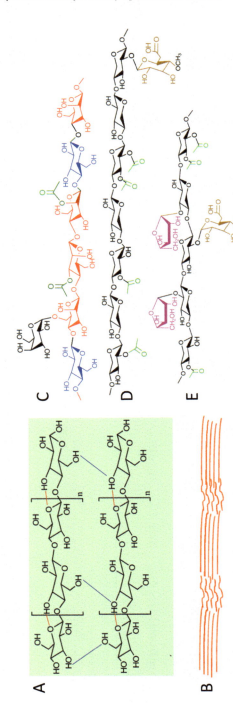

Figure 13.1 (A) Schematic representation of cellulose supramolecular structure; colored lines represent intra- (red) and intermolecular (blue) hydrogen bonds. (B) scheme showing crystalline (straight lines) and amorphous (wavy lines) regions in cellulose microfibrils. Examples of hemicelluloses from (C) softwood (O-acetyl-galactoglucomannan), (D) hardwood (O-acetyl-4-O-methylglucurono-D-xylan), and (E) *Gramineae* (arabino-(O-acetyl-4-O-methylglucurono)-D-xylan). Red, blue, and black hexapyranosic structures in (C) represent mannose, glucose, and galactose, respectively. Black pentapyranose and brown hexapyranose units in (D) and (E) are xylose and glucuronic acid units, respectively. Methyl groups are black (D, E), acetyl groups are green (C–E), and arabinose units are pink (E).

The third major lignocellulose biopolymer, lignin, is a polyphenol made of phenylpropanoid units linked by ether and carbon-carbon bonds forming a complex three-dimensional (3D) network (Fengel and Wegener, 1989; Ralph et al., 2019). The lignin content is higher in wood than in gramineous biomass, and it is higher in softwood than in hardwood (Table 13.1). As for hemicelluloses, the composition of lignin depends on the type of biomass. Although other subunits may also be present, the three predominant subunits in lignin are p-hydroxyphenyl, guaiacyl, and syringyl. Guaiacyl subunits are the basic units of softwood lignin, while hardwood lignin contains both guaiacyl and syringyl subunits (Fig. 13.2). Gramineous lignin contains substantial proportions of all three of the predominant phenylpropanoid subunits since p-hydroxyphenyl subunits are also present. Lignin is intimately associated with cellulose and hemicelluloses forming lignin-carbohydrate complexes, which affect the reactivity during chemical or enzymatic processing (Tarasov et al., 2018). Therefore, it is advantageous to remove lignin to facilitate enzymatic saccharification of cellulose.

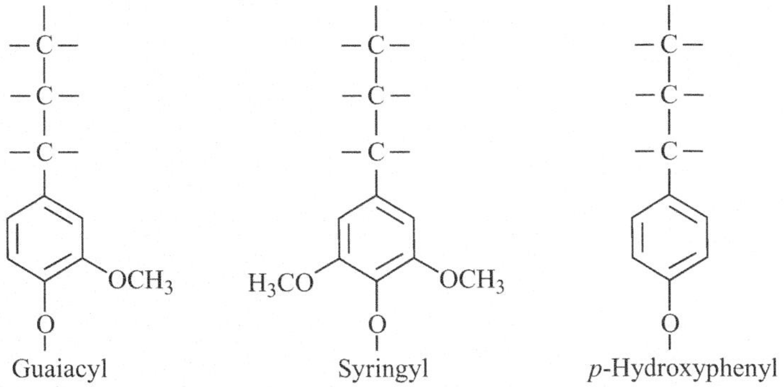

Figure 13.2 Predominant phenylpropanoid units in lignin.

Lignocellulosic biomass also contains small fractions of extractives and minerals (Fengel and Wegener, 1989). Extractives can be removed by extraction with solvents but exhibit high heterogeneity regarding both composition and chemical functionality. They represent a minor fraction of biomass dry weight, and that fraction will vary depending on the solvent(s) used and the extraction procedure. Low fractions of minerals are also present in plant biomass, and their content is lower in wood than in many *Gramineae* plants (Table 13.1). Despite being present in low amounts, extractives and minerals can affect biomass processing.

13.3 Biodegradation of Lignocellulose in Nature

Biodegradation of lignocellulosic polysaccharides is mainly an extracellular hydrolytic process, in which cellulose and hemicelluloses are degraded to oligosaccharides and disaccharides and further on to monosaccharides that are then ingested and metabolized by microbial cells. For several decades, the enzymic machinery of the soft-rot ascomycete *T. reesei* has been in the focus for the elucidation of the structure and function of hydrolases involved in the degradation of cellulose and hemicelluloses (Bischof *et al.*, 2016; Druzhinina and Kubicek, 2016). Fungal enzymes involved in these processes are typically glycoproteins that are sometimes equipped with a carbohydrate-binding module (CBM) that mediates interaction with substrates. CBMs are not necessary for the function of such enzymes but may be advantageous in environments with high water content (Várnai *et al.*, 2013).

Depending on their effects on the substrate, fungi growing on lignocellulosic substrates are often categorized as white rots, brown rots, or soft rots. Whereas all three of these groups of fungi degrade cellulose and hemicelluloses, white rots are the only microorganisms that efficiently mineralize lignin (Kirk *et al.*, 1975), an oxidative process that primarily occurs under aerobic conditions. The ability to modify lignin, partially degrade lignin, or metabolize low molecular mass lignin-degradation products is, however, widespread among several types of microorganisms (Cragg *et al.*, 2015). Cellulose degradation by brown-rot fungi is different as it involves a non-enzymatic process based on reactive oxygen species created through Fenton chemistry (Goodell *et al.*, 2017).

Whereas many free-living fungi involved in lignocellulose biodegradation prefer a slightly acidic pH, such as a pH around 5, there are exceptions, such as *Humicola insolens*. Like many bacteria, *H. insolens* prefers neutral or slightly alkaline conditions (Ben Hmad and Gargouri, 2017). Enzymatic saccharification reactions have typically been performed in the range of 45–50 °C (Viikari *et al.*, 2007). There are, however, cellulases that are relatively stable in the range of 50–80 °C (Patel *et al.*, 2019), at least for shorter periods.

Cellulose and hemicelluloses are present also in aqueous environments, which is due to the occurrence of cellulose and other polysaccharides in micro- and macro-algae but also the occurrence of detritus from vascular plants ending up in aqueous environments (Cragg et al., 2020). A wide variety of organisms are involved in cellulose degradation in aqueous environments (Barzkar and Sohail, 2020). As could be expected due to partially anoxic conditions, lignin degradation is typically slow in blue carbon ecosystems (Cragg et al., 2020).

Gut microbiomes of cellulose-degrading animals, insects, and other organisms are currently in the focus of intensive research efforts. This includes not only bacteria but also anaerobic fungi that inhabit the guts of herbivores (Haitjema et al., 2014).

As most enzymes involved in the saccharification of cellulose and hemicelluloses are hydrolases, they belong to Class 3 according to the Enzyme Commission (EC) system for classification of enzymes (IUBMB, 2021). However, as lignin biodegradation is an oxidative process involving oxidoreductases, and as certain oxidoreductases, notably lytic polysaccharide monooxygenase (LPMO), are involved in the degradation of lignocellulosic polysaccharides, EC Class 1 enzymes are also important for lignocellulose degradation. Synergism between different enzymes (Van Dyk and Pletschke, 2012), and amorphogenesis (Arantes and Saddler, 2010) to improve the accessibility to cellulose (Arantes and Saddler, 2011) are other significant features of enzymatic saccharification of cellulosic substrates.

The classification of enzymes involved in the biodegradation of lignocellulose is often based on the system for "Carbohydrate-Active enZYmes" (CAZy, 2021), which was introduced in 1991 (Lombard et al., 2014). The CAZy system is based on catalytic activity, protein sequence similarities, and predicted protein folding. According to this system, enzymes of relevance for degradation of lignocellulosic biomass are classified as belonging to glycoside hydrolases (GHs), glycosyltransferases (GTs), polysaccharide lyases (PLs), carbohydrate esterases (CEs), or auxiliary activities (AAs). The CAZy system also covers associated modules, which include CBMs. Enzymes belonging to the same class, for example, GH are divided into families and subfamilies. GH families sharing common protein fold and catalytic machinery are grouped into clans.

13.4 Fungal Enzymes

Enzymatic saccharification is achieved through the complementary and synergistic activities of multiple carbohydrate-active enzymes, such as cellulases, hemicellulases, and pectinases (Van Dyk and Pletschke, 2012). Whereas enzymes of most CAZy classes are involved in the degradation of glycosidic bonds, GTs are responsible for the assembly of complex carbohydrates by the formation of glycosidic bonds, and AA members are involved in reactions that support the activity of other CAZy enzymes. As this chapter is focused on the enzymatic saccharification of lignocellulosic biomass, it covers relevant GHs, PLs, CEs, and AAs, but not GTs.

13.4.1 Glycoside Hydrolases

GHs (EC 3.2.1.-) are a group of enzymes that hydrolyze glycosidic bonds between two or more carbohydrates or between a carbohydrate and non-carbohydrate component leading to the formation of a sugar hemiacetal or a hemiketal and the corresponding non-carbohydrate moiety. According to the CAZy database (http://www.cazy.org), there are currently 171 GH families (GH1-GH171) and 18 clans (GH-A to GH-R). Based on phylogenetic analysis, five of the GH families, have been divided further into subfamilies: GH5 with 56 subfamilies, GH13 with 43, GH16 with 27, GH30 with 9, and GH43 with 37 subfamilies. The number of modules in currently classified GH families amounts to >982 000, of which >19 000 are non-classified modules.

GH families contain multiple cellulolytic enzymes, which are widely distributed among bacteria, fungi, and plants. Unlike many other commonly studied enzymes, cellulases act on insoluble substrates and are sometimes multimodular, having both CBMs and linkers that make them into multifunctional enzymes. The substrate specificity and mode of action of GHs are mainly governed by their 3D structure (Davies and Henrissat, 1995). GHs involved in cellulose biodegradation may be endo-acting enzymes that hydrolyze long β-1,4-glucan chains (endoglucanase, EG), processive exo-acting enzymes that recognize either the reducing or the non-reducing end of the cellulose chain producing cellobiose or cellotetraose (cellobiohydrolase, CBH; exoglucanase), and enzymes that catalyze the hydrolysis of cellobiose or cellotetraose to monomeric units, viz. β-glucosidase (BGL) (also referred to as cellobiase) (Fig. 13.3).

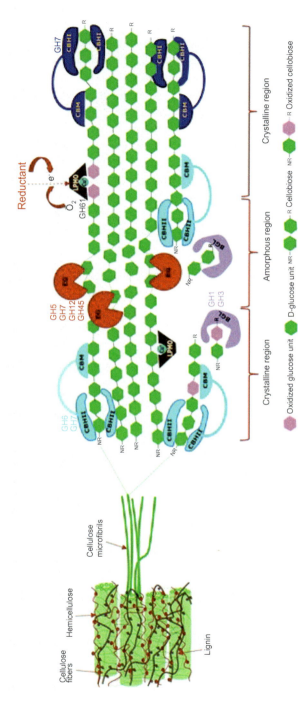

Figure 13.3 Schematic representation of enzymatic degradation of cellulose chains by the synergistic interaction of fungal cellulolytic enzymes (EG, endoglucanase; CBH, cellobiohydrolase/exoglucanase; CBM, carbohydrate-binding module; BGL, β-glucosidase; LPMO, lytic polysaccharide monooxygenase; NR, non-reducing end; R, reducing end).

Most GH enzymes contain multiple carbohydrate-binding sites in their catalytic domains (CDs). The non-reducing end subsite (−n) and the reducing end subsite (+n) are used for characterizing carbohydrate-binding sites (Davies et al., 1997; Davies and Henrissat, 1995). According to this system, the cleavage of glycosidic bonds by GHs occurs between the −1 and +1 subsites.

The enzymatic hydrolysis of glycosidic bonds by GH members follows an acid-base catalysis reaction in the presence of a proton donor and a nucleophile/base. Koshland (1953) found two reaction mechanisms in GHs giving rise to retaining or inverting mechanisms with regard to the configuration of the anomeric carbon. In both these mechanisms, the position of the proton donor is the same with regard to the hydrogen-bonding distance from the glycosidic oxygen atom.

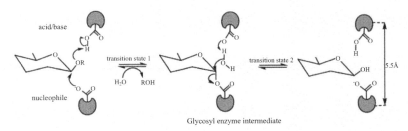

Figure 13.4 Retaining mechanism of GH enzymes.

The retaining mechanism is a two-step double displacement mechanism. A nucleophilic base is in close vicinity to the anomeric carbon of the saccharide. The glycosidic oxygen is protonated by the acid catalyst and the nucleophilic base, which is located at around 5.5 Å from the acid catalyst, assists the departure of the aglycon. Typically, Asp or Glu is a part of the active site of GH enzymes and is involved in catalyzing the reaction. Retention of the configuration of the anomeric carbon during hydrolysis is achieved through the formation of a covalently linked glycosyl-enzyme intermediate, which then undergoes hydrolysis (Fig. 13.4). To lower the energy barrier, each step passes through a transition state (1 and 2 in Fig. 13.4) by forming an oxocarbenium ion. The second nucleophilic substitution at the anomeric carbon generates a product with the same stereochemistry as that of the substrate (Fig. 13.4). Enzymes exhibiting the retaining mechanism account for around 60% of the

GH families. Although hydrolysis is typically the favored outcome, many retaining GHs exhibit transglycosylase activity resulting in the formation of glycoconjugates (Bissaro et al., 2015).

The inverting mechanism is a one-step, single-displacement mechanism involving an oxocarbenium-ion-like transition state which results in a product with opposite stereochemistry to that of the substrate. In this reaction, protonation of the glycosidic oxygen and departure of the aglycon is accompanied by a simultaneous attack of a water molecule that is activated by the nucleophilic base, which is 6–11 Å apart from the acid catalyst (Fig. 13.5).

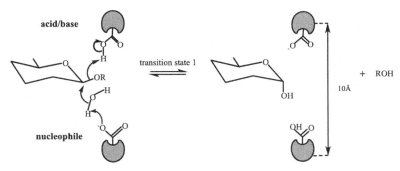

Figure 13.5 Inverting mechanism of GH enzymes.

Most fungal and bacterial cellulases follow the retaining or inverting mechanisms. Subfamilies of GH1 and GH3 (EC 3.2.1.21, BGLs), GH5 (EC 3.2.1.4, EGs), GH7 (EC 3.2.1.91 and 3.2.1.76, cellobiohydrolases CBHII and CBHI; EC 3.2.1.4, EGI), and GH12 (EC 3.2.1.151 and 3.2.1.4, EGIII) hydrolases exhibit the retaining mechanism. However, GH6 (EC 3.2.1.91, CBHII), GH45 (EC 3.2.1.4, EGV), and GH74 (EC 3.2.1.151, EG and xyloglucanase, XG) subfamily hydrolases exhibit the inverting mechanism. In addition, several variations on these mechanisms have recently been found. One fundamentally different mechanism, catalyzed by an NADH cofactor, has been discovered in GH families 4 and 109 (Varrot et al., 2005).

Fungal cellulolytic enzyme cocktails primarily contain enzymes from GH families 1, 3, 5, 6, 7, 12, and 45. Among well-studied fungi secreting cellulolytic enzymes, *T. reesei* has a central position with regard to enzymatic saccharification of lignocellulosic biomass. The *T. reesei* wild-type strain QM6a is known to produce at least 193 GHs, 93 GTs (glycosyltransferases), 5 PLs, 17 CEs, and 41 CBMs. For

T. reesei, the CAZy database lists two highly expressed CBHs in GH families 6 and 7, five characterized EGs within GH families 5, 7, 12, and 45, two LPMOs, and two characterized BGLs in GH families 1 and 3 (Martinez *et al.*, 2008). Even though *T. reesei* secretes a rather limited set of hemicellulases, pectinases, acetyl esterases, and other enzymes involved in the degradation of plant cell walls, its efficiency lies mainly in its high capacity to produce and secrete cellulases (Martinez *et al.*, 2008). In comparison, *Aspergillus niger* produces five EGs from GH families 5 and 12, four CBHs from families 6 and 7, and 13 BGLs from families 1 and 3. This is the reason why early commercial cellulase preparations based on enzymes from *T. reesei*, such as Celluclast 1.5, were typically fortified with Novozymes 188, a BGL-rich enzyme preparation from *A. niger* (Novozymes A/S, Bagsværd, Denmark).

Fungal cellulases from cellulase family A, also called GH5, is the largest of all the GH families, and are considered as key EGs (EGI and EGII) in enzyme cocktails used for biomass conversion (Aspeborg *et al.*, 2012). These are grouped in the GH-A clan and exhibit a $(\beta/\alpha)_8$ fold that is characteristic of enzymes that are capable of degrading equatorially oriented glycosidic linkages (Jenkins *et al.*, 1995; Pickersgill *et al.*, 1998). Cel5A (EGII) (PDB 3QR3) from *T. reesei* and EGI from *Schizophyllum commune* are commonly studied representatives of GH5 EGs. Most of the GH5 subfamilies are endo-active and multimodular. The multimodularity of these subfamilies is attributed to the presence of both binding and catalytic functions through the association of CBMs with the CDs by flexible linker peptides (Payne *et al.*, 2015). Enzymes from fungal GH5 subfamilies typically have the CBM1 module, either at the amino- or the carboxy-terminal end of the protein. However, bacterial enzymes in this family do not have CBM1 modules.

GH5 EGs exhibit broad substrate specificity. They act on various substrates, such as carboxymethylcellulose (CMC), phosphoric acid swollen cellulose (PASC), Avicel (microcrystalline cellulose), bacterial nanocellulose (BNC), pretreated corn stover, xyloglucan, wheat arabinoxylan, β-1,4-mannan, and galactomannan. They have several catalytic activities, such as β-1,4-glucanase, 1,6-galactanase, 1,3-mannanase, 1,4-xylanase, and xyloglucanase activity (Jenkins *et al.*, 1995; Pickersgill *et al.*, 1998). There are, however, exceptions, for instance, GH5 members of subfamily 5, which includes fungal and bacterial monospecific EGs with single catalytic activity (St John et al., 2010; Lombard et al., 2014).

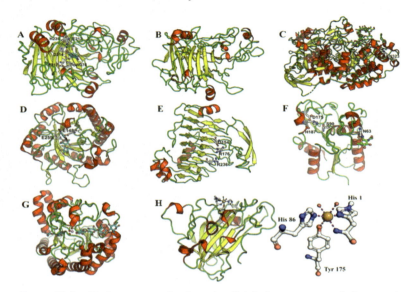

Figure 13.6 3D Structures of selected cellulolytic enzymes: α-helices, red; β-sheets, yellow; loops, green; ligands, cyan; active-site residues, gray with red oxygen atoms and blue nitrogen atoms; N-glycosylation, green carbon atoms. (A) CBHI from T. reesei (PDB 1CEL) with active-site residues and ligand IBTG (o-iodobenzyl-1-thio-β-D-glucose); (B) EGI from T. reesei (TrCel7B, PDB 1EG1) showing binding cleft and surface loops; (C) BGL from A. fumigatus (PDB 5FJI) showing active site, N-glycosylation at Asn323; (D) EGII from T. reesei (TrCel5A, PDB 3QR3) showing the active site and a substrate mimicking complex with 2,4-dinitrophenyl-2-deoxy-2-fluoro-β-D-cellobioside; (E) pectin lyase A from A. niger (PDB 1IDJ) showing the substrate-binding site and residues expected to play a role in catalysis (Asp154, Arg176, Arg236); (F) acetyl xylan esterase (AXE) from T. reesei (PDB 1QOZ) showing the catalytic triad Ser90-His187-Asp175, and a glycosylation site at Asn63; (G) Cel6A from the fungus Chaetomium thermophilum (PDB 4A05) showing the catalytic core with an active-center Li$^+$ ion; (H) structure of family AA9 LPMO from Thermoascus aurantiacus (PDB 2YET) and its catalytic site with key residues in ball-and-stick representation with carbon atoms in gray, nitrogen atoms in blue, and oxygen atoms in red. The copper atom is shown as a golden sphere and the coordinated water molecules are shown in red.

GH6 includes enzymes with endohydrolytic cellulase activity (EC 3.2.1.4) and cellobiohydrolase activity (EC 3.2.1.91). TrCel6A (CBHII) exhibits a distorted β/α barrel structure (PDB 3CBH, Fig. 13.6). GH6

CBHs are typically unidirectional, acting from the non-reducing end of cellulose chains and showing exo/endo synergism with EGs from the GH5 family (Henrissat et al., 1985). Similar to Cel5A enzymes, Cel6A enzymes do not hydrolyze cellobiosides.

GH7 cellulases are the predominant fungal cellulolytic enzymes involved in biomass degradation. Unlike other cellulase-containing GH families (5, 6, 12, and 45), GH7 cellulases are predominantly fungal rather than bacterial or archaean. *T. reesei* secretes a single GH7 EG and a single GH7 CBH, while *P. chrysosporum* encodes multiple GH7 CBHs and EGs (Martinez et al., 2004; Wymelenberg et al., 2006). In fact, *P. chrysosporum* was the first basidiomycete for which structural details of a GH7 CBH were elucidated. *Tr*Cel7A was the first member of GH7 for which the crystal structure of CBHI was revealed (PDB 1CEL, Fig. 13.6) (Divne et al., 1994). *Tr*Cel7A contains two antiparallel β-sheets forming a large β-sandwich. Furthermore, *Tr*Cel7A has a large substrate-binding tunnel (twice in length compared to *Tr*Cel6A) containing four Trp residues (unlike the corresponding structure of Cel6A, which contains three such Trp residues). *Tr*Cel7A employs the two-step retaining mechanism unlike the one-step inverting mechanism of *Tr*Cel6A. *Tr*Cel7A has two Glu residues positioned 5.5 Å apart in the active site. One of them acts as the nucleophile and the other acts as the acid/base proton donor. The ability to catalyze hydrolysis at the reducing end of cellulose chains differentiates this enzyme from Cel6A, which acts on non-reducing ends. *Tr*Cel7B (PDB 1EG1, Fig. 13.6), another member of the GH7 family, has endoglucanase activity (EGI). The crystal structure of *Tr*Cel7B revealed a resemblance of the overall fold with that of *Tr*Cel7A, except that it has a completely open substrate-binding cleft. This could be due to the absence of certain surface loops (B2, B3, B4, and A4) near the cellononaose ligand making EGs differ in functionality compared to CBHI of GH7 and making them less processive in the hydrolysis of cellulose chains. In addition, the presence of three Arg residues at a hydrogen-bonding distance from the +1/+2 glycosyl residues of the cellononaose ligand makes *Tr*Cel7A and other CBHs differ in functionality with EGs.

In addition, GH12 enzymes, being EGs (EC 3.2.1.4), also exhibit activity against β-1,3/1,4-glucan (EC 3.2.1.73), xyloglucan (EC 3.2.1.151), and xylan (EC 3.2.1.8) (Payne et al., 2015). *Tr*Cel12A (EGIII), which was the first well-studied EG from the GH12 family, is a small protein (218 amino acid residues) compared to other *T. reesei* cellulases and does not include any CBM (Foreman *et al.*, 2003).

Most BGLs belonging to the GH1 and GH3 families exhibit the retaining mechanism (Decker *et al.*, 2001). Two BGLs from *T. reesei* are produced at low levels (Reczey *et al.*, 1998) and are subject to strong product inhibition (Chen *et al.*, 1992). These characteristics prevent *T. reesei* from extensive *in vitro* saccharification of cellulose to glucose. In contrast, *aspergilli* typically produce high levels of BGL and are more glucose tolerant (Reczey *et al.*, 1998; Riou *et al.*, 1998).

There are two models for enzymatic depolymerization of cellulose, the free-enzyme model and the cellulosome model. Typical fungal cellulases, such as those from *T. reesei*, follow the free-enzyme model, in which cellulases diffuse as single catalytic units along with CBMs that are covalently attached to the CDs through linkers (Fig. 13.3). The primary catalytic process includes random cleavage of less ordered amorphous regions of cellulose chains by non-processive endo-acting endoglucanases (EGs; EC 3.2.1.4) (Fig. 13.3). *Tr*Cel5A (EGII) and *Tr*Cel7B (EGI) are the most abundantly produced EGs of *T. reesei* (Foreman *et al.*, 2003; Vlasenko *et al.*, 2010). Both EGs contain CBMs, which enhance the efficiency in the degradation of cellulose microfibrils by binding to cellulose (Beckham *et al.*, 2010; Guillen *et al.*, 2010). The secondary catalytic process includes the attack on ends of cellulose chains by exo-acting processive CBHs/exoglucanases which depolymerize cellulose chains to cellobiose (Fig. 13.3). The two highly expressed CBHs of *T. reesei*, CBHI (*Tr*Cel7A; EC 3.2.1.176) and CBHII (*Tr*Cel6A; EC 3.2.1.91), are considered to work synergistically and act in a unidirectional manner either from the non-reducing ends (*Tr*Cel6A) or from the reducing ends of cellulose chains (Nutt *et al.*, 1998) (Fig. 13.3). CBHs are also considered to be important for the hydrolysis of the crystalline parts of cellulose (Liu *et al.*, 2011). The CBHs of *T. reesei* are highly sensitive to product inhibition, particularly by cellobiose, which might explain the need for a high proportion of CBHs in effective fungal cellulase enzyme mixes (Bezerra and Dias, 2005). After endo- and exo-cleaving of cellulose, the tertiary catalytic process ensues. This is catalyzed by BGLs (EC 3.2.1.21) belonging to GH families GH1 and GH3, which degrade soluble oligosaccharides and cellobiose to monomeric glucose units (Fig. 13.3).

In addition to the cellulose backbone, common backbone structures of hemicelluloses, such as xylan, xyloglucan, and galactomannan, are hydrolyzed by enzymes in different GH families. Most of the xylan backbone is usually degraded during a hydrothermal pretreatment preceding the enzymatic saccharification, but residual xylan is degraded further during enzymatic saccharification by the action of β-1,4-endoxylanases (GH10 and GH11). Xylan is degraded to shorter oligosaccharides, which are further cleaved into xylose by β-1,4-xylosidases (GH3 and GH43). Fungal β-1,4-endoxylanases of the GH10 family are similar to enzymes from GH1, GH2, and GH5 (Polizeli et al., 2005). GH10 endoxylanases have a TIM-barrel fold in the catalytic domain. In contrast, GH11 endoxylanases have a β-jelly-roll structure in the catalytic domain (Pollet et al., 2010). GH10 and GH11 endoxylanases also differ from each other with regard to substrate specificity (Biely et al., 1997). In general, GH10 endoxylanases have broader substrate specificity. They degrade both linear and highly substituted xylan chains as well as smaller xylooligosaccharides (XOS). GH11 endoxylanases specifically hydrolyze linear xylan chains (Biely et al., 1997; Pollet et al., 2010). β-Xylosidases belonging to GH3 differ from BGL from the same family by the absence of an Asp residue in the active site.

EGs/XGs from GH12 and GH74 are involved in the hydrolysis of xyloglucan. These two families of XGs differ by retaining and inverting mechanisms (Gilbert et al., 2008). In addition, unlike GH74 XGs of *T. reesei*, GH12 enzymes of *A. niger* do not cleave branched glucose residues and prefer XOS with more than six glucose residues (Master et al., 2008; Desmet et al., 2007).

β-1,4-Endomannanase (GH5 and GH26) and β-1,4-mannosidase (GH2) are involved in the degradation of (galacto-)mannan (De Vries and Visser, 2001). *A. niger* and *T. reesei* GH5 fungal endomannanases show substrate specificity toward manno-oligosaccharides containing more than three D-mannose residues (Tenkanen et al., 1997; Do et al., 2009). Similar to most fungal carbohydrate-active enzymes, some endomannanases have a CBM domain (mainly CBM1) for enzyme-substrate association (Pham et al., 2010; Boraston et al., 2004). The released mannobiose and mannotriose are further degraded by β-1,4-mannosidases of the GH2 family (Ademark et al., 2001). However, xylans and mannans generally have several different substituents linked to the main backbone, such as arabinose units, acetyl groups, galactose units, and glucose units. For that reason, degradation requires many ancillary enzymes to remove these residues from the backbone to give access to enzymes that degrade the backbone. Some of these ancillary enzymes are α-L-arabinofuranosidase, α-glucuronidase, ferulic acid esterase (FAE), α-galactosidase, AXE, and acetyl mannan esterase. FAEs specifically cleave the linkages between hemicellulose and lignin. α-L-Arabinofuranosidases have different specificities. Some cleave 1,2-linkages or 1,3-linkages, while others are able to cleave double-substituted arabinose residues from arabinoxylan.

Enzymes in the same GH family usually share sequence similarities. Some families, such as GH5, cover different catalytic activities, such as exoglucanase, endoglucanase, and endomannanase activities (Dias et al., 2004). In addition, specific enzyme activity can be present in several CAZy families. Thermal stability, pH stability, and substrate specificity of cellulases can be altered or improved by mutagenesis, by introducing disulfide bridges, and by hyperglycosylation (Banerjee et al., 2012; Karp et al., 2014).

Degradation of the pectin backbone requires the action of GHs, CEs, and PLs. Fungal GHs involved in the degradation of pectin mostly belong to the GH28 family (Martens-Uzunova and Schaap, 2009). These GH28 enzymes can be endo- and exo-polygalacturonases depending on the specific region of degradation of the smooth region of pectin. They cleave α-1,4-glycosidic bonds between α-galacturonic acids and are subgrouped depending on their substrate specificity. *A. niger* encodes seven endo-polygalacturonases (PgaI–PgaVII) and four exo-polygalacturonases (PgaX, PgxA, PgxB, and PgxC) (Martens-Uzunova and Schaap, 2009). However, more intricate, so-called hairy regions, require the actions of endo- and exo-rhamnogalacturonases (GH28) (enzymes that cleave α-1,2-glycosidic bonds between D-galacturonic acid and L-rhamnose residues in the hairy regions) (Kofod et al., 1994), xylogalacturonases (GH28), α-rhamnosidases (GH78), unsaturated glucuronyl hydrolases (GH88), and unsaturated rhamnogalacturonan hydrolases (GH105).

13.4.2 Polysaccharide Lyases

PLs (EC 4.2.2.-) (PLs) include enzymes catalyzing the cleavage of uronic acid glycosides, such as those found in pectins, by a β-elimination reaction resulting in an unsaturated hexenuronic acid residue at the non-reducing end and the formation of a new reducing end at the cleavage site. Unlike GH enzymes, cleavage by PL enzymes typically occurs without the involvement of a water molecule. There are currently 41 PL families in the CAZy database. Some of these families (such as families 1–12, 14–15, 17, and 22) contain 1–13 subfamilies (Lombard et al., 2014). Gacesa (1987) proposed a mechanism for PL catalysis. This mechanism involves (*i*) proton abstraction at the C5 carbon atom of the sugar ring of a uronic acid or ester by a basic amino acid residue, (*ii*) stabilization of the resulting anion by charge delocalization, and (*iii*) β-elimination of the 4-*O*-glycosidic bond assisted by proton donation from a catalytic acid to yield a hexenuronic acid moiety at the non-reducing end (Fig. 13.7).

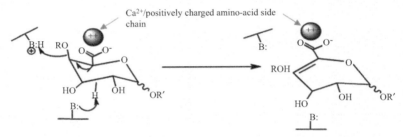

Figure 13.7 Mechanism of a PL enzyme acting on α-(1,4)-polygalacturonan (B:H, catalytic acid; B:, basic amino acid side chain).

PLs show similarity with GHs with regard to being multimodular in the sense that the catalytic module is connected to one or more ancillary modules, such as CBMs, additional PL modules, or CE modules. PLs exhibit a large variety of folds, ranging from β-helices to α/α barrels and the varying structure indicates that they have emerged from fundamentally different scaffolds (Lombard et al., 2010).

Pectin lyases (EC 4.2.2.10) and pectate lyases (EC 4.2.2.2) cleave α-1,4-linked D-galacturonic acid residues within smooth regions of pectin via a β-elimination mechanism (Lombard et al., 2010). Fungal pectin lyases characterized so far in the CAZy database all belong to the PL1 family, while pectate lyases belong to families PL1, PL3, and PL10. The occurrence of such lyases differs significantly in different species of fungi (Coutinho et al., 2009). For example, A. niger encodes six pectin lyases and only one pectate lyase (Benen et al., 2000), while A. nidulans encodes two pectin lyases, five identified pectate lyases, and six putative pectate lyases (Galagan et al., 2005). Structural similarities between pectin lyases and pectate lyases suggest that they descended from a common ancestor (Mayans et al., 1997). However, these two types of lyases exhibit important differences with respect to their active site. As a consequence, pectin lyases preferentially attack heavily methyl-esterified substrates and exhibit optima at around pH 5.5 (Mayans et al., 1997). In contrast, pectate lyases are more specific for demethylated or low degree esterified pectins, have optima at around pH 8.5, and require Ca^{2+} for their activity (Mayans et al., 1997). Pectin lyases and pectate lyases from A. niger (PDB 1IDJ, Fig. 13.6) exhibit parallel β-helix folds. Even though there are structural similarities between these two types of lyases, divergence in their substrate-binding cleft results in substantial differences in substrate specificity. The substrate-binding cleft of pectate lyase is rich in charged amino acid residues, contains no aromatic amino acid residues, and Ca^{2+} ions are involved in the activation of the C5 proton of pectate. Pectin lyase has a binding cleft that is rich in aromatic amino acid residues, and Asp154, Arg176, and Arg236 are potential catalytic groups. They do not require Ca^{2+} for catalysis, and instead, Arg176 plays a similar role with regard to the stabilization of negatively charged species. The way in which the active site assists bond cleavage is therefore different in pectin lyases and pectate lyases, and even if they share a common structure they diverge significantly with regard to the binding of carbohydrates (Mayans et al., 1997).

The hairy region of pectin is cleaved by rhamnogalacturonan lyases, which belong to families PL4 and PL11. These families of lyases differ substantially in their structure from pectin lyases and pectate lyases. In addition, PL4 lyases have a much lower pH optimum than PL11 lyases (Jensen et al., 2010), and the presence of acetyl groups in the backbone of rhamnogalacturonan affects cleavage by these enzymes (Mutter et al., 1998; De Vries et al., 2000). Hence, the cooperative action of rhamnogalacturonan acetyl esterases in addition to accessory enzymes, such as α-arabinofuranosidases (GH51 and GH54), β-galactosidases (GH2 and GH35), β-xylosidases (GH3, GH43), endoarabinanases (GH43), exoarabinanases (GH93), β-endogalactanases (GH53), and several different esterases (CE8, CE12, and CE13) (Martens-Uzunova and Schaap, 2009) is required for efficient degradation of xylogalacturonan and rhamnogalacturonan pectin structures (De Vries *et al.*, 2000).

13.4.3 Carbohydrate Esterases

CEs (EC 3.1.1- or 3.1.5-) are hydrolytic enzymes responsible for the removal of *O*-acetyl and *N*-acetyl moieties from polysaccharides. According to the CAZy database, CEs comprise 19 families that include multiple non-classified polypeptides. CEs involved in biomass degradation are mainly AXEs (EC 3.1.1.72), which are distributed in CE families 1–7 and 12, acetyl esterases (AEs; EC 3.1.1.6) in the CE16 family, feruloyl or FAE (EC 3.1.1.73) in the CE1 family, pectin methylesterase (PME; EC 3.1.1.11) in the CE8 family, pectin acetyl esterase (PAE; EC 3.1.1.-) in the CE12 and CE13 families, rhamnogalacturonan acetyl esterase (EC 3.1.1.-) in the CE12 family, and 4-*O*-methyl-glucuronoyl methyl esterase (EC 3.1.1.-) in the CE15 family. These enzymes are well studied, with regard to fungal and bacterial sources, and act as accessory enzymes by playing a synergistic role with cellulases for achieving efficient degradation of lignocellulosic biomass (Lombard *et al.*, 2014).

AEs and AXEs of CE families 1, 4, 5, 6, and 16 hydrolyze ester linkages of acetate residues in xylan chains (Biely *et al.*, 2011). This promotes the catalytic action of endoxylanases and β-xylosidase involved in the degradation of the xylan backbone. *Aspergillus* encodes four characterized AXEs, while *T. reesei* RUT-30 encodes one AXE and one AE (Lombard *et al.*, 2014). The main difference between the CE families is their preference for hydrolyzing different *O*-linked acetyl groups. Enzymes from CE families 1, 4, and 5 have a strong preference for 2-*O*-linked residues, the most common acetyl linkage in hemicellulose, while CE16 enzymes favor 3-*O*- and 4-*O*-linked residues (Li *et al.*, 2008; Biely *et al.*, 2011). For instance, expression of *An*AXE1 in hybrid aspen resulted in less acetylated xylan, especially at the C-2 position (Pawar *et al.*, 2017), indicating that AXE was targeted to the cell wall for post-synthetic xylan deacetylation and resulting in significant improvement in the accessibility of cellulose to cellulolytic enzymes (Pawar *et al.*, 2017). In addition, expression of *Hypocrea jecorina* (name sometimes used for *T. reesei*; Druzhinina and Kubicek, 2016) AXE (*Hj*AXE) from CE5 in hybrid aspen was targeted to the secretory pathway (Wang *et al.*, 2020). Due to the presence of a CBM at the C-terminus, *Hj*AXE was predicted to deacetylate xylan in the close vicinity of cellulose (Margolles-Clark *et al.*, 1996). Unlike CE1 AXEs, which exhibit broad substrate specificity acting on both poly- and oligosaccharides, CE5 AXEs are more specific for polymeric xylan (Biely *et al.*, 2011; Koutaniemi *et al.*, 2013). Some esterases, such as 4-*O*-methyl-glucuronoyl methyl esterase of CE15, were observed to reduce cross-links between cell wall biopolymers, thereby increasing the extractability of cell wall polymers and improving the accessibility of cellulases and xylanases to their substrates (Gandla *et al.*, 2015). Some AEs were found to hydrolyze acetyl residues attached to galactomannan chains (Tenkanen *et al.*, 1995). Typical serine esterases, such as AXEs and FAEs, contain an α/β-hydrolase fold and a catalytic core with an $\alpha/\beta/\alpha$ sandwich structure with a catalytic triad (typically Ser, His, and Asp), and an oxyanion hole. Biely and co-workers (Biely *et al.*, 1996; 1997) found that *Hj*AXE (PDB 1QOZ; Fig. 13.6) is capable of removing acetyl groups from both positions 2 and 3. The rate of hydrolysis is faster when there is a free hydroxyl group at the other position (Hakulinen *et al.*, 2000). If the xylopyranoside residue is double acetylated, both acetyl groups are removed by the catalytic triad by first removing one acetyl group, and then the residue is reoriented so that the nucleophilic oxygen of Ser can attack the second acetyl group. However, this enzyme cannot remove acetyl groups located close to large side groups, such as 4-*O*-methyl glucuronic acid. However, *Hj*AXE from family CE16 can catalyze deacetylation at positions 3 and 4 and the mode of deacetylation by *Hj*AXE differs from that of other fungal AXEs from the same family (Puchart *et al.*, 2016). The first deacetylation, at either position 3 or 4, by this enzyme is followed by the action of α-glucuronidase and β-xylosidase before the second deacetylation.

Esterified *p*-coumaric acid and ferulic acid, two cinnamic acids that are often found as esters in xylan, are removed by feruloyl/*p*-coumaroyl esterases. On basis of differences in substrate specificity, FAEs are classified into four types (types A to D). The four model substrates that are used for the classification include methyl *p*-coumaric acid (MpCA), methyl caffeic acid (MCA), methyl ferulic acid (MFA), and methyl sinapic acid (MSA) (Crepin *et al.*, 2004;

Benoit et al., 2008). These esterases have not been assigned any classification in the CAZy database, but some of them belong to the CE1 family even though substrate cross specificity was not observed for these enzymes (Puchart et al., 2007).

13.4.4 Auxiliary Activities

The so-called auxiliary activities, or AAs, are a more recent addition to the CAZy database. The AAs currently include 16 families, of which nine families contain ligninolytic enzymes and seven contain enzymes that act directly on polysaccharides. The latter families include LPMO and cellobiose dehydrogenase (CDH) (Levasseur et al., 2013).

CDHs (EC 1.1.99.18), are extracellular multi-domain hemoflavoenzymes produced under cellulolytic culture conditions by lignocellulose-degrading fungi (Zhang et al., 2011). CDH contains an amino-terminal cytochrome domain connected to a carboxy-terminal dehydrogenase domain, containing the FAD redox cofactor. The active site and a cellulose-binding region reside in the flavoprotein domain. This enzyme employs a wide spectrum of electron acceptors, such as quinones, Fe^{3+}, and Cu^{2+}, to oxidize soluble cellodextrins to the corresponding lactones (Henriksson et al., 2000).

LPMOs were initially associated with two families in the CAZy database, that is, glycoside hydrolase family 61 (GH61) and carbohydrate-binding module family 33 (CBM33). These were later renamed as auxiliary activity families AA9 and AA10 (Levasseur et al., 2013; Lombard et al., 2014). Today, LPMOs are divided into seven families (9–11, 13–15, and 16). AA9 LPMOs are of fungal origin and act on cellulose and cello-oligosaccharides (Isaksen et al., 2014), xyloglucan (Agger et al., 2014), chitin and xylan (Frommhagen et al., 2015). AA10 LPMOs are mostly found in bacteria and are active on both chitin and cellulose (Forsberg et al., 2014b; Vaaje-Kolstad et al., 2010). AA11 LPMOs are produced by the fungus *Aspergillus oryzae* and are involved in the cleavage of chitin chains (Hemsworth et al., 2014). Starch-active AA13 LPMOs exhibit activity on polysaccharides that contain α-1,4-linked units, such as amylose and amylopectin (Vu et al., 2014). AA14 LPMO enzymes act on xylan coated cellulose fibers (Couturier et al., 2018). Two AA15 enzymes generated by the insect *Thermobia domestica* showed activity with cellulose and chitin (Sabbadin *et al.*, 2018). AA16 LPMOs produced by the fungus *Aspergillus aculeatus* act on cellulose (Filiatrault-Chastel *et al.*, 2019).

Family AA9 LPMOs exhibit an immunoglobulin-like distorted β-sandwich fold, which contains antiparallel β-strands connected by loops and α-helixes (Fig. 13.6) (Eijsink *et al.*, 2019.). Unlike classic glycosidic hydrolases containing obvious substrate-binding grooves, LPMOs use a relatively flat binding surface to catalyze the degradation of cellulose (Fig. 13.3). A divalent copper atom coordinates two His residues in a histidine brace, one Tyr, and two water molecules (Quinlan *et al.*, 2011) (Fig. 13.6).

LPMO has emerged as an important tool in enzymatic saccharification of recalcitrant lignocellulosic biomass. LPMO breaks glycosidic bonds using an oxidative mechanism, thereby fragmenting cellulose chains into smaller pieces. This fragmentation boosts the activity of GHs in cellulolytic enzyme mixtures by creating more hydrolysis targets (Hemsworth *et al.*, 2015). Oxidation of cellulose by LPMO typically leads to chain cleavage at either the C1 or the C4 position of a sugar ring (Fig. 13.8). LPMO-mediated C1 oxidation leads to the formation of a lactone, and then the lactone dissociates in water into an aldonic acid residue at the reducing end. In comparison, C4 oxidation yields a ketoaldose at the non-reducing end, and, after hydration, a geminal diol (Fig. 13.8). LPMOs are classified into three types based on their C1/C4 regioselectivity, that is, PMO-1, PMO-2, and PMO-3. PMO-1 and PMO-2 enzymes only oxidize the C1 position and the C4 position, respectively. PMO-3 enzymes can oxidize both the C1 and the C4 position (Borisova *et al.*, 2015; Phillips *et al.*, 2011). There are also reports about the oxidation of the C6 position (Chen *et al.*, 2019).

LPMO oxidizes and breaks glycosidic bonds in the presence of molecular oxygen and an external electron donor. The catalytic reaction begins with the reduction of Cu (II) to Cu(I) (Fig. 13.8). Different reactive copper-oxygen intermediates, such as Cu (II)-superoxide or Cu (II)-oxyl, may be involved (Bertini *et al.*, 2018; Phillips *et al.*, 2011). Subsequently, the enzyme abstracts a hydrogen atom from C1 or C4 of the substrate, which is followed by hydroxylation of the resulting radical through an oxygen-rebound mechanism (Fig. 13.8). The hydroxylation causes a destabilization

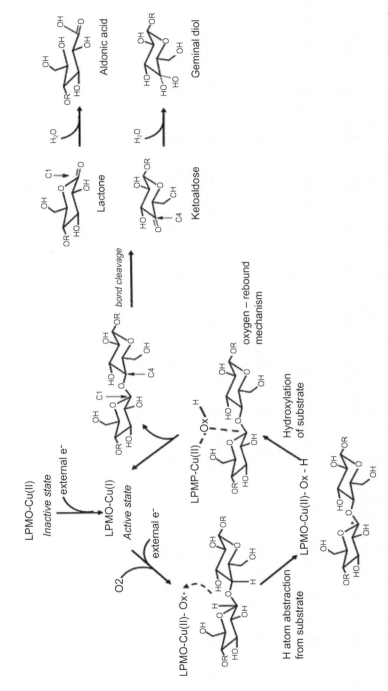

Figure 13.8 Schematic mechanism of LPMO-catalyzed reactions. "Ox" could tentatively refer to copper(II)-superoxide (LPMO-Cu(II)–O-O·) or copper(II)-oxyl (LPMO-Cu(II)–O·) intermediates.

of the glycosidic bond and the formation of the final product occurs via an elimination reaction (Bertini *et al.*, 2018; Kjaergaard *et al.*, 2014). Both small and large molecules might function as electron donors. Small molecules performing this function could be ascorbic acid and gallic acid, while large molecules could be fungal CDH (Phillips *et al.*, 2011). Moreover, other enzymes, such as polyphenol oxidase (Frommhagen *et al.*, 2017) or glucose-methanol-choline (GMC) oxidoreductase, could be involved as electron donors for LPMO (Kracher *et al.*, 2016). Lignin-derived substances might also serve as electron donors. The catalytic activity of LPMO depends on the availability of molecular oxygen. However, some studies suggest that hydrogen peroxide is the preferred co-substrate rather than molecular oxygen (Bissaro *et al.*, 2017). Therefore, the identity of the oxidants and reductants involved in LPMO catalysis in nature is still uncertain. Nevertheless, enzyme producers have improved their cellulolytic enzyme cocktails by adding LPMO (Müller *et al.*, 2015).

13.4.5 Associated Modules

CBMs are non-catalytic parts of carbohydrate-active enzymes and are usually connected to the catalytic core through flexible linkers (Gilbert *et al.*, 2013). CBMs were previously known as cellulose-binding domains (CBDs), but later, when additional carbohydrate-binding modules were found that could bind other carbohydrates than cellulose, a more comprehensive terminology was adopted (Boraston *et al.*, 2004). There are currently 88 CBM families in the CAZy database, and the majorities of these families have members that target constituents of the cell walls of plants. The classification mainly aims at identifying CBMs, predicting binding specificity, identifying functional amino acid residues, revealing evolutionary relationships, and predicting polypeptide folds. Most CBMs have a β-sandwich fold and show similarities with lectins with regard to structural features and binding mechanisms, but, as they are functionally distinct, they are separated into different families.

CBMs are classified into three types; A, B, and C. Type A CBMs bind to the surface of crystalline polysaccharides, such as cellulose and chitin, Type B CBMs bind internally on glycan chains (endo-type) and exhibit extended clefts that bind single carbohydrate chains of hemicellulose, pectin, and amorphous regions of cellulose or chitin. Type C CBMs bind to the termini of glycan chains (exo-type) and usually bind to mono-, di-, and trisaccharides (Gilbert et al., 2013).

Biomass-degrading fungi commonly employ family 1 CBMs for the degradation of plant cell walls. The presence of such modules was first reported by Van Tilbeurgh et al. (1986), who studied TrCel7A. The first structure of a GH1 CBM was determined by Kraulis et al. (1989) using NMR spectroscopy for studies of TrCel7A CBM, which forms a 36-residue irregular, triple-stranded, antiparallel β-sheet with amphiphilic character. It has a large, hydrophilic flat face exhibiting three Tyr residues and a large number of polar amino acid residues, and a hydrophobic face on the wedge portion of the CBM. The CBM contains four Cys residues that form two disulfide bonds. The three conserved Tyr residues on the flat, hydrophilic face of CBM (Tyr5, Tyr31, and Tyr32 in TrCel7A CBM) are involved in binding to crystalline cellulose. Studies of TrCel7A have indicated that the CBM is responsible for targeting the enzyme to crystalline regions, thereby increasing the concentration of the CD on the cellulose surface for enabling efficient catalytic performance (Payne et al., 2015). Several T. reesei cellulases lack CBM and linker, such as TrCel12A, TrCel61a, and TrCel61b (Foreman et al., 2003).

Some multimodular enzymes contain PTS linkers (containing Pro, Ser, and Thr residues) that connect CBMs to CDs. Linkers have been found to play a role in maintaining sufficient distance between the CBM and the CD and have been proposed to facilitate dynamic adsorption to the surface of cellulose (Srisodsuk et al., 1993). Studies of removal of linkers indicate that, as consequence, the activity of the cellulase toward both crystalline and amorphous cellulose can be reduced (Jang et al., 2012). Linkers in cellulases do not exhibit any greater extent of sequence homology. Fungal GH6 and GH7 cellulases exhibit differences in the length of their linkers, with GH6 and GH7 linkers having an average length of 42 and 30 amino acid residues, respectively (Sammond et al., 2012). Linkers of fungal and bacterial cellulases differ with respect to the composition of amino acid residues, as fungal linkers are rich in Ser and Thr, while bacterial linkers are rich in Pro.

13.5 Bacterial Enzymes

A wide range of bacteria has been investigated with regard to the potential occurrence of enzymes involved in the degradation of plant biomass. Cellulolytic bacteria are commonly found in phyla such as *Actinobacteria*, *Bacteroides*, *Fibrobacteres*, *Firmicutes*, and *Proteobacteria* (Gupta *et al.*, 2012; Koeck *et al.*, 2014). Many bacteria that produce cellulolytic enzymes are saprophytes (Mardanov *et al.*, 2012).

Clostridium thermocellum is an example of a well-studied anaerobic bacterium that is of interest for biofuel production (Olson *et al.*, 2015). Studies based on proteomics and transcriptomics have indicated that *C. thermocellum* relies heavily on enzymes from GH families 5, 8, 9, 11, and 48 for biomass deconstruction (Xu *et al.*, 2016). Meta-transcriptomic studies of the rumen of dairy cattle revealed an abundance of species of *Bacteroides*, *Fibrobacteres*, and *Firmicutes* producing cellulose-degrading enzymes from GH families 5, 9, 48, and 74, and hemicellulose-degrading enzymes from GH families 10, 11, and 43. High levels of GH94 (cellobiose phosphorylase) suggested a putative role for phosphorylation in the deconstruction of oligosaccharides (Comtet-Marre *et al.*, 2017).

Cel6A from the thermophilic filamentous fungus *Chaetomium thermophilum*, a GH6 enzyme, has an active site suited for endo-initiated attack (PDB 4A05, Fig. 13.6) (Thompson *et al.*, 2012). *Ct*Cel6A displays a typical GH6 family distorted β/α barrel including full-length active-site loops A and B. The enzyme shares 77% sequence identity with CBH of *Humicola insolens*, *Hi*Cel6A, and 63% with *Tr*Cel6A, suggesting it is a CBH. The enzyme has potential binding sites for cellobiose and cellotetraose. A tetrahedrally coordinated Li$^+$ ion in the active center mimics an oxocarbenium ion-like transition state that results in an inverting catalytic mechanism.

Many bacterial AA10 LPMOs are involved in the degradation of cellulose (Forsberg *et al.*, 2014a). The secretomes of aerobic biomass-degrading mesophilic and thermophilic bacteria, such as *Streptomyces coelicolor*, *Thermobifida fusca*, and *Cellvibrio japonicus*, produce cellulose-degrading LPMOs with active sites containing a copper ion in a histidine brace. Studies of *S. coelicolor* LPMOs (LPMO10B and CelS2) have resulted in the first 3D structures for bacterial cellulose-degrading LPMOs (Forsberg *et al.*, 2014a) (PDB

4OY6 and 4OY7). These enzymes exhibit distorted β-sandwich structures comprising two β-sheets with the copper atom at the active site showing octahedral geometry in a conserved histidine brace. CelS2 AA10B LPMOs from *C. japonicus* and *T. fusca* are C1 oxidizers. However, *Sc*LPMO10b and *T. fusca* LPMO10A, are both C1 and C4 oxidizers (Hemsworth et al., 2015).

Microbial enzyme systems involved in the decomposition of plant cell walls include multi-enzyme complexes (cellulosomes), free single enzymes, and multifunctional enzymes. Anaerobic microorganisms belonging to the phylum *Firmicutes* possess extracellular cellulolytic enzyme complexes, cellulosomes, which act on crystalline cellulose. Dockerin domains of enzymes in the cellulosome bind to cohesin domains of scaffoldins, which keep cellulosomes together and anchor them to bacterial cells. Scaffoldins contain CBMs that assist the binding of cellulosomes to their cellulosic substrate (Koeck et al., 2014). *C. thermocellum* has eight scaffoldin genes and the cellulosomal complex of this organism contains up to 63 enzymes. The seven-module *C. thermocellum* enzyme *Ct*-Cbh9A is a 140 kDa highly glycosylated protein. Glycosylation protects cellulosomes from proteases and contributes to protein-protein and protein-carbohydrate interactions (Blumer-Schuette et al., 2014).

Studies of gut microbiomes of humans, rodents, and ruminants have revealed a multitude of cellulase genes (Flint et al., 2012; White et al., 2014). *Firmicutes* dominate the microbiome with regard to GHs in the bovine rumen (Brulc et al., 2009). The CelI enzyme from buffalo rumen has been expressed in *E. coli* and found to be a typical GH5 cellulase (Dadheech et al., 2018). Metagenomic analysis of the porcine microbiome resulted in the detection of enzymes from 29 CAZy families presumably involved in the degradation of cellulose, xylan, and pectin (Yang et al., 2016). Metagenomic sequence data produced from the hindgut microbiome of the termite *Nasutitermes sp.* revealed that *Spirochetes* and *Fibrobacteres*, rather than *Firmicutes*, are major sources of GHs and accessory modules (Warnecke et al., 2007).

Metagenomic studies indicate that thermophilic bacteria, such as *Thermoanaerobacterium saccharolyticum* (T_{opt} 55 °C), *Thermoanaerobacter mathrani* (T_{opt} 70 °C), *Thermotoga maritima* (T_{opt} 80 °C), *C. thermocellum* (T_{opt} 60 °C), *Caldicellulosiruptor* sp. (T_{opt} 65–78 °C), *Acidothermus cellulolyticus* (T_{opt} 55 °C), and *T. fusca* (T_{opt}

50 °C), are involved in biomass degradation (Blumer-Schuette et al., 2014). They occur in a variety of environmental conditions, such as soil, hot springs, compost, and guts, and have gained attention for their ability to utilize a wide range of carbohydrates including cellulose. These organisms act as a source of genes encoding different carbohydrate-active enzymes that can withstand high process temperatures and often harsh process conditions (Olson et al., 2015; Blumer-Schuette et al., 2014).

13.6 Determination of Cellulolytic Activity

Cellulose is a water-insoluble substrate that can exist in different forms, and its degradation is a concerted effort involving several enzymatic activities. For these reasons, assaying cellulase activity is not a straightforward procedure.

Quantitative assays to determine cellulase activity can either be assays of individual enzymes, such as EG, CBH, and BGL, or assays of combined cellulolytic activity, such as the filter paper unit (FPU) assay or filter paper activity (FPA). Assays based on insoluble cellulosic substrates are usually nonlinear with regard to time and enzyme dosage. Cellulase activity assays can be based on the accumulation of products after saccharification (the most common approach), quantitation of reduction of substrate, or change in the physical properties of the reaction mixture (such as viscosity).

Determination of formation of reducing sugar using 3,5-dinitrosalicylic acid (DNS) is a commonly used spectrophotometric assay. DNS is reduced to 3-amino-5-nitrosalicylic acid by carbonyl groups at the reducing ends of sugars, which results in an increase in absorbance at 540 nm. (Miller, 1959). The DNS method is less sensitive at lower glucose concentrations (below 70 µg ml^{-1}) and the color develops only under alkaline conditions. The Nelson–Somogyi method (Nelson, 1944), which is more sensitive at lower sugar concentrations, can also be used to estimate reducing sugar.

Determination of total cellulase activity assay is based on the combined action of EG, CBH, and BGL on substrates such as filter paper, cotton fiber, or Avicel (microcrystalline cellulose). The FPA method is recommended by the International Union of Pure and Applied Chemistry (IUPAC) due to its uniformity and due to the availability of suitable filter paper substrate (Ghose, 1987). A 600 mm² piece of filter paper (Whatman No. 1) (50 mg) is incubated with citrate buffer (0.05 M, pH 4.8) at 50 °C for 60 min. The reaction is stopped by adding DNS reagent (3 ml) and the tubes are boiled in a water bath for 5 min. The absorbance at 540 nm is used to determine the concentration of reducing sugar. The method varies greatly depending on the amount of BGL in the cellulase preparation. The standard procedure (Ghose, 1987) suffers from drawbacks such as laborious dilutions of cellulase preparations, time consumption, and the use of large amounts of reagents. The standard FPA method has been supplemented with a more convenient microplate-based variant (Xiao et al., 2004a) and by a variant in which the assay volume is reduced tenfold compared to that of the standard method (Camassola and Dillon, 2012).

Substrates such as PASC, Sigmacell 20, and Avicel are used to determine the activity of CBH. Avicel (PH 101) (1% w/v) is suspended in water and incubated at 50 °C for 2 h. The released sugar can be estimated using the Nelson–Somogyi assay of reducing sugar or using the phenol-H_2SO_4 (total sugar) assay. Cotton fiber and CMC are not attacked to a significant extent by CBH, but PASC is hydrolyzed with a characteristic slow decrease in DP. Longer chain cello-oligosaccharides are hydrolyzed at a rate that increases with the DP. Highly crystalline Avicel is the preferred substrate for CBH due to its relatively low DP.

EGs are key enzymes for initiating saccharification of cellulose. They hydrolyze amorphous cellulose, CMC, hydroxymethyl cellulose (HEC), and trinitrophenyl-carboxymethyl cellulose (TNP-CM-cellulose). The rate of hydrolysis of longer chain cello-oligosaccharides increases with the DP. CMC and HEC are considered preferred substrates (Ghose, 1987). CMC is considered a selective EG substrate because of its steric hindrance to entering the tunnel-like structure of the catalytic center of CBH. CMC 7L2 2% (w/v) is dissolved in sodium citrate buffer (0.05 M, pH 4.8) and two dilutions of EG are used, where one releases less and the other releases more than 0.5 mg glucose. The reaction mixtures are incubated at 50 °C for 30 min. The result can be estimated by using the DNS method, the Nelson-Somogyi method, or the viscosity method. A drawback is that there might be relatively large activity differences with different cellulases (Gilkes *et al.*, 1997). The filter paper assay has an advantage, as it is uniform and readily available.

BGL is a very important component of the cellulase system by completing the hydrolysis of short-chain cello-oligosaccharides and cellobiose to glucose. Cellulase systems containing low levels of BGL have poor saccharifying power because of the inhibition of EGs and CBHs by cellobiose. BGL hydrolyzes cello-oligosaccharides at a decreasing rate with increasing DP. Substrates such as p-nitrophenyl-β-D-glucoside and cellobiose are typically used to determine BGL activity. The substrate is dissolved in sodium acetate buffer (0.1 M, pH 4.8–5.0) and incubated with the enzyme at 50 °C for 30 min. Spectrophotometric measurement of p-nitrophenol at 420 nm or estimation of released glucose is used for the determination of BGL activity.

Commonly used commercial enzyme preparations include, for example, Celluclast 1.5 from *T. reesei* ATCC 26921, Novozyme 188 from *A. niger*, Cellic CTec2, and Cellic CTec 3 (from Novozymes), and Spezyme CP, Multifect xylanase, and Accellerase 1000 (from Genencor). Loadings and activities of commercial cellulase cocktails vary depending on the feedstock and the pretreatment conditions used. Monosaccharides are typically characterized using liquid chromatography, including HPLC (e.g. Bio-Rad Aminex HPX-87H and HPX-87P columns used with refractive index detection) and HPAEC (e.g. Dionex CarboPac PA1 column used with electrochemical detection), glucose-oxidase-based methods, and capillary electrophoresis (Gandla *et al.*, 2018).

13.7 Biorefining of Lignocellulosic Feedstocks

The abundance of lignocellulosic feedstocks positions them as the raw material of choice for the production of biobased energy carriers and a large number of the platform chemicals and materials that are today produced from fossil resources. The most rational way of converting lignocellulosic biomass into high-value products is by applying a biorefinery approach. A biorefinery operation is "the sustainable processing of biomass into a spectrum of marketable products and energy" (De Jong and Jungmeier, 2015).

In lignocellulose biorefining, biomass feedstocks are first subjected to a fractionation step, where cellulose, hemicelluloses, and lignin are selectively separated, and the resulting fractions are then directed to the production of relevant end products. A biorefinery can process all feedstock components into marketable products and energy in an analogous way as petroleum refineries do with crude oil. The range of products to be manufactured depends on multiple factors, for example, feedstock composition, reactions involved, separation technology, and operational conditions. Biorefining is not new, as many forest-industrial enterprises based on chemical pulping serve as biorefineries already today. However, as this chapter is about enzymatic saccharification, the focus will be on biochemical conversion technologies. Enzymatic saccharification is advantageous due to high selectivity and low by-product formation. Nevertheless, the raw material first needs to be fractionated.

Biomass polymers can be selectively separated by diverse methods, and different fractionation sequences can be applied. One approach is to first separate hemicelluloses from biomass, for instance, by hydrothermal treatment in aqueous media (Penín *et al.*, 2019). That leads to a liquid stream rich in oligosaccharides, monosaccharides, and other hemicellulosic components, such as acetic acid and uronic acids. After separation of hemicelluloses, the resulting biomass can be submitted to further fractionation by either lignin solubilization using solvents or cellulose hydrolysis using enzymes (Fig. 13.9A).

An alternative approach is recovering lignin as the first step of the fractionation sequence, and then processing the carbohydrate fractions (Matsakas *et al.*, 2019). Effective ways of separating lignin without damaging the polysaccharides include the use of an organic solvent in a process known as organosolv, or by using modern techniques based on chemical pulping (primarily Kraft pulping and sulfite pulping). Using the organosolv approach, lignin and hemicelluloses are solubilized and they end up in a liquid stream, which also contains the solvent (Fig. 13.9B). The latter is recovered by distillation, lignin is regenerated by precipitation, and a hemicelluloses-rich aqueous fraction will remain. Cellulose contained in the solid fraction and solubilized hemicelluloses is hydrolyzed for generating hexoses (mostly glucose and mannose) and pentoses (mostly xylose). The resulting sugars are processed by microbial fermentation or chemical-catalytic conversion to biofuels (ethanol, butanol) or different platform chemicals (furans, organic acids). Lignin can be processed into phenolic compounds, polymers, composites, and a wide spectrum of added-value specialty chemicals and fuels.

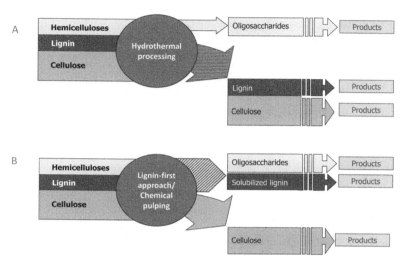

Figure 13.9 Simplified scheme of lignocellulosic biorefining following different fractionation sequences: Hemicellulose solubilization as the first step (A) and lignin first approach (B). The actual yields of lignocellulosic constituents in the resulting fractions would be lower than the theoretical yields indicated in the figure as fractionation would be partial rather than complete.

Implementation of additional large-scale biorefineries with circular bioeconomy strategies is expected to accelerate the transition to a sustainable society. In that sense, any initiative on launching commercial-scale biorefineries should thoroughly evaluate the environmental, economic, and social sustainability of the entire value chain. That includes potential impacts on water use, arable land availability, greenhouse gas emissions, biodiversity, and food production.

During the last years, there has been a dynamic investment toward the commercialization of lignocellulose-processing biorefineries. Although the gap between laboratory research and commercial-scale operation has caused the failure of many attempts of bringing R & D projects into the industrial scale (Chandel et al.,

2018), many demonstration initiatives have been implemented in several European countries, as well as in North America, Brazil, China, and India. Furthermore, there are some cases, where large-scale biorefineries have already been operating steadily for a long period. Borregaard (in Norway) and Domsjö Fabriker (in Sweden) are two examples of successful implementation of commercial-scale biorefineries. Currently, Borregaard (https://www.borregaard.com/) produces specialty cellulose, lignosulfonates, bioethanol, vanillin, and biogas, while Domsjö Fabriker (https://www.domsjo.adityabirla.com/) manufactures specialty cellulose, lignosulfonates, bioethanol, carbon dioxide, biogas, bioresin, and soil conditioners. Both Borregaard and Domsjö Fabriker have technical capacity for producing other products depending on the market scenario.

13.8 Pretreatment to Facilitate Enzymatic Saccharification

Enzymatic saccharification is a commonly used approach for selectively deconstructing cellulose to glucose, which can then be converted to end products of interest (Gandla *et al.*, 2018). The recalcitrance of lignocellulosic biomass, which is a consequence of intrinsic feedstock properties, is a major problem affecting saccharification. To reduce feedstock recalcitrance, pretreatment is performed as the first step of lignocellulose bioconversion. By removal of certain chemical components or by other actions on biomass chemistry, structure or morphology, pretreatment hits some of the barriers responsible for recalcitrance, so that cellulose reactivity toward bioconversion is enhanced. Removal of hemicelluloses or lignin, hydrolysis of acetyl groups, disruption of lignin–carbohydrate complexes, or decreasing of DP of cellulose are some chemistry-related factors behind the activating effect observed after different pretreatments. Decreasing cellulose crystallinity, increasing the porosity, and reducing the particle size are other effects associated with pretreatment (Zhao *et al.*, 2012; Wang *et al.*, 2018).

Several pretreatment methods with high innovative potential have been validated in demonstration-scale facilities, and some of them have been upscaled to commercial plants (Table 13.2).

Table 13.2 Examples of pretreatment methods of commercial relevance

Method	Range of operational conditions	Effect on lignocellulose constituents	Upscaling examples
Auto-catalyzed hydrothermal pretreatment	~170–230°C, ~5–30 min	Partial solubilization of hemicelluloses, slight removal of lignin	Inbicon, RE Energy (Denmark)
Hydrothermal pretreatment with dilute acid	~120–230°C, from a few min to ~1 h	Hydrolysis of hemicelluloses, disruption, redistribution and slight removal of lignin, partial depolymerization of cellulose	Iogen Corporation (Canada), POET-DSM (USA), Raízen Energia (Brazil)
Hydrothermal pretreatment with steam explosion	~160–230°C, ~1–30 min	Partial to complete solubilization of hemicelluloses, deacetylation, slight removal, and modification of lignin	Sekab (Sweden), Abengoa Bioenergy (USA)
Mild alkaline methods	~25–180°C, from a few min to several weeks	Significant removal of lignin, partial solubilization of hemicelluloses, deacetylation	DuPont (USA)
Chemical pulping-based methods (including sulfite and organosolv)	90–250°C, 30–60 min	Extensive removal of lignin, variable removal of hemicelluloses, decrease of degree of polymerization and crystallinity of cellulose	Borregaard (BALI process) (Norway), Chempolis (Finland)

Many other reported methods are so far only of academic interest. To be effective, a pretreatment method should result in greatly enhanced enzymatic digestibility of cellulose and high recovery of hemicellulosic sugars/oligomers (Jönsson and Martín, 2016). To be technically relevant for upscaling, pretreatment should allow handling high solids loads with minimal energy demand, low use of chemicals, and low capital and operational cost (Mankar *et al.*, 2021). Hydrothermal processes, in which moist feedstocks, either alone or in the presence of a chemical additive, are heated for a certain time, have a high potential for industrial application with different types of biomass. Different lignocellulosic materials have been used in pretreatment research, but since the effectiveness of a given method is feedstock-dependent, the response can diverge for different types of biomass (Martín, 2021).

Several approaches of hydrothermal pretreatment (HTP) are among the most technological-mature methods for different feedstocks (Ruiz *et al.*, 2020). The most basic approach is auto-catalyzed hydrothermal pretreatment (A-HTP), which is also known as liquid hot water pretreatment. In A-HTP, biomass is suspended in water and heated to around 200°C under high pressure, which keeps the water in a liquid state (Table 13.2). Under those conditions, water is autoionized into H_3O^+ and OH^-, which allows catalysis of deacetylation of hemicelluloses. The resulting acetic acid catalyzes the splitting of glycosidic bonds of hemicelluloses, which leads to further hydrolysis and solubilization. Uronic acids are released, and they also contribute to acid catalysis. A-HTP leads to an increase of biomass surface area, which results in the enhancement of enzymatic digestibility of cellulose. A major strength of A-HTP is that neither chemical additives, except water and alkali for pH adjustments, nor expensive anticorrosion materials are required. A drawback is its low effectiveness toward softwood and other highly recalcitrant feedstocks. Anyway, it is possible to optimize the efficiency of A-HTP for different types of biomass by tuning its severity by modifying the temperature or the reaction time (Ilanidis *et al.*, 2021a, b). A-HTP technology for wheat straw has been developed in the Inbicon demonstration plant in Kalundborg, Denmark, and a commercial-scale biorefinery, RE Energy, is now under construction (BEST, 2021).

An HTP variation is the so-called dilute acid pretreatment, or dilute acid-catalyzed hydrothermal pretreatment (DA-HTP), which is a technology with high commercialization potential (Solarte-Toro et al., 2019). DA-HTP involves heating a suspension of biomass in diluted acid to above 120°C for different periods (Table 13.2). Sulfuric acid is commonly used, but other acids are also of practical relevance. DA-HTP leads to almost full hydrolysis of hemicelluloses, some lignin removal, and a remarkable enhancement of the susceptibility of cellulose to enzymatic saccharification (Gandla et al., 2018). Major drawbacks compared to A-HTP are the requirement of sophisticated alloys for the equipment, as well as more formation of inhibitory compounds (Jönsson and Martín, 2016). Anyway, due to their effectiveness, ease of implementation, and relatively low capital expenditures, acid-based approaches are the options of choice in many upscaling initiatives (Silveira et al., 2015; BEST, 2021).

The effect of HTP can be enhanced by applying a sudden decompression at the end of the holding time in a process that is commonly known as steam explosion. Hydrothermal pretreatment with a steam explosion (HTP-SE) is a texturing-hydrolysis process (Smichi et al., 2020), where combined chemical and physical actions disrupt the plant cell wall structure, partially hydrolyze and remove hemicelluloses, and redistribute lignin due to partial depolymerization and condensation. As a consequence, the accessibility of enzymes to cellulose is enhanced, which leads to a high degree of saccharification even using a rather low enzyme loading. If HTP-SE is performed with no added chemicals, the process is catalyzed primarily by hydronium ions from water autoionization as it happens in A-HTP. HTP-SE can also be catalyzed by added acidic reagents, for example, sulfuric acid or sulfur dioxide, or by the addition of alkali. If the process is acid-catalyzed, substantial hydrolysis of hemicelluloses and formation of monosaccharide sugars will occur, whereas alkaline reagents lead to solubilization of hemicelluloses without causing complete hydrolysis to monosaccharides. Despite the high energy consumption for reaching the required temperature and pressure, the effectiveness of HTP-SE toward a wide variety of lignocellulosic feedstocks makes it attractive for commercial applications (Table 13.2).

Some mild alkaline methods are of interest for biomass pretreatment (Kim *et al.*, 2016). In those methods, ester bonds between hemicelluloses and lignin are split, and cellulose peeling reactions occur. That leads to lignin removal, partial solubilization of hemicelluloses, some cellulose depolymerization, and, consequently, to the improvement of cellulose digestibility in enzymatic saccharification. Mild alkaline methods require lower temperatures than those used for HTP methods (Table 13.2). In addition to using strong forms of alkali, such as sodium hydroxide, ammonia and lime can also be used.

Some methods, such as the BALI process of Borregaard (Table 13.2), are based on the sulfite process. The sulfite process removes lignin by the formation of lignosulfonates and solubilizes hemicelluloses. This results in a large improvement of the susceptibility of cellulose to enzymatic saccharification (Rødsrud *et al.*, 2012).

Organosolv pretreatment is another method based on an approach developed in the pulping industry. It is based on the use of organic solvents for solubilizing the lignin and part of the hemicelluloses, and it also causes a certain decrease in the DP and cellulose crystallinity. That results in an increase in the susceptibility of cellulose to enzymatic saccharification. Using acid catalysts in organosolv enhances the hydrolysis of hemicelluloses and lignin solubilization, which allows operation at lower temperatures than those typically required for uncatalyzed processes (Ferreira and Taherzadeh, 2020). Although the cost of solvent recovery is a drawback, the effectiveness of the organosolv process with respect to the selective separation of biomass constituents into high-quality streams makes it interesting from an industrial point of view. Organosolv pretreatment has been verified on a pilot scale, and a demonstration plant owned by Chempolis is in operation in Oulu, Finland (BEST, 2021).

Some methods in which oxidants are used for removing lignin, an approach inspired by the pulping industry, are also relevant with regard to lignocellulose pretreatment (Morone *et al.*, 2017). The oxidants disrupt the lignin-carbohydrate association and induce some solubilization of hemicelluloses, which results in enhanced enzymatic digestibility of cellulose. Oxidative methods can be combined with other approaches, and they typically require temperatures below 200 °C. It was recently shown that the addition of oxygen can modulate the severity of hydrothermal pretreatment under acidic conditions (Ilanidis *et al.*, 2021c).

Another method of interest is ammonia fiber expansion (AFEX), which is based on heating biomass with liquid ammonia, applying pressure, and then releasing it in a way comparable with HTP-SE. That results in decrystallization of cellulose, redistribution of hemicelluloses and lignin, and an increase of cell wall porosity, which leads to enhanced enzyme accessibility. Although AFEX does not cause any major degradation of biomass carbohydrates and does not require washing prior to enzymatic hydrolysis, the high energy requirement for ammonia recovery and its low effectiveness for lignin-rich feedstocks are obstacles for industrial implementation (Kim *et al.*, 2016).

Pretreatment using ionic liquids (ILs) has attracted interest recently. ILs are effective for solubilizing cellulose, which can then be regenerated using an antisolvent. Regenerated cellulose has low crystallinity, high surface area, and reduced interference by lignin and hemicelluloses, and it is prone to enzymatic saccharification. Commercialization of IL pretreatment is hindered by economic issues (Cao *et al.*, 2017), and by issues related to the handling of degradation products.

Physical and biological pretreatment methods are of some interest, but they face major drawbacks for implementation as stand-alone technologies. Physical actions, such as milling, extrusion, or irradiation, lead to structural disruption of biomass and reduction of cellulose crystallinity, which cause some enhancement of the susceptibility to enzymatic saccharification (Mankar *et al.*, 2021). High energy consumption is a major drawback for implementation. Biological pretreatment consists of lignin removal by lignin-degrading microorganisms. It has low energy consumption and low capital expenses, but the slow rate and some cellulose consumption are serious limitations. Combination with other methods or making it part of a multi-product system, for instance producing edible fungi or bioactive compounds (Xiong *et al.*, 2019), gives some relevance to biological pretreatment.

13.9 Inhibition of Enzymatic Saccharification

When lignocellulose is subjected to hydrothermal pretreatment under acidic conditions, a large variety of degradation products will be generated. These degradation products include oligosaccharides, disaccharides, monosaccharides, sugar acids, aliphatic carboxylic acids (such as acetic acid from acetyl groups in hemicelluloses), heteroaromatic substances (furan aldehydes and furanic acids), phenylic substances (phenolic and non-phenolic aromatics), benzoquinones, and aliphatic aldehydes (Jönsson and Martín, 2016). When enzyme preparations are then used for saccharification of pretreated lignocellulose, further degradation products will be created, primarily various saccharides. In addition to that, industrial cellulolytic enzyme preparations typically contain esterases that catalyze the formation of acetic acid and other degradation products.

Cellulolytic enzymes are affected by end-product inhibition (also referred to as feedback inhibition) (Xiao et al., 2004b). Oligosaccharides, disaccharides, and monosaccharides generated through hydrolysis of polysaccharides inhibit the hydrolytic enzymes that generate them. Recent studies on steam pretreated lignocellulose suggest that oligosaccharides exhibit relatively little influence compared to the inhibitory effects caused by monosaccharides (Zhai et al., 2016).

Aromatic substances, such as phenolics derived from various lignocellulosic feedstocks, have also been found to inhibit enzymatic saccharification of cellulose and hemicelluloses (Kim et al., 2013; Michelin et al., 2016; Zhai et al., 2018a). The role of aromatics in inhibition has been further supported by the finding that conditioning methods (such as sulfonation by sulfur oxyanions) causing hydrophilization of water-soluble aromatic by-products alleviate enzyme inhibition, whereas similar conditioning methods (such as treatment with sodium borohydride) that have no major impact on hydrophilicity do not (Cavka and Jönsson, 2013; Jönsson and Martín, 2016). Thus, the addition of sulfur oxyanions, such as sulfite and dithionite, offers a way to alleviate enzyme inhibition problems (Cavka and Jönsson, 2013). The research also indicates that hydrophobic interactions are involved in inhibitory effects of water-soluble aromatics on enzymatic saccharification (Cavka and Jönsson, 2013; Zhai et al., 2018b). Another mechanism of inhibition, exerted by aromatics with phenolic hydroxyl groups, is the denaturing effect that phenols have on proteins, a mechanism that has been exploited in the tanning industry for thousands of years.

Although there are reports in the literature about the inhibition of cellulolytic enzymes by carboxylic acids, this needs to be regarded with some caution. Saccharification of cellulose is a concerted effort depending on the synergistic actions of many different enzymes (Van Dyk and Pletschke, 2012), and enzymes sometimes have narrow pH optima. Firstly, in experiments with acids as potential inhibitors it is often unclear whether the pH was strictly controlled when acids were added to reaction mixtures, and, secondly, carboxylic acids, such as acetic acid, are frequently used in high concentrations in buffers, such as acetate buffer, seemingly without causing any problems.

Inhibition of enzymatic saccharification is also caused by substances in the solid fraction of pretreated lignocellulose. One such mechanism is the catalytically non-productive binding of carbohydrate-degrading enzymes to lignin (Nakagame *et al.*, 2010; Rahikainen *et al.*, 2013; Pareek *et al.*, 2013). Lignin affects recalcitrance in several ways including by physical shielding of cellulose from enzymatic saccharification, by preventing swelling of the substrate, and by retarding saccharification by adsorption of the enzyme (Nakagame *et al.*, 2010; Wu *et al.*, 2020). In addition, pseudo-lignin, an aromatic substance formed from carbohydrates during hydrothermal pretreatment, has a similar effect (Wang and Jönsson, 2018). Catalytically non-productive adsorption of cellulolytic enzymes can be alleviated by introducing charged groups on lignin (Wu *et al.*, 2020). This will decrease hydrophobic interactions between the lignin and the enzymes. Recent findings indicate that this effect can be achieved also under mild reaction conditions and using low concentrations of chemicals (Ilanidis *et al.*, 2021d).

13.10 Process Configurations

Enzymatic saccharification of lignocellulosic polysaccharides and fermentation of the resulting sugars are the basic steps in the production of advanced biofuels, such as second-generation ethanol (2G ethanol), and other sugar-platform bio-products. Saccharification and fermentation can be integrated with different configurations for maximizing yield and reducing costs (Fig. 13.10).

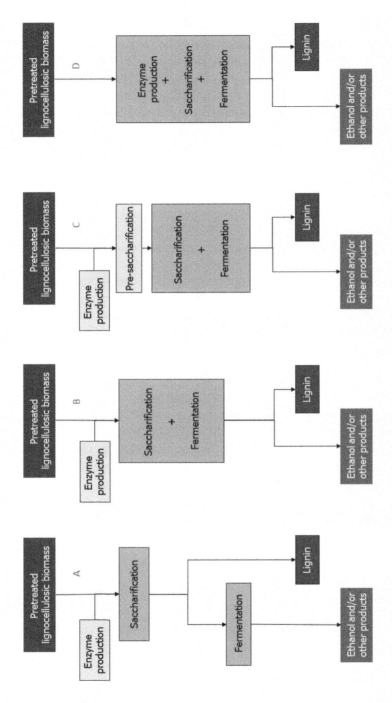

Figure 13.10 Different process configurations for bioconversion of pretreated lignocellulosic biomass (solid fraction after hydrothermal pretreatment) by enzymatic saccharification and microbial fermentation. SHF (A), SSF (B), hybrid hydrolysis and fermentation (C), and consolidated bioprocessing (D).

The simplest configuration is separate hydrolysis and fermentation (SHF), which consists of sequentially arranged process steps (Fig. 13.10A). In SHF, the pretreated feedstock is typically hydrolyzed in a bioreactor at around 45–55°C, which is the optimal temperature range for cellulase preparations, and then the produced hydrolysate is fermented at a lower temperature, which depends on the exact requirements of the fermenting microorganism. For the yeast *Saccharomyces cerevisiae*, the most commonly used microorganism, the temperature would be in the interval 28–40 °C, depending on the specific strain used (Favaro et al., 2019). Since *S. cerevisiae* is highly productive, and since it is tolerant to alcohols and inhibitors, it is the organism of choice for producing ethanol from cellulosic hydrolysates (Favaro et al., 2019). Other yeasts, for example, *Pichia stipitis*, *Candida shehatae*, and some bacteria are also of interest, especially if fermentation of pentoses is a relevant issue. A major problem of the SHF configuration is that sugar yield in the hydrolysis step is restricted by end-product inhibition of cellulases caused by glucose and cellobiose.

Hydrolysis and fermentation of hexoses can also be arranged simultaneously in a configuration known as simultaneous saccharification and fermentation (SSF) (Fig. 13.10B). Pentose fermentation, if relevant, could be performed separately. The main advantage of SSF over SHF is the avoidance of end-product inhibition. As a consequence, higher hydrolysis rate and ethanol concentrations are achieved using SSF compared to SHF. Further strengths are the avoidance of sugar losses in the separation of the hydrolysate after enzymatic hydrolysis and the decrease of the associated capital costs. It has been estimated that the capital investment is 20% lower in SSF than in SHF (Olofsson et al., 2008). Different from SHF, where process steps are performed under optimal conditions, in SSF, hydrolysis, and fermentation are performed under compromise conditions, which is a major weakness. The optimum temperature for most fermenting microorganisms is around 15–20 °C lower than that required by most enzyme cocktails for optimal saccharification. The optimum pH is also often slightly different for hydrolysis and fermentation stages (Dahnum et al., 2015). Another drawback is the difficulty in yeast recycling because of the problems of separating it from lignin after fermentation (Olofsson et al., 2008). Using thermotolerant yeasts, such as *Kluyveromyces marxianus* strains producing ethanol at 45°C

(Castro and Roberto, 2014), is a promising strategy to overcome the difficulties related to the optimum temperature.

In another configuration, referred to as hybrid hydrolysis and fermentation (HHF) (Fig. 13.10C), a pre-saccharification step is combined with an SSF process (Cassells *et al.*, 2017). Pre-saccharification is run under the optimal conditions for the used enzyme, which leads to a high rate of cellulose hydrolysis with a considerable reduction of the viscosity of the reaction suspension. After a relatively short period, the temperature is lowered to a compromise value, the fermenting microorganism is inoculated, and the process is resumed as SSF. In the second stage, the sugars produced during pre-saccharification are converted by the fermenting organism, and more sugar is produced and consumed simultaneously. Compared with a classical SSF, in the second stage of an HHF process, the initial slurry is significantly liquefied, which facilitates the mass transfer and reduces the cost of mixing.

In consolidated bioprocessing (CBP) a single organism is used for enzyme production, hydrolysis, and fermentation (Fig. 13.10D) (Van Zyl *et al.*, 2007). The advantage is that it simplifies the operation. Long fermentation periods, low ethanol yield due to diversion of carbon, alcohol sensitivity of microorganisms, and the limitation of the growth to the supernatant of the reaction mixture are issues that require more research (Olguin-Maciel *et al.*, 2020). The organisms to be used in CBP should be able to produce the enzymes required for efficient lignocellulose deconstruction, and for transforming the sugars to ethanol or other bio-products. Ideal microorganisms for implementing CBP as an efficient industrial process are yet to be introduced. Different ways that are considered for ethanol production using CBP are (*i*) identifying native microbes with cellulolytic and ethanologenic activities, (*ii*) using microbial co-cultures containing both cellulolytic and ethanologenic microorganisms, or (*iii*) genetic engineering of cellulolytic microorganisms to be ethanologenic or ethanologenic organisms to be cellulolytic (Salehi Jouzani and Taherzadeh, 2015).

Several bacteria and fungi with potential for application in CBP have been identified and characterized, and some of them are being subjected to in-depth investigations (Kroukamp *et al.*, 2018). However, since the most promising microbes are so far below the expectations, the co-cultivation of two or more organisms has gained some interest, while genetic engineering remains the main strategy. Intensive research is being devoted to developing genetically modified organisms satisfying the requirements for efficient CBP. It is expected that further investigations will lead to the development of microorganisms that will allow CBP to play an essential role in future biorefineries (Olguin-Maciel et al., 2020).

13.11 Future Outlook

Research and technological development of enzymatic saccharification of lignocellulosic substrates has made great progress during recent decades. Efforts in the area have resulted in the realization of demonstration-scale industrial biorefineries that include enzymatic saccharification as a key process step that enables the processing of thousands of tons of biomass. Renewed research efforts have resulted in findings such as thermostable cellulolytic enzymes, characterization of new key enzymes, such as LPMO, the discovery of new enzymes in environments such as animal guts, improved methods to produce enzymes, improved pretreatment methods, and new ways to make enzymes perform better in industrial environments by the conditioning of the pretreated lignocellulose. Issues that will likely be addressed in future research include, for example, methods for recirculating and reusing enzymes in industrial processes, and further elucidation of the biochemical mechanisms associated with lignin biodegradation. Despite recent progress, this dynamic area will likely continue to develop rapidly over the coming years.

References

Abas N., Kalair A., Khan N. *Futures,* **69** (2015), 31–49.

Ademark P., De Vries R. P., Hägglund P., Stålbrand H., Visser J. *Eur. J. Biochem.*, **268** (2001), 2982–2990.

Agger J. W., Isaksen T., Varnai A., Vidal-Melgosa S., Willats W. G. T., et al. *Proc. Nat. Acad. Sci. USA*, **111** (2014), 6287–6292.

Arantes V., Saddler J. N. *Biotechnol. Biofuels*, **3** (2010), 4.

Arantes V., Saddler J. N. *Biotechnol. Biofuels*, **4** (2011), 3.

Aspeborg H., Coutinho P. M., Wang Y., Brumer H., Henrissat B. *BMC Evol. Biol.*, **12** (2012), 186.

Banerjee G., Car S., Liu T., Williams D. L., Meza S. L., *et al*. *Biotechnol. Bioeng.*, **109** (2012), 922–931.

Bar-On Y. M., Phillips R., Milo R. *Proc. Nat. Acad. Sci. USA*, **115** (2018), 6506–6511.

Barzkar N., Sohail M. *Appl. Microbiol. Biotechnol.*, **104** (2020), 6873–6892.

Beckham G. T., Matthews J. F., Bomble Y. J., Bu L., Adney W. S., *et al*. *J. Phys. Chem. B*, **114** (2010), 1447–1453.

Ben Hmad I., Gargouri A. *J. Basic Microbiol.*, **57**, (2017), 653–658.

Benen J. A., Kester H. C., Parenicova L., Visser J. *Biochemistry*, **39** (2000), 15563–15569.

Benoit I., Danchin E. G., Bleichrodt R. J., De Vries R. P. *Biotechnol. Lett.*, **30** (2008), 3873–3896.

Bertini L., Breglia R., Lambrughi M., Fantucci P., De Gioia L., *et al*. *Inorg. Chem.*, **57** (2018), 86–97.

BEST, https://demoplants.bioenergy2020.eu/, Accessed on June 24, 2021.

Bezerra R. M., Dias A. A. *Appl. Biochem. Biotechnol.*, **126** (2005), 49–59.

Biely P., Cote G. L., Kremnicky L., Greene R. V., Dupont C., *et al*. *FEBS Lett.*, **396** (1996), 257–260.

Biely P., Mastihubova M., Tenkanen M., Eyzaguirre J., Li X. L., *et al*. *J. Biotechnol.* **151** (2011), 137–142.

Biely P., Vrsanska M., Tenkanen M., Kluepfel D. *J. Biotechnol.*, **57** (1997), 151–166.

Bischof R. H., Ramoni J., Seiboth B. *Microb. Cell Fact.*, **15** (2016), 106.

Bissaro B., Monsan P., Fauré R., O'Donohue M. J., *Biochem. J.*, **467** (2015), 17–35.

Bissaro B., Røhr A. K., Müller G., Chylenski P., Skaugen M., *et al.*, *Nat. Chem. Biol.* **13** (2017), 1123–1128.

Blumer-Schuette S. E., Brown S. D., Sander K. B., Bayer E. A., Kataeva I., *et al*. *FEMS Microbiol. Rev.*, **38** (2014), 393–448.

Boraston A. B., Bolam D. N., Gilbert H. J., Davies G. J. *Biochem. J.* **382** (2004), 769–781.

Borisova A. S., Isaksen T., Dimarogona M., Kognole A. A., Mathiesen G., *et al*. *J. Biol. Chem.*, **290** (2015), 22955–22969.

Brulc J. M., Antonopoulos D. A., Miller M. E., Wilson M. K., Yannarell A. C., *et al*. *Proc. Nat. Acad. Sci. USA*, **106** (2009), 1948–1953.

Camassola M., Dillon A. J. P. *Sci. Reports,* **1** (2012), 125.

Cao Y. J., Zhang R. B., Cheng T., Guo J., Xian M., *et al. Appl. Microbiol. Biotechnol.,* **101** (2017), 521–532.

Cassells B., Karhumaa K., Sànchez i Nogué V., Lidén G. *Appl. Biochem. Biotechnol.,* **181** (2017), 536–547.

Castro R. C. A., Roberto I. C. *Appl. Biochem. Biotechnol.,* **172** (2014), 1553–1564.

Cavka A., Jönsson L. J. *Bioresour. Technol.,* **136** (2013), 368–376.

CAZy, http://www.cazy.org, Accessed June 15, 2021.

Chandel A. K., Garlapati V. K., Singh A. K., Antunes F. A. F., da Silva S. S. *Bioresour. Technol.,* **264** (2018), 370–381.

Chen H., Hayn M., Esterbauer H. *Biochim. Biophys. Acta,* **1121** (1992), 54–60.

Chen J., Guo X., Zhu M., Chen C., Li D. *Biotechnol. Biofuels,* **12** (2019), 42.

Ciolacu D., Ciolacu F., Popa V. I. *Cellulose Chem. Technol.,* **45** (2011), 13–21.

Comtet-Marre S., Parisot N., Lepercq P., Chaucheyras-Durand F., Mosoni P., *et al. Front Microbiol.,* **8** (2017), 67.

Coutinho P. M., Andersen M. R., Kolenova K., Van Kuyk P. A., Benoit I. *et al., Fungal Genet. Biol.,* **46** (2009), S161–S169.

Couturier M., Ladeveze S., Sulzenbacher G., Ciano L., Fanuel M., *et al. Nat. Chem. Biol.,* **14** (2018), 306–310.

Cragg S. M., Beckham G. T., Bruce N. C., Bugg T. D. H., Distel D. L., *et al. Curr. Opin. Chem. Biol.,* **29** (2015), 108–119.

Cragg S. M., Friess D. A., Gillis L. G., Trevathan-Tackett S. M., Terrett O. M., *et al. Annu. Rev. Mar. Sci.,* **12** (2020), 469–497.

Crepin V. F., Faulds C. B., Connerton I. F. *Appl. Microbiol. Biotechnol.,* **63** (2004), 647–652.

Dadheech T., Shah R., Pandit R., Hinsu A., Chauhan P. S., *et al. Int. J. Biol. Macromol.,* **113** (2018), 73–81.

Dahnum D., Tasum S. O., Triwahyuni E., Nurdin M., Abimanyu H. *Energy Procedia*, **68** (2015), 107–116.

Davies G. J., Wilson K. S., Henrissat B. *Biochem. J.,* **321** (1997), 557–559.

Davies G., Henrissat B. *Structure,* **3** (1995), 853–859.

De Jong E., Jungmeier G. Biorefinery concepts in comparison to petrochemical biorefineries, in *Industrial Biorefineries and White Biotechnology* (Pandey A., Höfer R., Taherzadeh M., Nampoothiri K.M., Larroche C., eds), Elsevier, Amsterdam, 2015.

De Vries R. P., Kester H. C., Poulsen C. H., Benen J. A., Visser J. *Carbohydr. Res.*, **327** (2000), 401–410.

De Vries R. P., Visser J. *Microbiol. Mol. Biol. Rev.*, **65** (2001), 497–522.

Decker C. H., Visser J., Schreier P. *Appl. Microbiol. Biotechnol.*, **55** (2001), 157–63.

Desmet T., Cantaert T., Gualfetti P., Nerinckx W., Gross L., et al. *FEBS J.*, **274** (2007), 356–363.

Dias F. M., Vincent F., Pell G., Prates J. A., Centeno M. S., et al. *J. Biol. Chem.*, 279 (2004), 25517–25526.

Divne C., Ståhlberg J., Reinikainen T., Ruohonen L., Pettersson G., et al. *Science*, **265** (1994), 524–528.

Do B. C., Dang T. T., Berrin J. G., Haltrich D., To K. A., et al. *Microb. Cell Fact.*, **8** (2009), 59.

Druzhinina I. S., Kubicek C. P. *Adv. Appl. Microbiol.*, **95** (2016), 69–147.

Eijsink V. G. H., Petrovic D., Forsberg Z., Mekasha S., Røhr Å. K., et al. *Biotechnol. Biofuels*, 12 (2019), 58.

Favaro L., Jansen T., Van Zyl W. H. *Crit. Rev. Biotechnol.*, **39** (2019), 800–816.

Fengel D., Wegener G., (eds). *Wood: Chemistry, Ultrastructure, Reactions*; Walter de Gruyter, Berlin, 1989.

Ferreira J. A., Taherzadeh M. J. *Bioresour. Technol.*, **299** (2020), 122695.

Filiatrault-Chastel C., Navarro D., Haon M., Grisel S., Herpoël-Gimbert I., et al. *Biotechnol. Biofuels*, 12 (2019), 55.

Flint H. J., Scott K. P., Duncan S. H., Louis P., Forano E. *Gut Microbes*, **3** (2012), 289–306.

Foreman P. K., Brown D., Dankmeyer L., Dean R., Diener S., et al. *J. Biol. Chem.*, **278** (2003), 31988–31997.

Forsberg Z., Mackenzie A. K., Sorlie M., Rohr A. K., Helland R., et al. *Proc. Natl. Acad. Sci. USA*, **111** (2014a), 8446–8451.

Forsberg Z., Rohr A. K., Mekasha S., Andersson K. K., Eijsink V. G. H., et al. *Biochemistry*, **53** (2014b), 1647–1656.

Frommhagen M., Mutte S. K., Westphal A. H., Koetsier M. J., Hinz S. W. A., et al. *Biotechnol. Biofuels*, **10** (2017), 121.

Frommhagen M., Sforza S., Westphal A. H., Visser J., Hinz S. W., et al. *Biotechnol. Biofuels*, **8** (2015), 101.

Gacesa P. *FEBS Lett.*, **212** (1987), 199–202.

Galagan J. E., Calvo S. E., Cuomo C., Ma L. J., Wortman J. R., et al. *Nature*, **438** (2005), 1105–1115.

Gandla M. L., Derba-Maceluch M., Liu X., Gerber L., Master E. R., *et al. Phytochem.*, **112** (2015), 210–220.

Gandla M. L., Martín C., Jönsson L. J. *Energies*, **11** (2018), 2936.

Ghose T. K. *Pure Appl. Chem.*, **59** (1987), 257–268.

Gilbert H. J., Knox J. P., Boraston A. B. *Curr. Opin. Struct. Biol.*, **23** (2013), 669–677.

Gilbert H. J., Stålbrand H., Brumer H. *Curr. Opin. Plant Biol.*, **11** (2008), 338–348.

Gilkes N. R., Kwan E., Kilburn D. G., Miller R. C., Warren R. A. J. *J. Biotechnol.*, **57** (1997), 83–90.

Goodell B., Zhu Y., Kim S., Kafle K., Eastwood D., *et al. Biotechnol. Biofuels*, **10** (2017), 179.

Guillen D., Sanchez S., Rodriguez-Sanoja R. *Appl. Microbiol. Biotechnol.*, **85** (2010), 1241–1249.

Gupta P., Samant K., Sahu A. *Int. J. Microbiol.*, **2012** (2012), 578925.

Haitjema C. H., Solomon K. V., Henske J. K., Theodorou M. K., O'Malley M. A. *Biotechnol. Bioeng.*, **111** (2014), 1471–1482.

Hakulinen N., Tenkanen M., Rouvinen J. *J. Struct. Biol.*, **132** (2000), 180–190.

Hemsworth G. R., Henrissat B., Davies G. J., Walton P. H. *Nat. Chem. Biol.*, **10** (2014), 122–126.

Hemsworth G. R., Johnston E. M., Davies G. J., Walton P. H. *Trends Biotechnol.*, **33** (2015), 747–761.

Henriksson G., Johansson G., Pettersson G. *J. Biotechnol.*, **78** (2000), 93–113.

Henrissat B., Driguez H., Viet C., Schülein M. *Nat. Biotechnol.*, **3** (1985), 722–726.

Ilanidis D., Stagge S., Jönsson L. J., Martín C. *Agronomy*, **11** (2021b), 487.

Ilanidis D., Stagge S., Jönsson L. J., Martín C. *Ind. Crops Prod.*, **159** (2021a), 113077.

Ilanidis D., Wu G., Stagge S., Martín C., Jönsson L. J. *Bioresour. Technol.*, **319** (2021c), 124211.

Ilanidis D., Stagge S., Alriksson B., Cavka A., Jönsson L. J. *Front. Energy Res.*, **9** (2021d), 701980.

Isaksen T., Westereng B., Aachmann F. L., Agger J. W., Kracher D., *et al. J. Biol. Chem.*, **289** (2014), 2632–2642.

IUBMB, https://www.qmul.ac.uk/sbcs/iubmb/enzyme/rules.html, Accessed June 15, 2021.

Jang Y. S., Kim B., Shin J. H., Choi Y. J., Choi S., *et al. Biotechnol. Bioeng.*, **109** (2012), 2437–2459.

Jenkins J., Leggio L. L., Harris G., Pickersgill R. *FEBS Lett.*, **362** (1995), 281–285.

Jensen M. H., Otten H., Christensen U., Borchert T. V., Christensen L. L., *et al. J. Mol. Biol.*, **404** (2010), 100–111.

Jönsson L. J., Martín C. *Bioresour. Technol.*, **199** (2016), 103–112.

Karp E. M., Donohoe B. S., O'Brien M. H., Ciesielski P. N., Mittal A., *et al. ACS Sust. Chem. Eng.*, **2** (2014), 1481–1491.

Kim Y., Kreke T., Hendrickson R., Parenti J., Ladisch M. R. *Bioresour. Technol.*, **135** (2013), 30–38.

Kim J. S., Lee Y. Y., Kim T. H. *Bioresour. Technol.*, **199** (2016), 42–48.

Kirk T. K., Connors W. J., Bleam R. D., Hackett W. F., Zeikus J. G. *Proc. Nat. Acad. USA*, **72** (1975), 2515–2519.

Kjaergaard C. H., Qayyum M. F., Wong S. D., Xu F., Hemsworth G. R., *et al. Proc. Nat. Acad. Sci. USA*, **111** (2014), 8797–8802.

Koeck D. E., Pechtl A., Zverlov V. V., Schwarz W. H. *Curr. Opin. Biotechnol.*, **29** (2014), 171–183.

Kofod L. V., Kauppinen S., Christgau S., Andersen L. N., Heldt-Hansen H. P., *et al. J. Biol. Chem.*, **269** (1994), 29182–29189.

Koshland D. E. *Biol. Rev.*, **28** (1953), 416–436.

Koutaniemi S., Van Gool M. P., Juvonen M., Jokela J., Hinz S. W., *et al. J. Biotechnol.* **168** (2013), 684–692.

Kracher D., Scheiblbrandner S., Felice A. K. G., Breslmayr E., Preims M., *et al. Science*, **352** (2016), 1098–1101.

Kraulis J., Clore G. M., Nilges M., Jones T. A., Pettersson G., *et al. Biochemistry*, **28** (1989), 7241–7257.

Kroukamp H., Den Haan R., Van Zyl J.-H., Van Zyl W.-H. *Biofuels Bioprod. Bioref.*, **12** (2018), 108–124.

Kumar M., Campbell L., Turner S. *J. Exp. Bot.*, **67** (2016), 515–531.

Levasseur A., Drula E., Lombard V., Coutinho P. M., Henrissat B. *Biotechnol. Biofuels*, **6** (2013), 41.

Li X. L., Skory C. D., Cotta M. A., Puchart V., Biely P. *Appl. Environ. Microbiol.*, **74** (2008), 7482–7489.

Lindman B., Medronho B., Alves L., Norgren M., Nordenskiöld L. *Q. Rev. Biophys.*, **54** (2020), e3.

Liu Y. S., Baker J. O., Zeng Y., Himmel M. E., Haas T., *et al. J. Biol. Chem.*, **286** (2011), 11195–11201.

Lombard V., Bernard T., Rancurel C., Brumer H., Coutinho P. M., *et al. Biochem. J.* **432** (2010), 437–444.

Lombard V., Ramulu H. G., Drula E., Coutinho P. M., Henrissat B. *Nucleic Acids Res.*, **42** (2014), D490–D495.

Mankar A. R., Pandey A., Modak A., Pant K. K. *Bioresour. Technol.*, **334** (2021), 125235.

Mardanov A. V., Kochetkova T. V., Beletsky A. V., Bonch-Osmolovskaya E. A., Ravin N. V., *et al. J Bacteriol.*, **194** (2012), 4446–4447.

Margolles-Clark E., Saloheimo M., Siika-aho M., Penttilä M. *Gene*, **172** (1996), 171–172.

Martens-Uzunova E. S., Schaap P. J. *Fungal Genet. Biol.*, **46** (2009), S170–S179.

Martín C. *Agronomy*, **11** (2021), 924.

Martinez D., Berka R. M., Henrissat B., Saloheimo M., Arvas M., *et al. Nat. Biotechnol.*, **26** (2008), 553–560.

Martinez D., Larrondo L. F., Putnam N., Gelpke M. D. S., Huang K., *et al. Nat. Biotechnol.*, **22** (2004), 695–700.

Master E. R., Zheng Y., Storms R., Tsang A., Powlowski J. *Biochem. J.*, **411** (2008), 161–170.

Matsakas L., Raghavendran V., Yakimenko O., Persson G., Olsson E., *et al. Bioresour. Technol.*, **273** (2019), 521–528.

Mayans O., Scott M., Connerton I., Gravesen T., Benen J., *et al. Structure*, **5** (1997), 677–689.

Meents M. J., Watanabe Y., Samuels A. L. *Ann. Bot.*, **121** (2018), 1107–1125.

Michelin M., Ximenes E., De Lourdes Teixeira de Moraes Polizeli M., Ladisch M. R. *Bioresour. Technol.*, **199** (2016), 275–278.

Miller G. L. *Anal. Chem.*, **31** (1959), 426–428.

Morone A., Chakrabarti T., Pandey R. A. *Cellulose*, **24** (2017), 4885–4898.

Müller G., Varnái A., Johansen K. S., Eijsink V. G. H., Horn S. J. *Biotechnol. Biofuels*, **8** (2015), 187.

Mutter M., Beldman G., Pitson S. M., Schols H. A., Voragen A. G. *Plant Physiol.*, **117** (1998), 153–163.

Nakagame S., Chandra R. P., Saddler J. N. *Biotechnol. Bioeng.*, **105** (2010), 871–879.

Nelson N. *J. Biol. Chem.*, **153** (1944), 375–380.

Normark M., Pommer L., Gräsvik J., Hedenström M., Gorzsás A., *et al. Bioenerg. Res.*, **9** (2016), 355–368.

Normark M., Winestrand S., Lestander T., Jönsson L. *BMC Biotechnol.*, **14** (2014), 20.

Nutt A., Sild V., Pettersson G., Johansson G. *Eur. J. Biochem.*, **258** (1998), 200–206.

Olguin-Maciel E., Singh A., Chable-Villacis R., Tapia-Tussell R., Ruiz H. A. *Agronomy*, **10** (2020), 1834.

Olofsson K., Bertilsson M., Lidén G. *Biotechnol. Biofuels*, **1** (2008), 7.

Olson D. G., Sparling R., Lynd L. R. *Curr. Opin. Biotechnol.*, **33** (2015), 130–141.

Pareek N., Gillgren T., Jönsson L. J. *Bioresour. Technol.*, **148** (2013), 70–77.

Patel A. K., Singhania R. R., Sim S. J., Pandey A. *Bioresour. Technol.*, **279** (2019), 385–392.

Pawar P. M., Derba-Maceluch M., Chong S. L., Gandla M. L., Bashar S. S., *et al. Biotechnol. Biofuels*, **10** (2017), 98.

Payne C. M., Knott B. C., Mayes H. B., Hansson H., Himmel M E., *et al. Chem. Rev.*, **115** (2015), 1308–1448.

Penín L., Peleteiro S., Santos V., Alonso J. L., Parajó J. C. *Cellulose*, **26** (2019), 1125–1139.

Pham T. A., Berrin J. G., Record E., To K. A., Sigoillot J. C. *J. Biotechnol.* **148** (2010), 163–170.

Phillips C. M., Beeson W. T., Cate J. H., Marletta M. A. *ACS Chem. Biol.*, **6** (2011), 1399–1406.

Pickersgill R., Harris G., Leggio L. L., Mayans O., Jenkins J. *Biochem. Soc. Trans.*, **26** (1998), 190–198.

Polizeli M. L., Rizzatti A. C., Monti R., Terenzi H. F., Jorge J. A., *et al. Appl. Microbiol. Biotechnol.*, **67** (2005), 577–591.

Pollet A., Delcour J. A., Courtin C. M. *Crit. Rev. Biotechnol.*, **30** (2010), 176–191.

Puchart V., Agger J. W., Berrin J. G., Varnai A., Westereng B., *et al. J. Biotechnol.*, **233** (2016), 228–236.

Puchart V., Vrsanska M., Mastihubova M., Topakas E., Vafiadi C., *et al. J. Biotechnol.*, **127** (2007), 235–243.

Quinlan R. J., Sweeney M. D., Leggio L. L., Otten H., Poulsen J. C. N., *et al. Proc. Nat. Acad. Sci. USA*, **108** (2011), 15079–15084.

Rahikainen J. L., Moilanen U., Nurmi-Rantala S., Lappas A., Koivula A., et al. *Bioresour. Technol.*, **146** (2013), 118–125.

Ralph J., Lapierre C., Boerjan W. *Curr. Opin. Biotechnol.*, **56** (2019), 240–249.

Reczey K., Brumbauer A., Bollok M., Szengyel Z., Zacchi G. *Appl. Biochem. Biotechnol.*, **70–72** (1998), 225–235.

Reese E. T., Levinson H. S., Downing M. H., White W. L. *Farlowia*, **4** (1950), 45–86.

Riou C., Salmon J. M., Vallier M. J., Gunata Z., Barre P. *Appl. Environ. Microbiol.*, **64** (1998), 3607–3614.

Roberts A. W., Roberts E. M., Haigler C. H. *Front. Plant Sci.*, **3** (2012), 166.

Rocha G. J. M., Nascimento V. M., Gonçalves A. R., Silva V. F. N., Martín C. *Ind. Crops Prod.*, **64** (2015), 52–58.

Rødsrud G., Lersch M., Sjöde A. *Biomass Bioenerg.*, **46** (2012), 46–59.

Ruiz H. A., Conrad M., Sun S. N., Sanchez A., Rocha G. J. M., et al. *Bioresour. Technol.*, **299** (2020), 122685.

Sabbadin F., Hemsworth G. R., Ciano L., Henrissat B., Dupree P., et al. *Nat. Commun.*, **9** (2018), 756.

Salehi Jouzani G., Taherzadeh M. *Biofuel Res. J.*, **2** (2015), 152–195.

Sammond D. W., Payne C. M., Brunecky R., Himmel M. E., Crowley M. F., et al. *PLoS One*, **7** (2012), e48615.

Silveira M. H. L., Morais A. R. C., Lopes A. M. C., Olekszyszen D. N., Bogel-Łukasik R., et al. *ChemSusChem*, **8** (2015), 3366–3390.

Smichi N., Messaoudi Y., Allaf K., Gargouri M. *Bioprocess Biosyst. Eng.*, **43** (2020), 945–957.

Solarte-Toro J. C., Romero-García J. M., Martínez-Patiño J. C., Ruiz-Ramos E., Castro-Galiano E., et al. *Renew. Sustain. Energy Rev.*, **107** (2019), 587–601.

Srisodsuk M., Reinikainen T., Penttilä M., Teeri T. T. *J. Biol. Chem.*, **268** (1993), 20756–20761.

St John F. J., Gonzalez J. M., Pozharski E. *FEBS Lett.*, **584** (2010), 4435–4441.

Tarasov D., Leitch M., Fatehi P. *Biotechnol. Biofuels*, **11** (2018), 269.

Tenkanen M., Makkonen M., Perttula M., Viikari L., Teleman A. *J. Biotechnol.*, **57** (1997), 191–204.

Tenkanen M., Thornton J., Viikari L. *J. Biotechnol.*, **42** (1995), 197–206.

Thompson A. J., Heu T., Shaghasi T., Benyamino R., Jones A., et al. *Acta Crystallogr. F. Struct. Biol. Commun.*, **68** (2012), 875.

Vaaje-Kolstad G., Westereng B., Horn S. J., Liu Z. L., Zhai H., et al. *Science*, **330** (2010), 219–222.

Van Dyk J. S., Pletschke B. I. *Biotechnol. Adv.*, **30** (2012), 1458–1480.

Van Tilbeurgh H., Tomme P., Claeyssens M., Bhikhabhai R., Pettersson G. *FEBS Lett.*, **204** (1986), 223–227.

Van Zyl W. H., Lynd L. R., Den Haan R., McBride J. E., Consolidated bioprocessing for bioethanol production using *Saccharomyces cerevisiae*, in *Biofuels. Advances in Biochemical Engineering/Biotechnology* (Olsson L., ed), vol. 108, Springer, Berlin, Heidelberg, 2007.

Várnai A., Siika-aho M., Viikari L. *Biotechnol. Biofuels*, **6** (2013), 30.

Varrot A., Yip V. L. Y., Li Y., Rajan S. S., Yang X., et al. *J. Mol. Biol.*, **346** (2005), 423–445.

Viikari L., Alapuranen M., Puranen T., Vehmaanperä J., Siika-aho M. *Adv. Biochem. Engin./Biotechnol.* **108** (2007), 121–145.

Vlasenko E., Schulein M., Cherry J., Xu F. *Bioresour. Technol.*, **101** (2010), 2405–2411.

Vu V. V., Beeson W. T., Span E. A., Farquhar E. R., Marletta M. A. *Proc. Nat. Acad. Sci. USA*, **111** (2014), 13822–13827.

Wang Z., Jönsson L. J. *Bioresour. Technol.*, **268** (2018), 393–401.

Wang Z., Pawar P. M., Derba-Maceluch M., Hedenström M., Chong S. L., et al. *Front. Plant Sci.* **11** (2020), 380.

Wang Z., Winestrand S., Gillgren T., Jönsson L.J. *Biomass Bioenerg.*, **109** (2018), 125–134.

Warnecke F., Luginbuhl P., Ivanova N., Ghassemian M., Richardson T. H., et al. *Nature,* **450** (2007), 560–565.

White B. A., Lamed R., Bayer E. A., Flint H. J. *Annu. Rev. Microbiol.*, **68** (2014), 279–296.

Wu J., Chandra R. P., Takada M., Liu L.-Y., Renneckar S., et al. *Front. Bioeng. Biotechnol.*, **8** (2020), 608835.

Wymelenberg A. V., Minges P., Sabat G., Martinez D., Aerts A., et al. *Fungal Genet. Biol.*, **43** (2006), 343–356.

Xiao B., Sun X. F., Sun R. C. *Polym. Degrad. Stabil.*, **74** (2001), 307–319.

Xiao Z., Storms R., Tsang A. *Biotechnol. Bioeng.*, **88** (2004a), 832–837.

Xiao Z., Zhang X., Gregg D. J., Saddler J. N. *Appl. Biochem. Biotechnol.*, **115** (2004b), 1115–1126.

Xiong S., Martín C., Eilertsen L., Wei M., Myronycheva O., et al. *Bioresour. Technol.*, **274** (2019), 65–72.

Xu Q., Resch M. G., Podkaminer K., Yang S., Baker J. O., *et al. Sci. Adv.,* **2** (2016), e1501254.

Yang H., Huang X., Fang S., Xin W., Huang L., *et al. Sci. Rep.,* **6** (2016), 27427.

Zhai R., Hu J., Saddler J. N. *ACS Sustainable Chem. Eng.,* **4** (2016), 3429–3436.

Zhai R., Hu J., Saddler J. N. *ACS Sustainable Chem. Eng.,* **6** (2018a), 3823–3829.

Zhai R., Hu J., Saddler J. N. *Sustain. Energy Fuels*, **2** (2018b), 1048–1056.

Zhang R., Fan Z., Kasuga T. *Protein Expres. Purif.,* **75** (2011), 63–69.

Zhao X. B., Zhang L. H., Liu D. H. *Biofuels Bioprod. Bioref.,* **6** (2012), 561–579.

Chapter 14

Biological Biorefineries Based on Orange Peel Wastes

Alberto García-Martín,[a] Itziar A. Escanciano,[a]
V. Martin-Domínguez,[a] Álvaro Lorente-Arévalo,[a]
Jorge García-Montalvo,[a] Jesús Esteban,[b] Juan M. Bolívar,[a]
Victoria E. Santos,[a] and Miguel Ladero[a]

[a]*Materials and Chemical Engineering Department, Chemical Sciences School, Universidad Complutense de Madrid, 28040, Madrid, Spain*
[b]*Department of Chemical Engineering and Analytical Science at the University of Manchester, The Mill, Sackville Street, Manchester, M13 9PL, United Kingdom*
mladerog@ucm.es

Over the last two decades, integrated biorefinery has been defined as the application of structured and integrated processes to various types of biomass, emulating the complexity of refinery complexes and their processes. Among the various biomasses, many of which are lignocellulosic, others richer in starch or protein, food waste stands out, including citrus waste, especially from orange juice production. This chapter summarizes various products that can be obtained by applying biological processes from these orange wastes (peel, pulp, and seeds), also known as orange peel wastes (OPWs).

Agricultural Biocatalysis: Enzymes in Agriculture and Industry
Edited by Peter Jeschke and Evgeni B. Starikov
Copyright © 2023 Jenny Stanford Publishing Pte. Ltd.
ISBN 978-981-4968-47-8 (Hardcover), 978-1-003-31310-6 (eBook)
www.jennystanford.com

14.1 Introduction

According to data collected in FAOSTAT (FAO Statistical Databases; Food and Agriculture Organization of the United Nations) from 2016 to 2019, the area dedicated to the cultivation of citrus fruits has increased more than 6% (from 7883 to 8349 kilohectares, Kha), with a slight increase of the productivity per hectare reflected in a 9% increase of the global citrus production (from 131 to 143.5 million tons, Mt) (FAOSTAT, 2021). In the particular case of oranges, both sweet and bitter, a notable increase from 72 to 78 Mt happened in those years. Considering continents, Asia and the Americas countries were the leading regions in that period, accounting for the production of about 80% of world production of oranges, lemons. Asian countries dominated the production of tangerines, clementines, mandarins, and similar fruits, with nearly 70% of the world production in the period 2016 to 2019. A more in-depth vision of the evolution of citrus fruit production is given in Fig. 14.1. Orange is the main citrus crop (55% of total production) followed by tangerines and similar fruits (near 25%); while these latter are mainly dedicated to table fruit, about 20 Mt oranges are dedicated to juice production. Roughly, 60% of the orange mass dedicated to juice ends into wastes (OPWs). Therefore, peels, seeds, flesh, and stalks mean a potential yearly waste mass of 12 Mt that needs to be disposed of (usually, by landfilling; partially, by being mixed with inorganic salts and transformed into cattle feed). However, it is a rich source of essential oils (EOs), flavonoids and other phenolics, simple sugars, and soluble fiber (Mahato *et al.*, 2021). Although today only about 18% of citrus fruit is processed, 60 kilotons (Kt) of waste per year could be collected using suitable collection logistics (Zerva *et al.*, 2019).

As a part of the water-energy-food nexus, the production and consumption of citrus fruits can be envisaged as an opportunity for better use of resources (Mahato *et al.*, 2021; Patsalou *et al.*, 2020). Food waste and food losses (FWL) mean near 1.6 gigatons (Gt) with an estimated carbon footprint of 3.3 Gt of CO_2 eq., only behind the production of Greenhouse Gases (GHG) of China and the USA (Munesue *et al.*, 2015). It is also interesting to consider that FWL involves an energy loss near 2% of the global produced energy in the best of cases (Cuellar and Webber, 2010). Given that

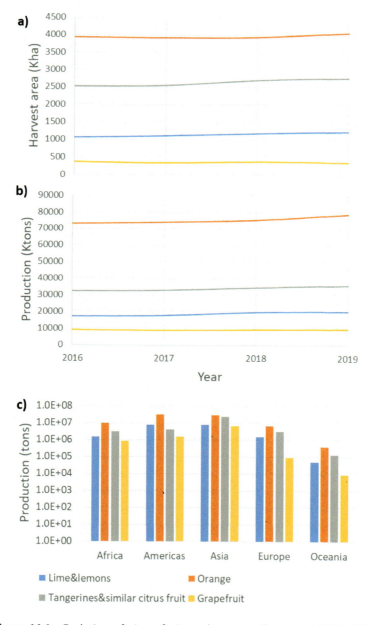

Figure 14.1 Evolution of citrus fruit production in the period 2016–2019. (a) Harvest surface (Kha); (b) fruit production (in Kt), and (c) production per continent (in tons; t) (FAOSTAT, 2021).

agriculture is the first water consumer sector in the world, it is simple to understand the enormous effect of FWL on water footprint (Mekonnen and Gerbens-Leenes, 2020). In this scenario, food waste biorefineries emerge as a key tool to valorize FWL and create a truly circular economy based on the use of biomass as a substitute for fossil resources, that is, circular bioeconomy (Mahato et al., 2021; Patsalou et al., 2020; Mak et al., 2020). These efforts are in line with the Sustainable Development Goals (SDGs) of the United Nations, in particular with Goal 2 (Zero Hunger) and Goal 13 (Climate Action), but also affecting, at least, Goal 9 (Industry, Innovation, and Infrastructures) and Goal 12 (Responsible Production and Consumption) (UN, 2021). A major idea is to reduce 50% FWL worldwide by 2030 (Jeong et al., 2021).

As briefly mentioned before, OPW and other wastes from citrus fruits (CPW) can be employed for the integrated and intensive production of several by-products in the food biorefinery. Usually, this type of residue is mainly constituted by peels, with outer layers rich in EOs, and inner layers rich in pectin (13–43% DS in CPW). Lignin (0.5–8% DS) is relatively scarce if compared to other lignocellulosic biomasses, while cellulose (9–31% DS) and hemicelluloses (4–31% DS) constitute a notable portion of dry CPW. They are also rich in protein (about 8% DS) (Jeong et al., 2021; Senit et al., 2019).

Most of these residues are used for cattle feed and composting. Incineration comes at a price, due to the higher water content of OPW (and CPW in general). Dumping and landfilling are also employed, though a cost due to waste disposal needs to be faced; moreover, directives 2006/12/CE and 2008/98/CE indicate that wastes such as CPW need to be recycled and valorized, reducing the impact on society of those components that can damage the environment (Negro et al., 2017). This is much in line with the EU's desire to reduce 60% food waste (FW) by 2030. When formulating cattle feed, only 4% w/w of these wastes can be used due to intestinal discomfort and other illnesses suffered by cattle fed with a high quantity/concentration of OPW (Negro et al., 2017). On the other side, OPW, as a feed ingredient, improves lactation and reduces fat in poultry (De la Torre et al., 2019). As for its use as a food ingredient, OPW (and CPW) is considered very rich in soluble fiber and functional ingredients, as antioxidants; thus, its use in low percentage in dough and meat is being studied in a way to improve organoleptic properties of the food and increase its shelf life due to the antimicrobial nature of these residues (Han et al., 2021). Indeed, as almost 40% of FW is originated in the food industry from vegetables and fruits, methods such as extrusion can be applied to obtain ingredients rich in fiber from food waste, such as OPW (Garcia-Amezquita et al., 2019). Another recycling strategy very linked to the food-industry composting, so the product can be employed as a natural fertilizer for several crops, being rich in nutrients and increasing water retention. The main drawback comes from the acidity of the waste, which could lead to unwanted fermentations (De la Torre et al., 2019). Another minority, yet interesting, use for OPW and CPW is as a source of materials (e.g., biochar) with some specific functions: bio-adsorbents to remove heavy metals, dyes, and other pollutants from wastewaters, support for metallic catalysts, and material for electrodes, to name a few (Ehsani and Parsimehr, 2020; De la Torre et al., 2019).

Biorefineries, as a concept, are refineries based on biomass, instead of fossil resources. As refineries, they are complex systems whose aim is to fractionate and transform biomass into fuels, chemicals, materials, food, and feed. To that aim, we can see two complementary approaches: the thermochemical transformation to intermediate complex fractions, and the biochemical fractionation to simple monomers and their derivatives, as platforms to obtain several value-added products and energy vectors (Ortiz-Sanchez et al., 2021). Although first-generation biorefineries are simpler from a technical perspective, they are based on food biomass, not plentiful enough and suitable for the particular purpose of feeding Humanity. Thus, FWL, lignocellulose, and algal biomasses emerge as feedstock for fuel, chemicals, and materials, and OPW (and CPW) satisfies these purposes of the second generation biorefinery (Ortiz-Sanchez et al., 2021; Mak et al., 2020; De la Torre et al., 2019).

Lignocellulosic biomass (LCB) is essentially structural. Based on amorphous and crystalline cellulose, hemicelluloses and lignin, these biomasses need harsh physical (milling, extrusion), chemical (acid and basic), and physicochemical (e.g., steam explosion, AFEX) treatments. New trends advocate for using ethanol-water solutions or mixing water with other solvents, either classical (glycerol, carboxylic acids) or new (ionic liquids, deep eutectic solvents), recycling the liquors to reduce energy consumption and increase lignin removal (Vergara *et al.*, 2019; Ozturk *et al.*, 2018; 2019). OPW and CPW are, in comparison to most lignocellulosic biomass, more porous and humid, less rich in lignin, and much richer in pectin, so, even if several common pretreatments for LCB can be applied, those based on solvents, acids, drying, grinding, and extrusion are the most successful (De la Torre *et al.*, 2019).

This chapter wants to emphasize different ways and strategies to valorize CPW, and OPW in particular, using biological processes. With a mention of pretreatments to be applied to get useful and high-value components, such as EO, the main objective is to describe enzymatic and microbiological processes to several key products, including chemicals and materials. The chapter ends with a visit to techno-economic studies in the CPW biorefinery and a section of future perspectives.

14.2 Upstream Processes in Biological Biorefineries from OPW

OPW valorization by biological processes needs specific pre-treatments to render the biomass more amenable to enzyme action while removing phenolics and other low molecular weight components, such as limonene (Ortiz-Sanchez *et al.*, 2021; De la Torre *et al.*, 2019). The enzymatic and fermentative processes can be driven either in series (separated hydrolysis and fermentation, SHF) or at the same time (simultaneous saccharification and fermentation, SSF), with particular enhancements either by recycling enzymes or microorganisms or having microorganisms able to grow and produced on pentoses and hexoses (co-fermentation) and/or produce depolymerizing enzyme while producing chemicals or materials of interest (Consolidated Bioprocessing, CBP) (Mahato *et al.*, 2021; De la Torre *et al.*, 2019).

14.2.1 Pretreatment of OPWs

Pretreatment of biomass involves a variety of different unitary operations. All of them aim to modify raw materials to improve the reaction steps and the downstream. However, some products of interest can be already obtained by pretreatment before the primary reaction stages. The improvement mentioned above is a consequence of two effects. First, biomass matrix suffers physicochemical modifications, such as increased surface area, reduction of polysaccharide crystallinity, and polymerization degree. Second, removing compounds that cause inhibitory effects on the subsequent steps is carried out. Mainly when biotransformation reactions are employed (Kumar et al., 2021; Mankar et al., 2021). The compounds that are extracted in these stages of the whole process for orange wastes are EO and natural phenolic compounds (NPCs), and also polysaccharides such as pectin. These molecules and polymers have value added by themselves. However, even though pretreatment comprises other operations (e.g., particle size reduction, acid or alkaline treatments to access the biopolymers easily), in this section, we focus on the stabilization of biomass by drying and in the extraction of EOs, NPCs, and pectins due to their interest.

In the case of EOs, they are a mixture of different hydrophobic and small volatile organic compounds. In the aromatic herbs and, in particular, on citrus peels, they accumulate on sacks-like structures called oil glands. Due to their aromatic, antimicrobial properties and their classification as Generally Recognized as Safe (GRAS), EOs are envisaged as products with broad applications and future perspectives. They are used in cosmetics, in the food industry, polymer manufacturing, etc. (Dosoky and Setzer, 2018). Additionally, NPCs are a wide group of aromatic-derived compounds that are synthesized as secondary metabolites on plants. Their most remarkable feature is their antioxidant activity and their antimicrobial attributes, as well as EOs. The application of these molecules is the bio-based packaging industry, food preservatives, nutraceuticals, among others (Sigh B. et al., 2020). To know how extraction processes or pretreatment operations affect EOs and NPCs some parameters show it, as EOs yield is in mass basis. Concerning NPC, two parameters show the concentration and their antioxidant capacity. These parameters are the total phenolic content (TPC) measured as mg of gallic acid equivalents (mg GAE) per mass of solid. For antioxidant activity mg of TROLOX equivalent antioxidant capacity (mg TEAC) per mass of solid or inhibitory concentration (IC) are measured.

Pretreatment operations are classified in physical, chemical, physicochemical, and biological. From a process perspective, one of the first operations that are employed is physical: due to the moisture content of orange waste, drying operations are employed to stabilize the biomass. Also, the high free sugar content produces that the shelf life of oranges wastes is compromised. In these conditions, the microorganisms overgrowth, producing biomass, declines and the consequent loss of biomolecules of interest. Sun and shadow drying are the most common and feasible ways of drying food and other biomass. They involve the drying of raw materials due to the effect of atmospheric conditions. However, other classical methods involve convection or force convection for drying, which use higher temperatures but less operational time than sun and shadow drying. However, in sun-drying, the direct effect of the sun can affect phenolic and EO content due to their degradation. Finally, freeze-drying is a way of drying at low temperatures preserving biomass characteristics such as TPC and EO.

Moreover, innovative ways of drying such as microwave and ultrasound drying heat more efficiently and disrupt biomass, promoting EO and NPC extractions. Some studies analyze the effect of drying. For example, the EO yield can vary from around 3.0% v/w for sun-drying to 4.5–5.0% (v/w) for shadow drying, and TPC of 3.23 mg GAE/100 g and 4.26 mg GAE/100 g, respectively. Compare to freeze-drying which achieved a higher EO yield (6.90% v/w of EO) and TPC 12.73 mg GAE/100 g (Farahmandfar *et al.*, 2020). Regarding convection drying, some authors analyze the optimal temperature to obtain a good TPC and TEAC. The moderate-high temperature employment of 60 °C yields 60.97% of DPPH scavenging activity (Afrin *et al.*, 2021) and for 65 °C 26.72 mg GAE/g of dry solid and DPPH scavenging activity of 32.89 mg TEAC/g (Deng *et al.*, 2018). Furthermore, some innovative techniques combine classical convection drying with ultrasounds, ultraviolet and pulsed electric fields (Onwude *et al.*, 2017).

Extraction of EO is carried out by distillation and extraction operations because of their chemical characteristics. The former is the classical way of extraction for these components from citrus peels and aromatic herbs. These operations employed steam to drag EO out of oil glands on the orange peels. Additionally, there are two ways of distillation: hydro distillation and steam distillation. However, they usually involve high-energy consumption and long times of operation. Due to these disadvantages, solid-liquid extraction is another common way of obtaining EO and NPC. In this case, the selected solvent is crucial for improving the yield and making the process cost-effective and environmentally friendly. Therefore, nowadays, a wide range of green and bio-based solvents are studied to replace classical petrochemical-derived solvents such as hexane which is highly toxic for the environment. In the case of orange residues, greener bio-based organic solvents have been tested (e.g., 2-methyl tetrahydrofuran and cyclopentyl methyl ether) manage to get higher extraction yields (1.78% and 1.37% on a dry basis, respectively) compared to hexane [0.99% (w/w)] (Ozturk et al., 2019). Deep Eutectic Solvents (DES) exhibit attractive qualities for both EO and natural phenolics extraction. For instance, choline chloride (ChCl)-based DES show an elevated selectivity toward some phenolics of orange peel. However, bio-based solvents (e.g., ethylene glycol (EG)) extract higher TPC than DES (5.84 mg GAE/g compare to 3.61 mg GAE/g for EG and EG:ChCl DES, respectively) but with lower selectivity for cinnamic and hydroxybenzoic acids (Ozturk et al., 2018). Another study shows the ability of ChCl glycerol-based DES to extract limonene from orange peel (3.84 mg g^{-1} fresh weight) and ChCl:EG for NPC extraction (45.7 mg GAE/g fresh weight) (Panić et al., 2021).

The physicochemical disruption of oil glands and the consequent release of EO and NPC is another way of recovering these chemicals. New methodologies combined with classical extraction and distillations have been studied in the last years to recover EO and NPC from wastes more efficiently. For example, ultrasound-assisted extraction (UAE) produces the disruption of the cellular structures due to cavitation forces. Sometimes in orange or other citrus wastes, hydro distillation could be combined with UAE as shown in a recent study (Heydari et al., 2020). In that sense, another methodology applied is microwave-assisted extraction (MAE). Microwave treatment enables a more efficient to break the orange structure improving the extraction of EO and NPC. Techno-economic analysis shows the viability of MAE with these extraction purposes. For instance, microwave steam diffusion achieves a yield of 1.5% (v/w) in less than one hour for EO (Razzaghi et al., 2019). As well as that happens in UAE, in MAE, other techniques such as hydrodistillation could be used together. Furthermore, the use of lignocellulolytic enzymes that hydrolyze cell walls enhances the release of EO (Gavahian et al., 2019).

Pectin is a complex heteropolysaccharide that is characteristic of citrus fruits. It interacts with cellulose, hemicellulose, and lignin on citrus peels. It is made up of galacturonic acid (GalA), rhamnose, arabinose, and galactose predominantly. These monosaccharides are combined in different ways, making three structural motifs: homogalacturonan (HG), rhamnogalacturonan-I, and (RhG-I) rhamnogalacturonan-II (RhG-II). The rheological characteristics that show this polymer give it a value added itself. However, it is usually modified to tune these characteristics.

Extraction of pectin is carried out in acidic conditions (pH = 1.0–3.0), moderate-high temperature (70–100 °C), and short time (0.5–2 h). Due to these conditions, the lignocellulosic matrix is disrupted and the interaction of the pectin with the other polymer is broken. Isolation of solubilized pectin accomplishes by precipitation with an organic solvent (ethanol or isopropanol commonly) and low temperature (4 °C). An optimization study obtains an extraction yield of 20% (w/w) employing acidic conditions (Senit *et al.*, 2019). However, other breaking technologies based on hydrodynamic cavitation (Meneguzzo *et al.*, 2019) and MAE recover a high percentage of pectin, in the last case up to 32.8% (w/w) (Su *et al.*, 2019). Also, the use of a combination of pressurized CO_2 and water treatment can be taken as an emerging technology in this field (Tsuru *et al.*, 2020). Figure 14.2 is a compilation of the mentioned pretreatments.

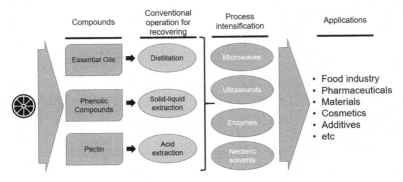

Figure 14.2 General scheme of the most common products of interest obtained among OPWs' pretreatment. The conventional obtention procedures and process intensification tecniques.

14.2.2 Enzymatic Saccharification of OPWs

OPWs are high porosity residues with a high polysaccharides content and a high proportion of free sugars like fructose, glucose, and sucrose. The main polysaccharides in the OPWs are cellulose or pectin and in minor proportion hemicellulose (Senit et al., 2019). Except for pectin, the other polysaccharides are formed of classic fermentable sugars like glucose, xylose, galactose, etc. Besides, OPW has a low content in lignin, a strong growth inhibitor of different microorganisms (de la Torre et al., 2020).

Acid hydrolysis of polysaccharides is a very usual two-step industrial process. The first step is a short acid treatment of sulfuric acid (H_2SO_4) [0.1–1% (w/w)] at 121 °C and 15 psi (1 atm) for 15 min after which the solid is separated by centrifugation. The remaining solid suffers another acid diluted hydrolysis step with H_2SO_4 1.0% (w/w). In this case, a longer treatment is applied, 30 min, to completely hydrolyze cellulose to glucose. This liquor can be used as a culture medium for different microbial production as bioethanol. Acid hydrolysis is fast, presents high yields and a minor cost if compared to its enzymatic counterpart, as it only needs inorganic acid and high temperature. But it has the drawbacks of low selectivity with the subsequent formation of toxic by-products like furfural and 5-hydroxymethylfurfural (5-HMF), which inhibits microorganisms' growth (Oberoi et al., 2010).

To avoid those by-products, the implementation of enzymatic saccharification has been studied for a long time. The main process catalyzed by the enzyme using OPW is the saccharification due to their optimal characteristics for the action of enzymes, like high porosity, low lignin content, and low crystallinity of cellulose. In addition, pectin extraction and partial hydrolysis to produce pectic oligosaccharides are subject to very promising research efforts (Cano et al., 2020; Cui et al., 2020). Different processes and optimal conditions are collected in Table 14.1.

Saccharification is the enzymatic hydrolysis of different lignocellulosic biomass for the obtention of fermentable sugars. To ensure close contact between enzymes and the solid substrate, the accessibility of the biocatalysts needs to be improved by disrupting the structure of the cell wall. In addition, product inhibition of the

Table 14.1 Operational conditions for exemplary hydrolysis processes of citrus wastes

Substrate	Hydrolysis Method	Conditions of the Process	Production	References
Fresh and homogenized OPW	Enzymatic hydrolysis	Acetate buffer 100 mM, pH 4.75, 50 °C, 4 h and 500 r.p.m. 1500 U g^{-1} sludge and 60 U g^{-1} sludge	79.24 +- 1.82 g L^{-1} of reducing sugars	(Kuo et al., 2019)
OPW + acid treatment	Hot diluted nitric acid hydrolysis + enzymatic hydrolysis	Acid hydrolysis: pH 1.8, 80 °C, and 3 h. Enzymatic hydrolysis: 1% (w/w) DS sodium citrate buffer 50 mM and pH 4.8. 4 FPU g^{-1} substrate of Cellic® CTec2, 50 °C, 120 r.p.m, 72 h	45% (w/w) glucose 2.5% (w/w) arabinose 1% (w/w) galactose 3% (w/w) xylose	(Satari et al., 2017)
OPW fresh and milled	Enzymatic hydrolysis	Celluclast 1,5 L: 24.3 FPU g^{-1} DS Novozym 188: 23 UI g^{-1} DS Pectinex Ultra SP-L: 1340 UI g^{-1} pectin	45 g L^{-1} glucose 30 g L^{-1} fructose 12 g L^{-1} GalA	(Velasco et al., 2017)
OPW dried	Acid hydrolysis prior removal EOs	0.5% (v/v) H$_2$SO$_4$, 125 °C and 120 min	21.9 g L^{-1} glucose 9.3 g L^{-1} fructose	(Ayala et al., 2021)
OPW dried	Enzymatic hydrolysis prior removal of essential oils	Citrate buffer pH 4.8 at 50 °C and 150 r.p.m. for 24 h. Biogazyme 2X: 112 FPU g^{-1} DS Pectinex Ultra-SP-L: 67 UI g^{-1} DS	40 g L^{-1} glucose 68 g L^{-1} reducing sugars	(Pocan et al., 2018)
OPW partial drying	Enzymatic hydrolysis	pH 5.2, 50 °C and 300 r.p.m. 3.18 FPU g^{-1} dry solid and 10% (w/w) DS	50 g L^{-1} glucose	(de la Torre et al., 2017)

free sugars that remains in the residue should be considered (de la Torre *et al.*, 2017). To increase the accessibility to enzymes two alternatives can be followed: physicochemical treatments such as a steam explosion at short times or relatively low temperature and pressure (to avoid by-products), or to treat the OPW mass with pectinases that break down this polysaccharide, thus improving the yields of saccharification with cellulases and hemicellulases (de la Torre *et al.*, 2017).

Pectin is a key ingredient in the food industry, but its main monosaccharide, the GalA, is not a classic fermentable sugar. Thus, if the pectin is removed before saccharification, the accessibility of cellulose is higher and mass-transfer issues due to the gelling properties of pectin (with concomitant high viscosity) are avoided. The other way around, for disrupting the cell network, the first step with cellulases can be performed, thus increasing cell permeability. In this way, pectin can be extracted by an enzymatic process with the bonus of an increase in the feasibility of the whole process. Moreover, this way GalA is avoided in the hydrolysis liquor after a second saccharification (Cui *et al.*, 2020).

Nowadays, instead of pectin extraction, a cocktail of pectinases is added to the saccharification reaction mixture. The action of pectinases results in a higher yield for saccharification as mass-transfer rates of all enzymes acting on the solid substrate increase, with the subsequent increase in monosaccharide yield and productivity (Kuo *et al.*, 2019). Furthermore, GalA is obtained as a by-product, although few microorganisms, if any, are capable of using it as a carbon source. To utilize this substrate, metabolic engineering has been applied to *Saccharomyces cerevisiae*, obtaining a strain able to grow in a glucose-GalA mixture to produce *meso*-galactaric acid directly from OPW (Protzko *et al.*, 2018).

As enzymatic saccharification is more expensive than acid hydrolysis some optimization work is needed to be done. The most important factors in the enzymatic saccharification are substrate concentration [% of dry solid (DS)], cellulase, and other auxiliary activities like xylanases and operational variables like stirring, pH, and temperature. A critical parameter to be optimized is the enzyme loading in the process as it is a key factor in the economic feasibility of the process. Substrate concentration should be also be considered as, usually, a high concentration of monosaccharides is sought and high-solid loadings in batch processes are needed, or they need to be added in several loads in a fed-batch process, reducing the high viscosity of the mixture. As the residue has a high content of free sugars, if the initial concentration is high, enzymes could be inhibited during the process due to product inhibition. Moreover, pH control is crucial as OPW is an acid waste due to its high content in galacturonic and citric acids, which can inhibit saccharification if very low pH values are reached (de la Torre *et al.*, 2017). In addition, the temperature in the 45–50 °C range should be sought, as higher temperatures inactivate fungal enzymes such as those from *Trichoderma*, *Aspergillus*, and *Penicillium* geni usual in this field. The last important operational variable is stirring and solid-liquid mixing, as a good mass-transfer rate is needed, especially in those residues that present high viscosity, such as OPW. However, a harsh agitation can inactivate enzymes, possibly due to air–liquid intimate contact, and agitation energy expenses are also to be considered, so a trade-off needs to be achieved (de la Torre *et al.*, 2017).

14.3 Biological Processes to Platform Chemicals and Materials

Once OPW is pre-treated, a biological biorefinery processing continues through a fermentative stage, with the obtained sugars undergoing biotransformation using different microorganisms (Satari and Karimi, 2018). OPW fermentative processes can focus on the production of energy conversion products, such as biogas or bioethanol, or higher value-added chemicals, such as organic acids or other specialties, and biocatalysts as, for example, several enzymes.

14.3.1 Bioethanol and Superior Alcohols

Ethanol production by fermentation has been the first target in what are now called biorefineries, as an alternative fuel to gasoline or fuel to mix with it (Ilhak *et al.*, 2019). Therefore, its production from numerous feedstock is of utmost interest; first of all, agricultural products used in food - corn, sugarcane, barley, wheat, sugar beet, and sweet sorghum - were used. The current focus is on the utilization of lignocellulosic biomass not for food purposes, particularly agricultural residues, such as straw and corn stubble, sweet sorghum and sugar beet bagasse; and wheat straw (Ayodele *et al.*, 2020). To move from starch- and free sugar-based ethanol to ethanol from lignocellulose is requiring more effort in the development of the pre-fermentation stages, but also in the development of strains prepared both to tolerate ethanol and to metabolize various types of sugars from those new pre-fermentation stages (Ayodele *et al.*, 2020; Sakar *et al.*, 2020).

In this sense, the use of OPW has been considered as an interesting feedstock for the development of ethanol production. The use of CPW has been demonstrated to be a very promising raw material to be used in biorefineries for valorization into fuels due to its low lignin content (Jeong *et al.*, 2021; Patsalou *et al.*, 2020; Choi *et al.*, 2015).

The production of ethanol from OPW has been usually studied by separating the different fractions of the residue, in particular, limonene (due to its antimicrobial properties) and pectin (because it has generally been considered as a non-fermentable material) and carrying out the necessary pretreatments and hydrolysis stages to obtain fermentable sugars from the other fractions, which would be used in alcoholic fermentation (Patsalou *et al.*, 2020; Choi *et al.*, 2015). The main microorganisms used in fermentation are *S. cerevisiae* and *K. marxianus*, which are being utilized at the industrial level, however, studies have been also carried out on the use of immobilized biochar thermotolerant organisms (P. kudriavzeni KMP10) to reduce operating costs due to the cooling required for fermentation, which may also entail a higher risk of contamination (Patsalou *et al.*, 2019).

The great interest in ethanol production within the biorefinery concept has led to the approach of the microbial process from various perspectives, even the introduction of cellulase expression in S. cerevisiae is studied to perform saccharification simultaneously with fermentation when using OPW (Yang, *et al.*, 2018). As discussed, ethanol production from OPW has been directed to the separation of polymer fractions and their separate valorization; in general, the cellulose fraction is used to obtain ethanol and the rest for obtaining other products, such as the production of biogas (Kyriakou *et al.*, 2020; Taghizadeh-Alisaraei *et al.*, 2017). However, emerging studies focus on the simultaneous production of lactic acid and ethanol from

OPW (Fazzino et al., 2021), including the possibility of performing an isopropanol-butanol-ethanol (IBE) fermentation from mandarin waste by combining two Clostridium strains that present tolerance to the presence of limonene (Tomita et al., 2019).

The integral utilization of this type of waste for ethanol production has to address aspects necessary to carry out a successful alcoholic fermentation from OPW. As mentioned throughout this chapter, the composition of OPW (or CPW in general), unlike the biomass waste studied so far for ethanol production, contains pectin in high proportions. The industrial strains of *S. cerevisiae* for ethanol production are not able to metabolize GalA and sugars from pectin hydrolysis (Jeong et al., 2020). Therefore, efforts are being made to achieve this goal by employing metabolic engineering.

The development of strains capable of fermenting GalA is still in its initial stages, identifying metabolic capabilities in several bacteria (*E. coli* and some species of *Lactobacillus*) and in aerobic metabolisms of fungi (*Trichoderma reseii*, *Botrytus cinerea*, and *Rhodosporium toruloides*), however, its heterologous expression in *S. cerevisiae* has produced unexpected results although the possibility of obtaining results from the route in fungi could be possible due to consumption of 1 g L^{-1} of GalA was observed, the main problem seems to lie in the transport of this acid through the cell membrane which is highly dependent on pH, so an expression of a GalA transporter is needed (Jeong et al., 2021). This is the focus of the work of Protzko et al. (2018), in which they succeed in expressing a heterologous transporter from *Aspergillus niger* in *S. cerevisiae* for the co-utilization of glucose and GalA to be used in the production of ethanol and meso-galactaric acid, respectively.

Besides, to ferment OPW completely, it is also necessary to consume other sugars that are found in smaller proportions, such as L-arabinose, L-rhamnose, galactose, and xylose. *S. cerevisiae* is able to consume galactose naturally, while the consumption of xylose would require the expression of a heterologous pathway, which has been extensively studied (Jeong et al., 2021). However, in the case of L-rhamnose, it seems that the expression of a specific heterologous transporter would be necessary (Jeong et al., 2021).

Finally, it should be noted that, although work on the production of alcohols from OPW or CPW has focused on obtaining ethanol, some work is beginning to focus on higher alcohols. As previously discussed, the simultaneous production of isobutanol-butanol-ethanol has been addressed (Tomita et al., 2019). The production of butanol has also been studied (Fiori da Silva et al., 2020), via ABE fermentation from orange bagasse pellets using a wild type of microorganism of *Clostridium beijerinkii*, demonstrating that this residue is very promising for this type of process, in this case using only the cellulose fraction of the residue.

14.3.2 Gas Energy and Material Vectors from OPW

From the point of view of energy intensity and environmental reasons, direct combustion of OPW or the generation of bioethanol is not necessarily the most efficient alternative. Thus, the anaerobic digestion (AD) to biogas, biomethane, or biohydrogen is also considered by the energy sector.

Biogas is a mixture mostly consisting of biomethane (CH_4) (45–75% v/v), a lesser amount of carbon dioxide (CO_2), and even lower quantities of other components generated in AD, with varying composition depending on the raw materials. This inevitably affects the lower heating value (LHV), which is around 16 to 28 MJ m^{-3}. From the upgrade and purification of biogas mainly by CO_2 removal, biomethane can be obtained, which has a higher LHV of 36 MJ m^{-3} and, advantageously, can use the supply chain and distribution channels currently in use by natural gas. For its part, hydrogen shows clear benefits as a fuel candidate and its production is being pursued in through multiple pathways. Not only does it provide a high-energy yield (142.4 kJ g^{-1}), but also water is the only product generated from its combustion, which gives it a very clean profile. For this reason, the production of biohydrogen (H_2) is also sought through AD. For these three products, significant growths in the share of energy supply have already been observed and are estimated to continue by 2030 and beyond (International Energy Association, 2021). This is partly due to the adoption of policies toward the security of more affordable and cleaner energy, particularly in the case in which it is produced from agriculture and FW as is the case of OPW. From AD processes, also short-chain organic acids, also known as volatile fatty acids (VFA) can be simultaneously produced. These are chemicals with intrinsic value owing to their application not only in technologies related to energy, such as generating electricity in microbial fuel cells but also in the formulation of products in the food or pharmaceutical sector, to mention a couple (Esteban and Ladero, 2018).

AD is a process that features a series of steps. First, hydrolysis of the feedstock takes place, after which lipids, carbohydrates, proteins, and other large components are broken down by anaerobic bacterial consortia, such as *Bacillus thermomonospora* or *Ruminococcus baceriodes*. The following stage is acidogenesis, where bacteria of the strains *Streptococcus* or *Lactobacillus* among others can transform the monomers previously generated into VFAs or short-chain alcohols. Next comes acetogenesis, whereby *Clostridium* or *Acetobacterium* can transform the latter into H_2, CO_2, and acetic acid. Last, methanogenesis is a reductive step that generates CH_4 as a product with *Methanolobus* or *Methanococcus* for example.

While advantageous, AD of OPW presents two main challenges. The first is the seasonality of the waste, which affects the amount and potentially the composition of the feedstock of the process. For this, ensiling is an option, which is based on the acidification of vegetal biomass that facilitates its conservation also thanks to the absence of oxygen (Calabrò and Panzera, 2018; Calabrò, Fazzino *et al.*, 2020). The second has to do with the antimicrobial and inhibitory effect of EO, which feature compounds like terpenes and terpenoids, highly present in OPW. Among these compounds, D-limonene is the most relevant owing to its relative presence. Thus, it is recommended to devise strategies to overcome the complications arising from their presence, such as their removal by solid-liquid extraction (Ozturk *et al.*, 2019), steam distillation, the use of activated carbon (Calabrò *et al.*, 2019), aeration, thermal and alkaline treatments (Calabrò, *et al.*, 2018). Many works in literature have explored the AD of OPW focusing on different aspects and following strategies to mitigate the pernicious effect of EO. Table 14.2 summarizes some relevant works for the production of biogas and their components biomethane, biohydrogen, or VFAs in a more pure quality employing OPW as raw material.

Table 14.2 Summary of the most relevant works on the valorization of OPW to biogas, biomethane, biohydrogen, and VFAs

Purpose of Study	Strategy Against EO	Operating Conditions	Main Results	References
Assess the viability of AD of OPW with glycerol as co-substrate	No pretreatment, but the addition of glycerol to reduce by dilution the inhibitory effect while supplying nutrients	Semicontinuous reactors (3.5 L) Mesophilic (35 C) and thermophilic (55 C) Anaerobic sludge inoculum: 7 g VS/L; OLR = 1.91 g VS/(m³ d) HRT = 8.5–30 d Substrate mixtures COD 1:1 (OPW:Gly); Nutrient ratios: COD:N:P (300:5:1)	Mesophilic conditions performed better overall. $Y_{CH4} = 330\ mL\ g^{-1}\ VS$	Martin et al., 2013
Study the effect of D-limonene removal on AD and elucidation of the kinetics to describe methane production, of which the best model is based on a logistic curve	D-Limonene extraction by steam distillation at lab scale	Batch experiments in stirred tank reactors (3.5 L) at thermophilic (52 C) conditions. 12 g VSS/L of granular sludge as inoculum HRT = 5 d 1–6 g COD/L over a 15-day period (1.21 g COD/L acclimatization)	$Y_{CH4} = 3800\ mL\ STP\ CH_4$ for 4.5 g COD/L	Martin et al., 2018

(Continued)

Table 14.2 (Continued)

Purpose of Study	Strategy Against EO	Operating Conditions	Main Results	References
Determine the biodegradability of citrus waste, assess the inhibitory effect of d-limonene on AD, characterize it and evaluate biomass adaptation	None. Also, the work studied different d-limonene concentrations on the digestion of microcrystalline cellulose (MCC)	Batch experiments in glass bottles (2 L) Mesophilic (38 C) (a) AD of OPW Inoculum: 26.9 gVS/L Inoculum to substrate ratio: 2.6 (b) AD of MCC No limonene added: Inoculum: 31.7 gVS/L ISR = 2 d-Limonene at 200 mg kg^{-1} Inoculum: 35.7 gVS/L ISR = 2.2	(a) Y_{CH4} = 357.3 mL g^{-1} VS CH_4 production rate = 39.9 mL/(gVS d) (b) No d-limonene added: Y_{CH4} = 441.6 mL g^{-1}VS CH_4 production rate = 204.9 mL/(gVS d) d-Limonene at 200 mg kg^{-1}: Y_{CH4} = 405.3 mL g^{-1}VS CH_4 production rate = 77.6 mL/(gVS d)	Ruiz and Flotats, 2016
Assess three different strategies for d-limonene removal and co-digestion with cow manure on methane production rate	(a) Solid-state fermentation with fungi (Penicillium genus), (b) steam distillation and (c) ethanol extraction	As in (Ruiz and Flotats, 2016) with the addition of cow manure, the OLR changed to 3 kgVS/(m^3 d)	(a) d-Limonene removal: 22% Y_{CH4} = 338 mL g^{-1}VS CH_4 production rate = 41 mL/(gVS d) (b) d-Limonene removal: 44% Y_{CH4} = 417 mL g^{-1}VS CH_4 production rate = 69 mL/(gVS d) (c) d-Limonene removal: 100% Y_{CH4} = 465 mL g^{-1}VS CH_4 production rate = 74 mL/(gVS d)	Ruiz et al., 2016

Purpose of Study	Strategy Against EO	Operating Conditions	Main Results	References
Analysis of concentration of D-limonene on AD co-digestion with kitchen waste and agro-waste.	None as part of the study refers to its influence on AD and CH_4 production	Batch experiments (0.5 L bottles) at (a) thermophilic (50 C) and (b) mesophilic (35 C) conditions; 1.1 L bottles for mesophilic. Different inocula with sludge, cow manure, or agro-waste with variable organic loads.	(a) Y_{CH4} = 300 mL g^{-1} VS (no limonene added, agro-waste inoculum) (b) Y_{CH4} = 370 mL g^{-1} VS (250 mg L^{-1} limonene added, agro-waste inoculum)	Calabrò et al., 2016
Study of D-limonene degradation to p-cymene by dehydrogenation		EO artificially added at different concentrations (240–2000 mg L^{-1}) HRT = 30 d		
Study the effect of ensiling OPW and adaptation of the inoculum to the substrates used	(a) Ensiling up to 37 days, (b) mixing inoculum consisting of sludge and OPW ensiled for 7 days	Batch experiments (1.1 L bottles) in mesophilic (35 °C) conditions. HRT = 30 d, (a) Inoculum: 6.3 gVS/L, ISR = 3; (b) Inoculum: 5.22 gVS/L, ISR = 3	(a) Y_{CH4} = 365 mL g^{-1} VS (b) Y_{CH4} = 513.7 mL g^{-1} VS	Calabrò and Panzera, 2018
Test the effect of four pretreatment methods of OPW, optimize their combination, and study the kinetics of CH_4 by AD	(a) Ensiling (37 days), (b) aeration (400 L h^{-1}), (c) thermal (70 °C) and (d) alkaline treatments (5 g $Ca(OH)_2$ /100 g OPW) and combinations	As in (Calabrò and Panzera, 2018) for volume, temperature, and HRT. Variable combinations of inoculum to substrate ratios (1.82 -3.44) and total solids in inocula as detailed in the publication	Y_{CH4} ranged from 322 to 499 mL g^{-1} VS, the latter obtained by aeration	Calabrò et al, 2018

(Continued)

Table 14.2 (Continued)

Purpose of Study	Strategy Against EO	Operating Conditions	Main Results	References
Reduce volatile solids loss during ensiling and lactic acid (LA) production with stimulated (LA) bacteria	No specific treatment. Ensiling is the method selected to produce LA	Ensiling at room temperature for 28 days. OPW supplemented with $MnCl_2$ at 0.005 g kg^{-1} OPW	$Y_{CH4} \approx 10$ mL g^{-1} VS $Y_{LA} = 55$ g kg^{-1} TS $Y_{AceticAcid} = 26$ g kg^{-1} TS $Y_{EtOH} = 120$ g kg^{-1} TS	Fazzino et al., 2021
Comparison of the potential of (a) two-stage AD (acidogenic and methanogenic) versus (b) single-stage process	No pretreatment, but the first of two stages to avoid inhibition by d-limonene	Batch experiments in CSTR (4.3 L) mesophilic conditions (35 °C) pH = 5–6 (acidogenic); 7–8 (methanogenic) HRT = 25.8 d OLR = 0.36 g COD/(L d) (two-stage reactor); 0.40 g COD/(L d) (one-stage reactor)	(a) $Y_{CH4} = 790$ mL g^{-1} VS $Y_{biogas} = 0.79$ L g^{-1} SVT CVFA, total ≈ 14 g L^{-1} (acidogenic stage) CVFA, total ≈ 25 g L^{-1} (methanogenic stage) (b) Single-stage process: $Y_{CH4} = 490$ mL g^{-1} VS $Y_{biogas} = 0.49$ L g^{-1} SVT CVFA≈30 g L^{-1} VFA: acetic, propionic, butyric, and isobutyric	Jiménez-Castro et al., 2020
Analyze biogas and biomethane production (a) removing EO by distillation and (b) then hydrolyzing citrus waste with Fenton's reagent	Removal of citrus oil by distillation	Batch experiments (125 mL) at mesophilic (35 °C) conditions. ISR = 2 HRT = 31 d	(a) $Y_{gas} = 262$ mL g^{-1} VS $Y_{CH4} = 122.48$ mL g^{-1} VS (a+b) $Y_{gas} = 332$ mL g^{-1} VS $Y_{CH4} = 100.33$ mL g^{-1} VS	Magare et al., 2020

Purpose of Study	Strategy Against EO	Operating Conditions	Main Results	References
Production of H_2 and VFA in acidogenic stage (I) and CH_4 in methanogenic stage (II). Kinetic analysis of H_2 production and understanding of microbial communities involved in the metabolic pathway	No pretreatment, but the first of two stages consume most D-limonene present	Batch experiments (250 mL) at mesophilic (30 C) conditions. (a) Stage I: 15 g L^{-1} OPW; 2.25 g TVS/L of autochthonous and 3 g TVS/L of allochthonous inocula, 5 g L^{-1} of NaCl, and pH = 8.5 HRT = 22 h (b) Stage II: 3 gTVS/L of allochthonous inoculum Supplemented with Zinder medium and vitamin solution HRT = 700 h	(a) Y_{H2} = 13.29 mmol/L C_{VFA} ≈ 1400 mg L^{-1} (b) Y_{CH4} = 50.2 mmol L^{-1} No VFA left	Camargo et al., 2021a
Experimental design to optimize operating conditions for the production of H_2 and VFA	No pretreatment	HRT = 30 d Variables studied in the following ranges: pH (5.5–8.5); temperature (30–44 C); autochtonous (0.75–2.25 g$_{TVS}$/L) and allochtonous inocula (1–3 g$_{TVS}$/L); OPW concentration (5–15 g L^{-1}); headspace (40–60%); nutritional medium components concentrations including yeast extract (0–1 g L^{-1}), $CaCO_3$ (0–5 g L^{-1}), NaCl (0–5 g L^{-1}) and peptone (0–5 g L^{-1})	Y_{H2} = 13.29 mmol L^{-1} C_{VFA} = 1340 mg L^{-1}	Camargo et al., 2021b

The group of Siles tested the use of glycerol as co-substrate for the AD of OPW as a means to mitigate the inhibitory effect of D-limonene by dilution while simultaneously supplying nutrients to the medium. This approach allowed to enhance the efficiency of biomethanization, although the OPW to glycerol ratio is an important variable to control as too high organic loads may lead to the accumulation of VFAs, hence leading to low pH and destabilization of the process. For this set of experiments, mesophilic conditions proved more efficient than thermophilic (Martín *et al.*, 2013). In further work, steam distillation was performed to remove up to 70% of D-limonene from the OPW matrix and evaluate the effect of this pretreatment on methane generation. A subsequent study using Logistic, Gompertz, and Sigmoid models as base equations revealed that the former describes the kinetics of the process best (Martin *et al.*, 2018).

Ruiz, Flotats *et al.* also conducted significant work on mandarin and orange waste valorization to gas energy vectors. In a first study, it was determined that from a concentration of 200 mg D-limonene per kg, AD is seriously hindered and the effect is more intense as this compound is transformed into cymene and other by-products by dehydrogenation (Ruiz and Flotats, 2016). In further work, biological removal with fungi (*Penicillium digitatum* and *P. italicum*) and removal by steam distillation or extraction with ethanol were conducted prior to AD showing increasing degrees of efficiency. In accordance with this removal efficiency, the biomethane production potential and its production rate showed increased values (Ruiz *et al.*, 2016).

Calabrò *et al.* have performed extensive studies on the AD of OPW. For example, the co-digestion of OPW with inocula containing kitchen or agricultural waste adding different amounts of EO to understand the behavior of AD and also the reaction mechanism that D-limonene underwent (Calabrò *et al.*, 2016). In a subsequent study, they employed ensiled OPW during 37 days as a substrate for biogas production to mitigate the effect of EO. Using this strategy at mesophilic conditions they were able to obtain methane at 365 mL g^{-1} VS, which was improved by 40% making the microorganisms adapt to the substrate by mixing the sludge with OPW subject to ensiling for 7 days (Calabrò and Panzera, 2018). The subject of D-limonene removal and adaptation of the microorganism to the medium was deepened in a subsequent study where different pretreatment methods and their combinations were tested using different inocula (Calabrò et al., 2018). More recently, the production of VFA like lactic and acetic acids as well as ethanol was approached by ensiling OPW in a process where lactic acid bacteria were stimulated by inexpensive $MnCl_2$, thus making it an attractive process for implementation (Fazzino et al., 2021).

Another approach to the pretreatment of citrus waste was distillation to remove EO followed by oxidation with Fenton's reagent, which has shown improvements in the yields to biogas owing to a better disruption of the pectin microstructure (Magare et al., 2020).

The AD to generate biogas was compared using a two-stage versus a single-stage process, whereby the first step is acidogenic and plays a part in reducing the amount of inhibitory compounds like D-limonene. Despite not being a pretreatment in itself, this step allowed a more productive methanogenic stage, increasing the yields of biogas and methane concentration significantly when using the two-stage process. Also, a configuration in two stages normally provides better control owing to an independent optimization of the conditions and control for each reactor (Jiménez-Castro et al., 2020).

Varesche's group has recently published a series of works with a focus on hydrogen generation with special emphasis on bacterial strains responsible for the metabolic pathways. AD produced H_2 and VFA first in an acidogenic stage and then CH_4 in a second methanogenic stage, where a metataxonomic characterization using next-generation sequencing approaches led to the conclusion that the genera *Escherichia, Clostridium, Paraclostridium*, and *Enterobacter* were the major contributors to hydrolysis and/or H_2 and VFA production in the first stage. In the methanogenic step, acetoclastic methanogenesis was regarded as the main mechanism with acetyl-CoA synthetase playing a major role (Camargo et al., 2021a). These authors also performed a comprehensive analysis through a Plackett–Burman design of experiments to optimize as many as 10 variables that affect H_2 and acetic acid production. The most relevant were pH (optimum at 8.5), allochthonous inoculum (3 g TVS/L), and substrate concentration (15 g_{OPW}/L) leading to productions of 13.29 mmol L^{-1} of H_2 and 1340 mg L^{-1} of acetic acid confirmed that *Escherichia* and *Clostridium* were the main strains responsible for H_2 generation (Camargo *et al.*, 2021b).

Considering the efforts from the studies mentioned above, the valorization of OPW by AD provides a good scenario to underpin a holistic valorization strategy of this residue. In fact, in addition to the recovery of D-limonene and other EO, by pretreatment of OPW, it is possible to obtain polyphenolics, pectin, and fermentable sugars for AD. Recent work shows a combination of experimental results and simulations to have a preliminary estimation of operation and capital expenses with the net profit over the life of the project (Mariana *et al.*, 2021).

14.3.3 Monomers and Other Organic Compounds

Due to the high content of water, sugars, fats, and polysaccharides in citrus wastes, spontaneous fermentations sometimes take place. From a biotechnological point of view, these reactions represent a great opportunity to carry out controlled processes through which to obtain basic value-added products, such as carboxylic acids (De la Torre *et al.*, 2019). These compounds have a high number of applications in the food, pharmaceutical, and chemical industries and are currently mostly generated by petrochemical processes Esteban and Ladero (2018). Table 14.3 shows some of the most representative citrus wastes fermentation processes in recent years.

Citric acid (CA) is an organic acid widely used as an acidulant, antioxidant, preservative, flavoring, or astringent, among other applications. Comparing the different microorganisms that produce CA, the *Aspergillus niger* fungus seems to be the best option due to its ease of handling and the low amount of by-products it generates (Abbas *et al.*, 2016; Dutta *et al.*, 2019). Abbas *et al.* (2016) performed surface culture fermentation with this microorganism from sweet OPW, managing to optimize the operating conditions to produce 14–16 g L^{-1} of CA. Later, Dutta *et al.* (2019) carried out batch fermentations of OPW with a yield of 0.44%, after observing how the selection of the appropriate conditions of pH, temperature, nitrogen source, inoculum size, and methanol concentration could increase the yield up to 11%.

Table 14.3 Organic compounds production processes from citrus wastes

Product	Substrate	Microorganism	Type of Operation	Production	References
CA	OPW	A. niger BM-12	Batch (flasks), 30 °C, pH 6 to pH 3.3, stirring, NH_4NO_3, 750 µL inoculum, 4% (v/v) methanol	0.44 g g^{-1}	Dutta et al. (2019)
CA	Sweet OPW	A. niger	Surface culture, 32 °C, pH 4, 2% inoculum, 25% sucrose	14–16 g L^{-1}	Abbas et al. (2016)
LA	OPW	L. delbrueckii ssp delbrueckii CECT 286	Batch (reactor), resting cells (from the reactor with pure hydrolysate), 40 °C, pH 5.8, 800 rpm	96.34 g L^{-1} 0.94 g g^{-1} 3.70 g (L h)$^{-1}$	De la Torre et al. (2020)
LA	OPW	L. delbrueckii ssp delbrueckii CECT 286	Batch (reactor), 37 °C, pH 5.8, 200 rpm	0.86 g g^{-1} 0.63 g (L h)$^{-1}$	Bustamante et al. (2020)
SA	CPW	A. succinogenes 130Z	Fed-batch (reactor), 37 °C pH 6.8, 0.5 vvm CO_2	22.4 g L^{-1} 0.73 g g^{-1} 0.45 g (L h)$^{-1}$	Patsalou et al. (2020)
SA	CPW	A. succinogenes 130Z	Batch (bottles), 37 °C, 100 rpm, 0.5 vvm CO_2	8.30 g L^{-1} 0.70 g g^{-1}	Patsalou et al. (2017)
AA	Citrus wastewater	Presents in wastewater	Fed-batch (reactor), pH 5 to pH 7, stirring, filling ratio 95%, C: N: P 200:0.1:0.1, COD < 5000 mg L^{-1}	2.85 g L^{-1}	Corsino et al. (2021)
EA	OPW	A. fumigatus MUM 1603	Submerged fermentation (flasks), 30 °C, 200 rpm, 2 × 10^7 spores g^{-1} inoculum, 6.2 g L^{-1} polyphenols	0.02 g g^{-1}	Sepúlveda et al. (2020)
DHA	OPW	Aurantiochytrium sp. KRS101	Batch (flasks), 28 °C, pH 5.5, 120 rpm, 1.2 g L^{-1} $NaNO_3$	0.63 g L^{-1}	Park et al. (2018)

LA is an important building block used, among other applications, as an acidulant, for the manufacture of lotions, cleaning agents, and polylactic acid (PLA). Its production through the biological route is especially interesting compared to the chemical route because it is possible to avoid the generation of racemic mixtures (Esteban and Ladero, 2018). The species *Lactobacillus delbrueckii* ssp. *delbrueckii* is a homofermentative producer of D-LA, due to this, Bustamante *et al.* (2020) compared different strains through batch-type fermentations. They obtained the best yields with the reference strain CECT 286 [0.86 g g^{-1}, 0.63 g (L·h)$^{-1}$], although they also achieved very close results with the strain CECT 5037 [0.84 g g^{-1}, 0.55 g/(L h)]. Using the CECT 286 strain, De la Torre *et al.* (2020) carried out OPW fermentations with growing and resting-state cells. Thanks to the deprivation of nutrients, they managed to double productivity, reaching values as high as 3.7 g/(L h).

Succinic acid (SA) is a very versatile carboxylic acid. It is one of the main chemical platforms and it is also a very promising compound for the bioeconomy era as a key compound for the generation of biodegradable polymers. Among the microorganisms capable of catalyzing the production of SA, it is worth highlighting those isolated from the rumen. One of the most promising is *Actinobacillus succinogenes* due to its ability to use CO_2 to produce high amounts of this acid Patsalou *et al.* (2020). Patsalou *et al.* (2017) carried out a preliminary study of the production of SA from citrus residues, obtaining 8.3 g L^{-1} through batch-type fermentation in the bottle. Subsequently, they increased the scale of the experiments by carrying out fermentation in batch, fed-batch, and SSF type reactors, concluding that the most suitable mode of operation was the second one, reaching 22.4 g L^{-1} of SA Patsalou *et al.* (2020).

Apart from these acids, other value-added compounds can be obtained by fermentation of citrus wastes. Corsino *et al.* (2021) took advantage of citrus wastewater to obtain acetic acid (AA) thanks to the fermentation of the microorganisms present in the waters themselves. After optimizing the C: N: P ratio, chemical oxygen demand (COD) and pH managed to produce 2.85 g L^{-1} of AA. Sepúlveda *et al.* (2020) studied the production of ellagic acid (EA), a polyphenol with anticancer activity, from OPW using *Aspergillus fumigatus* MUM 1603 as a biocatalyst. For this, they carried out a submerged fermentation process with which they reached a concentration of this compound of 18.68 mg g^{-1}. Finally, the experiments on the production of docosahexaenoic acid (DHA) by *Aurantiochytrium* sp. KRS101 should be highlighted. Park *et al.* (2018) investigated the use of OPW and several nitrogen sources to improve this process. They concluded that the addition of 1.2 g L^{-1} of sodium nitrate (NaNO$_3$) led to 0.63 g L^{-1} of DHA; in other words, an amount 2.5 times greater than with a conventional basal medium.

14.3.4 Production of Enzymes from OPWs

The production of enzymes is a key unit operation in bioprocess engineering and biotechnology. Cost-effective enzyme production is critical for the viability of enzyme applications in multiple areas as biosensing, biomedical applications, (bio)chemical technology, and across diverse industries such as detergents, paper industry, textile, food industry (Ferreira *et al.*, 2021; Tarafdar *et al.*, 2021; Fasim *et al.*, 2021). An ideal process for production involves the selection of an optimal microorganism, optimization of both conditions of cultivation, and the medium culture. Usually, the cost-effective production of pure and highly active enzymes is still a challenge (Ferreira *et al.*, 2021; Tarafdar *et al.*, 2021; Fasim *et al.*, 2021). Conditions of cultivation and the need for use of high purity substrates or specialized medium cultures increase excessively the cost of the biocatalyst (Ferreira *et al.*, 2021; Tarafdar *et al.*, 2021; Fasim *et al.*, 2021). In this regard, the use of low-cost plant-based biomasses as a sustainable substrate for enzyme production is a promising cost-effective approach (Sakhuja *et al.*, 2021). Given the composition, citrus fruit-based wastes such as OPWs are an excellent raw material to be used as a substrate for microorganism cultivation. Indeed, upgrading food waste for the production of enzymes as biotechnological products is considered very promising and of current importance (Freitas *et al.*, 2021; Sakhuja *et al.*, 2021). Although it requires suitable industrial development. Examples of application and development are shown as follows.

Recent studies involving enzyme production using agro- and food-industry wastes have primarily investigated the effect of pre-treatment to enhance enzyme production. This is because of the very heterogeneous nature of agricultural waste. The goal of the pretreatments is to make accessible nutrients of the citrus peel waste (Ravindran *et al.*, 2018; Teigiserova *et al.*, 2021b), usually for multipurpose strategy, for example, to liberate the carbohydrate fraction for the synthesis of bioethanol while the pectin fraction also can be utilized for the production of hydrolytic enzymes (Mathias *et al.*, 2019). Another important aspect is the evaluation and elimination of potentially toxic compounds for microorganism growth (e.g., phenolics derived from lignin degradation or furfurals) (Ravindran *et al.*, 2018; Teigiserova *et al.*, 2021b).

The next critical decision is the selection and strain development of the suitable microorganism (bacterial-, yeast- or fungi-based) able to grow on citrus peel derived medium and able to produce the desired protein, with suitable potential for industrial application and scale-up (Zhou *et al.*, 2019; Kc *et al.*, 2020). Microorganism and protein production biosystem (e.g., plasmid encoding the desired protein) selection can be performed by the screening of microorganisms naturally growing on the waste or/and genetic engineering (Zhou *et al.*, 2019). To perform cultivation, an efficient bioreactor set-up must be designed. There are two basic options: submerged fermentation (SF) strategies or solid-state fermentation. SF involves a liquid medium (water) that contains nutrients along with lignocellulose substrate for enzyme production, normally stirred tank reactors are used to control cultivation conditions. In solid-state fermentation the substrate not only acts as an energy and nutrients source but also as a support material. Solid-state fermentation is highly apt for citrus peel substrates and fungi cultivation, but development and operation are a bit more complex (Ravindran *et al.*, 2018).

Literature offers multiple examples of the use of several plant biomass (e.g., sugar cane bagasse, wheat straw, OPW, pineapple waste, rice bran, wheat bran, raw potato starch, raw coffee pulp, and grapes) as substrates for enzyme production. (Ravindran *et al.*, 2018; Aslam *et al.*, 2020). Different enzymes classes have been produced with citrus peel and particularly with OPW as cellulases, mannase, β-glucanase, invertase, pectinase (Athanázio-Heliodoro *et al.*, 2018; Ravindran *et al.*, 2018; Ohara *et al.*, 2018; Mathias *et al.*, 2019; de la Torre *et al.*, 2019; Prajapati *et al.*, 2021), recent examples are compiled in Table 14.4. One key family of enzymes are the lignocellulose degrading hydrolytic enzymes since they are naturally related to the enzymatic system naturally degrading OPW and therefore these enzymes are key players in integrated biorefineries

(Ahmed *et al.*, 2016; Srivastava *et al.*, 2017; 2021; Ravindran *et al.*, 2018; Marín *et al.*, 2019; de la Torre *et al.*, 2019).

Table 14.4 Recent examples of enzyme production using citrus (orange) peel waste

Enzyme Produced	Relevant Aspects of Process	References
Diverse enzymes: hydrolytic enzymes: pectinase, phytase, amylase lipases	Examples until 2016	Ravindran *et al.*, 2018; Marín *et al.*, 2019; de la Torre *et al.*, 2019
Lipase	Solid-state fermentation of OPW with different fungi to study suitable enzyme production	Athanázio-Heliodoro *et al.*, 2018
Cellulase	Solid-state fermentation of *Emericella variecolor* NS3 of OPW. Study of conditions of cultivation	Srivastava *et al.*, 2017
Pectinase, amylase, cellulase, xylanase	Sold-state fermentation of *B. licheniformis* KIBGE-IB3 from fruit waste	Aslam *et al.*, 2020
Pectinase	Identification of strain producing pectinases by using citrus pectin	Kc *et al.*, 2020
Pectinase	Isolation of strain producing pectinase using citrus peel waste and study of the cultivation conditions	Prajapati *et al.*, 2021
Pectinase	SF of *A. Niger*. Optimization of cultivation conditions: purification and characterization of the enzyme	Ahmed *et al.*, 2016
Simultaneous production of lipase, CMCase, α-amylase, and β-glucosidase	Solid-state fermentation using diverse agro-waste, either individually or combined in different formulations,	Ohara *et al.*, 2018

14.3.5 Biopolymers, Exopolysaccharides, and High Molecular Weight Active Ingredients

Other products of high interest can be obtained from OPW fermentation, such as biopolymers and high molecular weight monomers for the chemical or food industry (Table 14.5). These compounds have gained considerable attention due to their biodegradability, biocompatibility, and as substitutes for polymers based on fossil sources. Dual production of two commercially important biopolymers, poly(3-hydroxybutyrate) [P(3HB)] and poly-γ-glutamic acid (γ-PGA), in a single batch from OPWs, was studied. The production from OPWs of 20 g L^{-1} of glucose during 79 h under control of pH and saturation of air yielded 0.2 g L^{-1} of both biopolymers using *Bacillus subtilis* (Sukan, Roy, and Keshavarz, 2017). Another study demonstrates the production of bioflocculants from citrus peel wastes, with an optimal fermentation yield of 3.49 g L^{-1} of bio-flocculant from 38.8 g L^{-1} of CPW, 35 °C, and pH = 4.5 (Qi *et al.*, 2020).

Exopolysaccharides are playing an important role in the exploitation of OPW. Enhanced green production of xanthan gum has been achieved by utilizing OPW. The variables acid hydrolysis, carbon source, and temperature were optimized to obtain a xanthan production and a reduced sugar conversion of 30.2 g L^{-1} and 69.3%, respectively, with the strain of *Xanthomonas campestris* (Mohsin *et al.*, 2018). Curdlan, a linear β-1,3-glucan with several applications as a gelling agent, has been produced in concentrations of 23 g L^{-1} by using *Alcaligenes faecalis* using orange peels. Firstly, fermentation medium was obtained via saccharification and detoxification and then, curdlan fermentation was conducted in detoxified orange peel hydrolysate followed by optimization of batch culture (Mohsin *et al.*, 2019). In another research, a novel approach for the valorization of OPW for the removal of aqueous organic pollutants is presented. The orange peel is combined with silk fibroin to obtain alcogels, which are successfully converted into highly porous biocomposite foams upon supercritical CO_2 drying (Campagnolo *et al.*, 2019).

Cellulose production is being investigated from OPW due to its great versatility as a product of interest. The synthesis of cellulose nanocrystals from OPW and lychee peel has been the object of study. Cellulose nanocrystals (CNC) possess many advanced applications such as enzyme immobilization, synthesis of antimicrobial drugs, and drug carriers in therapeutic and diagnostic medicine. In the study by Thulasisingh, Kannaiyan, and Pichandi (2021), a CNC yield from OPW and lychee wastes of 23.9% and 37.2%, respectively, has been achieved. In the work by Kuo *et al.* (2019), the saccharification of OPW with cellulases and pectinases was optimized, obtaining 81 g L^{-1} of reduced sugars. In addition, OPW was used as a culture medium for *Gluconacetobacter xylinus* during the production of bacterial cellulose (BC), obtaining a 4.2–6.3 times higher yield compared to the usual Hestrin & Schramm broth.

Table 14.5 Summary of recent processes to obtain biopolymers or exopolysaccharides

Product	Process	References
Poly(3-hydroxybutyrate) (P(3HB)), Poly glutamic acid (PGA)	Fermentation with *Bacillus subtilis* + extraction with cloroform and sodium hypochlorite (NaClO)	Sukan, Roy, and Keshavarz, 2017
Bioflocculants	Fermentation with *Alcaligenes faecalis* + limonene removal	Qi *et al.*, 2020
Xanthan	Fermentation with *Xanthomonas campestris* + precipitation with ethanol	Mohsin *et al.*, 2018
Curdlan	Saccharification and detoxification + fermentation with *Alcaligenes faecalis* + precipitation	Mohsin *et al.*, 2019
Bacterial cellulose	Cellulases and pectinases + fermentation with *Gluconacetobacter xylinus*	Kuo *et al.*, 2019
Pectin, polyphenols, essential oils	Extraction by hydro distillation	Fidalgo *et al.*, 2016; Hilali *et al.*, 2019

The extraction of pectin, polyphenols, and EOs is also receiving renewed attention due to its multiple applications in the food, chemical, and medical industries. Pectin, the partial methyl esters of polygalacturonic acid and its salt, obtained by extraction in an aqueous medium, is an exceptional polymer whose large and increasing use as hydrocolloid by the food industry is rapidly expanding into other industrial sectors. Pectin and D-limonene were extracted from waste orange and lemon peel by an innovative eco-friendly process using only water as dispersing medium and microwaves as an energy source and with a yield of 15% and 0.05%, respectively (Fidalgo et al., 2016). In another study, EOs, polyphenols, and pectins were extracted from orange peels employing solar energy. It was noted from this study that TPC, total flavonoid content (TFC), hesperidin, narirutin, and pectin are still present in the peels after extraction with high preservation amounts, particularly after solar hydro distillation, this may be because a longer distillation time is required (Hilali et al., 2019).

Also, an integrated biorefinery has been developed using OPWs derived from catering services. Free sugars, EOs, and a phenolic-rich extract were initially separated from the orange peels. The phenolic-rich extract contained mainly quinic acid followed by hesperidin and hesperetin. Pectin was extracted via dilute HCl or CA treatment and sugars derived from orange peels were used in *Komagataeibacter sucrofermentans* cultures to produce BC. The proposed biorefinery led to the production of 1.5 kg EOs, 1.3 kg phenolic-rich extract, 34 kg pectin-rich extract, and 68 kg BC from 1 t of OPW (Tsouko et al., 2020).

14.4 Techno-Economic and Environmental Impact Studies

Some years ago, most biorefinery studies and techno-economic approaches were focused on using OPW as a source of value-added products throughout extractions, proposing centralizing models of production (Ortiz-Sanchez et al., 2021). Despite this fact, in recent years, these production models have been complemented with revalorizations through fermentative processes with a wide variety of products or energetic vectors (Negro et al., 2017).

Nowadays, OPW biorefineries proposals are focused on the first stages of extraction of EOs and even pectin, followed by a final revalorization of extracted solid with saccharification and later fermentation to obtain value-added products (Cristobal *et al.*, 2018).

New production models are based on regionalization and dispersion of biorefineries specialized on particular wastes, providing specific solutions and process design, depending on the waste of interest and market conditions, contextualizing the process inside the region where is going to be implemented (De Bari *et al.*, 2020).

To implement these new trends on biorefineries, certain tools are required, such as the development of *in situ* experimental procedures for adapting specifically to available wastes; these techniques must be complemented with simulation and optimization approaches to provide facilities in economic and environmental contexts, combining high profits with LCA to minimize the environmental impact (Ortiz-Sanchez *et al.*, 2021).

Classically, OPW has been mainly employed as the source of EOs to be used in fine chemistry, cosmetic or feeding industries, however, Davila *et al.* in 2015 proposed a biorefinery model where OPWs were revalorized energetically, using extracted EOs for *p*-cymene and hydrogen production and later biogas production with remaining solids (Davila *et al.*, 2015). These authors also comment on the possibility of pectin extraction, which permits to reach a more consolidated process on the proposed OPW biorefineries (Davila *et al.*, 2015).

Valorization of OPW after EO and pectin extractions has been largely studied, using a fermentative process to obtain a great number of different products, such as chemicals as D-lactic acid (de la Torre *et al.*, 2019), fumaric acid (Martin-Dominguez *et al.*, 2020), and different energetic vectors, being biogas the most widely studied (Cristobal *et al.*, 2018).

Ortiz-Sanchez *et al.* proposed in 2012 a biorefinery for revalorizing OPW as EO and pectin source, being complemented through biogas production using AD, resulting that study on conclusions spotting and advancing tendencies referenced in last years, about regionalization and contextualization of biorefineries.

Better economic viabilities were reached at low scales (under 240 tons per day) with the need of reducing thermal requirements on the process, due to steam production on EO extraction (Ortiz-Sanchez *et al.,* 2012).

Revalorization studies have been completed in 2021 by Ortiz-Sanchez *et al.* (2021), embodying contextualization of biorefineries on specific scenarios (Colombia in this case) to achieve an optimal method with specific solutions to improve economic feasibility, combining this with commonly applied strategies for design and optimization (Ortiz-Sanchez *et al.,* 2021). This study reinforces the initial idea about EOs as the most profitable product obtained by OPW, complemented with the production of biogas to achieve a higher economical profit.

Biogas production has been tried to complement energy generation, but, according to some authors (Davila *et al.,* 2015), it is not convenient, having lower profitability due to production costs, while it is not environmentally friendly, having worse results on impact studies.

Apart from these studies, a multi-scenario LCA has been performed, including classical operations for wastes management such as incineration or landfill, but adapting all these different possibilities on the context of the European Union (Southern Italy); leading one more time, biogas produced through co-digestion, as a most profitable and eco-friendly way to revalorize OPW (Negro *et al.,* 2017). Despite this advantage, eutrophication has been spotted as the main inconvenience caused by biogas revalorization, which must be considered for removal, in a way to have the lowest environmental impact process (Joglekar *et al.,* 2018; Negro *et al.,* 2017).

14.5 Conclusions

In the last decades, a huge effort has been done to discover, intensify and/or optimize operations and processes to valorize FWL and, in particular, wastes from citrus fruits, including those of oranges. This circular economy approach is within the European Green Deal, being, in fact, one of the main tools to create value out of waste. A circular economy targets the conservation of the value of products reducing waste generation, and, as such a tool, promotes sustainability. Bioeconomy search for novel processes based on biomass, or optimize those existing yet, thus substituting fossil for resources that are renewable by nature. A general tool that merges circular economy and bioeconomy is the biorefinery, a complex production system that turns biomass into most products and materials needed by Humanity. Second and third-generation biorefineries are based on LCB, FWL, and algal biomass, renewable and plentiful resources. However, their use needs step-by-step complex processing, enhancement, and discovery of classic and new upstream operations: feedstock pretreatment and enzymatic/acid depolymerization, and also of downstream thermal, catalytic, and biocatalytic processes to final products. As LCB, FWL and algal biomass are relatively recalcitrant to any physicochemical change, challenges in all mentioned operations exist to achieve economically feasible processes and products. Techno-economic integrated studies and tools such as LCA/LCC are needed for the careful design and optimization of biorefinery processes.

OPW and CPW, in general, are disposed of and used for cattle feed and energy recovery. Those applications can cope with part of the resource, although they are of low, if any, value added. Dumping creates notable problems in soil, if there is any leakage, due to the acidic nature of the wastes, so it is a solution to be avoided and, at least in EU, could be banned or only permitted under strict conditions in the following years, in the framework of an ever-reducing policy for FWL.

As a solution, CPW integrated biorefinery emerges. In the case of CPW (and OPW) step-by-step valorization means the recovery of EOs, phenolic compounds, and other low molecular weight components to avoid inhibition of the following steps while contributing to the economy of the biorefinery. Intensification promoted by microwaves, ultrasounds, cavitation, pulsed electric fields, and sudden depressurization, can dramatically shorten processing times while maintaining or increasing product quality (Senit *et al.*, 2019). Further processing via anaerobic fermentation to biogas seems a simple, yet plausible, approach (Ortiz-Sanchez *et al.*, 2021; Negro *et al.*, 2017), but new materials such as biochar, nanoparticles, BC, and exopolysaccharides are also promising. For example, obtaining bioethanol from OPW is being enhanced through metabolic engineering, aiming to use all monosaccharides and derivatives for the production of this biofuel (Jeong *et al.*, 2021). Thus, for classical biorefinery products, this approach to wholly used OPW as a resource through CBP and/or co-fermentation is a present trend, so it is the search for novel and modified enzymatic steps to obtain new products, such as mucic acid, out of GalA, the most abundant monomer of pectin, the main polysaccharide in CPW (and OPW) (Jeong *et al.*, 2021).

References

Abbas N., Safdar W., Ali S., Choudhry S., Elahj S. *Int. J. Scient. Eng. Res.*, **7** (2016), 868–872.

Afrin S. M., Acharjee A., Sit N. *J. Food Sci. Technol.*, (2021). https://doi.org/10.1007/s13197-021-05108-2.

Ahmed I., Zia M. A., Hussain M. A., *et al. Radiat. Res. Appl. Sci.*, **9** (2016), 148–154.

Aslam F, Ansari A, Aman A, *et al.*, *J. Genet. Eng. Biotechnol.*, **18** (2020), 46.

Athanázio-Heliodoro J. C., Okino-Delgado C. H., Fernandes C. J. da C., *et al. Prep. Biochem. Biotechnol.*, **48** (2018), 565–573.

Ayodele B. V., Alsaffar M. A., Mustapa S. I. *J. Clean. Prod.*, **245** (2020), 118857.

Bustamante D., Tortajada M., Ramón D., Rojas A. *Fermentation*, **6** (2020), 1.

Calabrò P. S., Fazzino F., Folino A., Scibetta S., Sidari R. *Biomass Bioenergy*, **129** (2019), 105337.

Calabrò P. S., Fazzino F., Sidari R., Zema D. A. *Renew. Energy*, **154** (2020), 849–862.

Calabrò P. S., Panzera M. F. *Thermal Sci. Eng. Progress*, **6** (2018), 355–360.

Calabrò P. S., Paone E., Komilis D. *J. Environ. Manag.*, **212** (2018), 462–468.

Calabrò P. S., Pontoni L., Porqueddu I., Greco R., Pirozzi F., Malpei F. *Waste Manag.*, **48** (2016), 440–447.

Camargo F. P., Sakamoto I. K., Bize A., Duarte I. C. S., Silva E. L., Varesche M. B. A. *Int. J. Hydrogen Energy*, **46**(11), (2021b), 7794–7809.

Camargo F. P., Sakamoto I. K., Duarte I. C. S., Silva E. L., Varesche M. B. A. *Biomass Bioenergy*, **149** (2021a), 106091.

Campagnolo L., Morselli D., Magrì D., Scarpellini A., Demirci C., Colombo M., Athanassiou A., Fragouli D. *Adv. Sustain. Sys.*, **3** (2018), 1800097.

Cano M. E., García-Martín A., Morales P. C., Wojtusik M., Santos V. E., Kovensky J., Ladero M. *Fermentation*, **6** (2020), 1–27.

Choi I. S., Lee Y. G., Khanal S. K., Park B. J., Bae H.-J. *Appl. Energy*, **140** (2015), 65–74.

Corsino S. F., Di Trapani D., Capodici M., Torregrossa M., Viviani G. *Water Resour. Ind.*, **25** (2021), 100140.

Cristóbal J., Caldeira C., Corrado S., Sala S. *Bioresour. Technol.*, **259** (2018), 244–252.

Cuéllar A. D., Webber M. E. *Environ. Sci. Technol.*, **44** (2010), 6464–6469.

Cui J., Zhao C., Zhao S., Tian G., Wang F., Li C., Wang F., Zheng J. *Food Hydrocoll.*, **108** (2020), 106079.

Dávila J. A., Rosenberg M., Cardona C. A. *Waste Biomass Valor.*, **6** (2015), 253–261.

De Bari I., Giuliano A., Petrone M. T., Stoppiello G., Fatta V., Giardi C., Razza F., Novelli A. *Processes*, **8** (2020), 1585.

De la Torre I., Martin-Dominguez V., Acedos M. G., *et al. Appl. Microbiol. Biotechnol.*, **103** (2019), 5975–5991.

De la Torre I., Ladero M., Santos V. E. *Ind. Crops Prod.*, **146** (2020), 112176.

De la Torre I., Martin-Dominguez V., Acedos M. G., Esteban J., Santos V. E., Ladero M. *Appl. Microbiol. Biotechnol.*, **103** (2019), 5975–5991.

De la Torre I., Ravelo M., Segarra S., Tortajada M., Santos V. E., Ladero M. *Bioresour. Technol.*, **245** (2017), 906–915.

Deng L. Z., Mujumdar A. S., Yang W. X., Zhang Q., Zheng Z. A., Wu M., Xiao H. W. *J. Food Process. Preserv.* **44** (2019), e14294.

Dosoky N. S., Setzer W. N. *Int. J. Mol. Sci.* **19** (2018), 1196.

Dutta A., Sahoo S., Mishra R. R., Pradhan B., Das A., Behera B. C. *Environ. Exp. Biol.*, **17** (2019), 115–122.

Ehsani A., Parsimehr H. *Chem. Record*, **20** (2020), 820–830.

Esteban J., Ladero M. *Int. J. Food Sci. Technol.*, **53**(5), (2018), 1095–1108.

FAOstat, (2021). Consulted on 4th July 2021. Available online: http://www.fao.org/faostat/es/#data/QC.

Farahmandfar R., Tirgarian B., Dehghan B., Nemati A. *J. Food Meas. Charact.* **14** (2020) 862–875.

Fasim A., More V. S., More S. S. *Curr. Opin. Biotechnol.*, **69** (2021), 68–76.

Fazzino F., Mauriello F., Paone E., Sidari R., Calabrò P. S. *Chemosphere*, **271** (2021), 129602.

Ferreira R. G., Azzoni A. R., Freitas S. *Biofuels Bioprod. Biorefin.*, **15** (2021), 85–99.

Fidalgo A., Ciriminna R., Carnaroglio D., Tamburino A., Cravotto G., Grillo G., Ilharco L. M., Pagliaro M. *ACS Sustain. Chem. Eng.*, **4** (2016), 2243–2251.

Fiori da Silva G., Leite Mathias S., Junior de Menezes A., Pereira Vicente J. G., Palladino Delforno T., Amancio Varesche M. B., Silveira Duarte I. C. *Curr. Microbiol.*, **77** (2020), 4053–4062.

Freitas L. C., Barbosa J. R., da Costa A. L. C., et al. *Resour. Conserv. Recycl.*, **169** (2021), 105466.

Garcia-Amezquita L. E., Tejada-Ortigoza V., Pérez-Carrillo E., Serna-Saldívar S. O., Campanella O. H., Welti-Chanes J. *LWT*, **111** (2019), 673–681.

Gavahian M., Chu Y. H., Khaneghah A. M. *Int. J. Food Sci. Technol.* **54** (2019) 925–932.

Han L., Zhang J., Cao X. *Food Sci. Nutr.*, **9** (2021), 1061–1069.

Heydari M., Rostami O., Mohammadi R., Banavi P., Farhoodi M., Sarlak Z., Rouhi M. *J. Food Process. Preserv.* **e15585** (2021).

Hilali S., Fabiano-Tixier A.-S., Ruiz K., Hejjaj A., Ait Nouh F., Idlimam A., Bily A., Mandi L., Chemat F. *ACS Sustain. Chem. Eng.*, **7** (2019), 11815–11822.

Ilhak M. I., Tangoz S., Akansu S. O., Kahraman N. Alternative fuels for internal combustion engines, in *The Future of Internal Combustion* Engines (Carlucci A. P., ed), IntechOpen, 2019.

International Energy Association. Outlook for biogas and biomethane: prospects for organic growth. World Energy Outlook Special Report (2021), Accessed on January 2021: https://www.iea.org/reports/outlook-for-biogas-and-biomethane-prospects-for-organic-growth/an-introduction-to-biogas-and-biomethane.

Jeong D., Park H., Jang B. K., Ju Y., Shin M. H., Oh E. J., Lee E. J., Kim S. R. *Bioresour. Technol.*, **323** (2021), 124603.

Jeong D., Ye S., Park H., Kim S. R. *Bioresour. Technol.* **265** (2020), 122259.

Jiménez-Castro M. P., Buller L. S., Zoffreo A., Timko M. T., Forster-Carneiro T. *J. Environ. Chem. Eng.*, **8**(4), (2020), 104035.

Joglekar S. N., Pathak P. D., Mandavgane S. A., Kulkarni B. D. *Environ. Sci. Pollut. Res.*, **26** (2019), 34713–34722.

Kc S., Upadhyaya J., Joshi D. R., et al. *Fermentation*, **6** (2020), 59.

Kieliszek M., Piwowarek K., Kot A. M., Pobiega K. *Open Life Sci.*, **15** (2020), 787–796.

Kumar B., Bhardwaj N., Agrawal K., Chaturvedi V., Verma P. *Fuel Process. Technol.*, **199** (2020), 106204.

Kuo C.-H., Huang C.-Y., Shieh C.-J., David Wang H.-M., Tseng C.-Y. *Waste Biomass Valor.*, **10** (2019), 85–93.

Lukitawesa B., Eryildiz A., Mahboubi R., Millati M., Taherzadeh M. J. *Innov. Food Sci. Emerging Technol.*, **67** (2021), 102545.

Magare M. E., Sahu N., Kanade G. S., Chanotiya C. S., Thul S. T. *Waste Biomass Valor.* **11**(1), (2020), 165–172.

Mahato N., Sharma K., Sinha M., Dhyani A., Pathak B., Jang H., Park S., Pashikanti S., Cho S. *Processes*, **9** (2021), 220.

Mak T. M., Xiong X., Tsang D. C., Iris K. M., Poon C. S. *Bioresour. Technol.*, **297** (2020) 122497.

Mankar A. R., Pandey A., Modak A., Pant K. K. *Bioresour. Technol.* **334** (2021), 125235.

Mariana O.-S., Camilo S.-T. J., Ariel C.-A. C. *Bioresour. Technol.*, **325** (2021), 124682.

Marín M., Sánchez A., Artola A. *J. Clean. Prod.*, **209** (2019), 937–946.

Martin M. A., Fernandez R., Gutierrez M. C., Siles J. A. *Process Saf. Environ. Protec.*, **117** (2018), 245–253.

Martín M. A., Fernández R., Serrano A., Siles J. A. *Waste Manag.*, **33** (7), (2013), 1633–1639.

Martin-Dominguez V., Bouzas-Santiso L., Martinez-Peinado N., Santos V. E., Ladero M., *Processes*, **8** (2020), 108.

Mathias D. J., Kumar S., Rangarajan V. *Biocatal. Agric. Biotechnol.*, **20** (2019), 101259.

Mekonnen M. M., Gerbens-Leenes W. *Water*, **12** (2020), 2696.

Meneguzzo F., Brunetti C., Fidalgo A., Ciriminna R., Delisi R., Albanese L., Zabini F., Gori A., Mohsin A., Sun J., Khan I. M., Hang H., Tariq M., Tian X., Ahmed W., Niazi S., Zhuang Y., Chu J., Mohsin M. Z., ur-Rehman S., Guo M. *Carbohydr. Pol.*, **205** (2019), 626–635.

Mohsin A., Zhang K., Hu J., ur-Rehman S., Tariq M., Qamar Zaman W., Khan I. M., Zhuang Y., Guo M. *Carbohydr. Pol.*, **181** (2019), 793–800.

Munesue Y., Masui T., Fushima T. *Environ. Econ. Policy Stud.*, **17** (2015), 43–77.

Nascimento L. B. S., Carlo A., Ferrini F., Ilharco L. M., Pagliaro M. *Processes*, **581** (2019), 1–24.

Negro V., Ruggeri B., Fino D., Tonini D. *Resour. Conser. Recycling*, **127** (2017), 148–158.

Oberoi H. S., Vadlani P. V., Madl R. L., Saida L., Abeykoon J. P. *J. Agric. Food Chem.*, **58** (2010), 3422–3429.

Ohara A., dos Santos J. G., Angelotti J. A. F., et al. *Food Sci. Technol.*, **38** (2018), 131–137.

Onwudea D. I., Hashim N., Janius R., Abdan K., Chenc G., Oladejo A. O. *Innov. Food Sci. Emerg. Technol.*, **43** (2017) 223–238.

Ortiz-Sanchez M., Solarte-Toro J. C., Cardona-Alzate C. A. *Bioresour. Technol.*, **325** (2021), 124682.

Ortiz-Sanchez M., Solarte-Toro J. C., Orrego-Alzate C. E., Acosta-Medina C. D., Cardona-Alzate C. A. *Biomass Conv. Bioref.*, **11** (2021), 645–659.

Ozturk B., Parkinson C., Gonzalez-Miquel M. *Sep. Purif. Technol.*, **206** (2018), 1–13.

Ozturk B., Winterburn J., Gonzalez-Miquel M. *Biochem. Eng. J.*, **151** (2019), 107298.

Panić M., Andlar M., Tišma M., Rezić T., Šibalić D., Bubalo M. C., Redovniković I. R. *Waste Manage.*, **120** (2021), 340–350.

Park W. K., Moon M., Shin S. E., Cho J. M., Suh W. I., Chang Y. K., Lee B. *Algal Res.*, **29** (2018), 71–79.

Patsalou M., Menikea K. K., Makri E., Vasquez M. I., Drouza C., Koutinas M. *J. Clean. Prod.*, **166** (2017), 706–716.

Patsalou M., Chrysargyris A., Tzortzakis N., Koutinas M. *Waste Manag.*, **113** (2020), 469–477.

Patsalou M., Samanides C. G., Protopapa E., Stavrinou S., Vyrides I., Koutinas M. *Molecules*, **24** (2019), 2451.

Pocan P., Bahcegul E., Oztop M. H., Hamamci H., *Waste and Biomass Valor.*, **9** (2018), 929–937.

Prajapati J., Dudhagara P., Patel K. *Biocatal. Agric. Biotechnol.*, **35** (2021), 102063.

Protzko R. J., Latimer L. N., Martinho Z., De Reus E., Seibert T., Benz J. P., Dueber J. E. *Nat. Commun.*, **9** (2018), 1–10.

Qi X., Zheng Y., Tang N., Zhou J., Sun S. *Sci. Total Environ.*, **715** (2020), 136885.

Ravindran R., Hassan S., Williams G., Jaiswal A. *Bioengineering*, **5** (2018), 93.

Ruiz B., de Benito A., Rivera J. D., Flotats X. *Waste Manag. Res.* **34** (12), (2016), 1249–1257.

Ruiz B., Flotats X., *Biochem. Eng. J.*, **109** (2016), 9–18.

Sakar P., Mukherjee M., Goswami G., Das D. *J. Ind. Microbiol. Biotechnol.*, **47** (2020), 329–341.

Sakhuja D., Ghai H., Rathour R. K., et al. *Biotech*, **11** (2021), 280.

Satari B., Palhed J., Karimi K., Lundin M. *Bioresources*, **12** (2017), 1706–1722.

Senit J. J., Velasco D., Gomez Manrique A., Sanchez-Barba M., Toledo J. M., Santos V. E., Garcia-Ochoa F., Yustos P., Ladero M. *Ind. Crops Prod.*, **134** (2019), 370–381.

Sepúlveda L., Laredo-Alcalá E., Buenrostro-Figueroa J. J., Ascacio-Valdés J. A., Genisheva Z., Aguilar C., Teixeira J. *Electronic J. Biotechnol.*, **43** (2020), 1–7.

Singh B., Singh J. P., Kaur A., Singh N. *Food Res. Int.* **132** (2020), 109114.

Srivastava N., Srivastava M., Alhazmi A., *et al. Environ. Pollut.*, **287** (2021), 117370.

Srivastava N., Srivastava M., Manikanta A., *et al. Appl. Biochem. Biotechnol.*, **183** (2017), 601–612.

Su D. L., Li P. J., Quek S. Y., Huang Z. Q., Yuan Y. J., Li G. Y., Shan Y. *Food Chem.*, **286** (2019), 1–7.

Sukan A., Roy I., Keshavarz T. *J. Chem. Technol. Biotechnol.*, **92** (2017), 1548–1557.

Taghizadeh-Alisaraei A., Hosseini S. H., Ghobadian B., Motevali A. *Renew. Sustainable Energy Rev.,* **69** (2017), 1100–1112.

Tarafdar A., Sirohi R., Gaur V. K., *et al. Bioresour. Technol.,* **326** (2021), 124771.

Teigiserova D. A., Bourgine J., Thomsen M. *Sustain. Prod. Consum.,* **27** (2021a), 845–857.

Teigiserova D. A., Hamelin L., Thomsen M. *Resour. Conserv. Recycl.,* **149** (2019), 413–426.

Teigiserova D. A., Tiruta-Barna L., Ahmadi A., *et al. J. Environ. Manag.,* **280** (2021b), 111832.

Thulasisingh A., Kannaiyan S., Pichandi K. *Biomass Conv. Bioref.*, **10** (2021), 1–14.

Tomita H., Okazaki F., Tamaru Y. *AMB Expr.* **9** (2019), 1.

Tsouko E., Maina S., Ladakis D., Kookos I. K., Koutinas A. *Renew. Energy*, **160** (2020), 944–954.

Tsuru C., Umada A., Noma S., Demura M., Hayashi N. *Food Bioproc. Tech.*, **14** (2021), 1341–1348.

United Nations Sustainable Development Goals, (2021). Consulted on 4th July 2021. https://www.un.org/sustainabledevelopment/sustainable-development-goals/.

Velasco D., Senit J. J., De La Torre I., Santos T. M., Yustos P., Santos V. E., Ladero M. *Fermentation*, **3**(3), (2017), 37.

Vergara P., García-Ochoa F., Ladero M., Gutiérrez S., Villar J. C. *Bioresour. Technol.*, **280** (2019), 396–403.

Yang P., Wu Y. W., Zheng Z., Cao L., Zhu X., Um D., Jiang S. *Front. Microbiol.*, **9** (2018), 2436.

Zerva I., Remmas N., Ntougias S. *Water*, **11** (2019), 274.

Zhou Y.-M., Chen Y.-P., Guo J.-S., *et al. J. Clean Prod.*, **213** (2019), 384–392.

Index

AA *see* auxiliary activity
acetyl xylan esterase (AXE) 427,
    431, 434, 435
acid 99, 103, 310, 449, 451, 455,
    475–477, 481, 482, 486, 492,
    498
  abscisic 171, 285, 286
  acetic 446, 450, 454, 455, 488,
    495, 496, 498
  alkanoic 253, 254
  3-amino-5-nitrosalicylic 443
  ascorbic 163–165, 168, 173,
    176, 439
  aspartic 97
  caprylic 26, 28
  carboxylic 455, 475, 496, 498
  catalytic 432
  chicoric 143
  cinnamic 435
  coumaric 435
  cysteic 354
  2,4-dichlorophenoxyacetic 253
  3,5-dinitrosalicylic 443
  3,6-dichloro-2-methoxy benzoic
    257
  3,6-dichlorosalicylic 258
  docosahexaenoic 499
  ellagic 498
  fatty 6, 26, 29, 167, 169, 171,
    228, 230, 234, 236, 355
  ferulic 435
  fumaric 505
  furanic 454
  galactaric 483
  galacturonic 342, 431, 432, 480,
    484
  gallic 439
  glucuronic 435
  glutamic 502
  hydroxybenzoic 479
  indole-3-acetic 228
  indole-3-butyric 230
  inorganic 481
  jasmonic 60, 225, 228, 231, 236
  lactic 485, 492, 495, 505
  linolenic 231
  meso-galactaric 486
  methyl caffeic 435
  methyl sinapic 435
  mucic 508
  nucleic 75, 77, 117, 122, 137,
    167, 170, 349
  organic 121, 384, 447, 484, 487,
    496
  pectic 342, 343
  phosphoric 351, 353
  phytic 119, 128, 147
  polygalacturonic 504
  polylactic 498
  quinic 504
  ribonucleic 119
  salicylic 60, 285, 286
  sulfenic 162
  sulfuric 451, 481
  tricarboxylic 228
  uric 169, 233
  uronic 432, 446, 450
  vanillic 341
adenosine diphosphate (ADP) 119,
    132, 141, 142, 351
adenosine triphosphate (ATP) 76,
    119, 123, 130, 132, 142, 147,
    228, 351
ADP *see* adenosine diphosphate
agroecosystem 336, 355, 356
Alcaligenes faecalis 502, 503

Index

alcohol 8, 11, 30, 68, 351, 457, 486–488
alkaloid 163, 164, 173
AlkB domain *see* alkylation B domain
alkylation B domain (AlkB domain) 272, 275, 284, 285, 288
AMF *see* Arbuscular mycorrhizal fungi
APX *see* ascorbate peroxidase
Arabidopsis thaliana (*A. thaliana*) 40, 41, 44, 48–50, 78–80, 89, 90, 97, 100–102, 109, 110, 122–128, 132–138, 140–143, 179–182, 184–189, 192–194, 196–198, 200, 201
Arbuscular mycorrhizal fungi (AMF) 349, 355
Arepavirus 270, 272
artificial intelligence 23, 31
aryloxyphenoxy-propionate (FOP) 253, 255
ascorbate peroxidase (APX) 141, 164, 174–176, 206, 207, 232, 233
Aspergillus niger 52, 395, 426, 486, 496
Aspergillus oryzae 436
assays 251, 278, 443, 444
 APase activity 138
 biochemical 251
 cellulase activity 443
 filter paper 445
 immobilization 17
 sensitive screening 20
 spectrophotometric 443
A. thaliana see *Arabidopsis thaliana*
ATP *see* adenosine triphosphate
AtPAP10 93, 128, 135, 138, 141, 142, 146, 147
AtPAP12 123, 128, 135, 138, 139, 141–143, 145, 146
AtPAP15 104, 127, 128, 142, 146

AtPAP17 96, 123, 135, 136, 141, 144–146
AtPAP23 133, 135, 136, 144
AtPAP26 93–95, 123, 128, 134, 138–147
autoinhibition 276, 278, 286, 287
auxiliary activity (AA) 421, 422, 436, 483, 498
AXE *see* acetyl xylan esterase

Bacillus subtilis 502, 503
bacteria 6, 9, 41, 353, 355, 382–384, 390–393, 395–397, 401, 403, 404, 420–422, 441, 457, 458, 486, 488
 anaerobic 392
 cellulolytic 441
 lactic acid 495
 potato 60
 thermophilic 441, 442
bacterial cellulose (BC) 441, 503, 504, 507
BC *see* bacterial cellulose
benzene 369, 372, 374
Bevemovirus 270, 272, 275
BGL *see* β-glucosidase
binding 108, 254, 280, 288, 316, 426, 429, 433, 440, 442
 cation 51
 factor 189
 metal-ion 98
 non-productive 455
 substrate 254
bioaugmentation 383, 391, 395
biocatalyst 17, 23, 404, 481, 484, 498, 499
biochar 388, 475, 507
biochemical characterization 7, 17, 19, 24, 232
biodegradation 15, 378, 383, 394, 397, 400, 403, 415, 420, 421
biodiesel 8–12, 16, 23, 236
biodiversity 6, 311, 447

bioethanol 448, 481, 484, 487, 500, 507
bioflocculant 502
biofuel 23, 414, 447, 507
biogas 448, 484, 485, 487–489, 492, 494, 495, 505–507
biohydrogen 487–489
biomass 139, 142, 368, 369, 375, 376, 386, 387, 389, 414–417, 419, 445, 446, 450, 451, 453, 471, 474–478, 506, 507
  algal 475, 507
  fungal 401
  gramineous 419
  lignocellulosic 413, 415, 416, 421, 434, 437, 445, 448, 456, 474–476, 481, 484
  maize 389, 403
  microbial 306, 309, 316, 325, 403
  nitrogen-related 313
  plant-based 499
  spinach 386
  terrestrial 414
  vegetal 488
biomethane 487, 489, 492
biomolecule 108, 117, 119, 163, 478
biopolymer 477, 502, 503
biorefineries 446, 459, 475, 484, 485, 504–507
  first-generation 475
  food waste 474
  industrial 459
  integrated 471, 500, 504, 507
  lignocellulose-processing 447
  third-generation 507
bioremediation 16, 367, 368, 370–404
biostimulation 383, 402
biosynthesis 60, 130, 225, 228, 231, 235, 236, 249, 260
biota 367, 374, 380, 381, 383
Brachypodium sylvaticum 86, 87

Brambyvirus 270, 272, 274, 276, 278, 279, 285, 288
Brassica napus 142, 386
buprofezin 322–325
Bymovirus 270, 272, 275

Calvin–Benson cycle 229
carbohydrate-binding module (CBM) 420–423, 425, 426, 429, 430, 432, 435, 439, 440, 442
carbohydrates 229, 231, 384, 422, 433, 439, 443, 455, 488
carboxymethylcellulose (CMC) 426, 444
carotene 165, 167, 174
carotenoids 164, 165, 173, 174
cassava brown streak virus (CBSV) 271, 276, 285
CAT *see* catalase
catalase (CAT) 141, 164, 174–176, 200, 207, 226, 229, 232–234, 316–318
catalysis 77, 160, 176, 178, 195, 259, 316, 427, 433, 450
catalytic activity 77, 98, 100, 101, 104, 106, 124, 186, 421, 426, 427, 431, 439
CAZy database 422, 426, 432, 434, 436, 439
CBH *see* cellobiohydrolase
CBM *see* carbohydrate-binding module
CBP *see* consolidated bioprocessing
CBSV *see* cassava brown streak virus
CCS *see* copper chaperone for SOD
Celavirus 270, 272, 275
cell 7, 18, 19, 138, 139, 145, 147, 162, 164, 169, 171, 172, 192, 195, 203, 204, 306–309, 312
cell membrane 96, 119, 139, 168, 169, 200, 339, 486

cellobiohydrolase (CBH) 422, 423, 426, 428, 429, 441, 443–445
cellobiose 339, 422, 429, 441, 445, 457
cellular compartment 167, 168, 173–175, 177, 179, 180, 185, 187, 201–204, 226
cellular function 161, 170, 172, 173, 175, 181, 204
cellulase 324, 338, 339, 420, 422, 426, 429, 431, 434, 435, 440, 445, 483, 500, 501, 503
  bacterial 425, 440
  extracellular 339
cellulose 48, 337, 339, 341, 413–416, 419–421, 423, 429, 434–437, 439, 440, 443, 444, 446, 448–455, 480, 481, 483
  amorphous 440, 444
  bacterial 503
  crystalline 440, 442, 475
  degradation of 420, 421, 437, 441, 442
  hydroxymethyl 444
  microcrystalline 426, 443
  saccharification of 429, 455
  susceptibility of 451, 452
  trinitrophenyl-carboxymethyl 444
cellulose chains 339, 416, 422, 423, 428, 429, 437
cellulosomes 442
chemical oxygen demand (COD) 489, 492, 497, 498
chickpea 59–67, 69, 90, 128, 133
chitin 140, 345, 346, 436, 437, 439, 440
chitinase 61, 337, 345
chlorophyll 174, 247, 248
chloroplast 125, 129, 131, 146, 163–166, 168–171, 173, 175, 177, 179–181, 185–187, 226, 228, 229, 257, 259, 260

chromosome 18, 79, 93, 95, 98, 100, 181
chrysene 372, 374, 379, 380, 394, 401
circadian rhythm 189, 191
cistron 272, 276, 279, 280, 289
citrus fruit 472, 474, 480, 506
citrus peel 477, 478, 480, 499, 500
clay 306, 309, 316, 377
cleavage 19, 97, 191, 276, 281, 353, 424, 431–433, 436
  bond 433, 438
  hydrolytic 353
  random 429
clone 7, 17–20, 23–25, 30, 31
  chimeric 280
  positive 20
  triolein-hydrolyzing 25
  viral 276, 286
Clostridium thermocellum (*C. thermocellum*) 441, 442
CMC *see* carboxymethylcellulose
coat protein (CP) 100, 272, 277, 289
COD *see* chemical oxygen demand
combustion 369, 375–377, 487
compound 23, 24, 30, 111, 118, 121, 249, 253, 368, 373, 374, 380, 496, 502
  aromatic-derived 477
  bioactive 453
  carcinogenic 373–375, 380
  chemical 304, 309, 315
  chiral 5, 30
  inhibitory 451, 495
  inorganic 77, 118, 342
  lipid 371
  lipophilic 368
  organophosphorus 350
  PAH 369, 370, 374, 384, 387, 391, 396
  pectic 53
  pectin-derived 50
  pharmaceutical 23

phenolic 69, 174, 447, 507
synthetic auxin herbicide 254
toxic 380, 396, 500
value-added 498
consolidated bioprocessing (CBP) 456, 458, 459, 476, 508
constitutive splicing (CS) 192, 193, 209
copper chaperone for SOD (CCS) 192, 195–198, 202
cosmetics 477, 505
CP *see* coat protein
CPW 474–476, 485–486, 502, 507, 508
cropping system 252, 260, 263, 310
crop 118–120, 146, 246, 252, 288, 290, 304, 310, 355, 356, 381, 383
   citrus 472
   glufosinate tolerant 246
   herbaceous energy 415
   phosphorous-use-efficient 78
   transgenic 141
crosstalk 171, 188, 198
CS *see* constitutive splicing
C. thermocellum see *Clostridium thermocellum*
cucumber vein yellowing virus (CVYV) 276, 278, 280, 285, 286
cultivation 5, 368, 402, 472, 499–501
CuZn SOD 160, 177, 178, 180, 185–187, 191, 192, 194–198, 203–207
CVYV *see* cucumber vein yellowing virus
cyanobacteria 177, 179
cypermethrin 319, 320
cysteine 165, 178, 200, 232, 354
cytoplasm 137–139, 145, 164, 180, 181, 308

cytosol 120, 160, 163, 166, 168, 169, 177, 185, 187, 226

degree of polymerization (DP) 416, 444, 452
dehydroascorbate (DHA) 175, 176, 499
dehydrogenase 163, 165, 305, 306, 310, 316, 317, 337
   activity of 309, 317
   lactone 169, 209
   malate 230, 231, 234
deoxyribonucleic acid (DNA) 7, 17, 18, 22, 108, 121, 122, 132, 165, 167, 170, 171, 349, 374, 380
dephosphorylation 90, 146
depolymerization 337, 342, 429, 449, 451
detergent 7, 23, 499
detoxification 502, 503
DHA *see* dehydroascorbate
dicamba monooxygenase (DMO) 258–260
dicots 94–96, 98, 106, 110, 182, 189, 201
disaccharides 420, 454
disease 60, 61, 270, 355
   bacterial leaf spot 61
   bacterial speck 61
   neurological 381
   reproductive 380
   soft rot 61
   viral 50, 290
   wilt 59
DMO *see* dicamba monooxygenase
DNA *see* deoxyribonucleic acid
domain 22, 26, 41–43, 91, 94–96, 101, 122, 124, 195–197, 272, 275
   amino-terminal cytochrome 436
   carboxy-terminal dehydrogenase 436
   catalytic 97, 275, 424, 430

cellulose-binding 439
chaperone 196
cohesin 442
core 124
flavoprotein 436
metallophosphatase 96
metallophosphoesterase 96
prokaryotic lipoprotein 95
protease 272, 273, 275, 277, 279, 286
proteolytic 278
serine peptidase 271
terminal 123
trans-membrane 96
DP *see* degree of polymerization
drought 160, 167, 172, 182, 185, 194, 204–207, 231, 309, 310

earthworm 7, 355, 384
EC *see* emerging contaminants
E. coli see *Escherichia coli*
ecosystem 304, 306, 311, 336, 356
effluent 320, 322
    industrial 325
    paper mills 320
    tanning 319
    urban waste storage depot 319
    wastewater treatment plant 319
EG *see* endoglucanase
electron paramagnetic resonance (EPR) 232
electron transport chain (ETC) 168
emerging contaminants (EC) 5, 60, 77, 100, 102, 123, 125, 126, 174, 175, 318, 421, 422, 425, 427–429, 431, 432, 434, 436
enantioselectivity 20, 23, 27, 30
encoding genes 49, 93–95, 98, 102, 110, 139, 443
endoglucanase (EG) 422, 423, 425–429, 431, 444, 445
endoplasmic reticulum 166, 168, 170, 209

endosymbiosis 106, 160, 162, 179, 201
environment 311, 312, 314, 318, 367, 368, 370, 371, 374–377, 380, 381, 383, 385, 391, 414, 474, 479
    aerobic 309
    aquatic 253
    aqueous 421
    biotic 304
    cellular metabolic 168
    forest 312
    industrial 459
    natural 127, 304
    physiological 208
    polluted 315
    terrestrial 414
    unnatural 7
    volcanic 5
enzymatic saccharification 419, 421, 422, 430, 446, 448, 451–456, 459, 481, 483
enzyme 4–7, 18, 19, 21–24, 77, 78, 125–128, 173–175, 245–247, 251–257, 303–310, 315–317, 322–325, 335–339, 347–351, 413–416, 420–428, 430, 431, 433–437, 439–443, 483, 484, 499–501
    accessory 433, 434
    active 4, 20, 499
    adaptive 307
    ancillary 431
    antioxidant 174, 185
    arylsulphatase 310
    bacterial 426, 441
    biotechnological 248
    bypass 121
    carbohydrate-degrading 455
    cellulolytic 422, 425, 428, 434, 441, 454, 455, 459
    cellulose-degrading 441
    commercial 31, 126
    conserved 125

copper-containing 175
cytosolic 187
deactivation 260
demethylase 258
depolymerizing 476
dioxygenase 245, 247, 249, 253–256, 260–262, 392
downstream 260
dual-targeted 139
endo-acting 422
exo-acting 422
extracellular 307, 312, 313, 339, 342, 349, 395
flavoprotein oxidoreductase 175
functional 19
fungal 396, 420, 422–439, 484
hemicellulose-degrading 441
homologous 89
housekeeping 307
hydrolytic 127, 434, 454, 500, 501
inducible 307
intracellular 344
isolating 24
lignocellulolytic 479
lipolytic 4–7, 19, 21–23, 31
metagenomic 23, 31
microbial PPO 248
mitochondrial 183
monomeric 96
multifunctional 175, 422, 442
multimodular 440
native 256
nuclear-encoded 60
paralogous 96
peroxidase 400
phosphatase 79, 345, 348, 349
phosphinothricin acetyltransferase 246
phosphoamidase 353
phosphodiesterase 350
phosphotriesterase 350
plant 384
polyphosphatases 351
polysaccharide-hydrolyzing 307
prokaryotic 104
prokaryotic SAP 106, 127
single PAP 78
soil 303–320, 322–326, 335, 336
soil proteolytic 345
tetrameric 174
vacuolar 95
versatile 5
EO *see* essential oil
EPR *see* electron paramagnetic resonance
Escherichia coli (*E. coli*) 18, 19, 24, 25, 106, 107, 288, 442, 486, 495, 496
essential oil (EO) 472, 474, 476–479, 488, 491, 494–496, 503–507
esterase 4–6, 16, 23, 24, 30, 434–436, 454
　acetyl 426, 434
　acetyl mannan 431
　acetyl xylan 427
　carbohydrate 41, 421, 434
　coumaroyl 435
　ferulic acid 431
　N-methyl-glucuronoyl methyl 434, 435
　pectin acetyl 434
　pectin methyl 52, 342
ester 5, 6, 8, 12, 14, 15, 351, 432, 435
　methyl 504
　nitrophenyl 16
　organic sulfate 310
　phosphoric 146
ETC *see* electron transport chain
ethanol 10, 25, 26, 29, 30, 447, 455, 457, 458, 480, 485, 486, 494, 495, 503
ethanol production 458, 485, 486
eukaryote 102, 124, 125, 185, 188, 192, 196, 208, 262

evolution 78, 79, 108, 159–162, 178, 179, 185, 201, 270, 290, 472
   convergent 76, 177
   divergent 76, 111
exoglucanase 422, 431
exons 76, 78, 80–88, 109, 192, 193, 209
exopolysaccharides 502, 503, 507
expression 18–21, 25, 98, 100, 133, 134, 136, 138, 160, 188–191, 194, 288, 289, 434, 486
   cellulase 485
   differential 191
   heterologous 20, 24, 142, 486
   heterologous peptide 289
   protein 18
   transgenic 288
expression level 25, 49, 124, 136, 137, 140, 251
expression pattern 46, 118, 133–135, 140, 141, 143–145, 194
extract 64, 479, 493
   crude 27
   pectin-rich 504
   phenolic-rich 504
   root and shoot 64, 66, 67
   whole-cell 143
extraction 7, 419, 478–480, 489, 494, 503, 504
   classical 479
   microwave-assisted 479
   solid-liquid 488
   ultrasound-assisted 479

FAE *see* ferulic acid esterase
FCM method 145
feedstock 445, 450, 475, 484, 485, 488
   lignin-rich 453
   lignocellulosic 445, 447, 451, 454
   moist 450
   pretreated 457
Fenton's reagent 382, 492, 495
fermentation 455–458, 475, 476, 484–486, 490, 498, 503, 505
   anaerobic 507
   batch 496
   batch-type 498
   curdlan 502
   optimal 502
   solid-state 500, 501
   spontaneous 496
   submerged 497, 500
   surface culture 496
ferredoxin 258–260
fertility 335, 336
fertilization 148, 314, 319
fertilizer 313, 318, 355, 356
   ammonia-based nitrogen 309, 315
   natural 475
   nitrogen-based 313
   Pi-containing 146
ferulic acid esterase (FAE) 431, 434, 435
feruloyl 434, 435
Fe SOD 177–184, 187, 189, 194, 198, 205, 206
filter paper unit (FPU) 443, 482
flavonoids 163–165, 167, 173, 174, 472
flower 40, 95, 120, 123, 133, 144, 146, 147, 225
fluoranthene 372–374, 379, 380, 400, 401, 403
fluorene 372, 373, 400, 402
fluorescent protein (FP) 100, 289
fly ash 377, 379, 388, 390
Foc *see Fusarium oxysporum* f.sp. *ciceris*
foldase 24, 25, 27, 30
food chain 325, 379, 384
food industry 27, 475, 477, 483, 499, 502, 504

food waste (FW) 471, 472, 474, 475, 487, 499
food waste and food losses (FWL) 472, 474, 475, 506, 507
FOP *see* aryloxyphenoxy-propionate
FOP herbicides 253, 256, 257
fossil resources 413, 414, 445, 474, 475
FP *see* fluorescent protein
FPU *see* filter paper unit
Francisella tularensis 106, 107
fructose 314, 342, 481, 482
fruit ripening 48, 77, 225, 227, 231, 234
fuel 31, 245, 413, 447, 475, 484, 485
fungal infection 68, 123, 140
fungi 40, 41, 61, 62, 341, 342, 353, 355, 382, 383, 387, 395–398, 401, 403, 404, 420, 422, 436, 437, 486, 494
  anaerobic 421
  brown-rot 420
  edible 453
  free-living 420
  ligninolytic 367, 395–397, 401, 402
  lignocellulose-degrading 436
  mycorrhizal 387
  necrotrophic 50, 52
  non-ligninolytic 395, 397
  pathogenic 235
  thermophilic filamentous 441
  white-rot 341, 397, 403
fungicides 319, 321, 373
Fusarium oxysporum f.sp. *ciceris* (Foc) 59–65, 67–69
FW *see* food waste
FWL *see* food waste and food losses

galactolipids 119, 121, 126, 139
galactomannan 426, 430

galactose 416, 418, 480–482, 486
galactosidases 431, 433
gel 52, 53, 60, 64, 66–68
gene 18, 20–22, 40, 41, 45, 48, 49, 78, 79, 98, 100, 102, 122, 124, 125, 133–136, 140–145, 182, 188, 192, 203, 204, 246, 261
  annotated 122
  bacterial 393
  cellulase 442
  cloned 21
  fungal-induced 140
  intron-containing 192
  intron-containing plant 193
  methanol-inducible 51
  plant disease resistance 110
  scaffoldin 442
  stress-responsive 173, 201
gene duplication 79, 93, 98, 111
gene expression 20, 45, 47, 80, 108, 135, 136, 145, 182, 188, 191, 289
genetically modified organism (GMO) 246, 394, 459
genome 6, 78, 79, 88, 122, 125, 187, 201, 285
  annotated 76
  nuclear 179, 259, 260
  potyvirid 272
  single-stranded RNA 272
genome duplication 201, 203, 208
genotype 61, 63, 65, 68
  antisense 60
  resistant 59–61, 64, 68
  susceptible 59–61, 63, 64, 68, 69
germination 46, 48, 95, 120, 130, 146
  pollen 128
  seed 48, 49, 77, 225, 227, 229, 231, 234, 387
GH *see* glycoside hydrolase
glucose 314, 337–339, 342, 416, 418, 429, 444–446, 448, 457, 481, 482, 486

β-glucosidase (BGL) 305, 307, 310, 338, 339, 422, 423, 425–427, 429, 430, 443–445
glutathione (GSH) 163–165, 173, 175, 176, 233, 288
glycerol 9, 475, 489, 494
glycoside hydrolase (GH) 421, 422, 424, 425, 432, 437, 442
glycosylation 18, 135, 198, 442
GMO *see* genetically modified organism
GOE *see* Great Oxygenation Event
Golgi membrane 129, 146
Great Oxygenation Event (GOE) 159, 161
GSH *see* glutathione
GSNO *see* S-nitrosoglutathione

HAD-related phosphatase (HRP) 97, 98, 108, 110, 124, 139
HAP *see* histidine acid phosphatase
HC-pro *see* helper component proteinase
heavy metal 185, 204, 309, 317, 344, 369, 389, 394, 475
helper component proteinase (HC-pro) 272, 276, 278, 279, 287, 288, 290
hemicellulase 339, 341, 422, 426, 483
hemicelluloses 40, 341, 414–416, 418–421, 430, 431, 434, 440, 446, 448–454, 474, 475, 480
 hardwood 416
 hydrolysis of 449, 451
 partial solubilization of 449, 452
 softwood 416
 solubilization of 447, 451, 452
 solubilized 446
herbicide 245–249, 253, 256–258, 260, 262, 263, 309, 319–321
herbicide tolerance traits 245–253, 259–263
herbivores 60, 67, 124, 421

hexoses 416, 446, 457, 476
high-throughput method (HT method) 17, 20, 31, 53, 192, 251, 290
H. insolens see *Humicola insolens*
histidine 77, 101, 178, 180, 183, 277
histidine acid phosphatase (HAP) 102–104, 108, 110, 122, 126
homogalacturonan 40, 41, 45, 480
homologs 100, 170, 182, 194, 272, 277–280, 286
HRP *see* HAD-related phosphatase
HT method *see* high-throughput method
Humicola insolens (*H. insolens*) 420, 441
hydrolase 5, 306, 354, 420, 421, 425
 glucuronyl 431
 glycoside 421, 422
 glycosidic 437
 metal-containing acid 123
 parathion 350
 phosphamide 353
 rhamnogalacturonan 431
hydrolysate 260, 457, 497, 502
hydrolysis 25, 122, 123, 132, 276, 277, 310, 314, 349–351, 353, 422, 424, 425, 428–430, 444, 445, 450–454, 456–458, 481–483
hydrolysis halo 19, 25, 30
hydrothermal pretreatment 430, 449–451, 453–455

indicators 140, 143, 305, 338, 345
 ecological 315
 physical 336, 356
 sensitive 325, 337, 348
industry 4, 474
 agricultural 53
 bio-based packaging 477
 biofuel 23

dairy processing 24
detergent 23
pharmaceutical 5, 23, 373
pulping 452
tanning 455
infection 69, 272, 280, 283, 286, 288
inhibition 190, 234, 278, 287, 288, 304, 310, 315, 324, 445, 454, 455, 457
inhibitors 50, 62, 119, 316, 455, 457, 481
inhibitory effects 233, 319, 320, 454, 477, 488, 489
insecticides 309, 318–321, 323, 325, 373
insects 50–52, 110, 174, 263, 342, 421, 437
invertase 314, 324, 342, 500
Ipomovirus 270, 276, 278–280, 284
isocitrate lyase 230, 231, 234
isoforms 61, 64, 67, 126, 128, 162, 163, 174, 175, 178, 179, 183, 185, 186, 193–196, 200, 201, 203
  SOD 176–179, 183, 189, 194, 198, 200, 201, 204
isozymes 60, 67, 132, 138, 143

laccase 60–69, 342, 387, 397, 400
Lactobacillus 486, 488
lignin 48, 341, 342, 397, 414–416, 419, 420, 423, 446–449, 451–453, 455, 457, 474–476, 480, 481
lignocellulose 414, 415, 420, 421, 454, 455, 459, 475, 485, 500
limonene 476, 485, 486, 490, 491
lineage-specific expansion (LSE) 76, 94, 98
lipase 4–6, 11, 16, 23–25, 27, 30, 31, 501
lipid 28, 75, 77, 122, 125, 126, 139, 167, 229, 369, 488

Lolium perenne 386, 387
LPMO *see* lytic polysaccharide monooxygenase
LSE *see* lineage-specific expansion
lyase 421, 431–433
lytic polysaccharide monooxygenase (LPMO) 421, 423, 426, 436, 437, 439, 441, 459

Macluravirus 270, 272, 275
MAE *see* microwave-assisted extraction
maize 133, 136, 139, 256, 386, 388, 389, 400, 401
material 311, 416, 445, 475, 476, 484, 485, 487–503, 507
  abiotic 310
  anticorrosion 450
  genetic 22
  humus 306
  lignocellulosic 414, 415, 450
  non-fermentable 485
  organic waste 367, 391, 404
MDAR *see* monodehydroascorbate reductase
MDHAR *see* monodehydroascorbate reductase
mechanism
  autoinhibitory 286
  biochemical 279, 459
  oxidative 437
  oxygen-rebound 437
  physiological 168
  posttranscriptional 192
  posttranslational 208
  regulatory 189, 191, 278, 287
  retaining 424, 425, 428, 429
metabolism 131, 165, 168, 225, 258, 383, 486
  aerobic 159, 161, 168, 177
  carbon 141, 146

energy-efficient 161
fatty acid 307
lipid 169
nitro-oxidative 234, 235
oxidative 232
plant 128
polyamine 228, 231
versatile 227
metabolites 18, 168, 229, 374, 397, 400
  cytoplasmic Pi 139
  diol epoxide 374
  phosphorylated 102
  tricarboxylic acid cycle 141
  water-soluble 174
metalloprotein 161, 164, 185, 195
methanol 9–11, 13, 25, 30, 50, 51, 342, 497
microbes 179, 249, 253, 262, 304, 306, 309, 312, 314, 338, 339, 344, 348, 349, 355, 458
microbiome 390, 394, 442
microbiota 6, 7
microorganism 5, 6, 305, 308–310, 315, 316, 337, 355, 382–384, 420, 457–459, 476, 481, 483, 484, 494, 496, 498, 500
  autochthonous 383, 403
  cellulolytic 458
  cultivation of 5, 7, 499
  ethanologenic 458
  fermenting 457, 458
  lignin decomposing 341
  lignin-degrading 453
  non-culturable 24
  soil 305, 318, 342, 344, 381, 382
  symbiotic 41
microwave-assisted extraction (MAE) 479, 480
mitochondria 125, 138, 139, 145, 146, 160, 163, 164, 166, 168–171, 173, 177, 226, 228–230

Mn SOD (MSD) 169, 177, 178, 180, 183–186, 194, 200–203, 205, 206, 210
monocots 93, 98, 106, 110, 187, 189, 201
monodehydroascorbate reductase (MDAR, MDHAR) 175, 176, 232–234
monomers 259, 475, 488, 496, 508
monooxygenase 245, 247, 249, 258, 262, 392
monosaccharide 339, 420, 445, 446, 451, 454, 480, 483, 507
motif 21, 22, 45, 78, 92, 96, 97, 100–102, 104, 106, 125, 278, 280
  amino acid 124
  APase 80
  conserved 76, 77, 79, 89, 90, 98, 101, 104, 109, 261, 277
  dioxygenase 254
  hydrophobic 139
  metallophosphoesterase 90
  PAP 90
  peptide 280
  zinc-finger 279, 280
MSD *see* Mn SOD
mutants 51, 126, 143–145, 182, 185, 276, 286
mycoremediation 367, 395, 400–403

NADPH *see* nicotinamide adenine dinucleotide phosphate
naphthalene 371–373, 403
natural phenolic compound (NPC) 69, 477, 479
Nicotiana benthamiana 287, 289
Nicotiana tabacum 85, 128
nicotinamide adenine dinucleotide phosphate (NADPH) 119, 163, 170, 176, 233
nitrosation 232, 234

S-nitrosoglutathione (GSNO) 232, 233
NPC *see* natural phenolic compound
nuclease 121, 136, 146, 147, 350
nucleophile 104, 126, 424, 428
nucleophilic attack 93, 97, 108, 350, 368
nucleotides 76, 106, 121, 128, 170, 258, 380
nucleus 129, 138, 139, 145, 180, 181, 187, 199
nutrients 140, 303–305, 312, 314, 336, 337, 383, 384, 391, 397, 489, 494, 498–500

OC *see* organic carbon
oligosaccharide 339, 420, 429, 430, 435, 441, 446, 454, 481
olive oil 8, 10, 11, 26, 28, 30
OPW *see* orange peel waste
orange peel waste (OPW) 471, 472, 474–496, 498–508
organelles 102, 106, 164, 168, 169, 171, 177, 187, 226, 228, 232, 235, 236
organic carbon (OC) 305, 313, 316, 378
organic matter 305, 306, 308, 309, 312, 315, 316, 321, 336, 369, 374, 375, 377, 378, 383, 397
organic phosphorus 314, 345, 348, 349
organism 97, 160, 178, 179, 304, 309–311, 336, 339, 341, 385, 387, 401, 421, 457, 458
  aerobic 161
  aquatic 380
  biochar thermotolerant 485
  dead 314
  disease-causing 355
  ethanologenic 458
  fermenting 458

heterologous 20
marine 177
photosynthesizing 384
photosynthetic 226
primitive 179
sessile 75, 77, 111
soil 305, 310, 395
Oryza sativa 76, 80, 82, 89, 90, 96, 101, 109, 110, 179–181, 184, 186, 187, 193, 194, 196, 197
oxidants 166, 167, 382, 439, 452
oxidase 163–165, 209, 232, 354
  acyl-CoA 230
  copper-containing amine 231
  flavin 169
  glycolate 169, 229, 234
  oxalate 170
  protoporphyrinogen IX 247
  sarcosine 232
oxidation 69, 165, 169, 170, 175, 199, 200, 225, 228–231, 234, 369, 392, 437
oxidative damage 161, 166, 167, 169, 170, 172–174, 182, 195, 203, 204, 208
oxidoreductase 164, 165, 421, 439
oxygenase 245–249, 256–260, 262

PAH *see* polycyclic aromatic hydrocarbon
PAH biodegradation 387, 390, 391, 395, 396, 403
PAH removal 367, 368, 382, 383, 388, 389, 400, 401, 403
PAP *see* purple acid phosphatase
PAP member 127, 132, 133, 146, 147
PAP protein 90–92, 104, 128
PASC *see* phosphoric acid swollen cellulose
pathogen 50, 61, 62, 174, 232
pathway 6, 117, 139, 167, 170, 188, 198, 227–230, 234, 487, 493

biochemical 121, 225, 235
carotenoid biosynthetic 260
catabolic 393
cell secretory 133
fatty acid synthesis 248, 253
heme biosynthetic 247, 248
heterologous 486
plastoquinone biosynthetic 260
secretory 435
shikimate 128
signaling 119, 121, 253, 258, 286
signal transduction 80
stress-responsive 167
PCD *see* programmed cell death
pectin 39, 40, 50–53, 342, 343, 431–433, 440, 442, 474, 476, 477, 480–483, 485, 486, 501, 503–505, 508
pectinase 53, 342, 422, 426, 483, 500, 501, 503
pectin extraction 480, 481, 483, 504, 505
pectin methyl esterase (PME) 39–46, 48–53, 342, 343, 434
Penicillium 395, 484, 490
Penicillium digitatum 494
PEP *see* phosphoenolpyruvate
peptide 197, 257, 259, 260
peroxidase 164, 165, 167, 169, 175, 317, 318, 387, 397, 400
peroxisome 160, 163–166, 168–170, 174, 177, 180, 183, 185, 187, 225–236
peroxynitrite 162, 165, 176, 202, 210, 232, 233
pesticides 309, 317, 339, 350, 373
phenanthrene 372, 373, 386, 387, 393, 403
phosphatase 77, 100, 102, 126, 305–308, 310, 312, 314, 316, 317, 323, 337, 345, 347–349, 353

phosphate 99, 103, 108, 119, 147, 176, 314, 348, 351
phosphate ion (Pi) 75–79, 93, 97, 117–122, 124, 126, 128, 130, 135, 137–139, 144–146, 348, 351
phosphodiesterase 121, 146, 147, 348–352
phosphoenolpyruvate (PEP) 123, 128, 130, 147, 182
phospholipid 76, 102, 108, 117, 119, 128, 137, 139, 147, 349
phospholipid phosphatase (PLP) 100–102, 108, 110, 122, 125, 126, 139
phosphoprotein 76, 90, 108, 119, 137, 147
phosphoric acid swollen cellulose (PASC) 426, 444
phosphorylation 18, 119, 198–200, 441
phosphotriesterase 348, 350–352
photorespiration 169, 187, 225, 228, 234, 235
photosynthesis 76, 117, 119, 120, 163, 168, 177, 180, 182, 191, 228–230, 314
photosystem 168, 169, 187, 211
phylogenetic analysis 25, 27, 30, 80, 89, 100, 109, 422
phytase 94, 104, 126, 128, 501
phytate 95, 104, 124, 126–128, 130, 132, 137, 140, 142
phytoremediation 384, 386, 388–391, 395, 400–404
Pi *see* phosphate ion
Pi homeostasis 76, 78, 109, 111, 118, 134, 137, 139, 141, 145, 147
Pi scavenging 77, 118, 121, 123, 131, 132
Pi starvation 77, 95, 102, 122, 124, 125, 132, 137–139, 141, 143, 146

PL *see* polysaccharide lyase
plant 39–42, 45, 46, 49–51, 60–62, 67–69, 75–80, 100–102, 108–111, 117, 118, 122–124, 126–128, 132–134, 136–143, 160–210, 251–253, 304, 305, 309–314, 337, 378–387, 390, 391
  corn 256
  crop 245–247
  dead 314
  dicotyledonous 40, 41, 45, 78, 109, 253, 256, 260
  experimental 386
  flowering 78, 100
  maize 133, 368, 402
  monocotyledonous 41, 76, 260
  monocotyledonous rice 45
  mutant 182
  non-transgenic 142
  soybean 256, 257, 259
  starved 137
  tea 141
  transgenic 48, 52, 123, 142
  transgenic Arabidopsis 104
  transgenic potato 48
  vascular 414, 415, 421
  vegetable species 134
  wastewater treatment 379
  wild-type 48, 142, 144, 286
  willow 389
plasma 129, 131, 145, 164, 169
PLP *see* phospholipid phosphatase
plum pox virus (PPV) 271, 273, 274, 277, 280, 285, 286
PME *see* pectin methyl esterase
Poacevirus 270, 274, 276, 278–280, 285
pollutants 317–319, 370, 376, 378, 385, 388, 391, 397, 475
  organic 368, 369, 381, 383–385, 387, 391, 502

polycyclic aromatic hydrocarbon (PAH) 317, 342, 367–371, 373–397, 400–404
polymer 447, 477, 480, 502, 504
  biodegradable 498
  carbohydrate 342
  organic 397
  polyfluorene 373
  toxic condensed 60
polymerization 69, 373, 416, 449
polyphenol 342, 419, 497, 498, 503, 504
polyphenol oxidase (PPO) 59–69, 175, 211, 247, 248, 439
polyprotein 269, 272, 275, 276
polysaccharide 40, 48, 337, 339, 341, 342, 414, 421, 434, 436, 439, 477, 481, 483
polysaccharide lyase (PL) 119, 146, 421, 422, 425, 431, 432
posttranslational modifications (PTM) 18, 20, 135, 198–200, 203, 232, 233, 237, 278
potato 53, 60, 128, 141, 276, 285
potato virus A (PVA) 285, 287, 288
Potyviridae 269–273, 275, 290
potyvirids 269, 272, 276, 277, 288–291
Potyvirus 270–272, 276, 278–281, 286, 288, 291
Potyvirus Plum 274
PPO *see* polyphenol oxidase
PPV *see* plum pox virus
pretreatment 448–451, 453, 456, 476, 477, 480, 485, 489, 491–496, 499
  biological 453
  hot water 450
  organosolv 452
process
  bacterial/algal 376
  BALI 449, 452
  batch 484

biological 336, 471, 476, 484, 485, 487–503
biorefinery 507
biosynthetic 175
burning 376
cellular 45, 108, 162, 176, 193
de-esterification 51
defense-related 61
extraction 477
fed-batch 484
fermentative 476, 484, 504, 505
hydrothermal 450
industrial 4, 376, 378, 413, 458, 459, 481
lignification 68
metabolic 175
microbiological 476
non-enzymatic 420
organosolv 452
oxidative 420, 421
photosynthetic 415
physiological 120, 126, 160, 166, 168, 171, 173, 175, 177, 183, 225, 227, 234, 235
single-stage 492, 495
texturing-hydrolysis 451
uncatalyzed 452
programmed cell death (PCD) 166, 168, 169, 211
prokaryotes 78, 102, 106, 185, 188, 191, 192, 262
protease 41, 270, 271, 283, 307, 312, 324, 337, 344, 442
protein 44, 45, 60, 61, 66, 67, 75–77, 95–98, 102, 104–106, 119, 124, 125, 164, 165, 167, 170, 171, 197, 198, 200, 201, 232, 270–273, 275, 277–281, 283–286, 288
catalytic 179
cell wall 132
chloroplastic 201
coat 272, 289
dual-targeted 139

glycosylated 442
helix-loop-helix 189
mature 272
multifunctional 230, 236
mysterious 290
nuclear inclusion 272
PAP 123
pathogen-related 68
phosphorylated 119, 128
potyviral 277
potyvirid-encoded 290
vegetative storage 98, 125, 141
viral 270, 288
viral genome-linked 272
wild-type 286
proteinase 7, 269, 270, 272, 273, 275–279, 288, 289, 291, 307
proteolysis 171, 270, 276, 278, 286, 287, 306
PTM *see* posttranslational modification
purple acid phosphatase (PAP) 78, 90, 91, 93, 96, 104, 107, 108, 110, 111, 122, 123, 128, 133–136, 138, 141, 142, 145–147
PVA *see* potato virus A
pyrene 372–375, 377, 379, 380, 382, 384, 386, 394, 397, 399, 401, 403
pyrolysis 369, 375, 376
pyrophosphate 124, 129, 130, 147, 351

quizalofop 248, 253, 256, 257

RCS *see* reactive carbonyl species
reaction
  acid-base catalysis 424
  biocatalytic 24
  biochemical 312, 315, 336
  biotransformation 477
  catalytic 437
  cellular 117

cellulose peeling 452
Fenton 163, 164, 167, 169–171
fluorescein diacetate hydrolysis 317
Haber–Weiss 163, 167
kinetic resolution 30
lipid peroxidation 171
nonenzymatic 168, 170
nucleophilic substitution 97
oxidative 183
phosphoryl group transfer 124
photosynthetic 172
polymerase chain 21
radical addition 369
redox cycling 195
respiratory 119
reversible phosphorylation 80
synergistic 322
reactive carbonyl species (RCS) 162, 163, 167, 168, 171, 172, 175, 211
reactive nitrogen species (RNS) 162, 163, 166–172, 174, 175, 177, 200, 201, 225, 228, 232–234, 237
reactive oxygen species (ROS) 160–163, 166–169, 171–177, 201, 203, 204, 211, 225, 228, 232–234, 237, 319, 320, 337
reactive sulfur species (RSS) 162, 163, 167, 168, 171, 172, 175, 234
reductants 166, 174, 423, 439
reductase 164, 175, 176, 209, 229, 233, 234, 258, 317, 354
replication 89, 91, 283, 284, 286–288
residue 92, 97, 98, 100, 101, 104, 106, 108, 124, 303, 306, 431, 432, 434, 435, 437, 474, 475, 483–485, 487
  active 107
  agricultural 415, 485
  aldonic acid 437

animal 349
arabinose 431
arginine 133
basic amino acid 432
catalytic 110, 273, 277
catalytic site 180, 183
citrus 498
conserved 90, 92, 106
conserved arginine 101
d-mannose 430
glutamic-acid 277
glycosyl 428
hexenuronic acid 432
high porosity 481
histidine 19, 104, 126
hydrolyze acetyl 435
l-rhamnose 431
metal-ligating 90, 136
orange 479
organic 379
threonine/serine 200
tyrosine 90, 119, 200, 232
xylopyranoside 435
respiration 76, 117, 120, 128, 177, 306, 325
ribonucleic acid (RNA) 108, 119, 146, 191, 193, 194, 287, 349
rice 76, 78–80, 88, 90, 93, 95–97, 100, 111, 124, 126, 128, 132–134, 136, 142, 260
RNA see ribonucleic acid
RNase 121, 139, 146, 147
RNA silencing suppression 269, 279, 282–285
RNS see reactive nitrogen species
root 62–64, 66, 67, 104, 124, 127, 132–134, 136, 137, 140, 142, 143, 145–147, 310, 311, 385–387, 389
  dead 311
  hairy 132, 142
  maize 368, 389, 402, 403
  pathogen-infected 64, 66, 67
  willow 386

ROS *see* reactive oxygen species
ROS homeostasis 170, 172, 176, 177, 185, 188, 203, 208
ROS-mediated damage 171, 173, 203, 204
Roymovirus 270, 274, 276, 279
RSS *see* reactive sulfur species
rumens 7, 441, 442, 498
ryegrass 387, 388
Rymovirus 270, 276, 278, 279, 284

saccharification 413–415, 437, 443, 444, 448, 451, 454, 455, 457, 476, 481, 483–485, 502, 503, 505
Saccharomyces cerevisiae (*S. cerevisiae*) 195, 457, 483, 485, 486
SAP *see* SurE acid phosphatase
SAR *see* systemic acquired resistance
scavenging 75, 123, 125, 130, 131, 162–164, 172, 174, 175, 187
S. cerevisiae see *Saccharomyces cerevisiae*
sediments 12, 14, 368, 377
　coastal 7
　freshwater 319
　lake 377
　river 379
seed 48, 49, 79, 120, 132, 133, 146, 147, 471, 472
　barley 402
　esterified 49
　yellow cedar 46
seedling 63, 120, 123, 134–136, 144
senescence 53, 77, 123, 134, 139, 225, 227, 229, 231, 234
separate hydrolysis and fermentation (SHF) 457, 476
sequence 21, 22, 76, 79, 80, 90, 92, 93, 97–104, 111, 126, 127, 129, 272, 273, 275, 280

amino acid 5, 92, 133
consensus 89
crop rotation/crop 356
fractionation 446, 447
genomic 124, 273
heterologous 289
orthologous 104
phosphoprotein phosphatase 97
potyvirid 275
recombinant DNA 122
signal 24, 179, 187
serine 77, 119, 124, 277
SF *see* submerged fermentation
SHF *see* separate hydrolysis and fermentation
shoot 62–64, 66, 67, 120, 124, 134, 137, 140, 142, 145, 385, 389
shoot extract 62, 64, 66, 67
signaling 117, 168, 171, 174, 176, 177, 198, 204
　cellular 160, 166, 168, 177, 200, 203, 208
　environmental 45
　inter-organellar 169
　intracellular 169
　lipid 102
　organellar 169
　phytohormone 188
signal peptide 42, 94–96, 133, 184
signal transduction 76, 172, 189, 190
simulation 287, 496, 505
sludge 482, 489, 491, 494
SMV *see* soybean mosaic virus
SOD *see* superoxide dismutase
softwood 416, 418, 419, 450
soil 8–11, 118, 128, 137, 303–317, 321–323, 325, 335–339, 341–350, 353–356, 367, 368, 373, 374, 377–391, 393, 395–397, 400–404
　acidic 118, 142, 316, 348
　alkaline 118, 348
　anthropogenic 373

arable 379, 390
bare 389
bulk 348, 389
calcareous 316
compost 16
contaminated 381–384, 386–389, 391, 394, 396, 397, 400, 402
creosote-contaminated 401, 402
fat-contaminated 24
forbs-dominated 312
forest 7, 316, 378
metabolic processes of 336
mycoremediation of 401, 402
phosphorus-deficient 309
plant rhizosphere 7
polluted 367, 381, 383, 384, 386
rhizospheric 348
sandy 309
treated 322, 388
urease activity in 344
soil animals 303, 306, 325, 344
soil biodiversity 335, 336
soil colloids 345, 348
soil contaminants 317, 391
soil ecosystem 304, 305, 312, 314, 318, 325
soil environment 308, 311, 336, 338, 392, 395, 397
soil fertility 323, 325
soil health 311, 312, 355
soil invertase 314, 320, 322, 323, 342
soil system 318, 336, 350, 353
Solanum tuberosum 42, 85, 95, 206, 207
solvent 8, 13, 15, 25, 26, 416, 419, 446, 475, 476, 479
  organic 4, 5, 8, 11, 12, 15, 16, 19, 23–25, 27, 29–31, 369, 452
soybean 92, 125, 128, 132, 133, 135, 137, 142, 247, 256, 257
soybean mosaic virus (SMV) 285, 286

species 42, 45, 62, 78, 96, 162, 167, 177, 203, 205–207, 311
  bacterial 123
  dominant 309, 311
  fungi 396, 397, 433
  grass 45, 312
  oxidant/nitrating 171
  plant 90, 104, 125, 127, 132, 135, 137, 196, 227, 259, 312
  potyvirid 280
  reactive 160–163, 165, 167–176, 203
  rotation woody 415
SPFMV *see* sweet potato feathery mottle virus
SPMMV *see* sweet potato mild mottle virus
starch 337, 471, 485, 500
stress 136, 140, 161, 204, 205, 207, 235, 314
  abiotic 49, 61, 167, 172, 231
  biotic 49, 51, 61, 69, 118, 160, 172, 303
  cellular nitro-oxidative 234
  cold 188
  environmental 126
  heat 123, 140, 188, 191
  heavy metal 160
  oxidative 95, 123, 171, 182, 185, 194, 203, 205–208
  ozone 205
  salt 181
stress response 39, 127, 168, 171, 173–175, 177, 183, 188, 189, 191, 193
stress tolerance 177, 192, 204, 205, 231, 236
submerged fermentation (SF) 497, 498, 500
substrate 8–16, 19, 20, 76, 118, 121, 122, 126–128, 262, 307, 348, 350, 420, 424–426, 435–438, 443–445, 482, 483, 494, 499, 500

aromatic 259
citrus peel 500
dicamba 259
electrophilic 175
extracellular 145
filter paper 444
fungal 400
lignocellulosic 420, 459
long-chain 23
methyl-esterified 433
nitrophenyl phosphate 100
organic 128, 249, 395
polyprotein 270
sugar-phosphate 146
water-insoluble 5, 443
wood 368
wood chip 396, 400
substrate specificity 62, 68, 77, 128, 135, 342, 348, 422, 426, 430, 431, 433, 435
sucrose 136, 191, 230, 314, 342, 481, 497
superoxide dismutase (SOD) 159–163, 170, 171, 174–180, 183, 185, 188–209, 232, 318
SurE acid phosphatase (SAP) 104, 108, 110, 127
sweet potato feathery mottle virus (SPFMV) 272, 279, 280, 285
sweet potato mild mottle virus (SPMMV) 276, 279, 280, 285
system
   enzymatic 500
   immune 380
   integrated weed control 246
   intensive root 120
   multi-product 453
   rabbit reticulocyte lysate translation 277
   solvent-free 26–28
   three-component enzyme 258
systemic acquired resistance (SAR) 62, 63

TEV *see* tobacco etch virus
tissue 45, 49, 51, 52, 68, 69, 132, 133, 136, 182, 185, 228, 229, 251, 252, 380, 384, 385
   plant 52, 68, 133, 173, 251, 341, 342, 387
TMV *see* tobacco mosaic virus
tobacco 50, 68, 94, 122, 128, 137, 259, 260, 374
tobacco etch virus (TEV) 277, 285
tobacco mosaic virus (TMV) 50, 272
tobacco vein mottling virus (TVMV) 277, 280, 285, 287, 288
tocopherol 163–165, 167, 173, 174
total phenolic content (TPC) 477, 478, 504
toxicity 185, 318, 370, 371, 373, 380, 390
TPC *see* total phenolic content
traits 120, 245, 246, 248, 249, 252
transesterification 11, 12, 23, 27, 29
transgene 251, 256
triacylglycerol 5, 6, 25, 27, 30, 31
Tritimovirus 270, 276, 278–280, 285
TVMV *see* tobacco vein mottling virus
tyrosine nitration 164, 165, 232, 233

UAE *see* ultrasound-assisted extraction
UCBSV *see* Ugandan cassava brown streak virus
Ugandan cassava brown streak virus (UCBSV) 271, 276, 279, 285
ultrasound-assisted extraction (UAE) 479